Professional Nursing
Concepts & Challenges

Professional Nursing
Concepts & Challenges

3rd Edition

Kay Kittrell Chitty
RN, EdD, CS

Adjunct Faculty
College of Nursing
Medical University of South Carolina

W. B. SAUNDERS COMPANY
An Imprint of Elsevier Science
Philadelphia   London   New York
St. Louis   Sydney   Toronto

W. B. SAUNDERS COMPANY

An Imprint of Elsevier Science

The Curtis Center
Independence Square West
Philadelphia, Pennsylvania 19106

Library of Congress Cataloging-in-Publication Data

Professional nursing : concepts and challenges / [edited by] Kay Kittrell Chitty.—3rd ed.

p. ; cm.

Includes bibliographical references and index.

ISBN 0–7216–8711–3 (alk. paper)

1. Nursing—Vocational guidance. 2. Nursing—Social aspects. I. Chitty, Kay Kittrell.
[DNLM: 1. Nursing. 2. Vocational Guidance. WY 16 P9644 2001]

RT82 .P755 2001
610.7390699–dc21

00–024856

Vice President, Nursing Editorial: Sally Schrefer
Editorial Manager: Thomas Eoyang
Developmental Editor: Fran Murphy

PROFESSIONAL NURSING: Concepts and Challenges   ISBN 0–7216–8711–3

Printed in the United States of America

Last digit is the print number: 9   8   7   6   5   4   3

*The third edition of this book is dedicated
to professional nurses everywhere.
They devote their lives to the care of strangers.*

Contributors to Earlier Editions

Pamela J. Holder, RN, DSN
Director, School of Nursing
Middle Tennessee State University
Murfreesboro, Tennessee

Jennifer Jenkins, RN, MBA, CNAA
Vice President, Clinical Solutions
HealthMagic, Inc.
Columbia, South Carolina

Carolyn Maynard, RN, PhD, CS
Assistant Professor
University of North Carolina at Charlotte
Charlotte, North Carolina

Barbara R. Norwood, RN, ED, CNS
Assistant Professor
University of Tennessee at Chattanooga
Chattanooga, Tennessee

Cheryl A. Peterson, RN, MSN
Senior Policy Fellow, Health and Economic Policy
American Nurses Association
Washington, DC

Robert V. Piemonte, RN, EdD, CAE, FAAN
Consultant and
President Elect
New York State Nurses Association

Barbara K. Redman, RN, PhD, FAAN
Dean, College of Nursing
Wayne State University
Detroit, Michigan

Frances I. Waddle, RN, MSN
Retired Health Facilities Consultant
Oklahoma State Department of Health
Oklahoma City, Oklahoma

Contributors

Martha Raile Alligood, RN, PhD
Professor and Chair, MSN Program
College of Nursing
University of Tennessee
Knoxville, Tennessee

Virginia Trotter Betts, RN, MSN, JD
Associate Director for Health Policy Initiatives
Center for Health Policy
Professor of Nursing
University of Tennessee Health Sciences Center
Memphis, Tennessee

Carol T. Bush, RN, PhD
Adjunct Professor
Emory University
Nell Hodgson Woodruff School of Nursing
Atlanta, Georgia
and
Regional Executive Director
DeKalb Regional Board
Georgia Division of Mental Health, Mental
    Retardation, and Substance Abuse
Georgia Department of Human Resources
Decatur, Georgia

Cathy Campbell, RN, MN, PhD
Doctoral Candidate
Georgia State University
Atlanta, Georgia

Pamela S. Chally, RN, PhD
Dean and Professor
College of Health
University of North Florida
Jacksonville, Florida

M. Catherine Hough, RN, PhD
Assistant Professor
Department of Nursing
College of Health
University of North Florida
Jacksonville, Florida

Arlene W. Keeling, RN, PhD
Associate Professor
Director ANCP Program
Associate Director, Center for Nursing
    Historical Inquiry
Virginia School of Nursing
University of Virginia
Charlottesville, Virginia

Judith K. Leavitt, RN, MEd, FAAN
Associate Professor
School of Nursing
The University of Mississippi Medical Center
Jackson, Mississippi

Diane J. Mancino, RN, EdD, CAE
Executive Director, National Student Nurses'
    Association and the Foundation of the
    National Student Nurses' Association
New York, New York

Frances A. Maurer, RN, MS
Community Health Educator and Consultant
Baltimore, Maryland

Elaine F. Nichols, RN, EdD
Associate Professor of Nursing
Associate Dean of Academic Affairs
College of Nursing
University of Akron
Akron, Ohio

Karen J. Wisdom, RN, MHA
Vice President, Patient Care
Hamilton Medical Center
Dalton, Georgia

Preface to the Third Edition

Professions exist to serve society. When society changes, professions must also change to maintain their relevance and dynamism. So it is with nursing. As we embark on the first decade of the new millennium, nurses must possess a skill set far more complex than ever before in the history of the profession.

To be effective in the twenty-first century, nurses must be good leaders and good team members; they must think critically and creatively; they must communicate and collaborate with a diverse array of patients, families, and health care colleagues; they must be caring and businesslike; they must grapple with ethical and legal dilemmas not dreamed of even a decade ago; and they must practice their profession in both traditional settings and in nontraditional community settings. Needless to say, to be an effective nurse today is a daunting undertaking.

The third edition of this text is designed to assist students to understand what it means to be a professional; to appreciate the history of nursing; to understand and prize nursing's values, standards, and ethics; to recognize and deal effectively with the social and economic factors that influence how the profession is practiced; and to appreciate the need to be lifelong learners. It addresses concepts underlying the elements of the American Association of Colleges of Nursing's latest (1998) document, *The Essentials of Baccalaureate Education for Professional Nursing Practice.*

Feedback from users of earlier editions reveal that this text is used in RN to BSN "bridge" courses, in early courses in generic baccalaureate curricula, and as a resource for practicing nurses and graduate students. Students in nursing programs are increasingly second-degree students, midcareer adults, and others who bring considerable life experience to the learning situation. Accordingly, every effort has been made to present material that is comprehensive enough to challenge users at all levels without overwhelming the novice. The text has been designed to be "student friendly," and care has been taken to keep jargon to a minimum yet to provide a comprehensive glossary to assist in developing and refining a professional vocabulary. The visual features of the book have been carefully improved with today's visual learner in mind.

To faculty who have used the book before, this edition should feel and look familiar, with many of the successful features maintained and updated. For example, assisting users of all levels to greater self-awareness has been a goal of all three editions of this text. Therefore self-assessment exercises were retained and expanded in this revision. Upon close examination, however, differences from the previous edition will emerge. In some instances chapter headings have been modified to reflect current emphases. In addition to updating, new content has been added to every chapter. New content includes the following:

- The history and theory chapters have been completely rewritten by authorities in those fields.
- An emphasis on critical and creative thinking and clinical decision making has been added.
- The focus on men in nursing has been expanded.
- Cultural competence has been emphasized.
- Managed care content has been expanded.
- The impact of violence in society and the workplace has been added.
- An introduction to qualitative research and classification systems (NIC and NOC) have been added.
- Content on communication and collaboration have been improved and expanded.
- New roles in the community, such as parish nursing and nursing informatics, have been added.
- Where appropriate, clinical examples and vignettes have been added.
- Interviews with practicing nurses and other experts have been increased.
- The challenge of creating and maintaining a healthy work environment has been emphasized.
- Appendices have been added including the *Code for Nurses,* lists and e-mail addresses of state boards of nursing, and other valuable resources.
- Web resources have been added to each chapter to assist students to do independent research using reliable, pertinent sites online.

The Instructor's Manual has been revised based on user feedback to contain activities for both small and large groups. It contains inclass and out-of-class activities designed to enhance students' learning and to enrich classroom experiences. The Instructor's Manual also includes chapter outlines, chapter objectives, suggested readings, and a comprehensive test bank. Contact your sales representative or call our Sales Support Team at 1-800-222-9570 to obtain copies of the Instructor's Manual.

As with earlier editions, it continues to be my heartfelt hope that the students and faculty who use this new edition will find it even more stimulating, enjoyable, and enlightening than the first and second editions and that it will continue to contribute to the positive development of our profession.

Kay K. Chitty

Acknowledgments

The successful completion of any major project brings both a sense of accomplishment and of relief. The completion of the third edition of *Professional Nursing: Concepts and Challenges* also brings overwhelming gratitude to the many individuals who participated in what has truly been a great team effort:

- To the faculty and students who used earlier editions and provided me with their suggestions for revisions, especially Kathleen Scharer, Suzanne Doscher, and their students;
- To Jim Quigley who took on the responsibility of research assistant even as he and his family were undertaking a move to another state;
- To the reference librarians at the Charleston County Library and the Medical University of South Carolina for their unselfish donation of time, talents, and energy;
- To Sylvia Rayfield and Sharon Cox, friends who freely shared their profound expertise and contacts;
- To Sylvia Hart who reviewed the managed care content in the book and suggested important revisions;
- To Richard Sowell who shared his balanced insights about being a man in a female-dominated profession;
- To Madeleine Leininger who evaluated the cultural components of the book and made invaluable suggestions for improvement;
- To the many nurses who shared their experiences and perceptions in interviews;
- To all who assisted in gathering photographs—Arlene Keeling, Elaine Nichols, Diane Mancino, Dawn Marks, Karen Wisdom, Ben Brazell, Ria Fisher, Will McDonald, Joyce Dick, Carol Dobos, and Vivica Poole;
- To all who contributed philosophies of nursing from their schools and hospitals—Pam Chally, Martha Sherman, Charlene Robertson, and Karen Wisdom;
- To Fran Murphy, Associate Developmental Editor at W. B. Saunders, for her patience, attention to detail, and willingness to listen to my grumbling.

Special thanks are due the contributors to this edition, who took on this extra responsibility in spite of already over-full personal and professional lives. Their recompense will not be tangible, for academia is sadly lacking in rewards for textbook writing. In an odd twist of values, publishing a research article in an arcane journal that will be read by few and used by even fewer is seen as more desirable in today's colleges and universities than writing a textbook that has the potential to influence literally thousands of future professional nurses. In spite of this obstacle, these contributors rose to the occasion. Their love of the nursing profession and commitment to its hopeful future will serve as their remuneration. I am deeply indebted to them, one and all.

Finally, I wish to express my deepest appreciation to Thomas Eoyang, a fully human editor, who shared my vision from the beginning, kept the faith when my spirits flagged, and inspired and motivated me by his commitment to the nursing profession, which he values and understands.

Contents

CHAPTER 13
The Health Care Delivery System 304
Karen J. Wisdom

CHAPTER 14
Nursing Roles in the Health Care Delivery System 335
Karen J. Wisdom

CHAPTER 15
Critical Thinking, The Nursing Process, and Clinical Judgement 360
Kay K. Chitty

CHAPTER 16
Financing Health Care 384
Frances A. Maurer

CHAPTER 17
Illness and Culture: Impact on Patients and Families 421
Kay K. Chitty

CHAPTER 18
Communication and Collaboration in Nursing 450
Kay K. Chitty

Professional Nursing Comes of Age: 1859–2000

Arlene W. Keeling

Key Terms

Clara Barton
Mary Ann ("Mother") Bickerdyke
Mary Breckinridge
Cadet Nurse Corps
Mary E. Davis
Dorthea L. Dix
Lavinia L. Dock
Lorretta Ford
Florence Nightingale
Adelaide Nutting
Sophia Palmer
Phoebe Pember
Isabel Hampton Robb
Margaret Sanger
Jesse Sleet
Sojourner Truth
Harriet Tubman
Lillian Wald

Learning Outcomes

After studying this chapter, students will be able to:

- Identify the social, political, and economic factors that influenced the rise of professional nursing in the United States.
- Describe the influence of Florence Nightingale on the development of the nursing profession in the United States.
- Discuss major medical events that affected the nursing profession.
- Identify early nursing leaders.
- Explain the effects of the Civil War, the Spanish American War, the World Wars, and the Korean and Vietnam Wars on the nursing profession.
- Describe the struggles and contributions of African-American and male nurses in the profession's development.
- Trace the rise of advanced practice nursing in the United States.

To understand the challenges facing professional nursing today, it is essential to know something of nursing's history. The rise of nursing as a profession in the United States is a complex story of opportunities, challenges, struggles, and the search for identity within the context of larger social forces. From the work of Florence Nightingale in the Crimea (1854) to the present, the profession has been influenced by the social, political, and economic climate of the times and by technological advances and theoretical shifts in medicine and science. Early in its development, nursing was influenced by the ideology of the Victorian and the Progressive eras. By the mid-twentieth century, its evolution was imbedded in an emerging context of change: in attitudes toward minorities, the women's movement, advances in technology and science, and the rise of medical specialization. Since the 1980s, health care reform, politics, the Internet, and an emphasis on global awareness have all played a part in shaping nursing's development. This chapter presents a brief overview of some of the highlights of nursing's history and of several of its leaders. The history of nursing education, discussed in Chapter 2, is only introduced in this section. Since an indepth analysis of nursing's history is beyond the scope of this text, the reader is encouraged to use the references at the end of the chapter for further reading.

Nursing in Early Nineteenth-Century America

Prior to 1873 when the first "training schools" for nursing opened in the United States, nursing care was provided in the home by mothers, wives, daughters, and sisters of the sick. From the earliest years of settlement in the colonies, and during the growth and development of the United States as it expanded westward, the care of the sick was directed by physicians and managed by family members outside, of hospitals. Only those who were destitute, orphaned, or chronically incapacitated were admitted to hospitals, which were essentially almshouses. Care in these places was of poor quality and provided by other inmates, who were equally destitute and untrained.

Mid-Nineteenth Century Nursing in England: The Influence of Florence Nightingale

Florence Nightingale, extolled as the most influential nurse in the history of modern nursing, was born into the aristocratic social sphere of Victorian England, a heritage that would become critical to her success. At an early age, Nightingale received a classic education directed by her father. This education, combined with her personal characteristics of sensitivity, compassion, and restlessness, along with the perspective she gained through extensive travel on the continent, provided her with the foundation for the role she would play in the future.

As a young woman, Nightingale (Fig. 1–1) often felt stifled by her privileged and protected social position in upper-class Victorian England. In addition, because she had often accompanied her mother on visits to the poor, Nightingale became aware of both the disease and disability caused by poverty and the horrible conditions in public hospitals. As a result, she took it upon herself to visit the sick in her community.

By 1850, rebelling against her strict Victorian culture and convinced that she wanted to be a nurse, Nightingale entered the nurses' training program at Kaiserworth, Germany, where she spent three years learning the basics of nursing under the guidance of the Protestant deaconesses. After completion of her training, Florence Nightingale studied under the Sisters of Charity in Paris. Only a year later she would have the opportunity to use her newly acquired skills when Britain went to war in the Crimea.

Nightingale in the Crimea, 1854–1856

On hearing of the horrible conditions suffered by the sick and wounded British soldiers in Turkey during the Crimean War, Nightingale took a small band of untrained women to the British hospital in Scutari. There she found a

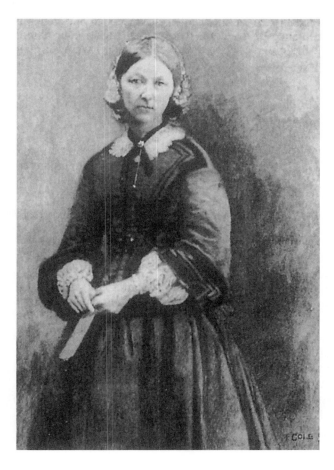

Figure 1–1
Florence Nightingale.

hospital "totally lacking in equipment. . . . There were no medical supplies. There were not even the basic necessities of life . . ." (Woodham-Smith, 1949, p. 162). With great compassion and in spite of the opposition of military officers, Nightingale set about the task of organizing and cleaning the hospital and providing care to the wounded soldiers. She boldly made use of her personal power and political and social connections, writing to influential government officials—including her dear friend Sir Sidney Herbert, the British Secretary of War. Armed with excellent training in statistics, Nightingale gathered data on morbidity and mortality of the soldiers in Scutari. Using this supportive evidence, Nightingale argued the case for reform of the entire British Army medical system.

The Nightingale School

Following the Crimean War, Nightingale founded the first training school for nurses at St. Thomas's Hospital, London (1860). This school would become the model for nursing education in the United States. Through the publication of numerous articles and papers, Nightingale promulgated her ideas about nursing and nursing education. In her most famous publication, the 1859 *Notes on Nursing: What It Is and What It Is Not,* Nightingale stated clearly for the first time that learning a unique body of knowledge was required of those wishing to practice professional nursing.

Nightingale held the firm belief that good nursing care was essential to the healing process and that the art of nursing included attention to the symptoms of the disease and factors in the environment. According to Nightingale, "[Nursing] has been limited to signify little more than the administration of medicines and the application of poultices. It ought to signify the proper use of fresh air, light, warmth, cleanliness, quiet and the proper choosing and giving of diet—all at the least expense of vital power to the patient." (Nightingale [1859], (1946) (p. 6). Moreover, Nightingale specifically rejected the theory that microorganisms, rather than filth and dampness, caused disease (Nightingale, [1859], (1946) (p. 7), and held fast to this notion despite evidence to the contrary being provided by such notable scientists as Joseph Lister and Louis Pasteur in the latter part of the century.

These widely published beliefs, along with Nightingale's dedication to hospital reform, to upgrading conditions for the sick and wounded in the military, and to establishing training schools for nurses, greatly affected the development of nursing in the United States.

1861–1873 Seeds of Change: The Need for "Trained" Nurses

There were no professional nurses in America when the first shots were fired on Fort Sumter, South Carolina, in 1861, initiating the War between the States. Furthermore, there was no organized system of medical or nursing care in either the Union or the Confederacy and no plan to cope with the deluge of wounded men who poured into Washington and Richmond following the Battle of Bull Run on July 21, 1861. There had been no provision for field hospitals, and hospital tents were to the rear of the fighting, too far from the front. As a result, the conditions on the battlefield were horrible: everywhere wounded and dying men lay in agony while the stench of chloroform and blood-soaked blankets filled the air (Young, 1959, p. 134).

Mary Livermore, writing about conditions at the front after the Battle of Bull Run in northern Virginia, related:

Mrs. Hoge and myself were sent to the hospitals and to medical headquarters at the front—with instructions to obtain any possible information that would lead to better preparations for the wounded of another great battle (Livermore, 1867, p. 187).

Immediately the appeal for nurses was made, and women on both sides responded. Most significant perhaps was the response by the Catholic orders, particularly the Sisters of Charity, the Sisters of Mercy, and the Sisters of the Holy Cross, who had a long history of providing care for the sick (Wall, 1995). Doubtless the most skillful and devoted of the women who nursed in the Civil War, these religious sisters were highly disciplined, organized, and efficient.

Union Nursing: 1861-1865

As word of the shocking conditions spread, northern women responded immediately. The Women's Central Relief Committee, formed in New York City early in the Civil War, sent a committee to Washington, D.C., to mobilize volunteer support and to pressure the government to provide care for the soldiers. An entire medical system was needed. President Lincoln heeded their recommendations and created the United States Sanitary Commission (Fig. 1–2), immediately appointing **Dorthea L. Dix,** an avid reformer of care for the mentally ill, as superintendent of Women Nurses of the Army. Unfortunately, Dix had no official corps of trained nurses to lead. She was faced with the task of supplying nurses when there were none, for in 1861 there were no training schools for nurses in the United States. As a substitute for professional training, Dix focused on the criteria of good health, high moral character, and a matronly, "plain" appearance as qualifications for service. She soon enlisted 100 women to train for a month under physicians at Bellevue Hospital and New York Hospital to prepare them to supervise the care of the sick and wounded throughout the Union.

As the year progressed, thousands of women volunteered to help, challenging social mores and the Victorian ideology that a woman's place was in the home. Black and white, rich and poor, and married and single women left their homes to care for soldiers in hospital tents and in hastily converted schools, churches, and warehouses. Among the African-American women who served were **Sojourner Truth,** a famous abolitionist, and **Harriet Tubman,** a former field slave who had escaped to the north in 1849. Defying the boundaries of time, place, gender, and race, both women not only cared for the soldiers but also smuggled slaves to freedom using the complex Underground Railroad system.

Meanwhile, Soldier's Aid Societies sprang into existence as women used their social organizations to serve the war effort. Employing their domestic skills, they stitched garments, rolled bandages, made blankets, knitted socks, and prepared boxes of food and supplies to be sent to the front.

SANITARY COMMISSION.

No. 39.

THIRD REPORT

CONCERNING THE

Aid and Comfort given by the Sanitary Commission

TO

SICK SOLDIERS PASSING THROUGH WASHINGTON.

BY FREDERICK N. KNAPP, Special Relief Agent.

WASHINGTON, *March* 21, 1862.

TO FRED. LAW OLMSTED,

Secretary Sanitary Commission:

SIR:—My last report bore date of October 21. Since that time to the present, the work upon our hands has steadily increased. More room, more money, more time, more medical attendance, have all been demanded. Fewer new regiments have arrived of late, but the regiments already in the field having become more generally acquainted with our plans for rendering help, are now in the habit of sending directly to our care sick and discharged men, who come to the city from the various regimental hospitals to obtain their pay and to start for home.

During the last two months quite a number of men have been sent to us thus, even from the more distant regiments at Poolsville and at Budd's Ferry, with letters from their surgeons, or other officers, requesting us to receive them and render them such assistance as they might demand. These men frequently reach here just at night, and are much exhausted, and need, peculiarly, the shelter and the helping hand which we give to them.

A large number of men have also come to us from the hospitals at Philadelphia, Baltimore, and Annapolis. These hospitals receive by hundreds the convalescents from the general hospitals in and around Washington. When these convalescents are well enough to join their regiments, or else, while partially recovered, they are so far diseased as to call for their discharge from the service, they return to Washington, all needing more or less care; some of them almost entirely helpless.

Figure 1–2

Sanitary Commission–Third Report. (Reproduced with permission of the Keeling Collection, the Center for Nursing Historical Inquiry, University of Virginia, School of Nursing.)

The Western Front

In the early months of the war, the deplorable conditions in the Washington, D.C. camps were repeated everywhere troops were stationed, and accounts of outbreaks of pneumonia and typhoid fever, poor food, and numerous deaths from injuries, amputations, and gangrene soon reached families back home.

In response to one letter reporting such chaos to a church in Illinois, the congregation sent **Mary Ann Bickerdyke,** an uneducated, widowed housekeeper known locally for her nursing ability, to the Western Front to investigate the situation. Bickerdyke found appalling conditions. Cairo was filled with thousands of previously robust soldiers, now suffering from fevers, dying of measles and dysentery, and living in filth. Undaunted by her lack of authority and over the strong objections of the surgeons in the camp, "Mother Bickerdyke" rallied the men, ordering them to chop kindling, build fires, and heat large kettles of water. In a whirlwind of activity, Bickerdyke arranged for many tasks to be done: the clothes washed, the soldiers bathed, the bedding fumigated, and the garbage removed. In fact, she made such an impact in so short a time that one surgeon complained that "a cyclone in calico" had struck the camp (Young, 1959, p. 92).

Other nurses who served on the Western Front included Mary Safford, a rich, frail, educated woman, and Emily Haines Harrison, a young widow who served as a nurse in Ohio from 1861 to 1865 (Ganger, 1988). Like Bickerdyke, these young women worked tirelessly to attend to the needs of the sick and injured, ignoring the opposition of the surgeons (Livermore, 1867).

Clara Barton

Soon after the Civil War broke out in 1861, **Clara Barton,** a Massachusetts woman who was working as a copyist in the U.S. Patent Office, began an independent campaign to provide relief for the soldiers. Appealing to the nation for supplies of woolen shirts, blankets, towels, lanterns, camp kettles, and other necessities (Barton, 1862), she established her own system of distribution, refusing to enlist in the military nurse corps headed by Dorthea Dix (Oates, 1994). Working outside of the government's official organization, Barton did not receive her first army pass authorizing her to take supplies to the battlegrounds of Virginia until August 12, 1862. Then, having taken a leave of absence from her patent job, she made her way to Culpeper, Virginia. At the scene of the battle, she set up a makeshift field hospital and cared for the wounded and dying. During this battle, Barton gained her famous title "Angel of the Battlefield." Her efforts did not end with the war. She went on to found an organization whose name is synonymous with compassionate service: the American Red Cross.

Nursing in the Confederacy

Like their sisters in the North, the women of the South responded to the news of war with an outpouring of support for the soldiers. Among those who served were Kate Cumming, Phoebe Pember, and Sally Thompkins. However, unlike the women in the North, southern women worked without the benefit of an official government organization. In contrast to Lincoln's rapid response to organize the provision of medical care, the Confederate government did not assume control and partial support of all southern military hospitals until the last months of 1861 and early 1862. Until this time, many hospitals were staffed only with lady volunteers or wounded soldiers. With the advent of government control, some aspects of hospital organization changed dramatically, and several women were appointed as superintendents of hospitals. Superintendent Sallie Thompkins, who had earlier established a private hospital in Richmond, Virginia, was commissioned a "captain of calvary, unassigned" by President Davis, and was the only woman in the Confederacy to hold military rank.

While thousands of women supported the war effort, only a few were appointed as matrons of hospitals. One of the earliest to be placed in charge was **Phoebe Pember.** When she was assigned to Chimborazo Hospital, a sprawling government-run institution on the western boundary of Richmond, Virginia, in September 1862, Pember noted that the care was provided by "sick or wounded men, convalescing and placed in that position, however ignorant they might be—until strong enough for field duty" (Pember, 1959, p. 18). Not only was there inadequate help, but there were also shortages in supplies throughout the South due to blockaded seaports. In Chimborazo, fuel was inadequate, food was skimpy, soap was unavailable, and bandages were reused without being cleansed (Pember, 1959). Pember remedied this situation as best she could, imposing order, discipline, and cleanliness on hospital operations.

Change in the American Military Medical System

By the end of the Civil War both the physical and the administrative structure of the military hospitals had been transformed. In both the North and South, women volunteers, religious orders, and newly appointed matrons and superintendents had made a significant impact. The hospitals were orderly, clean, and well ventilated, and the death rate was surprisingly low. Moreover, it had become clear that women as nurses and organizers had played a major role in these reforms. The Civil War, for all of its horror, had helped to advance the cause of professional nursing. The success in the reform of military hospitals would open the doors for reform of civilian hospital facilities throughout the country (Rosenberg, 1987).

1874–1900: The Roots Take Hold

During the years following the Civil War, a number of events exerted a positive influence on the founding of training schools for nurses. In 1869, Dr. Samuel Gross, a progressive physician, recommended to the American Medical Association that large hospitals should begin the process of developing training schools for nurses. He proposed that the students in these schools be taught by medical staff and resident physicians. Simultaneously, members of the United States Sanitary Commission, who had served during the war and learned its lessons, began to lobby for the creation of nursing schools. Support for their efforts gained momentum as advocates of social reform reported the shockingly inadequate conditions that existed in many hospitals. Another voice for nursing's cause belonged to Sarah J. Hale, editor of the popular and widely read *Godey's Lady's Book and Magazine.* Hale advocated formal training for nurses in an editorial entitled "Lady Nurses" in February 1871:

> Much has been lately said of the benefits that would follow if the calling of the sick nurse were elevated to a profession which an educated lady might adopt without a sense of degradation, either of her own part or in the estimation of others. . . . There can be no doubt that the duties of the sick nurse, to be properly performed, require an education and training little, if at all, inferior to those possessed by members of the medical profession. To leave these duties to untaught and ill-trained persons is as great a mistake as it was to allow the office of surgeon to be held by one whose proper calling was that of a mechanic of the humblest class. The manner in which a reform may be effected is easily pointed out. Every medical college should have a course of study and training especially adapted for ladies who desire to qualify themselves for the profession of nurse; and those who had gone through the course, and passed the requisite examination, should receive a degree and a diploma, which would at once establish their position in society. The "graduate nurse" would in general estimation be as much above the ordinary nurse of the present day as the professional surgeon of our times is above the barber-surgeon of the last century (Donahue, 1996).

Together, these influential men and women paved the way for the formal establishment of nurse training schools.

The First Training Schools for Nurses and the Feminization of Nursing

The first three training schools for nurses, modeled after Nightingale's famous school at St. Thomas's Hospital in London, were Bellevue Training School for Nurses in New York City, Connecticut Training School for Nurses in New Haven, Connecticut, and the Boston Training School for Nurses at Massachusetts General Hospital in Boston (Dock, 1907). The widely held Victorian belief in women's innate sensitivity and high morals led to the early requirement that applicants to these programs be female, for it was thought that only these feminine qualities could improve the quality of nursing's care. Thus, sensitivity, breeding, intelligence, and ladylike behavior, including submission to authority, were highly desired personal characteristics for applicants. The feminization of the profession took root. The number of training schools increased steadily during the last decades of the nineteenth century, and by 1900 they played a critical role in providing hospitals with a stable, subservient, female workforce, as hospitals came to be staffed primarily by students (Fig. 1–3). According to historian Rosenberg, "no single change transformed the hospital's day to day workings more than the acceptance of trained nurses and nurse training schools, which brought a disciplined corps of would-

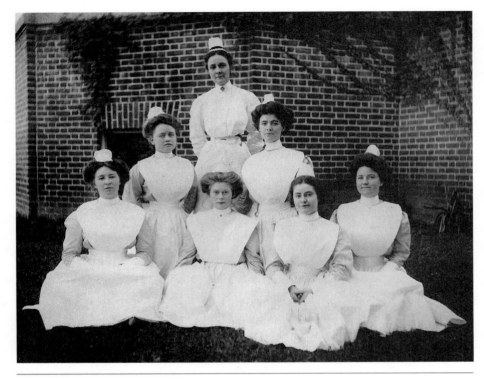

Figure 1–3
University of Virginia student nurses, circa 1910. (Reproduced with permission of the Brodie Collection, the Center for Nursing Historical Inquiry, University of Virginia, School of Nursing.)

be professionals in the wards. . . ." (Rosenberg, 1987, p. 344). (You will find a thorough description of the history of nursing education in Chapter 2.)

The 1893 Chicago World's Fair Promotes Professionalization

The 1893 Chicago World's Fair, a shining monument to the ideals of the Progressive Movement, was the setting for dramatic steps in the professionalization of nursing. There, some of the most influential nursing leaders of the century, including Isabel Hampton, Lavinia Dock, and Bedford Fenwick of Great Britain, gathered to share ideas and discuss issues pertaining to nursing education. In this setting, **Isabel Hampton Robb,** organizer of the Johns Hopkins School of Nursing and one of the greatest early leaders of nursing, presented a paper "protesting the lack of uniformity in nursing school curricula and the inadequacy of nursing education." A paper by Florence Nightingale addressing the need for scientific training of nurses was also read. The very next day, these visionary women began to transform ideas into action, establishing the American Society of Superintendents of Training Schools for Nurses to begin to address issues in nursing education. The society changed its name in 1912 to the National League of Nursing Education (NLNE); in 1952 it was again reorganized and given its current name, the National League for Nursing (NLN) (Christy, 1984).

Isabel Hampton Robb, a visionary and influential leader, recognized the need "to unite practitioners of nursing" as well as nursing educators. In 1896 she founded the Nurses' Associated Alumnae of the United States and Canada, which in 1911 became officially known as the American Nurses Association (ANA) (Christy, 1969, p. 38).

At the close of the decade, in 1899, this small group of American nursing leaders along with nursing leaders from abroad, collaborated again with Bedford Fenwick of Britain to found the International Council of Nurses (ICN). The ICN was dedicated to uniting nursing organizations of all nations, and, fittingly, the first meeting was held at the World Exposition in Buffalo, New York, in 1901. At that meeting, a major topic of discussion was the need for state registration of nurses.

Visiting Nursing: The Henry Street Settlement

It was also during this last decade of the century that urbanization, immigration, and industrialization had begun to create huge social problems. Chief among these were the overcrowding and filth of cities, the emergence of sweat shops and child labor, and the spread of infectious diseases. Typically, immigrant families lived in crowded, suffocating, rat-infested tenements, with the central air chutes filled with garbage. Responding to the needs of the immigrant communities, **Lillian Wald** and her colleague Mary Brewster moved into a tenement on New York's Lower East Side and, with the help of private philanthropists, established the Henry Street Settlement. This highly organized agency provided both visiting nursing care and civic and social services, including playgrounds and country camps, to inner city residents. Lillian Wald, writing in July 25, 1893, noted some aspects of the care and services she provided:

> My first call was on the Goldberg baby whose pulse and improved condition had been maintained after our last night's care. After taking the temperature, washing and dressing the child, I called on the doctor who had been sum-

moned before, told him of the family's tribulations and he offered not to charge them for the visit. Then I took Hattie Issacs, the consumptive, a big bunch of flowers and while she slept I cleaned out the window of medicine bottles. Then I bathed her . . . made the bed, cooked a light breakfast of eggs and milk which I had brought with me, fed her and assisted the mother to straighten up and then left. . . . After luncheon, I saw the O'Brien's and took the little one, with whooping cough, to play in the back of our yard. On the next floor, the Costra baby had a sore mouth for which I gave the mother borax and honey and little cloths to keep it clean . . . (Wald, 1893).

Lavinia Lloyd Dock

Lavinia Lloyd Dock, a fiery political and social activist who became a central figure in American and international nursing history during the Progressive Era (Estabrooks, 1995), soon joined the Henry Street Settlement to work with her colleagues.

Dock (Fig. 1–4) was not only a nurse but also a militant suffragist who linked the future of nursing to the greater women's movement. In one early article she wrote:

> As the modern nursing movement is emphatically an outcome of the original and general woman's movement . . . it would be a great pity for them [nurses] to allow one of the most remarkable movements of the day to go on under their eyes without comprehending it. . . . Unless we possess the ballot we shall not know when we may get up in the morning to find all that we had gained has been taken from us (Dock, 1907, p. 897).

War Crystallizes the Need for Nurses: Spanish American War—1898

In 1898 the United States Congress declared war on Spain, and once again, as in the Civil War, nursing would have a major role to play. Immediately, Cuban camps were devastated by typhoid fever and other infectious diseases, and a call for nurses was sent out. In response, Isabel Hampton Robb, president of the Nurses' Associated Alumnae of the United States and Canada, offered the services of trained nurses (Wall, 1995). Instead of accepting this offer, the sur-

---

HISTORICAL NOTE

In describing Lavinia Dock, Isabel M. Stewart, a colleague, said ". . . this suffrage thing—it was the whole thing for her; she wanted not only to work for it, but really to suffer for it. . . . [S]he was a member of the advanced wing of the Suffrage Party, and they were having a meeting in Washington at the time that Wilson was beginning to think of the possibility of war . . . and Lavinia got up and seized the flag and on she marched, out of the door, and they followed her . . . and they picketed the White House . . . ! Anyway, they all went into the cooler [jail] for the night. I think it just pleased her no end" (Stewart, 1961).

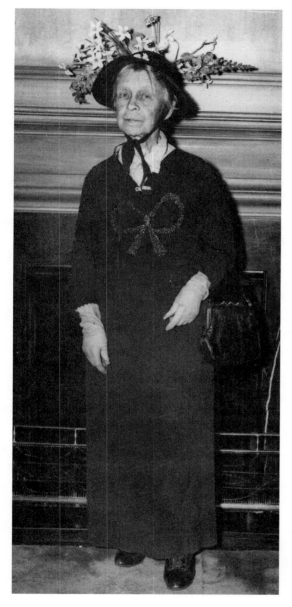

Figure 1–4
Lavinia L. Dock (Reproduced with permission of the Special Collections, Milbank Memorial Library, Teachers College, Columbia University.)

geon general appointed an ad hoc Hospital Corps, formed by the Daughters of the American Revolution (DAR) to recruit nurses. Anita N. McGee, a physician and DAR member, was granted the authority to head this group. McGee required that only graduates of nurse training schools be recruited as contract nurses for the army. However, when typhoid fever became epidemic and there were thousands of soldiers who needed care, others, including the

Sisters of the Holy Cross and untrained African-American nurses who had had typhoid fever in the past, were accepted for service (Wall, 1995). Significant for the first use of trained nurses in war, the Spanish–American War would set the stage for the development of a permanent Army Nurse Corps (1901) and Navy Nurse Corps (1908) in the future.

1900–1917: A Young Profession Faces New Challenges

In October 1900, after years of dedicated work by Isabel Hampton Robb, Mary Adelaide Nutting, Lavinia L. Dock, Sophia Palmer, and **Mary E. P. Davis,** the first issue of the *American Journal of Nursing* was published (Christy, 1984). **Sophia Palmer,** the director of nursing at Rochester City Hospital, New York, was appointed as the first editor. Nurses now had both a professional organization and an official journal through which they could communicate with each other. According to the editorial in the first issue:

> It will be the aim of the editors to present month by month the most useful facts, the most progressive thought and the latest news that the profession has to offer in the most attractive form that can be secured . . . (Palmer, 1900, p. 64).

State Licensure: A Milestone for the Profession

In 1903, state legislatures in North Carolina, New Jersey, New York, and Virginia passed licensure laws for nursing, all within a span of two months. Lavinia Dock noted the significance of these laws:

> We all understand that these little bills are only an opening wedge. We all know that the idea for which we are working is a state examination, to be passed, fixed upon a stated basis of work. I think our ideal bill would demand a specified time for graduates, I mean a certain amount of work to be done before they enter upon the study of nursing; then a specified time for practice in the work constituting the nurses' work . . . and make a compulsory examination before practice . . . (New York State Nurses Association, 1903).

Within the next decade, many other states followed with a plan for licensure of professional nurses (Fig. 1–5). The roots of professional nursing had taken hold.

HISTORICAL NOTE

The state of the art of medicine grew dramatically after the turn of the century. Science was well respected, and data were being collected on patients' conditions. Temperature graphs were routinely kept, the microscopic examination of urine and blood was an established procedure, and the x-ray was now widely available in hospitals (Howell, 1996).

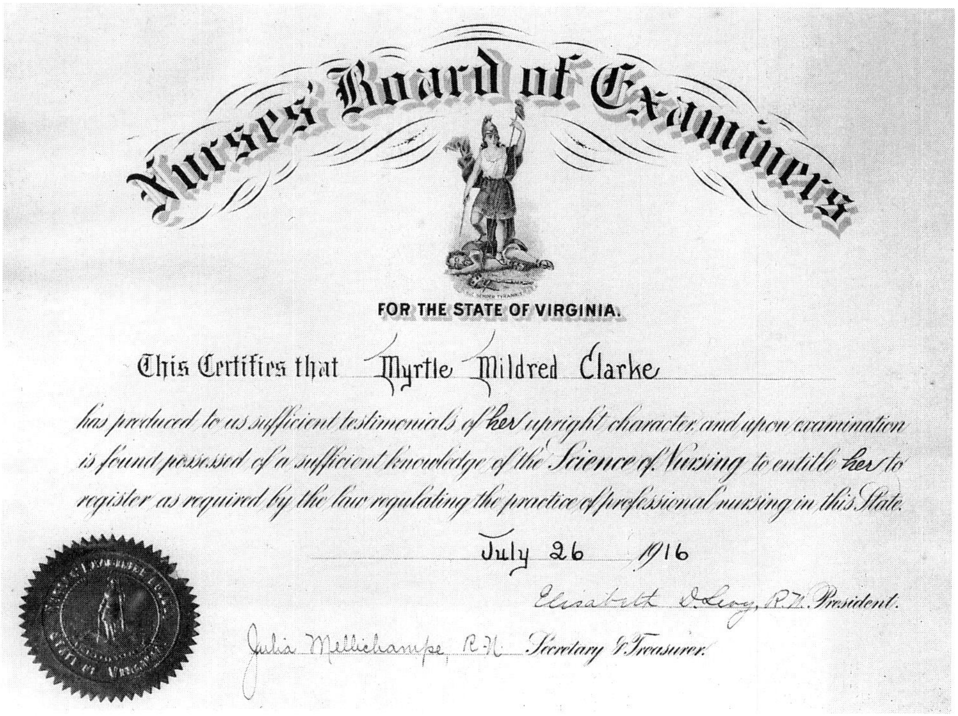

Figure 1–5
Early nursing license, circa 1906. (Reproduced with permission of School of Nursing Collection, The Center for Nursing Historical Inquiry, University of Virginia, School of Nursing.)

"A Successful Experiment": African–American Clinic Nursing in New York City

At the same time that nursing was addressing these professional issues, tuberculosis was a major health problem in the teeming slums of the newly developing cities. Dr. Edward T. Devine, president of the Charity Organization Society, noted the high incidence of tuberculosis among New York City's African-American population. Aware of racial barriers and cultural resistance to seeking medical care, Dr. Devine determined that a "Negro" district nurse should be hired to work in the African-American community to persuade people to accept treatment. **Jesse Sleet,** an African-American nurse who had been trained at Providence Hospital in Chicago, a hospital exclusively for colored people, was chosen to work on a trial basis. Her report to the Charity Organization Society was published in the *American Journal of Nursing* in 1901, entitled "A Successful Experiment":

> I beg to render to you a report of the work done by me as a district nurse among the colored people of New York City during the months of October and

November. . . . I have visited forty-one families and made 156 calls in connection with these families, caring for nine cases of consumption, four cases of peritonitis, two cases of chickenpox, two cases of cancer, one case of diphtheria, two cases of heart disease, two cases of tumor, one case of gastric catarrh, two cases of pneumonia, four cases of rheumatism, and two cases of scalp wound. I have given baths, applied poultices, dressed wounds, washed and dressed newborn babies, cared for mothers . . . (Sleet, 1901, p. 729).

Jesse Sleet (Fig. 1–6) was in fact so successful in community health work that she became legendary (Mosley, 1996). Sleet later recommended to Lillian Wald that Elizabeth Tyler, a graduate of Freedmen's Hospital Training School

Figure 1–6
Jessie Sleet Scales. (Reproduced with permission of the E. M. Carnegie Collection, Archives of Hampton University.)

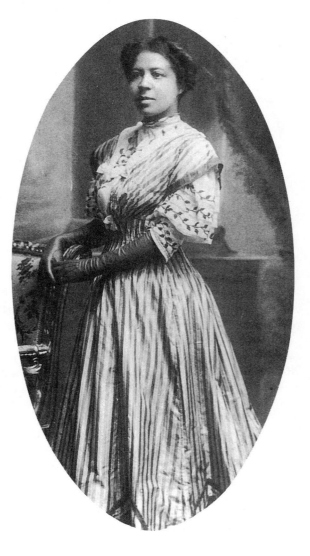

for Nurses, work with African-American patients at the Henry Street Settlement. Working within the confines of a racist society, she and Tyler established the Stillman House Branch of the Henry Street Settlement for "Colored People" in a small store on West Sixty-first Street.

For community health nursing, the addition of these pioneer African-American nurses to the ranks of the Henry Street Settlement signified activism, expansion, and growth. Despite the everpresent racial barriers and deplorable living and health conditions, these courageous young women succeeded in providing excellent nursing care to underserved families with spiraling health care needs.

In 1912, the ideas associated with the Henry Street Settlement won widespread acceptance. District and visiting nursing services proliferated, and national standards were needed. As a result, the National Organization of Public Health Nursing (NONPHN) was established with Lillian Wald as its first president.

1917: The Flu Epidemic and World War I Bring New Challenges to a Young Profession

Two significant events coincided in 1917 to provide nursing with new challenges. The United States entered World War I, and an influenza epidemic swept across the country. The concept of using trained female nurses to care for soldiers had been proved on the field of battle and accepted (Fig. 1–7). So, when the United States entered the war in Europe, a Committee on Nursing was formed under the Council of National Defense (Dock and Stewart, 1920). This committee was chaired by **Adelaide Nutting,** Professor of Nursing and Health, Columbia University (see Chapter 2 for further discussion of Nutting, a leader in nursing education) and included Jane A. Delano, Director of Nursing in the American Red Cross, among others. Charged with supplying an adequate number of trained nurses to U.S. Army hospitals abroad, the committee initiated a national publicity campaign to recruit young women to enter nurses training, established the Army School of Nursing with Annie Goodrich as dean, introduced college women to nursing in the Vassar Training Camp for

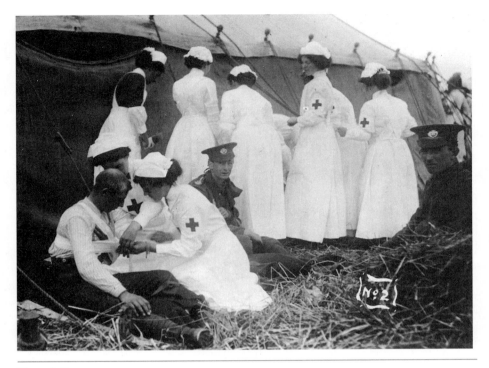

Figure 1–7
World War I Red Cross Nursing. (Reproduced with permission of the Keeling Collection, the Center for Nursing Historical Inquiry, University of Virginia, School of Nursing.)

Nurses, and began widespread public education in home nursing and hygiene through Red Cross nursing.

On the home front, the flu epidemic of 1917 to 1919 increased the public's awareness of the necessity of public health nursing. Across the nation, the public health service, American Red Cross, and Visiting Nursing Associations mobilized to provide care for the thousands of citizens struck with influenza. In Richmond, Virginia, in 1918, the burden of home visits fell to the Instructive Visiting Nurse Association (IVNA). According to the director, Nannie Minor, RN:

> For many days our office was a nightmare . . . from early morning until late at night we sat at the telephone with the receiver rarely out of our hands, listening to heartrending stories and appeals for aid to which we could so inadequately respond. For about two weeks we were receiving about 180–250 calls a day and the nurses were manning between 450–500 visits (Minor, 1918).

In spring 1919, the second wave of the flu epidemic struck the east coast and swept across the country. Although not as lethal as the first, widespread illness among Americans reclosed businesses, schools, and churches and made increased demands for nursing services.

1920–1930: The Roaring Twenties

By the time World War I ended, nursing again had demonstrated the effectiveness of using young, trained, professional nurses to care for soldiers during war. Moreover, the profession had also made clear the need for nursing to have both the responsibility for and the authority to manage the care of their patients. As a result, in 1920 Congress passed a bill that provided nurses with military rank (Dock and Stewart, 1920). This bill followed on the heels of the passage of the Nineteenth Amendment to the U.S. Constitution, a bill that granted women the right to vote. Both acts of Congress opened the decade of the "Roaring Twenties" and the beginning of unheard freedom for American women. Shortened hairstyles, rising hemlines, and the use of cosmetics, all a part of the "flapper" era, reflected these new-found freedoms.

The twenties also saw increased utilization of hospitals and an acceptance of the scientific basis of medicine. Most major surgical procedures were now being done in hospitals, and penicillin was discovered in 1928. This drug profoundly affected the treatment of infection, and antibiotic use for the prevention of postoperative infections became routine.

In the early part of the decade, Congress passed the Shephard-Towner Act to provide services for mothers and children in cities and counties throughout the nation. Amidst all of these changes, nursing was progressing in two divergent areas. The Goldmark Report, a study of nursing education, advocated the establishment of collegiate schools of nursing rather than hospital-based diploma programs (see Chapter 2), and programs in rural midwifery were being organized.

1925: The Frontier Nursing Service

In 1925, **Mary Breckinridge,** a nurse and certified midwife who had family social connections with Kentucky's health commissioner, established the Kentucky Committee for Mothers and Babies, later to be known as the Frontier Nursing Service (FNS). This service provided the first organized midwifery program in the United States. Nurses of the FNS worked in Leslie County, Kentucky, an isolated rural area in the Appalachian Mountains. There, they traveled by horseback to reach the families of each district. In 1930 alone, the FNS reported 22,347 visits to 8,563 families and 10,459 visits to their nursing centers (Pletsh, 1981). Serving the health needs of the poverty-stricken mountain community, the FNS nurses delivered babies and provided pre- and postnatal care, educated mothers and their families about nutrition and hygiene, and cared for the sick. Through this rural midwifery service, Breckenridge demonstrated that nurses could play a significant role in providing primary rural health care.

HISTORICAL NOTE

The concept of the postoperative recovery room staffed by graduate nurses, introduced in the late 1930s, would set the precedent for the development of intensive care units in the future (Lynaugh & Fairman, 1992).

1931–1945: The Profession Responds to the Great Depression and World War II

The crash of the stock market in 1929 with the resulting economic depression and unemployment was to have a profound impact on the nursing profession. Until this time, most nurses worked as private duty nurses in patient's homes, for hospitals were largely staffed by nursing students. As businesses failed and unemployment spread, families without incomes could no longer afford private duty nurses when they needed them, and many nurses joined the growing ranks of the unemployed. The creation of the Civil Works Administration (CWA) in 1933 by President Roosevelt was specifically important for unemployed nurses, particularly for public health nurses. Under the CWA, nurses participated in providing rural and school health services and took part in specific projects conducting surveys to determine service needs related to communicable disease and nutrition of children (Fitzpatrick, 1975).

During these economically shattered times, many hospitals were forced to close their schools of nursing. As a result, they no longer had a reliable, cheap student workforce and faced a shortage of staff to care for patients. At the same time there was a dramatic increase in the numbers of patients who needed charity care. The solution soon became apparent: The unemployed graduate nurses, willing to work for minimum pay, could be recruited to work in the hospitals rather than in private duty. This change in staffing hospitals with graduate nurses rather than students would have lasting implications for the profession.

World War II: New Opportunities for Nursing

By 1938 German and Italian expansionism in Europe threatened to involve the United States in war. Organized nursing began to prepare to meet the need for nurses should the United States become involved. The Army Nurse Corps increased its numbers, and in 1940 Julia C. Stenson, the ANA president, convened a meeting of representatives of the major nursing organizations to coordinate the efforts of the profession to prepare for war (Bullough, 1976). By 1941, when the Japanese bombing of Pearl Harbor drew the United States into war, nurses were vigorously recruited to serve at the battlefront.

Nurses who a few months earlier had not even thought of wartime nursing found themselves accompanying troops to Europe, landing in Normandy

---

HISTORICAL NOTE

From Tressa Cates' diary, Sternberg General Army Hospital in Manila, in the days immediately following the attack on Pearl Harbor: "Today was a ghastly dream. Beds that were empty yesterday were now occupied by mangled and horribly burned patients. In a few hours, the simple routine of our lives was completely changed. We worked twelve to fourteen hours at a time and felt no exhaustion—only numbness. We couldn't quite believe what happened . . . our wounded and dying continued to fill the beds (Cates, 1957, p. 18–19).

---

a few days after the invasion. Dressed in army fatigues, they cared for troops in field and evacuation hospitals in North Africa, Italy, France, and the Philippines, while Navy nurses gave care aboard hospital ships.

While soldiers were receiving care on the front, there were severe shortages of nurses at home. One of the most significant programs initiated as a result of the shortage of nurses for the war effort was the **Cadet Nurse Corps,** founded by Frances Payne Bolton, the congresswoman from Ohio. The Bolton Act became law on June 15, 1943. Headed by Lucile Petry Leone, the Cadet Corps sought to recruit 65,000 new students in 1944 and another 60,000 in 1945, about twice the number entering schools in peacetime (Petry, 1945). Admission to the Cadet Corps could not be refused because of race or marital status. Of further note, the Corps had minimum educational standards. These policies, combined with federal assistance to nursing schools and the requirement that schools have budgets that were separate from the hospitals, had a significant impact on the profession's growth and development as it sought to integrate African-American students and to break from the hospital-affiliated apprenticeship model of nursing education. By the end of the war, the Cadet program had subsidized the education of about 179,000 nursing students (Fig. 1–8). The Bolton Act also provided funds to graduate nurses for advanced study in order to increase the number of nursing instructors and prepare nurses to practice in psychiatry and in public health nursing.

Over 100,000 nurses volunteered and were certified for military services in the Army and Navy Nurse Corps (Nurses' Contribution, 1945, p. 683). Nursing made great strides in its professional development during the war and immediately afterward. In the field hospitals at the front, nursing and medical boundaries blurred as both professions worked together to save as many of the wounded as they could. As a result, nurses took on new responsibilities and learned new skills. As Virginia G. Shannon of the U.S. Army recalled:

In October 1944 we were ready for the invasion of Southern France. . . . We expected to be based at Lyon but just kept going until we were only 10 miles behind the lines. Again, we were in a hospital that had not been finished but had a big red cross on it. . . . There were so many casualties from the battles. Wounded and injured were brought in from the Rhine, and as fast as we could evacuate them, more were brought in. We had to learn a lot of things right on the spot. When there wasn't a doctor to do it, the nurses did it. I did

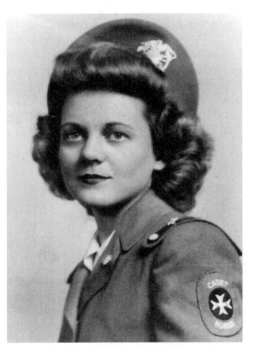

Figure 1–8
Cadet nurse Norma E. Shrewsbury, 1943–1944.
(Reproduced with permission of the School of
Nursing Alumni Association Collection, the Cen-
ter for Nursing Historical Inquiry, University of
Virginia, School of Nursing.)

blood transfusions, intravenous medications and even sewed up secondary
closure wounds (Fessler, 1996, p. 185).

After the war, further progress toward professionalization was made. In
1947, military nurses were awarded full commissioned status and segregation
of African-American nurses was ended. In 1948, The Brown Report recommended establishing schools of nursing in universities and colleges, enhancing the educational standards for professional nurses (Fig. 1–9) (see Chapter 2). By 1954 discrimination against male nurses was also reduced when
men were finally admitted into military nursing (Bullough, 1976).

1945–1960: The Rise of Hospitals—Bureaucracy, Science, and Shortages

There were numerous technological and scientific advances in medicine in
the period from 1945 to 1960. Following World War II, federal budget appropriations for medical research increased enormously, resulting in a surge of
research in many of the specialized areas. Dramatic innovations in medical
care followed. Sulfa drugs transformed the care of infectious diseases. New
cardiac drugs were developed. Cardiac surgeries were performed, and in 1941
Dr. Claude S. Beck, a surgeon at Western Reserve School of Medicine in
Cleveland, Ohio, reported the first two attempts of defibrillation for ventricu-
lar fibrillation during surgery.

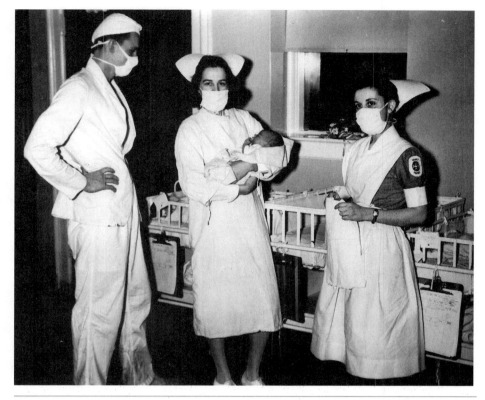

Figure 1–9
Cadet student with newborns and instructor, circa 1947. (Reproduced with permission of the School of Nursing Alumni Association Collection, the Center for Nursing Historical Inquiry, University of Virginia, School of Nursing.)

At the same time postwar economic resurgence, an expansion in private health care insurance, and the "baby boom" made an impact on the medical system (Fig. 1–10). In 1946, the Hill Burton Act, providing funds to construct hospitals, led to a surge in the growth of new facilities. This rapid expansion in the number of hospital beds resulted in an acute shortage of nurses and increasingly difficult working conditions for those who were employed. Long hours, inadequate salaries, and increasing patient loads made many nurses unhappy with their jobs, and threats of strikes and collective bargaining ensued. For years, there would be heated debates about whether or not professional nurses should go on strike.

In response to the shortages, "team nursing" was introduced. This method of care delivery utilized licensed practical nurses (LPNs), nursing assistants, and nurses aides under the supervision of a registered nurse. While efficient, the method fragmented patient care and removed the registered nurse from the bedside. Another response to the shortage was the institution of the associate degree program, an abbreviated two-year program designed by Mildred Montag (see Chapter 2).

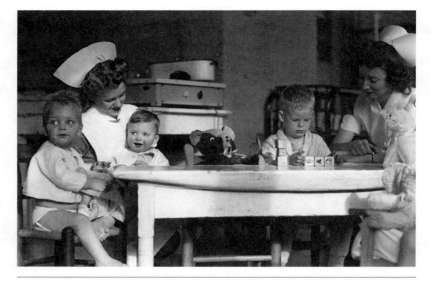

Figure 1–10
Student nurses in pediatrics, circa 1945. (Reproduced with permission of the School of Nursing Collection, the Center for Nursing Historical Inquiry, University of Virginia, School of Nursing.)

The 1950s saw other changes in health care. It was also during this decade that the profession advocated clinical nursing research, and the *Journal of Nursing Research* was first published. Military corpsmen entered nursing programs, and the number of male nurses increased. More nurses sought advanced degrees. State units of the American Nurses Association accepted African-American nurses for membership, as did the national organization, thereby ending racial discrimination in nursing organizations. The National Association of Colored Graduate Nurses was dissolved in 1951 (to be replaced in 1972 by the formation of the National Black Nurses Association). In 1957, challenged by the launch of Sputnick to keep up with the Russians in science and technology, America moved swiftly toward the development of space-age technology. The accompanying scientific advances in medical and nursing research would continue to revolutionize nursing and medical care for the remainder of the twentieth century.

HISTORICAL NOTE

MASH units in Korea: In 1950, when the Korean War broke out, nurses were once again required for combat. This time, Army nurses were stationed as close to the front as possible in Mobile Army Surgical Hospital (MASH) units that could be set up quickly to provide emergency trauma care. Once again, nurses at the front faced new challenges as the injured were flown in by helicopter only minutes after being wounded in combat.

1961–1985: New Roles for Nurses

While the first nursing specialists—nurse anesthetists at the Mayo Clinic and public health nurses in New York City—date back to the late 19th century, the 1960s is more often noted as the era of the rise in specialty care and clinical specialization for nurses. The impressive development of the clinical specialist role in psychiatric nursing in the early sixties, combined with the rise of intensive care units and technological advances of the period, fostered the growth of clinical specialization in other areas of nursing, including cardiac-thoracic surgery and coronary care.

Coronary Care Nursing

One of the most significant events of this period was the establishment of the coronary care unit (CCU), a subspecialty unit, created by Dr. Hughes Day in Kansas City and Dr. Lawrence Meltzer in Philadelphia, working independently in 1962–63. Several factors culminated in the development of this subspecialty care. Electrocardiograms were available, the defibrillator had recently been shown effective in saving lives, the concept of intensive care had been established and was already in place in many hospitals, and physicians were interested in subspecialty care. Furthermore, during the recent wars, nurses had accepted new responsibilities and roles as the need arose.

In the coronary care units (Fig. 1–11), nurses began to share with

Figure 1–11
Student nurse in Coronary Care Unit, 1969. (Reproduced with permission of the Keeling Collection, the Center for Nursing Historical Inquiry, University of Virginia, School of Nursing.)

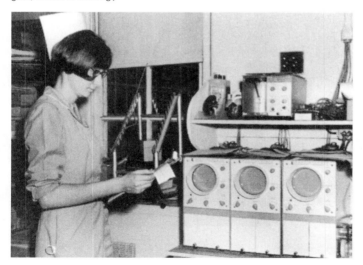

physicians the emerging medical knowledge about the diagnosis and treatment of cardiac arrhythmias. Soon they began to be recognized for their expertise in the care of critically ill cardiac patients and were permitted to administer intravenous drugs and defibrillate patients according to written protocols. Gaining acceptance as colleagues, the CCU nurses set the stage for more autonomous practice in a variety of specialty areas, including burn, dialysis, and oncology units as well as in medical and surgical ICUs.

Nurse Practitioners

The rise in medical specialization in the sixties, with the concurrent shortage of primary care physicians and the public demand for improved access to health care that grew out of Lyndon Johnson's "Great Society" reforms, also fostered the emergence of the nurse practitioner in primary care. In 1965, **Lorretta Ford,** RN, and Henry Silver, MD, opened the first pediatric nurse practitioner program at the University of Colorado. This collaborative project, designed to prepare professional nurses to manage common childhood illnesses and provide well-child care, demonstrated that nurse practitioners were competent in managing 75 percent of pediatric patients in community clinics (Ford and Silver, 1967). Their research subsequently attracted considerable attention across the United States and led to federal support for the nurse practitioner role. By the mid-1980s nurse practitioner programs had been developed in schools of nursing throughout the country and nurse practitioners were employed in a wide variety of outpatient settings. By the mid-1990s, there were also programs for acute care nurse practitioners, and jobs became available in tertiary care settings (Fig. 1–12).

Nursing in Vietnam

The war in Vietnam, one of America's longest and most controversial wars, provided nurses once again with opportunities to stretch the boundaries of the discipline as they did whatever needed to be done to provide immediate care to the massive numbers of casualties coming into the field hospitals. Working in inflatable medical units in the jungles of Vietnam, these nurses fought to save lives. They performed emergency tracheotomies, inserted chest tubes, administered blood, and gave morphine without orders when there were not enough physicians to meet the demands. One nurse wrote of how terrified and helpless she felt while transporting the critically ill:

HISTORICAL NOTE

In 1965, Medicare and Medicaid became law, ensuring access to health care for elderly, poor, and disabled Americans.

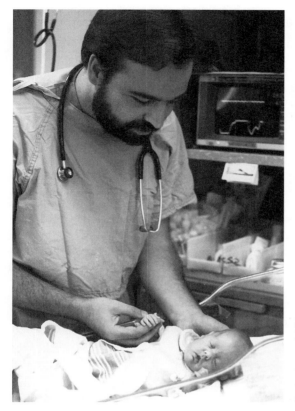

Figure 1–12
Tom Buckley, RN, BSN, Clinician V., circa 1990. (Reproduced with permission of the School of Nursing Collection, the Center for Nursing Historical Inquiry, University of Virginia, School of Nursing.)

Whenever we had someone who had a bad head injury, we'd have to send them to one of the hospitals on the coast, like the 85th Evac. Most of the time, the Air Force would do our evaking for us, but if it was just one person going down, then a lot of times the dust-off choppers would take him and they'd have one of us nurses ride along to take care of him. I went very often, because I was assigned to the emergency room. I remember just how desperate I used to feel during these nights; there was really nothing in the helicopter to take care of them with in case anything should happen. We did have a suction apparatus we could work with our foot, but that was about the only thing that we could really use. I remember praying all the way down that they

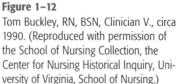

HISTORICAL NOTE

The concept of primary care nursing, introduced by Manthey in 1968, was implemented in many hospitals during the 1970s and 1980s. This method of care delivery advocated "total patient care" done by the registered nurse. It was a "return to the bedside" for experienced nurses and an attempt to combat the depersonalization of the bureaucratic delivery system of care (Lynaugh & Brush, 1996).

wouldn't die before they got there and feeling so afraid that something was going to happen. There was so little I could do (Walker, 1985).

Another nurse described the stress of the war:

> I still remember my baptism into the realities of war: the nausea and revulsion that spilled all over me; my shaking hands as I examined the wounded, took vital signs, and fought to get control of my brain. I still see the face of the first soldier I reached: brown eyes staring wide in death, the back of his head and neck blown away (Boulay, 1989, p. 272).

At the same time that the nurses faced these external challenges, they fought the emotional battles that rose within themselves as they struggled to comprehend the lack of support for their work from large segments of the American public. By 1967, after a massive military build-up by President Johnson, demonstrations against the war were a common occurrence throughout the United States. Later, after the nurses returned home, the trauma of the battlefield would be intensified by this lack of support, and many suffered posttraumatic stress disorder (PSTD).

1986–Present: Managed Care and its Challenges for Nursing

With the advent of managed care in the late 1980s, and the current emphasis on health care reform as a way to continue to cut the costs of medical care, nursing has recently been caught up in the whirlwind of change. Determined to take a proactive stance in the reform effort, the profession wrote its *Agenda for Health Care Reform* in 1992. The plan for reform, discussed more fully in Chapter 4, was comprehensive and focused on restructuring the health care system in the United States to reduce costs and improve access to care. Challenges for nursing in the managed care era include (1) providing quality, cost-effective care; (2) continuing to care, in a culture that has yet to value caring (Reverby, 1987); (3) obtaining third-party reimbursement for nurses in advanced practice roles in both primary and acute care; and (4) preparing to deal with the predicted nursing shortages in the future as both Americans and American nurses age and retire.

Lessons of History

The nursing profession cannot meet the challenges of the twenty-first century without an accurate understanding of its past. The classic reason for studying history is to avoid repeating it. However, there are issues and problems facing the profession that could be addressed using "recycled" solutions.

For example, today there are challenges in providing care to inner city communities. Earlier in this century, this challenge was met quite aptly by

Lillian Wald in the creation of the Henry Street Settlement, in which she addressed not only the physical but also the psychological needs of children and their families (Buhler-Wilkerson, 1993).

Today we are faced with the challenges of relating to a global community. Dock's emphasis on maintaining a world perspective and addressing nursing issues within the context of global women's issues may be instructive. We recognize the need for culturally sensitive care. In the past, African-American nurses met the needs of their patients by being sensitive to cultural differences while challenging racial barriers.

Today, the nursing profession often struggles to explain how nurse practitioners differ from physician's assistants. Yesterday's answer, by Lavinia Dock and Maitland Stewart, might be considered:

> The nurse often acts as the physician's assistant, but she has many duties apart from this function, the most important being her own distinct art of nursing. In this field it is she, and not the physician, who is expert (Dock and Stewart, 1920, p. 340).

The profession must adjust to the continually changing roles for nurses and expectations of what duties nurses can assume. In the past, especially during war, nurses have demonstrated flexibility and competence in the face of change. Cognizant of our heritage, we look to meet the challenges of the present and plan for the future.

Summary of Key Points

- In 1860 Florence Nightingale founded a school for nurses at St. Thomas's Hospital, London, that would become the model for nursing education in the United States.
- Civil War nurses played a major role in reform of military hospitals, thereby opening the door for reform of civilian hospitals nationwide and advancing the cause of professional nursing.
- Formal educational programs for U.S. nurses were established in 1873 in hospitals in New York City, New Haven, and Boston.
- American nursing's first professional organization, the American Society of Superintendents of Training Schools for Nurses, was founded during the 1893 Chicago World's Fair. This organization became the National League for Nursing Education (NLNE) in 1912 and the National League for Nursing (NLN) in 1952.
- The forerunner of the American Nurses Association (ANA) was founded in 1896 by Isabel Hampton Robb.
- In 1899 the International Council of Nurses (ICN) was formed to unite nursing organizations of all nations.
- The development of nursing and the general women's movement, including the right to vote, paralleled each other.
- The initiation of state licensure in 1903 heralded standardization of nursing education programs that, until this time, had varied widely.

- The establishment of the Henry Street Settlement and the rise of community health nursing played a major role in the widespread public acceptance of nurses, particularly African-American nurses.
- World War I and the influenza epidemic of 1917–1919 created a strong demand for nursing services. Many schools were opened in response, mostly in hospitals.
- The Great Depression and World War II created new opportunities for nurses, including the Cadet Nurse Corps, which added 179,000 new registered nurses to the profession by the end of the war.
- Since World War II, hospital expansion, technological advances, and social changes have created new and progressively autonomous roles for nurses, especially advanced practice nurses.

Critical Thinking Questions

1. Florence Nightingale is often credited with being the first nurse researcher. Why do you think this is so?
2. Discuss the significance of the events that occurred during the Chicago World's Fair, 1893, to the advancement of the nursing profession.
3. Do you agree with L. L. Dock's view that nursing is inevitably tied to the greater issues of the women's movement throughout the world? Why or why not?
4. Wars have often been the driving force in creating social change. How did wars influence the profession of nursing?
5. What are some emerging trends in health care that will impact the practice of professional nursing?

Web Resources

American Association for the History of Nursing, http://www.aahn.org/index.html

Black Nurses in History, http://www4.umdnj.edu/camlbweb/blacknurses.html

Canadian Association for the History of Nursing, http://members.xoom.com/bchn

Center for Nursing Historical Inquiry, http://www.nursing.virginia.edu/centers/history.html

Center for the Study of the History of Nursing, http://www.nursing.upenn.edu/history

History of Men in Nursing, http://www.geocities.com/Athens/Forum/6011

References

American Journal of Nursing (1945a). Army nurses in ETO. 45(9), 386–387.

American Journal of Nursing (1945b). The Nurses' contribution to American victory, facts and figures from Pearl Harbor to VJ Day. 45(9), 683–686.

Barton, C. (1862). *Diary. The papers of Clara Barton (1812–1912)*. Washington, D. C. Library of Congress, Manuscript Division.

Boulay, D. M. (1989). A Vietnam tour of duty. *Nursing Outlook,* 37(6), 271–273.

Buhler-Wilkerson, K. (1993a). Guarded by standards and directed by strangers. *Nursing History Review,* 1, 139–154.

Buhler-Wilkerson, K. (1993b). Bringing the care to the people: Lillian Wald's legacy to public health nursing. *American Journal of Public Health,* 83(12), 1778–1786.

Bullough, B. (1976). The lasting impact of WWII in nursing. *American Journal of Nursing,* 76(1), 118–120.

Carnegie, M. E. (1986). *The path we tread: Blacks in nursing, 1854–1984.* Philadelphia: J. B. Lippincott.

Cates, T. R. (1957). *The drainpipe diary.* New York: Vantage Press.

Christman, L. (1965). The influence of specialization on the nursing profession. *Nursing Science,* 3(6), 446–453.

Christman, L. (1971). The nurse specialist as a professional activist. *Nursing Clinics of North America,* 6(2), 231–235.

Christy, T. E. (1969). Portrait of a leader: Lavinia Lloyd Dock. *Nursing Outlook,* 17(6), 72–75.

Christy, T. E. (1975). The fateful decade: 1890–1900. *American Journal of Nursing,* 75(7), 1163–1165.

Dock, L. L. (1900). What we may expect from the law. *American Journal of Nursing,* I: 8–12.

Dock, L. L. (1907). Some urgent social claims. *American Journal of Nursing,* 7, 895–901.

Dock, L. L. (1908). Mountain medicine. *American Journal of Nursing,* 9, 181–183.

Dock, L. L., and Stewart, I. M. (1920). *A short history of nursing.* New York: Putnam.

Donahue, M. P. (1996). *Nursing: The finest art.* 2d ed. Philadelphia: Mosby.

Eastabrooks, C. A. (1995). Lavinia Lloyd Dock: The Henry Street years. *Nursing History Review,* 3, 143–72.

Fessler, D. B. (1996). *No time for fear: Voices of American military nurses in World War II.* East Lansing, Mich.: Michigan State University Press.

Fitzpatrick, M. L. (1975). Nursing and the Great Depression. *American Journal of Nursing,* 75(12), 2188–2190.

Ford, L. C. (1979). A nurse for all settings: The nurse practitioner. *Nursing Outlook,* 27(8), 516–521.

Ford, L. C., and Silver, H. K. (1967). The expanded role of the nurse in childcare. *Nursing Outlook,* 15(8), 43–45.

Ganger, C. W. (1988). A sketch of Emily Haines Harrison: Civil War nurse, spy and nurse on the Kansas prairie. *Journal of Nursing History,* 3(2), 22–35.

Griffon, D. P. (1995). Crowning the edifice: Ethel Fenwick and state registration. *Nursing History Review,* 3, 201–212.

Howell, J. (1996). *Technology in the hospital.* Baltimore: The Johns Hopkins University Press.

Kennedy, D. (1970). *Birth control in America: The career of Margaret Sanger.* New Haven: Yale University Press.

Livermore, M. (1867). *My story of the war.* Hartford, Conn.: S. S. Scranton.

Lynaugh J., and Fairman, J. (1992). New nurses, new spaces: A preview of the AACN history study. *American Journal of Critical Care,* 1(1), 19–24.

Lynaugh, J., and Brush, B. (1996). *American nursing: From hospitals to health systems.* Cambridge, Mass.: Blackwell Publishers.

Mayo, A. (1944). Advanced courses in clinical nursing. *American Journal of Nursing,* 44, 580.

Minor, N. (1918). Instructive Visiting Nurses Association papers. In Chauf, K., Richmond, Virginia, Nursing and the Influenza Epidemic of 1918. Charlottesville, Va.: University of Virginia, Center for Nursing Historial Inquiry manuscript collection.

Mosley, M. (1996). Satisfied to carry the bag. *Nursing History Review,* 4, 65–82.

New York State Nurses Association (1903). *Remarks made by Lavinia Dock* [Jan. 20]. New York: New York State Nurses Association.

Nightingale, F. [1859]. (1946) *Notes on nursing: What it is and what it is not.* Reprint, Philadelphia: J. B. Lippincott.

Norman, E. M. (1986). A study of female military nurses in Vietnam during the years 1965–1973. *Journal of Nursing History,* 2(1), 43–60.

Nurse's contribution. (1945). *American Journal of Nursing,* 45(12), 683.

Oates, S. B. (1994). *A woman of valor.* New York: The Free Press.

Palmer, S. (1900). The editor. *American Journal of Nursing,* 1(1), 64.

Pember, P. Y. (1959). *A Southern woman's story.* Atlanta: Bill Wiley.

Petry, L. (1945). The U.S. Cadet Nurse Corps: A summing up. *American Journal of Nursing,* 45(12), 1027–1028.

Pletsch, P. K. (1981). Mary Breckinridge: A pioneer who made her mark. *American Journal of Nursing,* 81(12), 2188–2190.

Reverby, S. M. (1987). *Ordered to care: The dilemma of American nursing,* 1850–1945. Cambridge: Cambridge University Press.

Reiter, F. (1966). The nurse clinician. *American Journal of Nursing,* 66(2), 274–80.

Rosenberg, C. E. (1987). *The care of strangers.* New York: Basic Books.

Sandelowski, M. (1997). Making the best of things: Technology in American nursing, 1870–1940. *Nursing History Review,* 5, 3–22.

Sarnecky, M. T. (1997). Nursing in the American Army from the Revolution to the Spanish-American War. *Nursing History Review,* 5, 49–69.

Simpkins, F., and Patton, J. (1936). *The women of the Confederacy.* Richmond, Va.: Garrett & Massis.

Sleet, J. (1901). A successful experiment. *American Journal of Nursing,* 2, 729.

Smoyak, S. A. (1976). Specialization in nursing: From then to now. *Nursing Outlook,* 24(11), 676–681.

Starr, P. (1982). *The social transformation of American medicine.* New York: Basic Books.

Smith, F. T. (1981). Florence Nightingale, early feminist. *American Journal of Nursing,* 81(5), 1021–1024.

Stevens, R. (1989). *In sickness and in wealth: American hospitals in the twentieth century.* New York: Basic Books.

Stewart, I. M. (1961). *Reminiscences of Isabel M. Stewart.* New York: New York Oral History Research Office, Columbia University.

Wald, L. D. (1893). *Letter to Jacob Schiff,* July 25. New York: L. D. Wald Collection, Manuscript Division, New York Public Library.

Walker, K. (1985). A piece of my heart: The story of twenty-six American women who served in Vietnam. New York: Ballantine.

Wall, B. M. (1995). Courage to care: The sisters of the holy cross in the Spanish-American War. *Nursing History Review,* 3, 55–77.

Woodham-Smith, C. (1951). Florence Nightingale. New York: McGraw-Hill.

Woodham-Smith, C. (1949). Florence Nightingale, London: Constable & Company LTD.

Young, A. (1959). *The women and the crisis: Women of the north in the Civil War,* New York: McDowell, Oblensky.

Educational Patterns in Nursing

Elaine F. Nichols

Key Terms

Accreditation
Advanced Degrees
Advanced Practice Nurses (APNs)
Alternative Educational Programs
American Association of Colleges
  of Nursing (AACN)
American Nurses Association
  (ANA) Position Paper
American Nurses Credentialing
  Center (ANCC)
Articulation
Associate Degree in Nursing
  (ADN)
Baccalaureate Degree
Bachelor of Science in Nursing
  (BSN)
Basic Programs
RN-to-BSN Education (BRN)
Brown Report
Certification
Commission on Collegiate
  Nursing Education (CCNE)
Contact Hour
Continuing Education (CE)
Diploma Program
External Degree
Generic Master's Degree
Generic Nursing Doctorate (ND)
Goldmark Report
Licensure
Lysaught Report

Mandatory Continuing Education
Mildred Montag
National Council Licensing
  Examination for Practical
  Nursing (NCLEX-PN)
National Council Licensing
  Examination for Registered
  Nurses (NCLEX-RN)

National League for Nursing
  (NLN)
National League for Nursing
  Accreditation Commission
  (NLNAC)
Pew Health Professions
  Commission
Practical Nurses

Learning Outcomes

After studying this chapter, students will be able to:

- Trace the development of basic and graduate education in nursing.
- Discuss the influence of early nursing studies on today's nursing education.
- Discuss traditional and alternative ways of becoming a registered nurse.
- Discuss program options for registered nurses and students with baccalaureate degrees in nonnursing fields.
- Differentiate between licensed practical nurses and registered nurses.
- Explain the difference between licensure and certification.
- Define accreditation and its influence on the quality and effectiveness of nursing education programs.
- Discuss the significance of the 1965 American Nurses Association position paper to today's types of nursing programs.
- Discuss similarities and differences among three reports projecting nursing education for the twenty-first century.
- Identify current and future issues in nursing education.

iversity is the major characteristic of nursing education today. Influenced by a variety of factors—societal changes, efforts to achieve full professional status, women's issues, historical factors, public expectations, professional standards, legislation, national studies, and constant changes in

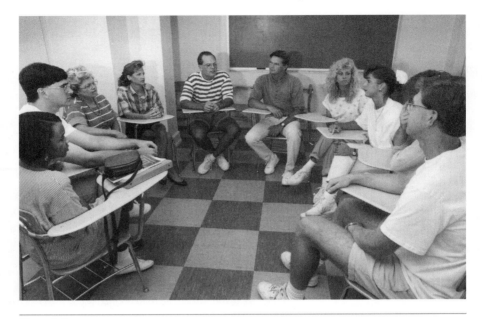

Figure 2–1
In 1996, there were 1,526 programs preparing beginning registered nurses. Students entering nursing to-day are widely diverse in terms of age, culture, and gender (Photo by Fielding Freed).

the health care system—many different types of nursing education programs currently exist.

In 1998, there were 1,526 basic programs preparing beginning registered nurses (RNs) in the United States (Fig. 2–1). Of these, 58.6 percent were associate degree programs, 34.9 percent were baccalaureate programs, and 6.5 percent were diploma programs (National League for Nursing, 1999c). In addition to the basic registered nurse programs, there were also 325 master's programs, 66 doctoral programs, and 1,107 practical nursing programs (National League for Nursing, 1997c, 1997d, 1999b). Also included in the educational system of nursing are a large number of continuing education programs and advanced-practice certification programs.

This chapter provides an orientation to the multiple nursing educational pathways in existence today. It covers the history behind educational programs, descriptions of the various programs, and trends and future issues.

Development of Nursing Education in the United States

As mentioned in Chapter 1, Florence Nightingale is credited with founding modern nursing and creating the first educational system for nurses. After hospitals came into existence in western Europe, and before the influence of

Florence Nightingale, hospital care was given by women prisoners and prostitutes, who were held in low regard by society. These women had no formal preparation in giving care because there were no organized programs to educate nurses until the late 1800s.

Nightingale stressed that nursing was not a domestic, charitable service but a respected occupation requiring advanced education. She opened a school of nursing at St. Thomas's Hospital, London, in 1860 and established the following basic principles for the school:

1. The nurse should be trained in an educational institution supported by public funds and associated with a medical school.
2. The nursing school should be affiliated with a teaching hospital but independent of it.
3. The curriculum should include both theory and practical experience.
4. Professional nurses should be in charge of administration and instruction and should be paid for their instruction.
5. Students should be carefully selected and should reside in nurses' houses that form discipline and character.
6. Students should be required to attend lectures, take quizzes, write papers, and keep diaries. Student records should be maintained (Notter and Spalding, 1976).

Nightingale also believed that the nursing schools should be separate financially and administratively from hospitals where the students trained. This was not the case, however, when nursing schools were first established in the United States.

As mentioned in Chapter 1, the first training schools for nurses in the United States were established in 1872. Located at Bellevue Hospital in New York, the New England Hospital for Women and Children in New Haven, Connecticut, and Massachusetts General Hospital in Boston, the course of study was one year in length. These schools became known as the "famous trio" of nursing schools. In October 1873, Melinda Anne (Linda) Richards became the first "trained nurse" in the United States. By 1879 there were 11 training schools in the United States. Other schools rapidly developed, and by 1900, there were 432 hospital-owned and hospital-operated diploma programs in the United States (Donahue, 1985). These early training programs differed in length from six months to two years, and each school set its own standards and requirements. The primary reason for the schools' existence was to staff the hospitals that operated them. The education of student nurses was not always a primary concern.

Early Studies of the Quality of Nursing Education

Nursing leaders of the early 1900s were concerned about the poor quality of the nurse training programs. They initiated studies about nursing and nursing education to prompt changes. October 1899 marked the culmination of some four years of work by the American Society of Superintendents of Training

Schools for Nurses. Isabel Hampton Robb chaired a committee to investigate a means to prepare nurses better for leadership in schools of nursing. Teachers College, which had opened in New York 10 years earlier for the training of teachers, seemed the logical location for the leadership training of nurses. The program was originally designed to prepare administrators of nursing service and nursing education and began as an eight-month course in hospital economics (Donahue, 1985).

Mary Adelaide Nutting came to Teachers College in 1907 to be the first nursing professor in the world. Under her direction, the department progressed and became a pioneer in education for nurses. The school became known as the "Mother-House" of collegiate education because it fostered the initial movements toward undergraduate and graduate degrees for nurses (Donahue, 1985). In 1912, Nutting conducted a nation-wide investigation of nursing education, "The Educational Status of Nursing," which focused on the living conditions of students, the material being taught, and the teaching methods being used (Christy, 1969).

One of the first major studies on the status of nursing education was published in 1923. Titled "The Study of Nursing and Nursing Education in the United States" and referred to as the **Goldmark Report,** it focused on the clinical learning experiences of students, hospital control of the schools, the desirability of establishing university schools of nursing, the lack of funds specifically for nursing education, and the lack of prepared teachers (Kalisch and Kalisch, 1995).

The year 1924 marked another first in nursing education when the Yale School of Nursing was opened as the first nursing school to be established as a separate university department with an independent budget and its own dean, Annie W. Goodrich. The school demonstrated its effectiveness so markedly that in 1929 the Rockefeller Foundation ensured the permanency of the school by awarding it an endowment of $1 million (Kalisch and Kalisch, 1995).

In 1934, another study entitled "Nursing Schools Today and Tomorrow" reported the number of schools in existence, gave detailed descriptions of the schools, described their curricula, and made recommendations for professional collegiate education (National League of Nursing Education, 1934). In 1937, *A Curriculum Guide for Schools of Nursing* was published outlining a three-year curriculum. This document influenced the structure of diploma schools for many years after its publication (National League of Nursing Education, 1937).

Although published over a 30-year period and undertaken by different groups, these early studies consistently made five similar recommendations:

1. Nursing education programs should be established within the system of higher education.
2. Nurses should be highly educated.
3. Students should not be used to staff hospitals.
4. Standards should be established for nursing practice.
5. All students should meet certain minimum qualifications upon graduation.

These studies set the stage for the development of the educational programs that exist today.

Educational Pathways to Becoming a Registered Nurse

Today, preparation for a career as a registered nurse can begin in one of three ways: in an associate degree program, in a baccalaureate degree program, or in a hospital-based diploma program. All the programs vary in the courses offered, the length of study, and cost.

Following the completion of a basic program for registered nurses, graduates are eligible to take the **National Council Licensing Examination for Registered Nurses (NCLEX-RN).** Upon successful completion of the licensing examination, graduates may legally practice as registered nurses and use the initials RN after their names. Employment and career advancement vary depending on the basic program attended.

Having three different educational routes to **licensure** for registered nurses is confusing to the public and even to nurses themselves. Each type of program is described in the following sections with its history, unique characteristics, and special issues. The basic programs are discussed in the order in which they appeared in nursing education history.

Diploma Program

The hospital-based **diploma program** was the first type of nursing education in the United States. At the peak of diploma education in the 1920s and 1930s, approximately 2,000 programs existed, with numerous programs in almost every state. Diploma programs produced many outstanding nurses, but since the peak in the first third of the century, their numbers have decreased steadily (Conley, 1973).

In the last 30 years, there has been a dramatic decline in diploma programs as nursing education began to move rapidly into collegiate settings. In 1960, there were approximately 800 diploma programs in the United States. By 1980, that number had decreased to approximately 300. By 1997, fewer than half of the states had diploma programs with only 100 diploma programs remaining in 20 states (National League for Nursing, 1999c).

In 1997, the largest number of diploma schools (28) remained in Pennsylvania, along with two other states, New Jersey and Ohio, having 14 and 11, respectively (National League for Nursing, 1999c). Although the number of diploma programs has significantly decreased, many nurses practicing today received their basic nursing education in diploma programs.

In the late 1800s and early 1900s, diploma programs provided one of the few avenues for women to obtain formal education and jobs. Most of the early programs followed a modified apprenticeship model. Lectures were given by physicians, and clinical training was supervised by head nurses and nursing directors. Nursing courses paralleled medical areas and included surgery, obstetrics, pediatrics, and operating room experience. Students were sometimes sent to affiliated institutions where they could obtain experiences that were not available at the home hospital.

The schedule was demanding, with classes being held after patient care assignments were completed. Critics charged that students were used as inexpensive labor to staff the hospitals and that education was a low priority. The truth of those charges varied, depending on which hospital was scrutinized, but there is no question that early nursing students literally ran the hospitals. Programs lasted three years, and at graduation, students were awarded diplomas in nursing. Today, most diploma programs are about 24 months in duration.

A problem that many diploma graduates have faced is that hospitals are not part of the higher education system in the United States. Therefore, most colleges and universities do not recognize the diploma in nursing as an academic credential and have often refused to give college credit for courses taken in diploma programs, regardless of the quality of the courses, students, and faculty. In recent years, diploma schools have established agreements with colleges and universities that enable students to earn college credit in courses such as English, psychology, and the sciences or to attain advanced standing in a baccalaureate program upon completion of the diploma program.

The decline in the number of diploma programs is due to several factors: the growth of associate degree and baccalaureate degree programs in nursing, the inability of hospitals to continue to finance nursing education, accreditation standards that have made it difficult for diploma programs to attract qualified faculty, and the increasing complexity of health care, which has required nurses to have greater academic preparation. Today, diploma programs represent fewer than 7 percent of the total number of basic nursing education programs in the United States (Fig. 2–2).

During nursing shortages, diploma programs generally have experienced increased enrollments. When the nursing profession has faced periods of job shortages, however, diploma graduates have found it necessary to return to school for further education to advance within today's complex health care system.

Baccalaureate Programs (BSN)

Armed with the early studies of nursing education, nursing leaders continued to push for nursing education to move into the mainstream of higher education, that is, into colleges and universities where other professionals were educated. Their belief was that nurses needed the **baccalaureate degree** to qualify nursing as a recognized profession and to provide leadership in administration, teaching, and public health.

By the time the first baccalaureate nursing program was established in 1909 at the University of Minnesota, diploma programs were numerous and firmly entrenched as the system for educating nurses. This first baccalaureate program was part of the School of Medicine and followed the three-year diploma program structure. Despite its many limitations, it was the start of the

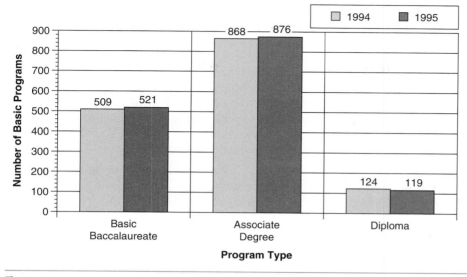

Figure 2–2

The number of diploma programs continue to decline (National League for Nursing Center for Research, *Nursing data review,* 1997. NLN Press and Bartlett Publishers, Sudbury, MA).

movement to bring nursing education into the recognized system of higher education.

Seven other baccalaureate programs in nursing were established by 1919 (Conley, 1973). Most of the early baccalaureate programs were five years in duration. This structure provided for three years of nursing education and two years of liberal arts. The growth in the numbers of these programs was slow both because of the reluctance of universities to accept nursing as an academic discipline and because of the power of the hospital-based diploma programs. The theoretical, scientific orientation of the baccalaureate program was in marked contrast to the "hands-on" skill and service orientation that was the hallmark of diploma education.

Influences on the Growth of Baccalaureate Education

National studies of nursing and nursing education stated and restated the need for nursing education and practice to be based on knowledge from the sciences and humanities. Chief among these studies was Esther Lucille Brown's report *Nursing for the Future.* Published in 1948, the **Brown Report** as it was called, recommended that basic schools of nursing be placed in universities and colleges and that efforts be made to recruit men and minorities into nursing education programs. This report, sponsored by the Carnegie Foundation, was widely reviewed, discussed, and debated.

Another major influence on the growth of baccalaureate education occurred in 1965, when the **American Nurses Association (ANA)** published a **position paper** entitled *Educational Preparation for Nurse Practitioners and Assistants to Nurses.* This paper, which subsequently created conflict and division within nursing, represented a significant influence on the growth of baccalaureate education in nursing. In preparing the position paper, the ANA studied nursing education, nursing practice, and trends in health care. It concluded that baccalaureate education should become the basic foundation for professional practice.

The position paper made four major recommendations:

1. Education for all those who are licensed to practice nursing should take place in institutions of higher learning.
2. Minimum preparation for beginning professional nursing practice should be the baccalaureate degree in nursing.
3. Minimum preparation for beginning technical nursing practice should be the associate degree in nursing.
4. Education for assistants in the health service occupations should consist of short, intensive preservice programs in vocational education institutions rather than in on-the-job training programs (American Nurses Association, 1965).

Despite tremendous opposition from proponents of diploma and associate degree education, in 1979 the ANA further strengthened its resolve by proposing three additional positions:

1. By 1985, the minimum preparation for entry into professional nursing practice should be the baccalaureate degree in nursing.
2. Two levels of nursing practice should be identified (professional and technical) and a mechanism to devise competencies for the two categories established by 1980.
3. There should be increased accessibility to high-quality career mobility programs that use flexible approaches for individuals seeking academic degrees in nursing (American Nurses Association, 1979).

The controversy created by the initial ANA position paper and the additional 1979 resolutions continued for many years. Practicing nurses across the United States, who were mainly diploma program graduates, as well as hospitals that supported diploma programs, vehemently protested the recommendations.

In 1970, the National Commission for the Study of Nursing and Nursing Education published its report entitled *An Abstract for Action* (Lysaught, 1970). Also known as the **Lysaught Report,** it made recommendations concerning the supply and demand for nurses, nursing roles and functions, and nursing education. Among the priorities identified by this study were (1) the need for increased research into both the practice and education of nurses and (2) enhanced educational systems and curricula (Lysaught, 1970).

In the early 1980s, the National Commission on Nursing published two reports that suggested that the major block to the advancement of nursing was the ongoing conflict within the profession about educational preparation for nurses. These studies recommended establishing a clear system of nursing education, including pathways for educational mobility and development of additional graduate education programs.

The latest major national nursing group to support the baccalaureate as the entry credential was the **National League for Nursing (NLN).** The organization's membership is made up of nurses, faculty members, health care agencies, all types of nursing programs, and nonnursing citizens who are supportive of nursing. In 1982, after much debate, the NLN board of directors approved the *Position Statement on Nursing Roles: Scope and Preparation,* which affirmed the nursing baccalaureate degree as the minimum educational level for professional nursing practice and the associate degree or diploma as the preparation for technical nursing practice (National League for Nursing, 1982).

Baccalaureate Programs Today

Today, baccalaureate programs provide education for both basic students who are preparing for licensure and registered nurses returning to school to obtain a **bachelor of science in nursing (BSN).** This section focuses on the program characteristics of prelicensure baccalaureate education, sometimes called **basic programs.** Baccalaureate programs for registered nurses are discussed later.

Basic baccalaureate programs combine nursing courses with general education courses in a four- or five-year curriculm in a senior college or university. Students may be admitted to the nursing program as entering freshmen or after completing certain liberal arts courses. Students meet the same admission requirements to the university as other students and often must meet additional requirements to be admitted to the nursing major.

Courses in the nursing major focus on nursing science, communication, decision making, leadership, and care to persons of all ages in a wide variety of settings. Because this education takes place in senior universities, nursing students interact with the larger student population, which promotes diverse thinking, cultural awareness, and broader socialization.

Faculty qualifications in baccalaureate programs are usually higher than in other basic nursing programs. A minimum of a master's degree and often a doctorate in nursing or a related field is required. The requirement of a doctorate ensures that nursing faculty are able to meet the teaching, research, and service requirements expected of faculty members in universities.

Baccalaureate graduates are prepared to take the National Council Licensing Examination for Registered Nurses and, after licensure, assume beginning practice and ultimately leadership positions in any health care setting, including hospitals, community agencies, schools, clinics, and homes (National League for Nursing, 1997b). Graduates with a BSN are also prepared to move into graduate programs in nursing and advanced practice certification programs. Programs granting a BSN are the most costly of the basic programs in terms of time and money, but such an investment results in long-term professional advancement. Today, there is great demand for BSN graduates, and they enjoy the greatest career mobility of all basic program graduates.

An early criticism of baccalaureate preparation involved the perception that new BSN graduates had fewer clinical skills than their diploma-educated counterparts. Contemporary BSN programs have responded to this concern by increasing students' time in clinical practice (Fig. 2–3). Additional time spent in clinical settings and preceptorships, in which students are paired with practicing registered nurses and work intensively in clinical settings, have been successful in enhancing the clinical skills of BSN students.

Associate Degree Programs (ADN)

Associate degree in nursing (ADN) education represents the newest form of basic preparation for registered nurse practice. Begun in 1952 as a result of research conducted by **Dr. Mildred Montag,** and fueled by the community college movement of the 1950s, associate degree programs are now the most common type of basic nursing education program in the United States and graduate the most registered nurses of all the basic programs.

In 1997, 894 programs (58.6 percent of all basic programs) offered the associate degree in nursing (National League for Nursing, 1999c). The popularity of this program is due to several features: accessibility of community col-

Figure 2–3
A nursing student enjoys working with her patient (Courtesy of the University of Akron).

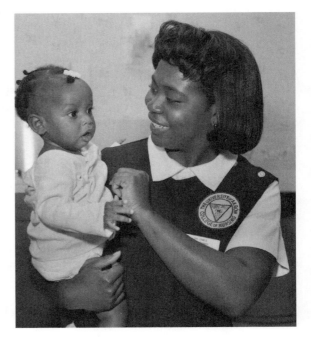

leges, low tuition costs, part-time and evening study opportunities, shorter duration of programs, and graduates' eligibility to take the licensure examination for registered nurses.

When first designed by Dr. Montag, associate degree programs were to prepare nurse technicians who functioned under the supervision of professional nurses. Associate degree nurses were to work at the bedside, performing routine nursing skills for patients in acute and long-term care settings. The original associate degree program, as outlined by Montag (1951), had general education courses in the first year and nursing courses in the second year. Montag originally viewed the associate degree as a final, end-point degree, not a stepping stone to the baccalaureate degree in nursing.

Today, Montag's original conceptions of associate degree programs have been greatly modified. Associate degree curricula now contain more nursing credits than she suggested. They also include content on leadership and clinical decision making, abilities that Montag did not foresee in technical nurses. Owing to additions to the curriculum, few students can complete associate degrees in only two years. Associate degree graduates are employed in a wide variety of settings and function autonomously alongside baccalaureate and diploma graduates. In the educational system of nursing today, the associate degree can be a step in the progression to the baccalaureate degree.

In 1990, the NLN Council of Associate Degree Programs prepared a document entitled *Educational Outcomes of Associate Degree Nursing Programs: Roles and Competencies*. This document was written in response to a national effort to differentiate the competencies of the associate degree nurse from those of the baccalaureate nurse. The document identified associate degree competencies in three roles: provider of care, manager of care, and member within the discipline of nursing. The further development of these competencies has had a direct effect on the associate degree programs that exist today.

External Degree Programs

External degree programs in nursing are different from traditional basic nursing education in that students attend no classes and follow no prescribed methods of learning. Learning is independent and is assessed through highly standardized and validated examinations. Students are responsible for arranging their own clinical experiences in accordance with established standards.

The New York Regents External Degree Nursing Program is the most well-recognized external degree model and has both general education and nursing requirements. General education requirements include humanities, social sciences, natural sciences, and mathematics. The nursing categories represent five areas: health, commonalities of nursing care, differences in nursing care, occupational strategies, and performance. The performance examination can be taken only after successful completion of the other four categories.

The New York Regents External Degree Nursing Program received NLN accreditation in 1981 through the Council of Baccalaureate and Higher Degree

Programs. In that same year, the California State University Consortium instituted a statewide external degree baccalaureate program in nursing. In contrast to the prelicensure program in New York, the California program is for registered nurses holding current licenses to practice in the state.

Articulated Programs

In response to the demand for educational mobility, **articulation,** or movement, between programs has become much more common in today's nursing education system. The purpose of articulation is to facilitate opportunities for nurses to move up the educational ladder. An example of a fully articulated system is the licensed practical nurse/associate degree in nursing/bachelor of science in nursing (LPN/ADN/BSN) program in which students spend the first year preparing to be an LPN and the second year completing the associate degree. If desired or necessary, students can "stop out" of the program at the end of the first year, take the licensure examination for practical nursing, and return to the associate degree program at a later time. Or they could continue study in the program after the initial two years to earn a baccalaureate degree (Rapson, 1987).

Multiple-entry, multiple-exit programs are difficult to develop. A tremendous amount of joint institutional planning is needed to work out equivalent courses and to keep the programs congruent with each other. A change in one curriculum dictates changes in all the others. These challenges explain why fully articulated programs are not common.

In increasing numbers, however, articulation agreements between BSN and ADN programs and ADN and LPN programs are being established that facilitate student movement between programs and accept transfer credit between institutions. These requirements often result in acceleration or advanced placement within the higher-degree school.

Alternative Educational Programs in Nursing

In addition to the basic programs leading to entry-level nursing practice, several **alternative educational programs** also exist.

Baccalaureate Programs for Registered Nurses (BRN, or RN-to-BSN Education)

After nursing organizations of the 1960s and 1970s publicly advocated for the baccalaureate degree to be the minimum education level for professional practice, the demand for the BSN degree increased. Employers of nurses recognized that broadly educated nurses matched well with the complexities of health care. As a result, they supported the BSN as a requirement for career mobility. Diploma and associate degree graduates returned to school in increasing numbers.

Registered nurses with diplomas and associate degrees were not always welcomed into baccalaureate programs. Many students were required to take courses that they believed they had already mastered. For a number of years, it was difficult for these nurses to complete their BSNs. In the past two decades, however, many baccalaureate programs have recognized the legitimacy of **RN-to-BSN education** and have developed alternative tracks to accommodate the unique learning needs of the registered nurse student. The abbreviation **BRN** is also used to refer to RN-to-BSN education in some parts of the country.

Baccalaureate programs for registered nurses are often offered by universities that also offer a basic baccalaureate program for nonnurses. The registered nurse students may be integrated with the basic students, or they may be in a separate or partially separate sequence. Some BSN programs for registered nurses are found in colleges that do not have a basic baccalaureate nursing program.

Programs containing RN-to-BSN education are increasingly offered owing to the demand for higher education by large numbers of associate degree nurses, many of whom enter ADN programs with plans to earn a BSN ultimately. In 1980 to 1981, 8,416 registered nurse students graduated from baccalaureate programs. There were 292 basic programs that also admitted registered nurses and 95 programs that admitted only registered nurses. During the period 1990 to 1995, the number of registered nurses graduating from baccalaureate programs decreased because there was a shortage of nurses, and nurses were staying in their jobs rather than returning to school. In 1995, however, the job shortage for registered nurses in hospital settings once again began forcing nurses back to school so they could become more marketable. A survey conducted in 1995 showed a marked increase, up 7.7 percent above a year earlier, in the numbers of registered nurses who were returning to school for the BSN degree (National League for Nursing, 1995b). In 1996, there were 521 basic baccalaureate programs and 144 BRN-only programs that enrolled registered nurse students with graduations of 12,000 (National League for Nursing, 1997c).

Most four-year colleges and universities allow the transfer of general education credits from associate degree nursing programs. With increasing frequency, transfer credit is given for nursing courses as well, or there is the option of receiving credit for previous nursing courses through a variety of advanced placement methods.

For diploma graduates, transfer credit is usually given for previous college courses, such as English, if they were included as part of the diploma program and taught by college faculty. Options for advanced placement of diploma graduates into BSN programs are extremely variable, and prospective registered nurse students should seek information from several BSN programs to select a program that fits individual needs and goals.

Unresolved issues surrounding BRN programs include the philosophy of some baccalaureate faculty that diploma and associate degree programs should not be stepping stones to baccalaureate degrees and that courses taken in those programs should not be transferable and be given baccalaureate credit. There are continuing concerns about maintaining standards and protecting the integrity of the baccalaureate degree while facilitating the progression of registered nurse students. There are also problems associated with evaluating previous learning, granting credit for that learning, and creating educational methods appropriate for the midcareer registered nurse student.

Fortunately, these issues are gradually being resolved, for it is clear that the demand for the BSN degree by large numbers of associate degree and diploma graduates is a continuing trend. More nurses are returning to school to prepare for the wider opportunities offered by the baccalaureate degree. With broad preparation in clinical, scientific, community health, and patient education skills, the BSN nurse is well positioned to move across settings such as home health care, outpatient centers, and neighborhood clinics, where opportunities are fast expanding.

Programs for Nonnursing Postbaccalaureate Students

A recent trend is a significant increase in the number of students with baccalaureate degrees in other fields entering nursing programs to make a career change. According to the 1996 survey *Profiles of the Newly Licensed Nurse,* close to one-fourth (25 percent) of the respondents had a college degree in another field before enrolling in a nursing program (Louden, Crawford, and Trotman, 1996). The educational system in nursing has responded to this group of students by offering options to the traditional basic baccalaureate education. Some baccalaureate programs offer these students an accelerated sequence, which results in a second baccalaureate degree. Many individuals with one degree, however, prefer to pursue a graduate degree.

This desire for graduate degrees led to the development of an accelerated master's degree in nursing for individuals with nonnursing bachelor's degrees. These programs, known as **generic master's degree** programs, usually require about three years to complete. Graduates take the registered nurse licensure examination after completing the generic master's program.

Another educational track for students with baccalaureate degrees in other fields is the **generic nursing doctorate (ND).** A program offering the ND as the first professional degree was begun at Case Western Reserve University in 1979. This program was based on that school's philosophy that professional nursing education should begin at the postbaccalaureate level. Following graduation, ND graduates take the registered nurse licensure examination. Graduates are prepared to function as advanced clinical specialists or nurse practitioners and to initiate clinical research utilization studies.

Practical Nursing Programs (LPN or LVN)

Nursing education includes a large number of programs preparing **practical nurses.** Practical nurses are differentiated from registered nurses by education and licensure and have a limited scope of practice. Licensed practical nurses (LPNs), or licensed vocational nurses (LVNs), are considered technical workers in nursing.

Practical nursing programs became a significant component of the nursing field during World War II. They were created to satisfy the demand for nurses and programs that could produce nurses quickly. The first planned curriculum for practical nursing was developed in 1942. While there is national accreditation available for practical nursing programs, the majority of the 1,107 LPN programs have had state approval rather than national accreditation.

Practical nursing education typically lasts 12 months and takes place in a variety of settings: vocational/technical schools, community colleges, and high schools. Many LPN programs now offer credit for prior learning to health care workers such as hospital aides, orderlies, paramedics, emergency medical technicians, and military corps personnel. These individuals often enter nursing through practical nursing programs.

Graduates of practical nurse programs must pass the **National Council Licensing Examination for Practical Nursing (NCLEX-PN)** to become licensed. The scope of their practice focuses on meeting basic patient needs in hospitals, long-term care facilities, and homes. They must practice under the supervision of a physician or registered nurse.

For many students enrolled in practical nurse programs, the goal is to become a registered nurse. Eighty-three percent of the newly licensed practical nurses in 1996 planned to become registered nurses, with the majority of these individuals either taking courses or planning to begin registered nurse courses in one to two years (Louden, Crawford, and Trotman, 1996). A significant number of newly licensed registered nurses were previously licensed as practical nurses. According to the third edition of *Profiles of the Newly Licensed Nurse,* 38 percent of all newly licensed registered nurses have practiced previously as licensed practical nurses (Louden, Crawford, and Trotman, 1996).

There are increasing pressures on LPN programs to expand and upgrade. These proposals are usually discussed during times when jobs in nursing are not readily available and include phasing out practical nurse programs or converting them to associate degree programs. When the demand for nurses is greater than basic registered nurse programs can meet, however, practical nurse programs flourish. In 1993, practical nurse programs experienced the highest number of admissions in 10 years. However, by 1995, there was a 6 percent decline in admissions (National League for Nursing, 1997c). Currently, there are significant employment opportunities for licensed practical nurses because their lower salaries fit well with the cost-containment requirements of today's health care system.

Accreditation of Educational Programs

The concept of **accreditation** of educational programs in nursing is important. Although all nursing programs must be approved by their respective state boards of nursing for graduates to take the licensure examination, nursing programs may also seek accreditation, which goes beyond minimum state approval. Accreditation refers to a voluntary review process of educational programs by a professional organization. The organization, called an accrediting agency, compares the educational quality of the program with established standards and criteria. Accrediting agencies derive their authority from the U. S. Department of Education.

Prospective nursing students should inquire about the accreditation status of any nursing program they are considering. Qualifying for certain scholarships, loans, and military service usually depends on being enrolled in an accredited program. Acceptance into graduate programs in nursing is also dependent on graduation from an accredited baccalaureate program. Employers of nurses are usually interested in hiring nurses who are graduates of accredited programs.

From 1952 through 1996, the National League for Nursing was the official professional accrediting organization for master's, baccalaureate, associate degree, diploma, and practical nursing programs in the United States. In 1997, due to a mandate from the U. S. Department of Education, a separate division of the NLN was created. The new division, the **National League for Nursing Accreditation Commission (NLNAC),** assumed responsibility for all national nursing program accrediting activity. The accrediting program is conducted through four NLNAC councils: the Council of Associate Degree Programs, the Council of Diploma Programs, the Council of Baccalaureate and Higher Degree Programs, and the Council of Practical Nursing Programs. Each council develops its own accreditation program and criteria and revises them periodically.

Accreditation of nursing schools grew out of concerns repeatedly expressed by members of the profession about the quality of and standards for nursing education. An accredited program voluntarily adheres to standards that protect the quality of education, public safety, and the profession itself. Accreditation provides both a mechanism and a stimulus for programs to initiate periodic self-examination and self-improvement. It assures students that their educational program is accountable for offering quality education. Program areas generally reviewed during accreditation include administration and governance, finances and budget, faculty, students, program effectiveness and outcomes, and resources. Criteria, or standards, are established in each area. In 1999, the NLNAC councils established standard outcome categories that are used to measure the program effectiveness for all types of nursing programs. Box 2–1 lists required and elective program outcome categories for all nursing programs.

Programs under review prepare reports, known as self-studies, that show how the school meets each criterion. The self-study is reviewed by a volunteer team composed of nursing educators from the type of program being reviewed, and an on-site program review is made by the same team. Following the site visit, the visitors' report and the program's self-study are reviewed by the appropriate NLN council, and a decision is made about the accreditation status of each nursing program.

BOX 2–1

National League for Nursing—Established Outcome Categories Used to Measure the Effectiveness of Each Type of Nursing Program[*]

Required Outcomes for All Nursing Programs
1. Critical thinking
2. Communication abilities
3. Therapeutic nursing interventions
4. Patterns of employment
5. Completion/graduation rates
6. Performance on NCLEX and certifying examinations

Elective Outcomes—Programs (Select Two)
7. Program satisfaction
8. Professional development
9. Employer satisfaction
10. Attainment of credentials
11. Organization or work environment
12. Scholarship
13. Service
14. Nursing unit defined

[*]NLNAC councils adopted the outcome categories June 1999. Data from the National League for Nursing Accreditation Commission office.

Once accredited and in good standing, continuing accreditation reviews take place every eight years. Programs that do not meet standards may be placed on warning and given a specific time period to correct deficiencies. Accreditation can be withdrawn if deficiencies are not corrected within the specified time.

In 1996, the **American Association of Colleges of Nursing (AACN)** organized the **Commission on Collegiate Nursing Education (CCNE)** after several years of discussion and planning and began the process of acquiring recognition from the U. S. Department of Education as the national accrediting body for baccalaureate and higher degree nursing programs. Officially, CCNE began operation in 1998 and has subsequently established an organizational structure, policies and procedures, and accreditation standards and criteria. In December of 1999, CCNE received a recommendation from the National Advisory Committee on Institutional Quality and Integrity, a panel of the U.S. Department of Education, that the Secretary of Education grant initial recognition of CCNE as a national agency for the accreditation of baccalaureate and graduate nursing education programs. The establishment of a second national accrediting body for nursing education represents a significant development in the evolution of the nursing profession.

Graduate Education in Nursing

A variety of economic, educational, and professional trends are fueling the demand for registered nurses with **advanced degrees.** The rapidly changing health care system requires nurses to possess increasing knowledge, clinical competency, greater independence, and autonomy in clinical judgments. Trends in community-based nursing centers, case management, complexity of home care, sophisticated technologies, and society's orientation to health and self-care are rapidly causing the educational needs of nurses to grow.

According to projections made by the federal government, 200,000 additional master's and doctorally prepared registered nurses will be needed by the year 2005 (U. S. Department of Health and Human Services, 1990). Nurses who have advanced education can become researchers, nurse practitioners, clinical specialists, educators, and administrators. Many open their own clinics where they provide direct care and serve as consultants to businesses and health care agencies. Chapter 5 describes some of the opportunities open to nurses with advanced degrees. Certainly, having highly educated nurses will further strengthen the profession.

Master's Education

The purpose of master's education is to prepare persons with advanced nursing knowledge and clinical practice skills in a specialized area of practice. Teachers College, Columbia University, is credited with initiating graduate education in nursing. Beginning in 1899, the college offered a postgraduate course in hospital economics, which prepared nurses for positions in teaching and hospital administration. From this limited beginning, there has been consistent growth in the number of master's programs in the United States.

Over the last 25 years, the growth in numbers of master's programs has been dramatic. In 1970, there were 70 programs; in 1980, 142 programs; in 1990, 212 programs, and in 1996, 321 programs. Enrollment of master's degree students nearly doubled during the 10-year period between 1986 and 1996 from 19,958 to 35,715 (National League for Nursing, 1999b).

Most individuals in the 1950s and 1960s viewed the master's degree in nursing as a terminal (final) degree. The master's degree was considered the highest degree nurses would ever need. Early master's programs were longer and more demanding than master's programs in other disciplines. Master's programs in the 1950s and 1960s prepared students for careers in nursing administration and nursing education.

With the rapid development of doctoral programs for nurses during the 1970s, however, the master's degree could no longer be considered as a terminal degree. Programs were shortened to the approximate length of master's study in most other disciplines, and advanced practice through clinical specialization became the emphasis. Master's programs in nursing are most often found in senior colleges and universities that have basic baccalaureate programs in nursing. These programs may also seek voluntary accreditation from the NLNAC's Council of Baccalaureate and Higher Degree Programs or, in the future, from the CCNE.

Entrance requirements to master's programs in nursing usually include the following: a baccalaureate degree from an NLN-accredited program in nursing, licensure as a registered nurse, completion of the Graduate Record Examination (GRE) or other standard aptitude test, a minimum undergraduate grade point average (GPA) of 3.0, at least one year's recent work experience as a registered nurse in an area related to the desired area of specialization, and specific goals for graduate study.

The average program length is 18 to 24 months of full-time study. The curriculum includes theory, research, clinical practice, and courses in other disciplines related to the student's selected area of specialization and role development. Students are often required to write a comprehensive examination or to complete a thesis or research project (or both). The majority of contemporary master's students are preparing for advanced clinical practice as nurse practitioners (Fig. 2–4). Fifty-one percent of 1996 master of science in nursing graduates were nurse practitioners, with 31 percent in clinical specialist roles, 12 percent in administration/management, and 6 percent in teaching (National League for Nursing, 1999b). Sixty-nine percent of master's students were engaged in part-time study.

Nine broad specialty areas are currently represented in nursing master's curricula: adult health, child health, community/public health, gerontology,

Figure 2–4
Nurse practitioner programs remained the specialty of choice for master's students. This is a change from 1993 when advanced clinical practice was the most common specialty. Teaching continued to be the specialty least often selected (NLN Center for Research, *Nurse practitioner programs remained the specialty of choice for master's students,* copyright 1997: NLN Press and Jones and Bartlett Publishers, Sudbury, MA).

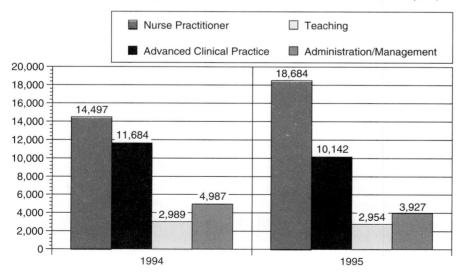

nurse anesthesia, nursing administration, nurse midwifery, and psychiatric/mental health. Newer options are being added. Recent additions include nursing informatics, oncology, early intervention, and neonatal nursing.

With the increasing demand for nurse practitioners, master's programs have expanded their practitioner tracks. Master's programs offering nurse practitioner options rose from 108 in 1992 to 240 in 1996, a 222 percent increase (National League for Nursing, 1999b). Nurse practitioners choose advanced practice areas such as family health, pediatrics, adult health, midwifery, anesthesia, women's health, gerontology, psychiatric/mental health, and school nurse concentrations.

The master of science (MS) and the master of science in nursing (MSN) are the two most common degrees offered. A new option in master's education is the RN/MSN track, which allows registered nurses prepared at the associate degree or diploma level, and who meet graduate admission requirements, to enter a program leading to a master's degree rather than a baccalaureate degree. Other newer graduate program options are the combined degrees such as the master of science in nursing/master of business administration (MSN/MBA) for nurse administrators or the master of science in nursing/doctor of law (MSN/JD) for nurse attorneys. As can be seen, diversity in nursing education extends to the graduate as well as the basic level.

Doctoral Education

Doctoral programs in nursing prepare nurses to become faculty members in universities, administrators in schools of nursing or large medical centers, researchers, theorists, and advanced practitioners. Doctoral programs in nursing offer several degree titles, the most common being the doctor of nursing science (DNS) and doctor of philosophy (PhD).

The DNS is viewed as a professional practice degree. Conceived as an advanced practice degree with an emphasis on clinical research, the DNS is intended to bridge the gap between practice and research (Allen, 1990). The PhD is considered an academic degree and prepares scholars for research and the development of theory.

A continuing issue is the relative merit of these two degrees. As currently structured in most universities, the two programs are more similar than different. In the major job market for nurses with doctorates, which is colleges and universities, the PhD is the more prestigious of the two degrees and therefore is favored by many doctorate-seeking nurses. Of 66 programs awarding doctoral degrees in 1996, 85 percent awarded the PhD (National League for Nursing, 1997a). Formal doctoral education began at Columbia University's Teachers College in 1910 with the creation of the Department of Nursing and Health. The first student completed her work for the doctor of education (EdD) with a major in nursing education and was awarded her doctorate in 1932. As of 1995, Teachers College was the only doctoral program in nursing education granting the EdD.

In 1934, New York University initiated the first PhD program for nurses. The programs at Teachers College and New York University provided many of the profession's early leaders who worked over the years for improvement in nursing education (Parietti, 1990).

From 1934 to 1954, no new nursing doctoral programs were opened. In 1954, the University of Pittsburgh opened the first PhD program in clinical nursing and clinical research in the United States. The ANA's *Facts About Nursing* (1961) reported that as the 1950s drew to a close, a total of only 36 doctoral degrees had been awarded in nursing (Parietti, 1990).

Owing to the limited number of nursing doctoral programs, most nurses in the 1950s and 1960s earned doctorates in nonnursing fields, such as education, sociology, and physiology. Doctoral education for nurses moved into a new phase when the federal government initiated nurse scientist programs in 1962. These programs were created to increase the research skills of nurses and provide faculty for the development of doctoral programs in nursing. The nurse scientist programs were discontinued in 1975 after more universities began offering doctoral programs in nursing.

The 1970s saw a major increase in the number of doctoral programs in nursing. Fifteen new doctoral programs were established in that decade alone. Between 1970 and 1980, the number of programs increased to 22. Between 1980 and 1990, the number more than doubled, from 22 to 48 (Parietti, 1990). In 1996, the number of doctoral programs stood at 66 (National League for Nursing, 1997a).

Enrollment trends indicate that there is strong support for doctoral education in nursing. During the 1990s, the number of requests for admission to these programs greatly increased. This trend has partially stemmed from the requirement of a doctorate for academic advancement and tenure for university nursing faculty. Nurses also desire the doctorate to become competent researchers and to advance the profession as a whole. Doctoral programs that prepare nurses predominantly for research and teaching reported 2,984 students enrolled in 1996. It is projected that large numbers of nurses with doctoral degrees will be needed in the future as positions requiring this degree expand in universities and throughout the health care system.

Certification Programs

Certification is a credential that has professional but not legal status. Specialized programs developed to recognize nurses for advanced practice often lead to certification. Some certification programs are part of degree-granting programs such as a master's program; others are considered part of continuing education.

Certification means that a certificate is awarded by a professional group as validation of specific qualifications demonstrated by a registered nurse in a defined area of practice. Certification programs that exist today include nurse practitioner preparation in programs such as pediatrics, gerontology, family health, women's health care, nurse midwifery, and nurse anesthesia.

These programs provide concentrated study in specific areas and last from several weeks to several months or even years. A comprehensive examination is required to become certified as well as documentation of experience, letters of reference, and other documents. Currently, more than 35 organizations offer advanced practice certification (Wise, 1999). Box 2–2 lists some of the professional associations that currently grant certification.

Certified nurses have greater earning potential, wider employment opportunities, status, and prestige and, in some states, are eligible for insurance reimbursement, just as physicians are. Requirements for admission to certification programs vary, with some requiring only registered nurse licensure and others requiring either a baccalaureate or a master's degree.

The **American Nurses Credentialing Center (ANCC),** a subunit of the ANA, provides a number of certification programs for registered nurses. **Advanced practice nurses (APNs)** certified by the ANCC must have master's degrees and demonstrate successful completion of a certification examination based on nationally recognized standards of nursing practice and designed to test their special knowledge and skills. For certain specialties, APNs also must show evidence of specified clinical practice experience. Once granted, certification is effective for three to five years, whereupon the individual must apply for recertification based on either a retest or demonstration of continuing education credits and evidence of ongoing clinical practice.

In response to the need to be more formally organized as a national peer review program for advanced practice nursing certification bodies, the ANCC and more than a dozen other certification boards formed the American Board of Nursing Specialties (ABNS). This umbrella board, established in 1991, approves membership of those APN-certifying bodies that have met the stan-

---

BOX 2–2
A Sample of Certifying Organizations in Nursing[*]

- American Association of Critical Care Nursing
- American Association of Nurse Anesthetists
- American Psychiatric Nurses' Association
- American College of Nurse Midwives
- American Nurses Credentialing Center
- Board of Certification for Emergency Nursing
- National Certification Board of Pediatric Nurse Practitioners
- National Certification Corporation for Obstetric, Gynecologic, and Neonatal Specialties
- National Board for Certification of School Nurses
- Rehabilitation Nursing Certification Board

[*]A complete list of certifying boards can be obtained from the *Journal of Continuing Education in Nursing,* Slack, Inc., 6900 Grove Drive, Thorofare, NJ 08086. Ask for the Annual Continuing Education Survey.

dards and principles of ABNS. One of the 12 standards that must be met is a requirement for uniform educational preparation (i.e., a master's degree in nursing).

Certification and licensure are both forms of regulation of a profession. Licensure refers to state regulation of the practice of nursing at the entry point to practice. Certification is a regulatory mechanism for advanced practice and is voluntarily pursued by individual nurses.

Nurses holding ANCC certification at the basic level can be identified by the initials RN, C. (registered nurse, certified) after their names. Those certified as clinical specialists use RN, CS. Box 2–3 lists the areas in which the ANCC offers certification.

Although certification is a desirable concept, there are many problems with the current methods of certification, such as lack of uniformity of programs, testing, and practice requirements. How to ensure certification standards and who should be responsible for certification of nurses are major issues in the nursing education system today. In October 1994, the American Association of Colleges of Nursing issued a position statement on the certification and regulation of advanced practice nurses. The position statement emphasized that the nursing profession must develop a standardized national advanced practice nursing certification process as expeditiously as possible. The statement recommended that all advanced practice nurses should hold a graduate degree in nursing and be certified in a manner standardized by one nationally recognized certifying board. This is particularly important because professional certification validates and standardizes the qualifications and practice competencies of advanced practice nurses (American Association of Colleges of Nursing, 1994).

Continuing Education

Continuing education (CE) is a term used to describe informal ways in which nurses maintain expertise during their professional careers. Continuing education for nurses takes place in a variety of settings: colleges, universities, hospitals, community agencies, professional organizations, and professional meetings. Continuing education appears in many forms, such as workshops, institutes, conferences, short courses, evening courses, telecourses, and instructional modules in professional journals.

The ANA Council on Continuing Education was established in 1973. This council is responsible for standards of continuing education, accreditation of programs offering continuing education, transferability of CE credit from state to state, and development of guidelines for recognition systems within states.

In the 1970s, the continuing education unit (CEU) was created as a method of recognizing participation in nonacademic credit offerings. One CEU was given for every 10 hours of participation in an organized, approved, continuing education offering. Today the **contact hour** has replaced the CEU, and nurses receive one contact hour of credit for each 50 or 60 minutes they spend in a continuing education course.

BOX 2–3

Areas of Certification Offered by the American Nurses Credentialing Center in 1999

Generalist Programs
- Cardiac rehabilitation nurse
- College health nurse
- Community health nurse
- General nursing practice
- Gerontological nurse
- Home health nurse
- Medical-surgical nurse
- Nursing continuing education/staff development
- Pediatric nurse
- Perinatal nurse
- Psychiatric and mental health nurse
- School nurse

Nurse Practitioner Programs
- Acute care nurse practitioner
- Adult nurse practitioner
- Family nurse practitioner
- Gerontological nurse practitioner
- Pediatric nurse practitioner
- School nurse practitioner

Clinical Specialist Programs
- Community health nurse
- Home health nurse
- Gerontological nurse
- Medical-surgical nurse
- Psychiatric and mental health nursing:
  Adult
  Child and adolescent

Nursing Administration Programs
- Nursing administration
- Nursing administration, advanced

Nursing Case Management
- Nursing case management/ambulatory care nursing

Informatics Nurse Certification

Data compiled from certification catalogs published by the American Nurses Credentialing Center (1999a, 1999b, 1999c, 1999d).

A major nationwide trend is **mandatory continuing education.** Before renewing their licenses in states with mandatory continuing education, nurses must provide evidence that they have met that state's contact hour requirements. This requirement is the government's way of ensuring that

BOX 2–4

States and Territories Requiring Continuing Education for Relicensure[*]

- Alabama
- Alaska
- California
- Delaware
- Florida
- Iowa
- Kansas
- Kentucky
- Louisiana
- Massachusetts
- Michigan

- Minnesota
- Nebraska
- Nevada
- New Hampshire
- New Mexico
- Ohio
- Puerto Rico
- Texas
- Virgin Islands
- West Virginia
- Wyoming

[*]A current list of states and territories requiring continuing education for relicensure can be obtained from the *Journal of Continuing Education in Nursing*, Slack, Inc., 6900 Grove Drive, Thorofare, NJ 08086. Ask for a reprint of their Annual Continuing Education Survey.

nurses remain up-to-date in their profession. In 1998, mandatory continuing education as a prerequisite for relicensure was required in 22 states and territories (Wise, 1999). Box 2–4 lists those states and territories.

Future Directions for Nursing Education

In 1993, three major organizations issued statements and reports about nursing education for the twenty-first century. Their reports addressed the new direction nursing education needed to take in the future. The reports included the NLN's "Vision for Nursing Education" (1993, 1995a), the AACN's "Nursing Education's Agenda for the 21st Century" (1993), and the Pew Health Professions Commission's "Health Professions Education for the Future: Schools in Service to the Nation" (O'Neil, 1993). Although the three organizations had somewhat different approaches and strategies, several common themes emerged in their reports. Common emphases included the following eight points:

1. Schools should recruit diverse students and faculties that reflect the multicultural nature of society.
2. Curricula and learning activities should develop student's critical thinking skills.
3. Curricula should emphasize students' abilities to communicate, form interpersonal relationships, and make decisions collaboratively with patients, their families, and interdisciplinary colleagues.

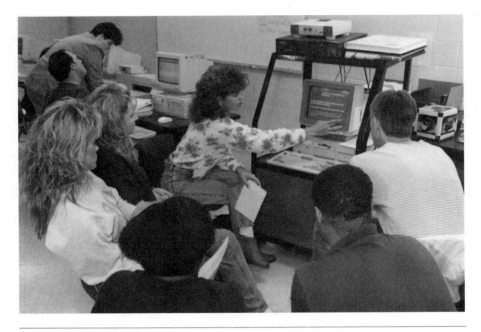

Figure 2–5
Information management is more important than ever in nursing. These nursing students are developing their computer skills to manage multiple sources of patient information successfully (Courtesy of the University of Akron).

4. The number of advanced practice nurses should be increased, and curricula should emphasize health promotion and maintenance skills for all nurses.
5. Emphasis should be placed on community-based care, increased accountability, state-of-the-art clinical skills, and increased information management skills (Fig. 2–5).
6. Cost-effectiveness of care should be a focus in nursing curricula.
7. Faculty should develop programs that facilitate articulation and career mobility.
8. Continuing faculty development activities should support excellence in practice, teaching, and research.

Issues in Nursing Education

There are several issues in nursing education that bear watching. They are closure of nursing programs, the impending faculty shortage, and the transformation of nursing education needed to meet the health care needs of the nation in the twenty-first century.

Closure of Nursing Programs

In 1995, the **Pew Health Professions Commission** recommended that the size and number of nursing education programs, especially associate degree programs, be reduced between 10 and 20 percent. This recommendation was based upon the Commission's projections that, as a result of managed care, there would be a loss of 60 percent of the nation's hospital beds and a resulting surplus of 200,000 to 300,000 nurses. In addition to an overabundance of programs, factors leading to school closures in the future may result from: job market fluctuations; diminishing clinical sites and increasing competition for clinical learning sites by all health profession schools; diminishing resources in institutions of higher education and the perception of the high cost of operating nursing education programs; and the inability of some nursing programs to meet new accreditation standards.

Faculty Shortage: A Looming Crisis

The nursing profession is aging, and along with it, so is the nurse faculty population. The mean age for faculty nationally is 49.7 years, which will result in increasing numbers of faculty retirements in the near future. The numbers of nurses with master's and doctoral degrees prepared for faculty roles has decreased dramatically over the last decade as graduate nursing programs have discontinued course offerings in role preparation in education in favor of advanced practice education. Only 3.3 percent of students in master's programs in 1998 were enrolled in education tracks (American Association of Colleges of Nursing, 1999). Compounding the situation is the fact that nurses with graduate preparation are not seeking faculty positions owing to the more favorable salary levels in the service sector. As a result, a severe faculty shortage is predicted to occur in the nation's schools of nursing by the year 2010.

Transformation of Nursing Education

In 1999, the National League for Nursing launched a five year project, "Transforming the Landscape for Nursing Education." The purpose of this project is to begin a national dialogue on skills and competencies, types of programs and curricula, academic and community partnerships, standards for future program types, and research initiatives for nursing education. Plans for this transformation include discovering the core knowledge needed to bridge education and practice; differentiating between knowledge and outcome competencies for a continuum of practice; identifying research on curricula, methods, and instructional strategies for core curricula common to basic preparation for health professions; developing seamless articulation along the continuum of nursing education; and creating infrastructures that provide for ongoing communication between leaders in education and practice (National League for Nursing, 1999). The transformation of nursing education over the next two decades will be significant. Box 2–5 contains the thoughts of a seasoned nurse educator about the factors prompting changes.

BOX 2-5
Education of Nurses Must Change

As we shift from the centrality of the hospital which remains notable for illness care, we soon recognize that the education of nurses must change to accommodate the increased expectations of nurses as practitioners, educators, researchers, managers and administrators as well as policy shapers. No longer must the professional nurse feel frustrated as the profession's independent function is compromised. The opportunity is now afforded to enhance collaborative and satisfying relationships between and among other health care providers and to form partnerships with those being served assuring their maximum independence and empowerment. As new partnerships are forged with the recipients of nursing services, the helping model so well known to nurses who practice in rehabilitation, mental health and substance abuse programs is replacing the medical model as more appropriate.

A variety of practice settings await tomorrow's nurse including the rapidly growing home care arena, nurse managed centers and integrated managed care systems. Programmatic emphasis on subacute and chronic care, primary prevention, family centered care, sophisticated information and communications technology, coupled with a culturally responsive care provider, offer unparalleled opportunities for nursing. With the diversity in nursing roles, we are challenged to think creatively as we make unprecedented contributions to improving the public's health at a time of great chaos and opportunity. Linking educational efforts and research priorities to reform goals can position nursing as an essential player in the change process.

Ferguson, V. L., *Educating the 21st century nurse,* Introduction, copyright 1997: NLN Press and Jones and Bartlett Publishers, Sudbury, MA.

Summary of Key Points

- The development of nursing education has been influenced by a number of factors leading to a diverse array of program offerings.
- First provided in hospitals, basic entry-level nursing education has evolved into three major types of programs: diploma, baccalaureate, and associate degree, each of which has both attractions and drawbacks.
- Alternatives such as baccalaureate degree programs for registered nurses, external degree programs, and accelerated options for postbaccalaureate students contribute to a complex educational picture for registered nurses.
- Voluntary accreditation is designed to provide assurance of the quality of nursing education programs.
- Programs in high demand in the 1990s included master's and doctoral preparation for nurses, specialty certification for advanced practice, and baccalaureate degree programs for registered nurses.
- Schools have had to restrict enrollments owing to fluctuating job markets, lack of clinical sites, and budget constraints.

- Life-long learning through continuing education is considered essential for all professionals, particularly in practice-based disciplines such as nursing. Twenty-two states and territories mandate continuing education as a prerequisite for relicensure, and the number is expected to increase.
- The problem of reduced resources in nursing education may soon reach crisis proportions, and weaker schools may close. This is a result of under-funding of higher education in general and, in particular, diminishing sources of federal funding for schools of nursing.
- Graduate programs in nursing are not preparing adequate numbers of nursing educators to meet current and future needs, and a severe faculty shortage is expected nationwide by 2010.
- In response to changes in higher education and the health care system, national organizations have suggested initiatives to revise educational re-quirements and program emphases for the twenty-first century that will enable future registered nurses at all levels to meet the changing health care needs of society.

Critical Thinking Questions

1. What factors did you use to determine the type of basic nursing program you entered?
2. How would you advise a high school student interested in nursing to select a program?
3. Should the nursing profession have only one basic program that leads to a career in nursing? Discuss the pros and cons. Where should this basic pro-gram be located? What academic credential should be awarded at the com-pletion of the program?
4. What content areas and skills should be included in basic nursing programs to prepare graduates for the twenty-first century?
5. Offering complete articulation of all levels of nursing education from practi-cal nursing through doctoral study seems like a logical course of action. Should states mandate articulation? Why or why not?
6. Discuss the merits and drawbacks of mandatory continuing education from the viewpoints of both nurses and consumers of nursing care.
7. What unique contributions to nursing are possible by nurses with a master's-level education? With a doctoral-level degree?

Web Resources

American Association of Colleges of Nursing, http://www.aacn.nche.edu

American Nurses Association/American Nurses Foundation Continuing Education Website, http://www.RNCE.org

American Nurses Credentialing Center, http://www.ancc.org

National Association for Practical Nurse Education and Service, http://www.napnes.org

National Center for Continuing Education, http://nursece.com

National Council of State Boards of Nursing, http://www.ncsbn.org

National League for Nursing, http://www.nln.org

New York State External Degree Program, http://www.regents.com

References

Allen, J., ed. (1990). *Consumer's guide to doctoral degree programs in nursing.* New York: National League for Nursing.

American Nurses Association (1979). *A case for baccalaureate preparation in nursing.* Kansas City, Mo.: American Nurses Association.

American Association of Colleges of Nursing (1993). *Position statement. Nursing education's agenda for the 21st century.* Washington, D. C.: American Association of Colleges of Nursing.

American Association of Colleges of Nursing (1994). *Position statement. Certification and regulation of advanced practice nurses.* Washington, D. C.: American Association of Colleges of Nursing.

American Association of Colleges of Nursing (1999). 1998–1999 *Enrollment and graduations in baccalaureate and graduate programs in nursing.* Washington, D. C.: American Association of Colleges of Nursing.

American Nurses Association (1965). *Educational preparation for nurse practitioners and assistants to nurses: A position paper.* Kansas City, Mo.: American Nurses Association.

American Nurses Credentialing Center (1999a). *1999 board certification catalog including clinical nurse specialist, nursing administration and generalist exams.* Washington, D. C.: American Nurses Credentialing Center.

American Nurses Credentialing Center (1999b). *Nurse practitioner board certification examination catalog.* Washington, D. C.: American Nurses Credentialing Center.

American Nurses Credentialing Center (1999c). *Informatics nurse certification catalog.* Washington, D. C.: American Nurses Credentialing Center.

American Nurses Credentialing Center (1999d). *Modular certification examination catalog.* Washington, D. C.: American Nurses Credentialing Center.

Brown, E. L. (1948). *Nursing for the future.* New York: Russell Sage Foundation.

Christy, T. (1969). Portrait of a leader: M. Adelaide Nutting. *Nursing Outlook,* 17(1), 20–24.

Conley, V. (1973). *Curriculum and instruction in nursing.* Boston: Little, Brown.

Donahue, M. P. (1985). *Nursing: The finest art: An illustrated history.* St. Louis: Mosby.

Ferguson, V. D. (1997). *Educating the 21st century nurse: Challenges and opportunities.* Sudbury, Mass.: NLN Press and Jones and Bartlett.

Kalisch, P., and Kalisch, B. (1995). *The advance of American nursing* (3rd ed.). Boston: Little, Brown.

Louden, D., Crawford, L., and Trotman, S. (1996). *Profiles of the newly licensed nurse* (3rd ed.). Sunbury, Mass.: NLN Press and Jones and Bartlett.

Lysaught, J. (1970). *An abstract for action.* New York: McGraw-Hill.

Montag, M. (1951). *The education of nursing technicians.* New York: Putnam.

National League for Nursing (1982). *Position statement on nursing roles: Scope and preparation.* New York: National League for Nursing.

National League for Nursing (1993). *A vision for nursing education.* New York: National League for Nursing.

National League for Nursing (1995a). Emerging environment for nursing education and practice examined during two-year vision campaign. *News from the National League for Nursing,* May 11. New York: National League for Nursing.

National League for Nursing (1995b). *Nursing data review 1995.* New York: National League for Nursing.

National League for Nursing, Center for Research in Nursing Education and Community Health (1997a). *Annual guide to graduate nursing education 1997.* Sudbury, Mass.: NLN Press and Jones and Bartlett.

National League for Nursing, Center for Research in Nursing Education and Community Health (1997b). *NLN guide to undergraduate RN education* (5th ed.). Sudbury, Mass.: NLN Press and Jones and Bartlett.

National League for Nursing, Center for Research in Nursing Education and Community Health (1997c). *1997 Nursing data review.* Sudbury, Mass.: NLN Press and Jones and Bartlett.

National League for Nursing, Center for Research in Nursing Education and Community Health (1997d). *Nursing datasource* 1997. *Volume I. Trends in contemporary RN nursing education.* Sudbury, Mass.: NLN Press and Jones and Bartlett.

National League for Nursing (1999). *Transforming the Landscape: Executive Summary.* Biennial Convention, June 5, 1999, Miami Beach, Florida.

National League for Nursing (1999a). *Nurse educators 1997: Findings from the RN and LPN faculty census.* Sudbury, Mass.: NLN Press and Jones and Bartlett.

National League for Nursing (1999b). *Nursing datasource 1997.* Volume II. *Graduate education in nursing: Advanced practice nursing.* Sudbury, Mass.: NLN Press and Jones and Bartlett.

National League for Nursing (1999c). RN *State-approved schools of nursing* 1998 (56th ed.). Sudbury, Mass.: NLN Press and Jones and Bartlett.

National League of Nursing Education (1934). *Nursing schools today and tomorrow.* New York: National League of Nursing Education.

National League of Nursing Education (1937). *A curriculum guide for schools of nursing.* New York: National League of Nursing Education.

Notter, L., and Spalding, E. (1976). *Professional nursing, foundations, perspectives and relationships* (9th ed.). Philadelphia: J. B. Lippincott.

O'Neil, E. H. (1993). *Health professions education for the future: Schools in service to the nation.* San Francisco: Pew Health Professions Commission.

Parietti, E. (1990). The development of doctoral education in nursing: A historical overview. In J. Allen (Ed.), *Consumer's guide to doctoral degree programs in nursing* (p. 1532). New York: National League for Nursing.

Pew Health Professions Commission (1995). *Critical challenges: Revitalizing the health professions for the twenty-first century.* Third Report. San Francisco: University of California, Center for the Health Professions.

Rapson, M. (Ed.). (1987). *Collaboration for articulation: RN to BSN.* New York: National League for Nursing.

U. S. Department of Health and Human Services (1990). *Seventh report to the president and congress on the status of health personnel in the United States.* Washington, D. C.: Government Printing Office.

Wise, P. (1999). Annual CE survey: State and association/certifying boards CE requirements. *Journal of Continuing Education in Nursing, 30*(1), 4–12.

The Social Context for Nursing

Kay Chitty and Cathy Campbell

3

Key Terms

Biomedical Technology
Caring Technology
Consumerism
Cultural Competence
Demographics
Dominant Culture
Feminism
Information Technology
Knowledge Technology
Medical Paternalism
Nursing Information System
Patient Acuity
Point of Care Technology
Role Strain
Sex Role Stereotypes
Socialization
Stereotypes
Transcultural Nursing
Woodhull Study

Learning Outcomes

After studying this chapter, students will be able to:

- Describe how individuals are socialized.
- Identify patterns of socialization and their effect on personal development.
- Analyze the traditional roles of women and how these have affected the development of the nursing profession.
- Discuss social trends affecting the development of nursing as a profession.
- Explain the impact of the media on the image of nursing.
- Evaluate the continuing development of technology and the implications for nursing.
- Describe the impact of societal violence on nursing.
- Describe the causes of imbalances in supply and demand for nurses in the United States.

Every profession is profoundly affected by the society it serves, and nursing is no exception. The social context has shaped nurses' attitudes, nursing practice, and the attitudes of the public toward nursing over the years. The social context also influences who chooses nursing as a career.

As you read this chapter, think about what drew you into the profession of nursing. What is the story of your individual journey into nursing? One individual's story is found in Box 3–1. This nurse entered nursing over 25 years ago. Can you identify some of the social forces that influenced her career choice? Are any of these forces still operating today? What are some of the social forces you are responding to as you enter or advance in nursing? Take a few minutes now to reflect on your own individual journey toward nursing.

Nurses need to understand how nursing is related to society as a whole. What impact does society have on the practice of nursing? Does the fact that nursing is a female-dominated profession have a bearing on the way the profession has developed? How have the women's movement and feminism in-

BOX 3–1
Critical Thinking Exercise: One Nurse's Journey Into Nursing

Instructions: Analyze the story below and determine the social forces behind this nurse's decision to enter the profession. What assumptions did she make about the profession prior to entering it? Were her assumptions accurate or inaccurate? How would her assumptions hold up today?

"I was always interested in the sciences and did quite well in those subjects during my early years of school. In junior high I had an excellent biology teacher and thought I would like to be a biology teacher someday. In about the ninth grade, however, I questioned how I could combine my love of sciences and teaching with another goal—having a husband and children. The answer for me was to become a nurse. I believed that I could have the "best of both worlds." I wanted a career, but I also definitely wanted to get married and have children.

Another motivation was my realization that my mother had wanted to become a nurse and never did. I know I entered nursing because of an intense interest in sciences, teaching, and doing something that would help my future family. But I believe my mother's unfulfilled wish to become a nurse also entered into my career choice."

fluenced the practice of nursing? Since greater numbers of men are entering nursing, what issues face them, and how has society reacted to their increasing presence in a traditionally female profession? How do **demographics** (population trends) affect nursing? How does the public view nurses? Should this public image be changed? If so, how? What causes periodic imbalances in supply of and demand for nurses? These questions are explored in this chapter.

Traditional Socialization of Women

Socialization is the process whereby values and expectations are transmitted from generation to generation. From birth, males and females are treated differently. Muff (1988a) asserts that:

Little girls learn to be "feminine," meaning passive, dependent, affectionate, emotional, and expressive. They learn that beauty and charm make one desirable to men, and that catching a man is the primary goal. Caring for him and his children is life's work. They learn, too, that the female role is less active, often less enjoyable, and certainly less valued than is the male role.

In Western society, women have generally been socialized to avoid risk taking, to avoid conflict, and to acquiesce to authority. Traditionally, feminine attributes included an orientation toward security, peacekeeping, and submission (Muff, 1988b).

Women have been socialized to be self-sacrificing to parents, husbands, and children. When women subordinate their own needs for the sake of others, they can avoid unpleasantness and conflict. They also avoid the appearance of aggressiveness, for which assertive behavior has often been mistaken in the past (Muff, 1988b).

Stereotypes are prejudiced attitudes developed through interactions with family, friends, and others in an individual's social and cultural system. **Sex role stereotypes** deal with prejudiced ideas of how men and women should behave in a cultural group. Some common sex role stereotypes of women identified by Cummings (1995) are found in Box 3–2.

An outcome of traditional female socialization was to prepare women for primary allegiance to families, not to succeed in careers. The socialized female traits of dependency, passivity, and need for approval unconsciously restrict women's choices in life to traditional family roles and certain "female" professions. Young girls have been encouraged to enter nursing because nursing was considered to be especially good training for marriage and motherhood. This attitude was reflected by the nurse whose story appears in Box 3–1.

In the early days of modern nursing, the roles assigned to women were healer, caretaker, and nurturer, none of which was highly valued by society. The first formal schools of nursing in the United States were developed to attract "respectable women" into nursing, which could have added to nursing's value. By replacing untrained hospital "nurses" with students who worked in the hospital in return for room, board, and training, however, one powerless labor pool was simply exchanged for another. Hospitals have been described as patriarchal "families," with nurses as obedient "daughters" to administrator

---

BOX 3–2
Common Sex Role Stereotypes of Women

Mother
- Subrogates own needs
- Freely gives advice
- Becomes the peacemaker
- Fosters dependence
- Is passive, wants recognition

Iron Maiden
- Is competitive versus collaborative
- Possesses the ability to "be in charge"
- Gives critical feedback
- Sets rigid interpersonal boundaries
- Can be unapproachable

Superwoman
- Demands perfection
- Will not delegate
- Overcommits her time
- Assumes multiple roles
- Feels isolated, not supported

Based on Cummings, S. H. (1995). Attila the hun versus Attila the hen: Gender socialization of the American nurse. *Nursing Administration Quarterly*, 19(2), 25.

"daddies," helpful "wives" to physician "husbands," and loving "mothers" to patient "children" (Muff, 1988a).

For decades, middle-class American women were raised expecting to be supported financially by their husbands. This expectation freed them from the need to choose a profession that offered long-term financial security. They could make a career choice with a focus on their present needs while realizing that, with any luck at all, they would not always need to support themselves. They entered nursing with a "now-but-not-necessarily-forever" attitude. This affected both salary expectations and commitment to nursing as a career (Cummings, 1995).

Approximately 95.7 percent of nurses in the United States are women. Like other traditionally female occupations, such as teaching and social work, nursing has been historically plagued with low status, low pay, and general subordination to higher-status men. Nurses faced, and still face, a double challenge of being predominately female and operating within the stereotypic boundaries of a traditionally "female" profession (Moss, 1995).

Nursing, Feminism, and Women's Movements

Nursing, **feminism,** and women's movements of the twentieth century have had an uneasy relationship. Contemporary feminists have often criticized nursing for failing to support women's movements. For example, the relatively young American Nurses Association (ANA) refused to endorse women's suffrage until 1915, although the fight for women's right to vote had been going on for the previous 40 years. Years later the more mature ANA chose not to endorse the passage of the Equal Rights Amendment (ERA) until the late 1970s because the ANA leadership believed that biological differences between men and women demanded special legislative attention that the more generic ERA did not address (Bunting and Campbell, 1990).

Nursing has been viewed by some feminists as a traditional and oppressive female occupation. There is some validity to this criticism because nurses have tended to build their own power bases on connections with governmental agencies and strong, male-dominated professions such as medicine rather than on identification with other nurses and other women's groups (Bunting and Campbell, 1990). Many nurses have inadvertently contributed to this stereotype by looking to others outside nursing to improve conditions in nursing rather than working with other nurses to strengthen the profession from within.

What exactly is feminism? There are several types, but Gray's (1994) explanation is helpful: "The primary focus of feminism is an examination of gender privilege, that is, privilege that accrues or is denied because of one's biologically determined sexual characteristics" (p. 506). Gray further explained that feminism values women, their experiences, knowledge, and ways of knowing in a **dominant culture** in which everyone lives, grows, and participates.

The feminist perspective is not the exclusive property of women. Feminism is concerned with the advancement of all people by eliminating the dominance-submission model of relating; placing value on the worth and dignity of all people; eliminating hierarchies based on one group's domination of others; eliminating health disparities based on gender, age, ethnicity, or social status; and creating a healthier and safer society (Gary, Sigsby, and Campbell, 1998). These are goals that can be embraced by every thoughtful person.

The women's movement that began in the 1960s has had a profound effect on society and has both hurt and helped the nursing profession. As women of the 1960s and 1970s sought career opportunities beyond the traditional female ones of teaching and nursing, bright and able women who formerly might have become nurses pursued careers in accounting, architecture, engineering, computer science, and a variety of other fields. This meant that nursing faced more competition for students than it once did.

Although this hurt nursing temporarily, the pendulum began to swing back in the late 1980s and 1990s as women realized how natural and good a "fit" nursing was for them. Currently, when women can freely choose any professional field of study, many are again choosing nursing. Deans and directors of schools of nursing in the United States report that applications are soaring from women who were originally educated to be attorneys, computer programmers, accountants, and other occupations more recently open to them. It seems that in spite of an almost unlimited array of career choices now available to men and women, nursing's appeal is strong to people of both genders who want to make a difference in the lives of others.

The women's movement helped nursing by bringing economic issues such as low salaries and poor working conditions into the open. The movement provoked a conscious awareness that equality and autonomy for women were inherent rights, not privileges, and stimulated the passage of legislation to assure those rights.

Nursing also benefited from the women's movement in more subtle ways. As nursing students were increasingly educated in colleges and universities, they were exposed to campus activism, protest, and organizations that were trying to change the status of women. Learning informal lessons about power and how to bring about change has had a positive effect on modern students, who later use this knowledge to improve the status of nursing.

Despite these positive directions, the nursing profession has been slow to internalize the women's movement message of self-determination and commitment. As mentioned earlier, many nurses have looked on nursing as a useful way to occupy themselves until marriage. To others, nursing was a "job" used to supplement the major breadwinner's income or to pay for a family vacation, new car, or camp for the kids. Sometimes nurses worked only to tide the family over temporarily rough economic waters, returning to home and family when the family's financial situation improved. This "stepping in" and "stepping out" of the profession has meant that these nurses' energies and loyalties were split. The result is that nursing has not prospered as it might have if all of its members were committed to long-term careers.

It is unfortunate that many registered nurses (RNs) have not fully accepted the necessity for long-term professional commitment, which not only enhances personal growth but also strengthens the profession from within. Feminism and women's movements have helped nurses learn that women can be autonomous and assertive. With the firm commitment of all its members, male and female, to lifelong full participation, nursing can grow to its maximum potential, expand opportunities for its members, and ultimately contribute to the advancement of society at large. Shea (1994) encouraged nurses to contribute to contemporary feminism in the following four areas (pp. 577–578):

1. By sharing their passionate conviction about feminism and nursing with family members, friends, co-workers, and community members, so the message reaches decision makers, and various changes take place.
2. By expressing themselves in public through letters to the editor in professional journals and daily newspapers; by telling nursing's stories that the public wants and needs to hear.
3. By creating good public role models in the main vehicle for change in American society, television. "Nursing needs another 'China Beach' series—updated and reflective of what nurses really do, and how they think and feel. . . . In order for these things to happen, some nurses will have to devote their full attention to 'nonnursing things' such as writing scripts, performing on the stage, taking photographs, developing artwork, and making feature-length films and documentaries featuring nurses" (p. 578).
4. By caring for nursing's young. Socialization into nursing has to change toward becoming a more empathic, nonhierarchial, mutually beneficial process. There must be tolerance of different learning styles and cultural values, reflecting the diversity of the population of nursing.

Even individuals who do not consider themselves feminists can agree that these are important goals for nursing.

Men in Nursing

In 1992, 4.3 percent (79,557) of practicing registered nurses in the United States were men. By 1996 that figure had risen to 5.4 percent (113,683) (U. S. Department of Health and Human Services 1996). This represents an increase of nearly 70 percent in only four years (Fig. 3–1). The male nurse, when compared with his female counterpart, is likely to be older, to be married, to have more education, and to choose nursing as a second career. Their motivations for entering nursing, however, are similar to those of their female counterparts. Most men enter nursing to help people (Villeneuve, 1994).

The American Assembly for Men in Nursing (AAMN) has developed a position statement on the role that gender should play in the nursing profession. Members of the AAMN believe that "Every professional nurse position and

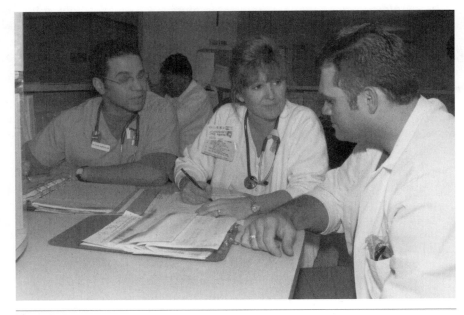

Figure 3–1
Male registered nurses are becoming more visible as their numbers increase.

every nursing educational opportunity shall be equally available to those meeting the entry qualifications regardless of gender" (Halloran and Welton, 1994, p. 690). The fact that the members of this organization thought this statement was necessary raises the question, "Have men in nursing suffered discrimination because of their gender?" Let us now examine how men have fared in a profession traditionally dominated by women.

Men are not new to the profession of nursing. They supplied much of the nursing care during the eleventh, twelfth, and thirteenth centuries. It was not until late in the nineteenth century that nursing became a predominately female profession.

Despite all the positive things she did, Florence Nightingale played a major role in excluding men from the profession by asserting that nursing was a female discipline. She worked hard to establish nursing as a worthy career for respectable women and largely ignored the historical contributions of men. She saw the male role as confined to supplying physical strength, such as lifting or moving patients, when needed.

The Industrial Revolution also influenced the exit of men from nursing. During those times, the accepted professions for men were science, technology, and business. Men chose medicine, and women chose nursing (Black and Germaine-Warner, 1995).

The first two schools of nursing for men were established in the late 1800s. They were the Mills School of Nursing for Men at New York's Bellevue Hospital and the McLean Asylum Training School. The purpose of these training programs was to prepare men for psychiatric nursing, a field that in those days often required physical stamina and strength.

In 1901, the U. S. Congress created the Army Nurse Corps for female nurses only. The Navy Nurse Corps followed seven years later and was also restricted to women (Black and Germaine-Warner, 1995). Because of the lack of training programs and the gender restrictions placed on military nurses, it was difficult for men to enter nursing before World War II. Cummings (1995) reported that in 1941 only 68 of the 1,303 schools of nursing accepted men.

After World War II, the GI Bill helped to increase the number of male nursing students by providing funding for education. Military corpsmen entered nursing schools in large numbers, as they have following every major military conflict since. Nevertheless, as late as 1990, 8.3 percent of American baccalaureate nursing programs still had no male students (Villeneuve, 1995).

Why Men Enter Nursing

In a study conducted by Perkins and colleagues (1993), the top three reasons men entered the profession of nursing were job security, career opportunity, and job flexibility. These responses were followed closely by a desire to nurture and to contribute. Traditionally, men tend to choose "aggressive" areas of nursing, such as intensive care units, cardiac care units, emergency departments, trauma units, flight nursing, or anesthesiology. These choices may also be due to a fear of being rejected in traditionally "feminine" areas of nursing, such as pediatric and obstetrical nursing (Boughn, 1994) or because they support a masculine indentity (Evans, 1997).

Men are frequently drawn to the technological aspects of acute care specialities and are challenged by the machines in those units. The typical dress in some areas may also affect practice choices of men. Nurses in acute care specialties typically wear "scrubs," and nurses in administrative and psychiatric settings wear street clothes. Scrubs or street clothes may be more acceptable to men than traditional white nursing uniforms.

Some men may look at nursing as a springboard to other professions. They may not stay in nursing long because of the low status and low pay (Williams, 1989). There are several issues facing the large number of men who do choose to stay in nursing. These men often feel **role strain,** an emotional reaction that may be felt by a person in a profession that has a social structure dominated by members of the opposite sex.

Attitudes Toward Men in Nursing

As mentioned earlier, in American society men interested in health care traditionally became physicians, whereas women became nurses. Men entering the profession of nursing have crossed over gender lines, and their masculinity may be questioned as a result. One negative assumption men in nursing encounter is that male nurses have problems with sex role identity (Kelly, Shoemaker, and Steele, 1996). The pervasive homophobia in society and the belief that nursing is strictly a feminine profession show some signs of changing; however, these attitudes are still pervasive enough to affect the decisions of teenage boys making career choices (Villeneuve, 1994).

Another issue men deal with is denial of the fact that men can be nurses. People commonly assume a man delivering health care is either a physician or a medical student. A male pediatric nurse commented (Williams, 1995, p. 68):

> It's very funny, working in pediatrics even today. I have 3-year-old patients and I always introduce myself as, "I'm Bill, and I'm going to be your nurse." And they say, "You can't be a nurse." And I say, "Well, why?" [And they say,] "Well because you're a guy."

Male nursing students often face discrimination from practicing nurses, physicians, and the public. Female nurses often ask male counterparts for assistance in lifting and turning patients, emphasizing physical strength rather than professional expertise. It is all too common for male students to find themselves unwelcome in prenatal clinics, delivery rooms, and other settings in which male physicians have free access.

One male obstetrician in a midsize southeastern community refused to allow a male nursing student in the delivery suite, explaining, "My patients are uncomfortable with a man in the room." The irony of one male health professional restricting the access of another male health professional student based on the student's gender did not escape the notice of the student. Unfortunately, the nurse in charge of the unit chose not to advocate for the student, and the student's clinical instructor was unsuccessful in doing so. He had to transfer to a different clinical group in another hospital to complete his clinical objectives. This type of incident is not uncommon, as evidenced by the accompanying News Note. Legal cases are being tried in the courts challenging these practices. Ketter (1994) interviewed a man involved in a recent court case who made the observation, "It makes no sense. Men doctors have been treating women for years. What's the difference if it's a doctor or a nurse?"

Countering with a positive perspective, Williams (1995), discussed some of what she termed "hidden advantages" for men in nursing. She asserted that men are preferred in hiring because of their strength and perceived potential for better leadership. According to Williams, because of their "renegade status" in a female-dominated profession, men are given more respect and encouraged to increase their education and enter the most prestigious specializations. She reported that men tend to earn more money than their female counterparts in nursing and that married male nurses are viewed as the traditional breadwinners of their families and are considered more permanent, reliable employees. Male physicians tend to treat male nurses as equals, as do men in management positions. This may serve as a hidden advantage to men in nursing (Evans, 1997).

How can the presence of men in nursing help women? Some women believe men might help them become more assertive. A male nurse commented

The Following Letter Appeared in Hundreds of U.S. Newspapers in February, 1999.

Dear Ann Landers: I read your column about the woman who needed a breast exam and was offended that the technician was male. The ignorance of the American public about male nurses is shameful.

I am a male nurse who chose this field because I want to make a difference in people's lives. I want to ease their suffering and do what I can for the sick and dying. Male nurses take the same classes as our female counterparts. We have the same training and lose the same amount of sleep, which is considerable. We work right alongside our female colleagues and are licensed by the same state board. When I am assigned to a female patient, it would never occur to me to make a pass or derive any sexual pleasure from that individual. Believe me, a hospital is not the romantic setting that the TV shows project. Please let all the female patients who read your column know that we are there only to make their hospital stay, medical tests and surgery as easy and comfortable as possible.—Everywhere, USA

DEAR EVERYWHERE: Thank you for speaking so eloquently about a subject that needs airing. TV has indeed portrayed hospitals as places where romances flourish and love affairs abound. The shows may romanticize the hospital setting, but the people who work there know it is serious business.

Reprinted with permission of Ann Landers.

on what he believes will have to happen for nursing to gain more respect (Williams, 1989, p. 126):

> Women will have to fight and stick up for who they are and what they do, and women do not do that. So many times women in nursing do not support each other, for one thing; more likely they tear each other apart . . . . I don't think women are strong enough, they're not vocal enough, they're not demanding enough. I'm sure that men are more demanding and will be over the years.

Another male nurse commented on the lack of career commitment of female nurses (Williams, 1989, p. 127):

> The reason I feel career conditions in nursing are so poor is because from the hospital's standpoint, nurses are short-term employees. They come and go. They have babies. They change careers. For whatever individual reason, they're not there long enough to treat them as permanent employees. . . . Until women as a group treat it [nursing] as a career and insist upon equal benefits as they have in other careers, it's going to stay as it is.

These attitudes were validated in a study of men in nursing by Cyr (1992). Most female respondents thought of nursing as a "job," while male respondents tended to view nursing as a "professional career."

Encouraging Men to Enter Nursing

What can be done to attract more men to nursing? Boughn (1994, p. 31) recommends the following strategies:

1. Correct public misconceptions about males' capacity for doing "caring work" such as nursing.
2. Re-educate high school guidance counselors to target appropriate populations for the rigors of nursing education and nursing practice not previously considered, such as academically capable male students.
3. Involve male nursing students in recruitment efforts and make them visible in recruitment materials.
4. Encourage national occupation publications to present nonsexist information regarding career options for males.
5. Encourage editors of professional journals and other literature to portray male nurses in advertisements depicting nurses.

In addition to these ideas, a male nursing professor pointed out that the absence of male role models for students in colleges and universities is a discouragement to potential students. He reported on an initiative to provide mentoring for male nursing students to prepare them for full participation in a profession overwhelmingly dominated by women (Sowell, 1999).

Whether men in nursing experience disadvantages or advantages or some of both, one thing is certain: The increasing number of men in nursing will make the profession different. This should be seen as a positive trend, for both feminine and masculine qualities and abilities are needed to strengthen the profession and to treat whole human beings (Fig. 3–2).

Figure 3–2
Steady increase in the percentage of men graduating from basic RN programs (Cummings, S. H., *NLN Center for research,* 1997: NLN Press and Jones and Bartlett Publishers, Sudbury, MA).

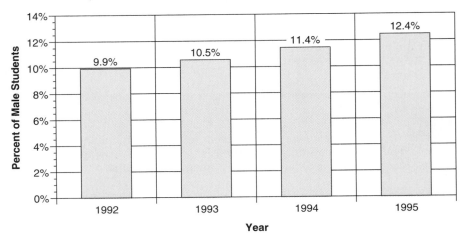

Image of Nursing

When you think of a nurse, what image comes to mind? Is it Florence Nightingale floating down the stairs carrying her lamp to attend the wounded soldiers? Perhaps you remember a humorous "get well" card depicting an unattractive woman carrying a bedpan under one arm and a huge hypodermic needle in the other hand? Or do you remember seeing heavily made-up soap opera nurses with big, blond hair and short, tight white dresses going about their work in high-heeled shoes? The image of nursing has been, and continues to be, colorfully presented and distorted in all forms of expression in society.

Why is image so important? First impressions say a lot about a particular group of people. These perceptions affect attitudes toward the profession of nursing. According to studies of public opinion, the public views nurses as nurturant and concerned for others but only moderately well educated. In the public's view, physicians cure diseases, whereas nurses are nice and caring (Campbell-Heider, Hart, and Bergren, 1994).

Caring is hard for the public to define. As part of a class project in 1998, prenursing students at Auburn University in Alabama surveyed over 800 nonnursing individuals on campus to evaluate their perceptions of nursing. The overwhelming majority of participants responded that nursing is a "caring, helping profession" performed by persons mainly in hospitals or doctors' offices. These global descriptors demonstrate that respondents' understanding of the exact nature of nursing and the qualities required to be a nurse is limited (Huffstutler et al., 1998).

Since most people come into contact with nurses from time to time, why does the public not better understand nursing? One problem is the difficulty in knowing who exactly are the registered nurses. Gone are the traditional white caps and uniforms:

> The nurse of today in many situations is unidentifiable by uniform. The stethoscope around the neck or tucked in a pocket serves to some degree as identification. In most regions of the country, caps are no longer worn and school pins have been replaced by hospital identification badges that may or may not include full names and titles (Mangum, 1994, p. 54).

Many nurses, especially with the entry of more men into the profession, are glad to see the demise of the traditional caps and white uniforms. Perhaps uniforms projected a stereotypic image rather than a realistic perception of nurses as autonomous providers with a high level of education and scientific expertise (Campbell-Heider, Hart, and Bergren, 1994). Uniforms, however, did help identify registered nurses and differentiate them from the everincreasing numbers of nonnursing assistive personnel.

Some hospitals and other health care organizations have contributed to the difficulty in identifying registered nurses by requiring all nursing staff to wear name badges with ambiguous titles such as "Patient Caregiver." This

Since the 1970s, nurses have largely given up the traditional white nurse's uniform and now wear various non-standardized attire including colors and patterns. This often renders them indistinguishable from a number of other health care workers. Nurses today seem to be unconcerned by patients' inability to recognize them, perhaps believing that what they know is more important than how they dress.

An interdisciplinary group of faculty at Brigham Young University in Provo, Utah examined the effect of a nurse's appearance on patients' perceptions of that nurse's professional image. They based their study on the assumption, supported by the literature, that people form impressions about another's competence and professionalism from appearance.

Over 1180 patients, ranging in age from 10 to >80, 918 nurses, and 332 administrators in 13 states were interviewed. Study participants were asked to look at nine pictures of a female nurse wearing different uniforms considered representative of today's nursing attire choices. They were then asked to rate each nurse on each of ten traits: confidence, competence, attentiveness, efficiency, approachability, caring, professionalism, reliability, cooperation and empathy. They were also asked to select the nurse they would most and least like to have care for them.

All participants rated the white pant uniform with stethoscope significantly higher than other uniforms. The white pant uniform with cap was second with all groups. Colored designer scrubs and white pants with colored top ranked lowest. Both patients and administrators

ranked colored designer scrubs significantly lower than did nurses. When asked by which nurse they would like to be cared for, all chose the nurse in white pant suit and stethoscope. Least preferred by patients and administrators were colored scrubs. Nurses least preferred street clothes with lab coat.

The researchers concluded that patients' first impressions, including the ability to recognize a nurse, have a strong impact. They encouraged nurses to consider the importance of patients' opinions in improving the image of nurses and questioned whether nursing should reestablish a traditional, easily identifiable appearance.

(From Mangum, S., Garrison, C., Lind, C., and Hilton, H. G. (1997). First impressions of the nurse and nursing care. *Journal of Nursing Care Quality*, 11(5), 39–47.)

trend coincided with cost cutting by reducing the number of registered nurses employed in direct patient care. This practice is seen by many thoughtful nurses as an attempt to obscure the relatively low number of registered nurses remaining in some settings by making everyone look the same.

Another area of concern for the image of nursing is the use of language and how health professionals address each other. Campbell-Heider and associates speak to this issue by noting that nurses often use their first names with patients, whereas physicians use their professional titles. These authors believe that this practice reinforces sex role stereotypes and promotes social distance and hierarchical relations between the two disciplines. If formal titles are used for physicians, they should be used for nurses. By using parallel styles of addressing each other, interdependence and mutual respect would be fostered. Campbell-Heider and associates (1994) conclude by stating, "Attention to personal symbols of language and dress advance the actuality and image of the professional nurse. Those who respect themselves will convey this attitude to their colleagues and patients" (p. 228).

Nurses cannot and should not attribute their image problems to any other group, including physicians. The nursing profession has major responsibility for improving its own image. Black and Germaine-Warner (1995) suggested a variety of things nurses can do, including recognizing that each nurse should work to improve nursing's image, participating in professional organizations, becoming politically active, writing for local media, providing technical assistance to the media, taking advantage of public speaking opportunities, and sharing positive aspects of nursing with others.

Influence of the Media on Nursing's Image

The influence of the media's portrayals of nurses is extremely powerful, and this causes great concern for nursing because the image portrayed has often been negative and demeaning.

Muff (1988b) identified six major nursing stereotypes commonly portrayed by the media:

- Angel of mercy
- Handmaiden to the physician
- Woman in white
- Sex symbol/idiot
- Battle-axe
- Torturer

Muff pointed out that almost all media choose to depict nurses as females. They are generally portrayed as unintelligent women in traditional, even obsolete, roles. One result of this misrepresentation of nurses in the media is probably a negative impact on the recruitment of future nurses (Muff, 1988b), especially when contrasted with the respectful treatment of physicians in the media.

Aber and Hawkins (1992) studied the portrayal of nurses in advertisements in medical and nursing journals. They found that in both profession's journals, nurses were portrayed in ways that were stereotypical and demeaning, wearing attire long outdated, or as sex objects and handmaidens to physicians. They concluded their report with the following thoughts (p. 293):

> If we continue to accept an image of nurses as portrayed in our print media as dependent, passive and minor figures in the health care system, then that is what we will continue to be. If we demand that the image be changed to that of active participants in the delivery of care, as independent and interdependent professionals and as major figures in the health care drama, then that is what we will become.

From 1988 to 1991, a grant from the Pew Charitable Trusts provided support for an organization known as Nurses of America (NOA). Nurses of America was sponsored by the four Quad-Council Organizations: the American Association of Colleges of Nursing (AACN), the ANA, the American Organization of Nurse Executives (AONE), and the National League for Nursing (NLN). Nurses of America initiated a multimedia project designed to inform the public, legislators, and business community about the contributions of contemporary nursing and nursing practice in the delivery of high-quality, cost-effective health care. A result of this project was publication of three *Media Watch* newsletters to over 200,000 readers.

Nurses of America also sponsored a 1991 study entitled "Who Counts and Who Doesn't in News Coverage of Health Care." The study found that nurses were "virtually silent" as sources of health care news. Even though nurses represented the largest profession in the health care system, persons in every other "occupational" category, out of 12 categories, were quoted more frequently than nurses about health care issues. Following physicians, the most frequently quoted persons were government officials, business people, patients, family members, other white-collar health professionals, and nonprofessional hospital workers.

According to the NOA report, this study has several implications for the nursing profession (Nurses of America, 1991, p. 17):

> In terms of nursing, it is difficult for a group to have influence in the development of public policy and the allocation of resources unless it can be seen and heard as part of the public discussion. The role of nursing as a contributor to the health care system is limited if the press, for whatever reason, does not consider nursing a legitimate or credible source or subject.

Another study of interest was a comparative analysis of nurse and physician characters in the entertainment media, made by Kalisch and Kalisch (1986). This study revealed that while the role of physicians was presented in an exaggerated, idealistic, and heroic light, "media nurses" were shown in substantially less desired roles (p. 185):

> Even basic intelligence, rationality, problem-solving abilities and clinical skills are absent in most nurse portrayals. Nurse characters are presented as generally unimportant in health care, largely occupying the background rather than playing an instrumental role in health care. Media nurses are viewed less positively than physicians by other characters, and show little commitment to their careers. The central and diverse role the nurse actually plays in the delivery of health care to the American public is virtually absent in the entertainment media.

The Kalischs asserted that these images of nurses not only affect consumers' opinions of nurses but also impact the images nurses hold of themselves. They called for an improvement in the manner in which nurses are portrayed in the media "even if this does require a diminishment of the intensity of the halo that the media physician has worn in recent decades" (p. 193).

Mikulencak gave mixed reviews to popular television shows in 1995, pointing out that nurses either loved or hated television medical dramas such as "ER" and "Chicago Hope." These shows had large audiences. A Neilsen survey in the *Wall Street Journal* on January 5, 1996, reported that "ER" ranked first in the top 10 prime-time programs with a 30 percent share of the viewing audience. This meant that 30 percent of all switched-on sets during that Neilsen Media Research survey period were tuned to "ER."

According to Buresh and Gordon (1995), "ER" received high positive reviews from nurses themselves. This was probably owing to the fact that a past president of the Emergency Nurses Association, consisting of 24,000 members, acted as a significant advisor for the producers of "ER." She conveyed feedback from nurses, suggested story ideas, and helped construct realistic scenarios.

This type of cooperation between nurses and television producers was new. In the past, organized nursing struggled with television producers over the image being portrayed. It was the unified power of nurses that launched a successful campaign to eliminate the television program "The Nightingales" in the late 1980s. This program outraged nurses by its depiction of nursing students as sex objects in demeaning situations. Pressure, in the form of a letter-writing campaign by nurses, was coordinated by NOA. This led the producers of this series to cancel the short-lived program.

Another 1980s television series, "China Beach," depicted nurses as intelligent, autonomous health professionals. This series, which received critical acclaim, was an award-winning drama about nurses in Vietnam. The program was widely praised by nursing groups, and its star became a media spokesperson and advocate for nursing. Unfortunately the series was canceled, and a letter-writing campaign by nurses calling for the renewal of the series was unsuccessful.

A recent comprehensive study of nursing in the print media was conducted in September 1997 by 17 students and 3 faculty coordinators from the University of Rochester (New York) School of Nursing (URSN). In this study, sponsored by Sigma Theta Tau International (STTI) and URSN, students examined approximately 20,000 articles from 16 newspapers, magazines, and trade publications. The **Woodhull Study on Nursing and the Media,** as it was called, was named in honor of the late Nancy Woodhull, a founding editor of *USA Today*. Woodhull became an advocate of nursing following her diagnosis of lung cancer when she was impressed with the comprehensive nursing care she received. She suggested the study and assisted in the design of the survey after she became concerned about the absence of media attention to nurses and nursing.

In December 1997, the students presented their findings and recommendations to a mixed audience of nurses and national media representatives at the STTI Biennial Convention. The key finding was "Nurses and the nursing profession are essentially invisible to the media and, consequently, to the American public" (Sigma Theta Tau, 1998, p. 8).

The purpose of the Woodhull Study, its major findings, and strategies to guide the nursing profession's collective response are found in Box 3–3.

Nursing organizations and associations are well-equipped to implement the recommended response strategies found in the Woodhull Report. But what

BOX 3–3

The Woodhull Study at a Glance: Purpose, Findings, and Recommendations

Purpose of the Study
The Woodhull Study was designed to survey and analyze the portrayal of health care and nursing in U.S. newspapers, news magazines, and health care industry trade publications.

Key Study Findings
Nurses and the nursing profession are essentially invisible in media coverage of health care and, consequently, to the American public.

1. Nurses were cited only 4 percent of the time in the over 2,000 health-related articles culled from 16 major news publications.
2. The few references to nurses or nursing that did occur were mostly just in passing.
3. In many of the stories, nurses and nursing would have been more germane to the story subject matter than the references selected.
4. Health care industry publications were no more likely to take advantage of nursing expertise, focusing more attention on bottom line issues such as business or policy.

Key Study Recommendations

1. Both media and nursing should take a more proactive role in establishing an ongoing dialogue.
2. The often repeated advice in media articles and advertisements to "consult your doctor" ignores the role of nurses in health care and needs to be changed to "consult your primary health care provider."
3. Journalists should distinguish researchers with doctoral degrees from medical doctors to add clarity to health care coverage.
4. To provide comprehensive coverage of health care, the media should include information by and about nurses.
5. It is essential to distinguish health care (the umbrella) from medicine as subject matter in the media.

Adapted from Sigma Theta Tau International (1998). *The Woodhull study on nursing and the media: Health care's invisible partner, final report.* Indianapolis, Ind.: STTI's Center Nursing Press.

about individuals? What can individual nurses do to improve the image of nursing portrayed in the media? Box 3–4 presents a checklist for monitoring media images of nurses and nursing. Use this checklist as you view television, watch movies, read books and newspapers, and look at advertisements. Then take action by writing those responsible for negative nursing images. Nurses themselves must reinforce positive images of nursing and, more importantly, speak out against negative ones.

BOX 3–4
Checklist for Monitoring Media Images of Nurses and Nursing

Prominence in the Plot

1. Are nurse characters seen in leading or supportive roles?
2. Are nurse characters shown taking an active part in the proceedings or are they shown primarily in the background (handing instruments, carrying trays, pushing wheelchairs)?
3. To what extent are nurse characters shown in professional roles, engaged in nursing practice?
4. Is it nurse characters or other characters who provide the actual nursing care?
5. In scenes with nonnurse professionals (physicians, hospital administrators), who does most of the talking?

Demographics

6. Does the portrayal show that men as well as women may aspire to a career in nursing?
7. Are nurse characters shown to be of varying ages?
8. Are some nurse characters single and others married?

Personality Traits

9. Are nurse characters portrayed as:

a. Intelligent	e. Sophisticated	i. Nurturant
b. Rational	f. Problem solvers	j. Empathic
c. Confident	g. Assertive	k. Sincere
d. Ambitious	h. Powerful	l. Kind

10. If other health care providers are included in the program, what differences are seen in their personality traits as compared with nurse characters?
11. When nurse characters exhibit personality traits 9a through 9h listed above, do such portrayals show them to be abnormal in some way?

Primary Values

12. Do nurse characters exhibit values for:
    a. Service to others, humanism   b. Scholarship, achievement
13. If other health care providers are included in the program, what differences are seen in their primary values as compared with nurse characters?
14. When nurse characters exhibit the primary values of scholarship and achievement, do such portrayals show them to be abnormal in some way?

Sex Objects

15. Are nurse characters portrayed as sex objects?
16. Are nurse characters referred to in sexually demeaning terms?
17. Are nurse characters presented as appealing because of their physical attractiveness or cuteness as opposed to their intellectual capacity, professional commitment, or skill?

(continued)

BOX 3–4
Checklist for Monitoring Media Images of Nurses and Nursing (*Continued*)

Role of the Nurse

18. Is the profession of nursing shown to be an attractive and fulfilling long-term career?
19. Is the work of the nurse characters shown to be creative and exciting?

Career Orientation

20. How important is the career of nursing to the nurse character portrayed?
21. How does this compare with other professionals depicted in the program?

Professional Competence

22. Are nurse characters praised for their professional capabilities by other characters?
23. Do nurse characters praise other professionals?
24. Do nurse characters exhibit autonomous judgment in professional matters?
25. Is there a gratuitous message that a nurse's role in health care is a supportive rather than central one?
26. Do nurse characters positively influence patient/family welfare?
27. Are nurse characters shown harming or acting to the detriment of patients?
28. How does the professional competence of nurse characters compare with the professional competence of other health care providers?
29. When nurse characters exhibit professional competence, are they shown to be abnormal in some way?

Education

30. Who actually teaches the nursing students?
31. Who appears to be in charge of nursing education?
32. Is there evidence that the practice of nursing requires special knowledge and skills?
33. What is actually taught to nursing students?

Administration

34. Are any roles filled by nurse administrators or managers or are all nurse characters shown as staff nurses or students?
35. Is there evidence of an administrative hierarchy in nursing or are nurses shown answering to physicians or hospital administrators?
36. Are nurse characters shown turning to other nurses for assistance or are they depicted as relying on a physician or other character (generally male) for guidance, strength, or rescuing?

Overall Assessment and Comments

37. Overall, is this a positive or negative portrayal of nursing? Why or why not?

From *The Changing Image of the Nurse* by Kalisch/Kalisch, © 1987. Adapted by permission of Prentice-Hall, Inc., Upper Saddle River, NJ.

Social Phenomena Affecting Nursing

Because nursing is an integral part of the social context in which it functions, it is affected by and responds to changes in that larger social environment. Over the course of American nursing history, nurses have responded as individuals to wars and other social phenomena. Contemporary nursing, however, seeks to respond as a profession to social changes that shape our nation.

Five major phenomena will be discussed: the aging population, the rise of consumerism, increasing cultural diversity, technological advances, and violence. Each profoundly affects nursing practice.

Graying of America

Growth in the number of elderly Americans is proceeding at a dramatic rate. In 1990, there were approximately 13 million people 75 years of age or older in the United States. By 1995, that number had risen to nearly 15 million, and in 2000 reached 16.5 million. Demographic projections of the U.S. Bureau of the Census anticipate the proportion of elderly will grow rapidly in the next few decades. The number of people 75 years of age or older in 2005 is expected to be 17.7 million, and by 2020, well within the working lives of most of today's nursing students, the number is expected to reach 21.8 million. In contrast, the number of 35- to 44-year-old Americans is expected to decline from 44.7 million in 2000 to 39.6 million by 2020. This phenomenon is often referred to as "the graying of America."

People over age 75 generally have fewer years of schooling and are more likely than younger people to be poor, widowed, female, living alone, and suffering from chronic disease. This elderly age group was young during the Great Depression and may have suffered from nutritional deficiencies and inadequate health care during their developmental years. As a consequence, this age group uses a disproportionately higher share of health services than other age groups.

The oldest "baby boomers," those Americans born between 1946 and 1964, will create a bulge in the aging population between the years 2010 and 2030. As these postwar babies age, their large numbers are expected to create an additional strain on the health care system. Up until this point in the history of the United States, the elderly population has always been vastly outnumbered by younger people. The disproportion between healthy, young adults and more fragile elderly adults expected in the next 20 years will create stress on the social systems of our nation. The graying of America will have a profound impact on the health care system and the nursing profession, which will stretch our already-challenged capacity to provide adequate medical and nursing care.

The nursing profession has responded to the aging population by increasing the number of courses offered in gerontological nursing to prepare nurses to care for elders more effectively. Gerontological nursing is now a full-fledged speciality, as evidenced by certification at the generalist, specialist, and nurse practitioner levels offered by the American Nurses Credentialing Center. Colleges of nursing now offer master's-level preparation for gerontological clinical specialists and nurse practitioners. In spite of these responses, much remains to be done to prepare nurses for the dramatic increase in the number of aging patients they will encounter in the next two decades.

Consumer Movement

Since the 1960s, there has been a movement by consumers to make the health care system more accountable for its actions. The American public, fueled by the principles of **consumerism,** criticized the dehumanization of health care. This led to the development in 1972 of the American Hospital Association's (AHA) document "A Patient's Bill of Rights," which guaranteed certain rights and privileges to every hospitalized patient. "A Patient's Bill of Rights" was revised in 1992 (Box 3–5).

Many people believe the AHA document was the first formal declaration of its kind. A little known fact is that in 1959, 14 years before the AHA action, the NLN issued a statement about patients' rights. Until the AHA's "A Patient's Bill of Rights" was published, however, the prevailing attitude in health care was that providers knew best and good patients simply followed directions without asking questions. This is known as **medical paternalism.**

The rise of consumerism in health care led to the involvement of consumers in pressing Congress for legislation protecting the public from inadequate care, experimental drugs, poor nutrition, and many other health-related issues. Consumer groups have demanded controls on spiraling health care costs and gained participation on boards of health planning agencies, accrediting bodies, and professional licensing boards. Most state boards of nursing have at least one consumer member.

The emphasis on consumerism is enhanced by the development of community partnerships designed to address health-related issues of concern to citizens. Farley (1994) stated that community partnerships are an outgrowth of an attempt to shift power from health professionals to citizens. The goal of community partnerships is not to eliminate all problems; the goal is to focus the community's energies toward those health-related problems that they are willing to work together to solve. Citizens in every community must be involved in their own health care decisions.

Nurses can play an instrumental role in taking the decision making closer to the consumer. Fagin and Binder (1994) remarked that the traditional physician-patient relationship has been a dominant-subordinate one, and the role of consumers in the health care system has been subordinate and passive. To change this traditional relationship, consumers must actively participate in the health care system, be responsible for their own health maintenance, and demand high quality and cost-effectiveness. In 1994 Fagin and Binder pointed out that this is the nursing model of care. They stated that for change to occur, a shift in the locus of control in health matters away from the

BOX 3–5
A Patient's Bill of Rights

Bill of Rights[*]

1. The patient has the right to considerate and respectful care.
2. The patient has the right to and is encouraged to obtain from physicians and other direct caregivers relevant, current, and understandable information concerning diagnosis, treatment, and prognosis.

   Except in emergencies when the patient lacks decision-making capacity and the need for treatment is urgent, the patient is entitled to the opportunity to discuss and request information related to the specific procedures and/or treatments, the risks involved, the possible length of recuperation, and the medically reasonable alternatives and their accompanying risks and benefits.

   Patients have the right to know the identity of physicians, nurses, and others involved in their care, as well as when those involved are students, residents, or other trainees. The patient also has the right to know the immediate and long-term financial implications of treatment choices, insofar as they are known.
3. The patient has the right to make decisions about the plan of care prior to and during the course of treatment and to refuse a recommended treatment or plan of care to the extent permitted by law and hospital policy and to be informed of the medical consequences of this action. In case of such refusal, the patient is entitled to other appropriate care and services that the hospital provides or transfer to another hospital. The hospital should notify patients of any policy that might affect patient choice within the institution.
4. The patient has the right to have an advance directive (such as a living will, health care proxy, or durable power of attorney for health care) concerning treatment or designating a surrogate decision maker with the expectation that the hospital will honor the intent of that directive to the extent permitted by law and hospital policy.

   Health care institutions must advise patients of their rights under state law and hospital policy to make informed medical choices, ask if the patient has an advance directive, and include that information in patient records. The patient has the right to timely information about hospital policy that may limit its ability to implement fully a legally valid advance directive.
5. The patient has the right to every consideration of privacy. Case discussion, consultation, examination, and treatment should be conducted so as to protect each patient's privacy.
6. The patient has the right to expect that all communications and records pertaining to his/her care will be treated as confidential by the hospital, except in cases such as suspected abuse and public health hazards when reporting is permitted or required by law. The patient has the right to expect that the hospital will emphasize the confidentiality of this informa-

(continued)

BOX 3–5
A Patient's Bill of Rights (*Continued*)

tion when it releases it to any other parties entitled to review information in these records.

7. The patient has the right to review the records pertaining to his/her medical care and to have the information explained or interpreted as necessary, except when restricted by law.

8. The patient has the right to expect that, within its capacity and policies, a hospital will make reasonable response to the request of a patient for appropriate and medically indicated care and services. The hospital must provide evaluation, service, and/or referral as indicated by the urgency of the case. When medically appropriate and legally permissible, or when a patient has so requested, a patient may be transferred to another facility. The institution to which the patient is to be transferred must first have accepted the patient for transfer. The patient must also have the benefit of complete information and explanation concerning the need for, risks, benefits, and alternatives to such a transfer.

9. The patient has the right to ask and be informed of the existence of business relationships among the hospital, educational institutions, other health care providers, or payers that may influence the patient's treatment and care.

10. The patient has the right to consent to or decline to participate in proposed research studies or human experimentation affecting care and treatment or requiring direct patient involvement, and to have those studies fully explained prior to consent. A patient who declines to participate in research or experimentation is entitled to the most effective care that the hospital can otherwise provide.

11. The patient has the right to expect reasonable continuity of care when appropriate and to be informed by physicians and other caregivers of available and realistic patient care options when hospital care is no longer appropriate.

12. The patient has the right to be informed of hospital policies and practices that relate to patient care, treatment, and responsibilities. The patient has the right to be informed of available resources for resolving disputes, grievances, and conflicts, such as ethics committees, patient representatives, or other mechanisms available in the institution. The patient has the right to be informed of the hospital's charges for services and available payment methods.

physician and to the consumer must occur. They recommended that consumers develop personal accountability for their health and medical choices. They further asserted that (p. 458)

> The time is ripe for transformation in the health care system that will bring consumers into the fold as equals in the delivery of health care and leaders in the promotion of their own care. It will be up to nurses and others to couple health promotion efforts and traditional public health messages with a campaign to empower consumers within the delivery system and expose the mythology of enforced passivity that many Americans believe is endemic to receiving health services. So far only nurses have stepped forward to promote such changes in the delivery of health care.

By 1999, these changes were already occurring. The 106th United States Congress, responding to the reaction of health care consumers to limited choices and restrictions brought about by managed care, debated a Federal Patient's Bill of Rights. This document, the result of lobbying efforts of nursing organizations, consumers, organized medicine, the American Association of Retired People (AARP), and many others, was designed to ensure that every American had a basic level of care. A version of this legislation is expected to receive Congressional approval early this century.

Cultural Diversity

Since its founding, the United States has been a "melting pot" of people from many cultures. At one time, people new to the United States were anxious to become assimilated and assumed American names, dress, manners, language, and ways as soon as possible. This is no longer the case. At the turn of the century, a more accurate description of the United States would be a "chunky stew" (Ahmann, 1994) or a "salad bowl" (Johnson, 1994). Instead of blending together, as in a melting pot, individuals from other countries are increasingly appreciated for the uniqueness and flavor they bring to the United States.

The population of most nondominant ethnic groups in the United States is growing. As the new millennium dawns, nondominant groups comprise an estimated 28.2 percent of the U.S. population. This figure is projected to increase to 37 percent by the year 2025 and to top 50 percent by 2080 (Andrews, 1992). In the states of California, Florida, and Texas, today's nondominant groups, most notably Hispanics, will become culturally dominant even sooner. Within the lifetimes of most students reading this book, the historically dominant Anglo-American (white) culture will become a minority culture. This represents a radical change in the demographics and cultural attitudes of the nation. Nursing must also change.

How well are nondominant cultures represented in the nursing profession? Despite dramatic increases in the nondominant population, in 1996 they represented only 10 percent of all registered nurses. This 10 percent consisted of 4.2 percent African-Americans, 3.4 percent Asian/Pacific Islanders, 1.6 percent Hispanics, 0.5 percent American Indian/Alaskan Natives, and 0.3 percent others (U. S. Department of Health and Human Services, 1996). As shown in Figure 3–3, the NLN (1997) reported that the percentage of minority students enrolled in basic RN programs increased only slightly from 1994 to 1995. To address the needs of a more culturally diverse society, nursing must increase its recruitment and retention of minority students. Barriers perceived by potential nursing students from groups known today as "minorities" must be eliminated so that the nursing profession can reflect the rich cultural diversity of the population. Nursing leaders recognize that it is necessary to increase the number of people in the profession who have world views different from those of the current dominant Anglo-American majority (Buerhaus and Auerbach, 1999).

What is nursing doing to respond to the increasing cultural diversity? The response actually began in 1955, when Dr. Madeleine Leininger, a visionary nurse and cultural anthropologist, founded the field of **transcultural nursing.** She defined transcultural nursing as a

> [H]umanistic and scientific area of formal study and practice in nursing which is focused upon differences and similarities among cultures with respect to human care, health (or well-being), and illness based upon the people's cultural values, beliefs, and practices. . . . [Nurses] use this knowledge to provide culturally specific or culturally congruent nursing care to people (Leininger, 1991, p. 60).

To participate fully in the celebration of diversity and the multicultural society we live in, individual nurses need to develop a sensitivity to and appreci-

Figure 3–3
Modest increase in percentage of minority students enrolled in nursing programs (National League for Nursing Research, *Nursing data review,* 1997. NLN Press and Jones and Bartlett Publishers, Sudbury, MA).

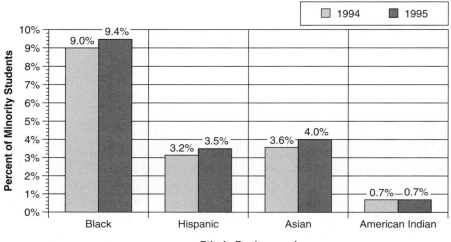

ation of the differences among cultures. More than ever before in the history of the profession, today's nurses must integrate knowledge, attitudes, and skills that enhance cross-cultural communication and appropriate interactions with others (Southern Regional Education Board, 1999). This is known as **cultural competence.** Attention to the development of culturally competent nurses has become an integral part of all progressive nursing education programs and is likely to become an even stronger influence in the future.

A more thorough discussion of the influence of culture on the family and nursing is found in Chapter 17.

Technological Advances

Technological advances have had a major effect on the practice of nursing. Between 1953 and 1979, medical specialization was increasingly supported by advances in technology, and the hospital business grew into a major technologically based industry. As medicine was transformed by technology, so was the practice of nursing as nurses assumed many of the responsibilities formerly performed by physicians.

Thompson and co-workers (1994) grouped health care technology into three major categories: biomedical, information, and knowledge. **Biomedical technology** involves complex machines or implantable devices used in patient care settings. This form of technology affected nursing practice because nurses often assume responsibility for monitoring the data generated from these machines and for assessing the safety and effectiveness of the equipment itself.

Information technology refers to hardware and software used to manage and process information. Nurses assumed much of the responsibility for data entry and retrieval with the advent of this technology. Simpson (1992, p. 28) described a **nursing information system** as a

> [s]oftware system that automates the nursing process, from assessment to evaluation, including patient care documentation. It also includes a means to manage the data necessary for the delivery of patient care, e.g., patient classification, staffing, scheduling and costs. The system can be either a stand-alone system or a sub-system of a larger hospital information system.

In a survey conducted by Simpson, 37 (29 percent) of 129 chief nurses reported that their nursing information systems had bedside capabilities. This means that nurses can enter data about the patient directly from the bedside. Some of the advantages of this **point of care technology** include (1) improvement in data accuracy and timeliness of documentation, (2) increase in nursing productivity because an electronic chart is always available for ready access, and (3) easy retrieval of patient clinical information (Happ, 1994).

Knowledge technology is described as a technology of the mind. It involves the use of computer systems to transform information into knowledge and to generate new knowledge. Through the creation of "expert systems," this form of technology will assist nurses with clinical judgments about patient management problems in the future. Deciding what expert knowledge to enter in these systems for clinical decision making, however, remains a challenge (Thompson, Amos, and Graves, 1994).

With so many kinds of technology, one might wonder, "Where is the patient?" One of the most widely debated issues is "high-tech" versus "high-touch" nursing. Technological advances now allow nurses to monitor their patients' conditions on computer screens at the nurses' station. Without even entering the patient's room, nurses can gather large amounts of information and make nursing decisions based on that information. Sometimes nurses seem to pay more attention to machines than to patients. They must actively guard against ignoring patients' needs for human interaction as a result of technological advances (Fig. 3–4). According to McConnell and Murphy (1990), nurses can be viewed as the "liaison between the machines" and their patients. These authors address the importance of technology in nursing by stating (p. 334):

Figure 3–4
Nurses in high-tech environments such as this coronary care unit must remember that the patient also needs human touch. Photo by Kelly Whalen.

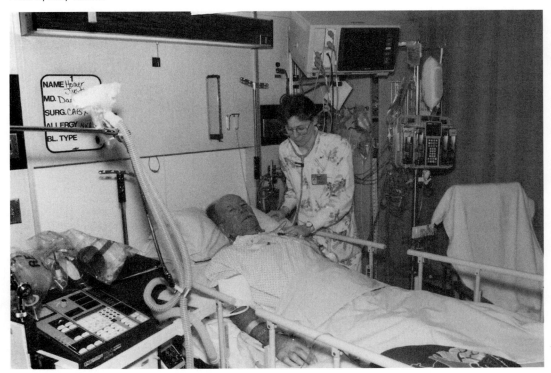

Nurses' knowledgeable use of technology, regardless of its sophistication, is imperative. But are nurses aware of the many opportunities being opened? Do nurses passively accept technology or actively shape it? Do they "react" to the transfer of technology or do they "act" to ensure that technology and medical device use is "appropriate?"

These are questions that bear thoughtful consideration by nurses. Locsin (1995) described a model of **caring technology.** Technology and caring coexist in nursing practice today, and Locsin's model is an attempt to explain the interconnectedness of technology and nursing. Successfully combining technology and caring requires sensitivity to patients' physical, emotional, and spiritual needs.

The high-technology environment encountered in hospitals is now moving into the home as health care becomes more community based. Technology can be viewed either as a "strategic opportunity" or a "strategic threat," according to Simpson (1993). His description of an innovative technological intervention that a nurse, Patricia Brennan, turned into a caring opportunity is found in Box 3–6.

Violence in America

Nurses are increasingly affected, both personally and professionally, by the rising tide of violence in this country. In spite of overwhelming media attention to the problem and congressional debates about gun control, little has been done to reduce the onslaught of violence. Perhaps this is because the root causes of violence are complex, multiple, and not readily changeable.

BOX 3–6
Combining Technology and Caring

Patricia Brennan, PhD, RN, FAAN, associate professor of nursing and systems engineering at the Frances Payne Bolton School of Nursing at Case Western Reserve University developed a telephone network that allowed caregivers of AIDS patients and Alzheimer's disease patients to communicate with each other and their medical center. Not only did this lead to tremendous participation and acceptance, but also the 24-hour access to electronic information and support was comforting for patients facing chronic illnesses. The network was also extremely effective in educating patients about potential clinical problems. In this case, technology was used strategically to reengineer service delivery, and not the other way around. This is as it should be. Whole new worlds can open as nursing's ability to deliver basic support, contact, and education to home-based patients is increased dramatically.

Modified with permission of Simpson, R. L. (1993). If you don't read this, you're missing out. Reproduced/adapted with permission from the September 1993 issue of *Nursing Management,* September 1993. Springhouse Corporation, Springhouse, PA.

Official concerns about violence were brought to the attention of the public as early as 1985 when the Surgeon General of the United States identified violence as a major public health issue (Cron, 1986). The resulting Surgeon General's Workshop on Violence and Public Health, held in 1985, brought together more than 100 health professionals to discuss violence-related issues. Since then, thousands of research studies have been done and millions of dollars have been spent in attempts to understand violent behavior, its causes and effects, and effective interventions. Little progress has been made. We have learned that the roots of violence extend deep into the historical, social, economic, and cultural soil of our society (Fairly, 1988).

Violence has been linked with poverty, family breakdown, racism, poor education, substance abuse, ready availability of weapons, the media, and a culture of tolerance for violence. Intervening in these problems has proved to be politically, economically, and strategically overwhelming.

There are three major types of violence: rape, domestic abuse, and other assaults. Victims of rape and domestic abuse are mostly young women and, increasingly, children and the elderly. Victims of other assaults are mainly young men. All three crimes are significantly correlated with poverty.

Assault by a spouse or intimate partner has for many years been the primary source of traumatic injuries to women in this country. The untold physical and emotional damage wrought by these three crimes has a profound effect on nursing practice. A new nursing role, the sexual assault nurse examiner (SANE), has been created to interview rape victims in a sensitive manner while collecting forensic evidence needed to prosecute perpetrators successfully. Dealing with battered women (and men) creates the need for nurses to be aware of the sometimes subtle signs of abuse that victims are often unwilling to report for fear of reprisal. Nurses must be able to determine if the injuries seen could have been caused by the "accident" reported. Firearm assaults are the leading cause of spinal cord injuries and ostomies in some cities (Pieper, 1992). Trauma units nationwide are filled with victims of gunshot wounds. Not only are more trauma nurses needed, but additional rehabilitation nursing care, including ostomy nursing care, is also necessary.

In addition to becoming clinically proficient in caring for the physical needs of victims of violence, the emotional and psychiatric needs of these people must be met. Victims of violence often experience posttraumatic stress disorder (PTSD). This entity was initially identified in Vietnam veterans but has since been diagnosed in victims of rape, incest, domestic violence, and other violence and even in witnesses to violence, including fire, police, and emergency personnel who respond to these crimes. Battered women's syndrome is another disorder created by violence in our culture, and there are others. School nurses must be alert to signs of abuse as well as potentially violent behavior in students themselves. Gerontological nurses, too, must be alert to signs of abuse. There is hardly a group of nurses today whose practices have not been affected by the increase in violent behavior in our society.

How has nursing responded? The Nursing Network on Violence and Abuse International (NNVAI) advocates for including spouse abuse content in nursing curricula and educating practicing nurses through continuing education. Individual nurses have qualified to be sexual assault nurse examiners, expert witnesses, trauma nurses, spinal cord rehabilitation specialists, and other violence-related specialty areas. But there is more that can be done.

First, nurses must become politically active in advocating for health policies that promote nursing research into violence, nursing interventions, and effective violence prevention strategies. Next, they can take leadership positions in ensuring that their communities have adequate shelters, rape crisis centers, prevention programs, and coalitions of people concerned with these issues. They may choose to advocate for gun control by writing, calling, faxing, e-mailing, and visiting their representatives and senators to support pending legislation. And they can contribute time and money to initiatives designed to reduce or prevent violence, whoever the victims may be.

Imbalance in Supply and Demand for Nurses

There is nothing new about periodic imbalances between the number of nurses working and available nursing positions. Society pays far more attention to nursing shortages than to oversupply, however, because the welfare of the general public is affected more by shortages.

The generic term *nursing shortage* is misleading because actual shortages are usually confined to institutional settings such as hospitals and nursing homes. Since World War II, hospitals have been plagued with periodic nursing shortages (Abdellah, 1990). Causes of shortages may be seen as either external or internal. Internal causes include salary issues, long hours, increased responsibility for unlicensed workers, and significant responsibility with little authority. External causes include changes in demand for nursing services, the increasing age of the American population, greater **patient acuity** (degree of illness) of hospitalized individuals, public perceptions of nursing as a profession, and widening career options for women.

In the past, each time a shortage of registered nurses became acute, two solutions were tried: increase the supply of nurses and create a new worker to supplement the number of nurses. Practical nursing programs, which produce graduates in only one year, were created to meet civilian and military needs of the United States during World War II. The nursing shortage of the 1950s stimulated a desire to shorten basic RN programs, and two-year associate degree programs were the result. In the 1960s, shortages led to the creation of the unit manager, whose job was to take over certain tasks to relieve nurses, who could then concentrate on providing patient care. The 1970s produced other new workers, such as emergency medical technicians (EMTs), physician's assistants, respiratory therapists, and others who took on various aspects of patient care formerly performed by nurses. The shortage of nurses in the late 1980s resulted in a proposal by the American Medical Association to create yet another "nurse extender" called the *registered care technician*. Tired of seeing "solutions" to nursing shortages that entailed substituting unlicensed personnel for nurses, nurses responded quickly and negatively, and that idea was dropped. This is an example of the collective power nurses have when they unite to act as a group.

A health care consulting firm, the Hay Group, conducted a study in 1998 that determined that 81 percent of 178 hospitals surveyed were either experiencing or predicting a nursing shortage. The nursing shortage of the late 1990s was different from previous ones and resulted from a combination of internal and external factors. One external factor was an increased demand for nurses because of the aging population. This is expected to continue, since both the general population and registered nurses themselves are getting older. The average age of registered nurses in 1996 was 44.3 years. As these nurses retire and withdraw from the profession for various reasons, a projected shortage of nurses to replace them is predicted (Peterson, 1999). This will occur at a time when the demand for nursing care is at an all-time high because of increasing numbers of elderly citizens, who generally use health care at a higher rate than young people.

Other external factors involve increased use of sophisticated technology and more educated consumers demanding better quality, affordable health care. Because nurses are identified as the ideal health care workers to provide care in a variety of settings, they are increasingly employed outside hospitals. Shortages are sometimes blamed on the phenomenon created by nurses leaving hospital work for nonhospital nursing positions. In reality, hospitals employ nearly the same proportion of the total pool of registered nurses, 60 percent, as they did decades ago, but the ratio of nurses to patients is higher. This is owing to three factors. First, more treatment is provided to hospitalized patients because they have illnesses and needs that demand greater attention. Less critical health problems are usually dealt with through outpatient services. Also, to control costs, patients are discharged to home care as soon as possible so there are fewer patients recuperating in the hospital. Second, technological advances, such as open heart surgery, organ transplants, and the like, have made special care units, staffed with specialized nurses, necessary. In these units, because patients are critically ill, one nurse cares for only one or two patients. And advances in technology prolong lives of chronically ill patients, which in turn creates more need for long-term nursing care (Peterson, 1999). Third, cost-containment measures have caused hospital consolidations, downsizing, and reengineering. There are more patients in fewer hospitals staffed with reduced numbers of personnel.

Although shortages are usually the focus of concern, a number of areas of the United States experienced an oversupply of nurses in the mid-1990s. This was due to many factors. A downswing in the national economy in the early 1990s resulted in an increase in applications to schools of nursing nationwide. Large numbers of graduates flooded the market a few years later, just as significant downsizing and reorganization occurred in traditional employment settings such as hospitals.

Although the U. S. Department of Labor forecasted in 1994 that 765,000 new registered nurse positions would be needed by 2005 (Fig. 3–5), a year

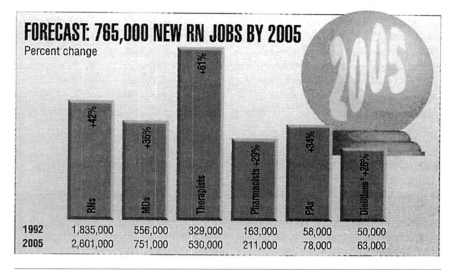

Figure 3–5

The health care industry will add 4.2 million jobs by the year 2005, growing at twice the rate of the total economy, says the U.S. Labor Department in its latest projection of employment prospects. The forecast is that registered nursing will see by far the largest numerical growth and will continue to dwarf the other health professions with the size of its work force—an estimated 2,601,000 in 2005. Industry trends will also boost employment for LPNs, aides, and techs; jobs for home health aides are expected to grow at the fastest rate—138 percent—to 827,000. *Includes nutritionists. (Source: Dietetics, Nursing, Pharmacy, and Therapy Occupations. Reprinted from *Occupational Outlook Handbook,* 1994–95 edition. U.S. Department of Labor, Bureau of Labor Statistics. Bulletin 2450-8 pp. 11–13. Washington, D. C.: Government Printing Office.)

later RN graduates in some parts of the United States were facing uncertain job prospects. This downturn occurred rapidly and unexpectedly, following as it did so quickly on the heels of a period of expansion in nursing education (AJN Newsline, 1995).

Recognizing that dramatic swings in the supply of and demand for registered nurses harm the profession, jeopardize patient care, and are costly, organizations inside and outside of nursing called for mechanisms to ensure more even distribution of the work force. In 1999, the ANA House of Delegates discussed the development of an integrated forecasting model that considers a variety of factors affecting supply and demand (Peterson, 1999). The Robert Wood Johnson Foundation (RWJF), a private foundation that funds innovative health care initiatives, has committed tens of millions of dollars to pursuing programs that help nursing schools, hospitals, and other health care agencies create regional work force development systems. Working with the American Association of Colleges of Nursing (AACN), the Robert Wood Johnson Foundation in 1996 began funding three-year projects addressing collaboration among all levels of nursing practice and education to ensure an adequate supply of registered nurses to meet the nation's health needs. This initiative was named "Colleagues in Caring."

To date there are no clear-cut solutions to the problem of periodic imbalances in the supply of and demand for nurses. It should be kept in mind that periods of oversupply may actually reflect poor distribution of nurses. Nurses who are willing to relocate away from major population centers have usually been able to find work easily. With dramatic demographic and health care system changes on the horizon, however, periodic shortages and oversupplies of nurses are likely to remain a recurring theme for the immediate future.

Summary of Key Points

- Women have traditionally been socialized to seek security and avoid risk and conflict.
- Because nursing is a female-dominated profession, the development of nursing has been affected by the traditional socialization of women in Western society.
- In the past, nurses themselves have unwittingly contributed to the stereotype by looking outside the profession for solutions rather than dealing with them responsibly within nursing.
- Social trends that have affected nursing include feminism, the women's movement, the consumer movement, the "graying of America," cultural diversity, men in nursing, violence, and technological advances in medicine.
- Powerful social influences, such as the media, project an image of nursing that is often distorted. This has led the public to develop misconceptions about nursing and nurses themselves.
- Individual nurses must take direct action when nursing is presented in an unfavorable light in any medium.
- The number of men in nursing is gradually increasing.
- Consumers, aided by information available on the Internet, are becoming more aware and demanding that they be treated as equal members of the health care team.
- Nurses are expected to become culturally competent in order to meet the needs of an increasingly diverse population.
- With the dizzying array of technology in use today, nurses must be always mindful of the human needs of patients.
- Imbalances in the supply of and demand for nurses arise periodically caused by changes in society and in health care itself. Recently there has been a concerted effort to ensure an adequate supply of registered nurses.

Critical Thinking Questions

1. Explain how being a female-dominated profession has affected the development of the nursing profession.
2. Analyze the social influences that affected your decision to enter the nursing profession. Did the media image of nursing and nurses play a positive or negative role? What other influences can you recall?

3. Describe your ideal nurse. What social stereotypes does your description reveal? Does your "ideal nurse" belong to a particular gender, race, or ethnic group?
4. What positive and negative impacts has the consumer movement had on health care in the United States?
5. List three social factors that have the potential to stimulate interest in nursing as a profession and explain their impact.
6. Describe three actions you personally can take to improve the public's image of nursing in your community.

Web Resources

American Assembly for Men in Nursing, http://www.freeyellow.com/members3/aamn

American Association of Retired People, http://www.aarp.org/indexes/health.html

American Hospital Association, http://www.aha.org

American Nurses Association fact sheets and position papers, http://nursingworld.org/readroom

Centers for Disease Control and Prevention, http://www.cdc.gov

Colleagues in Caring Project, http://www.aacn.nche.edu

Minorities, Facts, and Figures, http://www.census.gov/pubinfo/www.hotlinks.html

Mediawatch, http://www.mediawatch.com

U. S. Bureau of the Census, http://www.census.gov

References

Abdellah, F. G. (1990). Reflections on a recurring theme. *Nursing Clinics of North America,* 25(3), 509–515.

Aber, C. S., and Hawkins, J. W. (1992). Portrayal of nurses in advertisements in medical and nursing journals. *IMAGE: Journal of Nursing Scholarship,* 24(4), 289–293.

Ahmann, E. (1994). "Chunky stew": Appreciating cultural diversity while providing health care for children. *Pediatric Nursing,* 20(3), 320–322, 324.

AJN Newsline (1995). '95 RN graduates face uncertain job prospects. *American Journal of Nursing,* 95(4), 69, 72.

American Association of Colleges of Nursing. (1999). *Colleagues in caring project.* Available online at [http://www.aacn.nche.org].

Andrews, M. M. (1992). Cultural perspectives on nursing in the 21st century. *Journal of Professional Nursing,* 8(1), 7–15.

Black, V. L., and Germaine-Warner, C. (1995). Image of nursing. In G. L. Deloughery (Ed.), *Issues and trends in nursing* (pp. 455–473). St. Louis: Mosby.

Boughn, S. (1994). Why do men choose nursing? *Nursing & Health Care,* 15(8), 406–411.

Buerhaus, P. I., and Auerbach, D. (1999). Slow growth in the United States of the number of minorities in the RN workforce. *IMAGE: Journal of Nursing Scholarship,* 31(2), 179–183.

Bunting, S., and Campbell, J. C. (1990). Feminism and nursing: Historical perspectives.

In P. L. Chinn (Ed.), *Developing the discipline: Critical studies in nursing history and professional issues* (pp. 181–195). Gaithersburg, Md.: Aspen Publishers.

Buresh, B., and Gordon, S. (1995). Taking on the TV shows. *American Journal of Nursing,* 95(11), 18–20.

Campbell-Heider, N., Hart, C. A., and Bergren, M. D. (1994). Conveying professionalism: Working against the old stereotypes. In B. Bullough and V. Bullough (Eds.), *Nursing issues for the nineties and beyond* (pp. 212–231). New York: Springer.

Cron, T. (1986). The Surgeon General's workshop on violence and public health: Review of recommendations. *Public Health Reports,* 101, 8–14.

Cummings, S. H. (1995). Attila the hun versus Attila the hen: Gender socialization of the American nurse. *Nursing Administration Quarterly,* 19(2), 19–29.

Cyr, J. (1992). Males in nursing. *Nursing Management,* 23(7), 54–55.

Evans, J. (1997). Men in nursing: Issues of gender segregation and hidden advantage. *Journal of Advanced Nursing,* 26, 226–231.

Fagin, C. M., and Binder, L. F. (1994). Nursing and consumerism: How can we get decision making closer to the consumer? In J. C. McCloskey and H. K. Grace (Eds.), *Current issues in nursing* (pp. 450–459). St. Louis: Mosby.

Fairly, A. (1988). Family violence: A contemporary social phenomenon. *Proceedings: Family Violence; Public Health Social Work's Role in Prevention.* Washington, D. C.: Department of Health Services Administration.

Farley, S. (1994). Developing community partnerships: Shifting power from health professionals to citizens. In J. C. McCloskey and H. K. Grace (Eds.). *Current issues in nursing* (pp. 226–232). St. Louis: Mosby.

Gary, F., Sigsby, L. M., and Campbell, D. (1998). Feminism: A perspective for the 21st century. *Issues in Mental Health Nursing,* 19, 139–152.

Gray, D. P. (1994). Feminism and nursing. In O. L. Strickland and D. J. Fishman (Eds.), *Nursing issues in the 1990's* (pp. 505–527). Albany, NY: Delmar.

Halloran, E. J., and Welton, J. M. (1994). Why aren't there more men in nursing? In J. C. McCloskey and H. K. Grace (Eds.), *Current issues in nursing* (pp. 684–691). St. Louis: Mosby.

Happ, B. (1994). Point of care technology: Does it improve the quality of patient care? In O. L. Strickland and D. J. Fishman (Eds.), *Nursing issues in the 1990's* (pp. 254–266). Albany, NY: Delmar.

Huffstutler, S. Y., Stevenson, S. S., Mullins, I. L., Hackett, D. A., and Lambert, A. W. (1998). The public's image of nursing as described to baccalaureate prenursing students. *Journal of Professional Nursing,* 14(1), 7–13.

Johnson, M. H. (1994). Nursing care in a culturally diverse nation. In B. Bullough and V. Bullough (Eds.), *Nursing issues for the nineties and beyond* (pp. 187–198). New York: Springer.

Kalisch, P. A., and Kalisch, B. J. (1986). A comparative analysis of nurse and physician characters in the entertainment media. *Journal of Advanced Nursing,* 11(2), 179–195.

Kalisch, P. A., and Kalisch, B. J. (1987). *The changing image of the nurse.* Reading, Mass.: Addison-Wesley.

Kelly, N. R., Shoemaker, M., and Steele, T. (1996). The experience of being a male student nurse. *Journal of Nursing Education,* 35(4), 170–174.

Ketter, J. (1994). Sex discrimination targets men in some hospitals. *The American Nurse,* 94(1), 24.

Leininger, M. (1991). Transcultural nursing: The study and practice field. *Imprint,* 38(2), 55–66.

Locsin, R. C. (1995). Technology and caring in nursing. In A. Boykin (Ed.), *Power, politics, and public policy: A matter of caring* (pp. 24–36). New York: NLN Press.

Mangum, S. (1994). Uniforms and caps: Do we need them? In O. L. Strickland and D. J. Fishman (Eds.), *Nursing issues in the 1990's* (pp. 46–66). Albany, NY: Delmar.

McConnell, E. A., and Murphy, E. K. (1990). Nurses' use of technology: An international concern. *International Nursing Review,* 37(5), 331–334.

Mikulencak, M. (1995). Fact or fiction? Nursing and realism on TV's newest medical dramas. *The American Nurse,* 95(3), 31.

Moss, M. T. (1995). Developing glass-breaking skills. *Nursing Administration Quarterly,* 19(2), 41–47.

Muff, J. (1988a). *Women's issues in nursing: Socialization, sexism, and stereotyping.* Prospect Height, Ill.: Waveland Press.

Muff, J. (1988b). Of images and ideals: A look at socialization and sexism in nursing. In A. H. Jones (Ed.), *Images of nurses: Perspectives from history, art, and literature* (pp. 197–220). Philadelphia: University of Pennsylvania Press.

National League for Nursing. (1994). *Nursing data review* 1994. New York: National League for Nursing.

Neilsen Media Research. (1996). Top 10 prime-time programs. *The Wall Street Journal,* CCXXVII(3), Thursday, January 4, p. A8.

Nurses of America (1991). *Who counts and who doesn't in news coverage of health care.* A project of the Tri-Council of Nursing Organizations: Nurses of America.

Nurses of America (1991). *Summary Report and Recommendations*: Nurses of America.

Perkins, J. L., Bennett, D. N., and Dorman, R. E. (1993). Why men choose nursing. *Nursing & Health Care,* 14(1), 34–38.

Peterson, C. A. (1999). Nursing supply and demand. *American Journal of Nursing,* 99(7), 57–59.

Pieper, B. (1992). Persons who have a stoma: Victims of violence versus disease. *Journal of Enterostomal Therapy Nursing,* 19(1), 7–11.

Shea, C. A. (1994). Feminism: The new look in nursing. In J. C. McCloskey and H. K. Grace (Eds.), *Current issues in nursing* (pp. 572–579). St. Louis: Mosby.

Sigma Theta Tau International. (1998). *The Woodhull study on nursing and the media: Health care's invisible partner.* Indianapolis, Ind.: STTI's Center Nursing Press.

Simpson, R. L. (1992). What nursing leaders are saying about technology. *Nursing Management,* 23(7), 28–30.

Simpson, R. L. (1993). If you don't read this, you're missing out. *Nursing Management,* 24(9), 18.

Southern Regional Education Board, Council on Collegiate Education for Nursing. (1999). *Preparing graduates to meet the needs of diverse populations.* Atlanta: Southern Regional Education Board.

Sowell, R. (1999). Personal communication.

Thompson, C. B., Amos, L. K., and Graves, J. R. (1994). Knowledge technology: Costs, benefits, and ethical considerations. In J. C. McCloskey and H. K. Grace (Eds.), *Current issues in nursing* (pp. 746–751). St. Louis: Mosby.

U.S. Bureau of the Census. (1992). *Statistical abstract of the United States: 1992* (112th ed.). Washington, D. C.: Government Printing Office.

U.S. Bureau of the Census. (1994). *Statistical abstract of the United States: 1994* (114th ed.). Washington, D. C.: Government Printing Office.

U.S. Department of Health and Human Services, Division of Nursing. (1996). *Notes from the National Sample Survey of RNs, March 1996.* Washington, D.C.: Government Printing Office.

Villeneuve, M. J. (1994). Recruiting and retaining men in nursing: A review of the literature. *Journal of Professional Nursing, 10*(4), 217–228.

Williams, C. L. (1989). *Gender differences at work: Women and men in nontraditional occupations.* Berkeley: University of California Press.

Williams, C. L. (1995). Hidden advantages for men in nursing. *Nursing Administration Quarterly, 19*(2), 63–70.

Williams, M. B., and Cullen, K. V. (1994). Nurse shortages needn't be inevitable. *Modern Healthcare, 24*(33), 36.

Professional Associations

*Diane J. Mancino**

Key Terms

Association
Certification
Code for Nurses
Collective Action
Collective Bargaining
Contracts
Delegate
Economic and General Welfare
Grassroots Activism
Lobby
Members
Partnership
Professional Association
Professional Practice Advocacy

Resolution
Unlicensed Assistive Personnel

Whistle-blower
Workplace Advocacy

Learning Outcomes

After studying this chapter, students will be able to:

- Explain why professions have associations.
- Demonstrate an understanding of the complex role that associations play in the profession and in society.
- Analyze organized nursing's management of select issues, according to the values they depict, and the political stances or strategies used.
- Recognize the opportunities that associations offer to increase the leadership capacity of nursing students and registered nurses.

Associations are organizations of **members** with common interests. Merton defined a **professional association** as "an organization of practitioners who judge one another as professionally competent and have banded together to perform social functions which they cannot perform in their separate capacity as individuals" (1958, p. 50). Associations exist in all professions and in all parts of the world. Although state governments have legal control of nursing licensure, associations provide professional standards of practice and ethical conduct for their members to ensure the public of the availability of high quality services. Associations also serve their individual members through a variety of services and leadership development opportunities.

Work of Nursing Associations

Major nursing associations in Great Britain, Canada, and the United States all formed at about the same time in the late 1890s. Chapter 1 described the instrumental role played by Isabel Hampton Robb in establishing the forerun-

* The author wishes to acknowledge the contribution of the American Nurses Association in the preparation of this chapter.

ners of the American Nurses Association (ANA) and the National League for Nursing (NLN). Also mentioned was Lillian Wald's early leadership role in establishing the National Organization of Public Health Nurses.

Nursing association founders had two major concerns: (1) the need for laws to ensure the public of a standard of quality nursing care and protection from poorly prepared nurses and (2) lack of standardization in nursing education. The newly formed associations won those battles first by successfully lobbying for the establishment of state licensure laws and later by promoting accreditation of schools of nursing.

As society evolves, the nursing profession must change so that it continues to meet its responsibilities to the public. Professional associations provide a vehicle for nurses to meet present and future challenges and work toward positive, profession-wide changes that keep pace with society's complex health needs.

Whom Do Professional Associations Serve?

Nursing associations have three major constituents: the public, the nursing profession, and individual nurses. They serve each constituent group in different ways.

They serve the public by establishing codes of ethics and standards of practice, socializing new members to these codes and standards, and enforcing codes and standards in practice. These measures, when combined with state licensure laws, assure the public that nurses are competent professionals with safe standards of practice and appropriate ethical principles.

Associations serve the profession by being the organization through which the interests of its members are pressed collectively and focused politically (Aydelotte, 1990). **Collective action** is a frequently misunderstood term. It simply means that activities are undertaken on behalf of a group of people who have common interests. Professional associations help nurses use collective action to push for political responses to benefit recipients of health care and members of the profession.

Associations serve individual members by providing continuing education, recognizing skills in practice by offering credentials, and ensuring mechanisms for a professional workplace.

Associations address all these interests by advocating for adequate numbers of well-prepared registered nurses to serve the public, by forming **partnerships** with the public and other professions, and by ensuring that the profession's work is properly understood and supported by the public, government officials, and other health care professionals. Associations also provide an unparalleled influential national network of professionals at all levels and in all specialties who support each other. Belonging to a professional association helps to broaden and enhance professional knowledge and build leadership skills. Members are given the opportunity to work with, learn from, and become leaders.

Examples of Professional Association Activities

One of the most important activities of professional associations is communication. Most nursing associations have newsletters, journals, and websites, and some have all of these. Publications carry news stories, editorials, and articles of interest to members; information about pending legislation and political issues affecting nursing and health care; and notices of continuing education offerings.

The official newspaper of the ANA is *The American Nurse*, published six times each year. The *American Journal of Nursing* is the official journal of the ANA. Other associations' publications include *Nursing and Health Care Perspectives*, published bimonthly by the NLN; *Imprint*, published quarterly by the National Student Nurses Association (NSNA); and *Image, Journal of Nursing Scholarship*, published quarterly by Sigma Theta Tau International. There are many others. Some journal subscriptions, such as NSNA's *Imprint* magazine, are included in the association's dues, and others must be subscribed to separately. Students can subscribe to *The American Nurse* for a nominal fee.

In addition to communicating with members, there are many other activities of professional associations. The following examples offer greater insight into how collective action by association members addresses the needs of members and influences policy development.

Example A

Nursing students who are members of a school chapter of the NSNA were concerned about adequate educational preparation to practice in complex health care delivery systems when they graduate from nursing school. A group of students became aware that in the practice setting registered nurses are expected to know the basics of intravenous administration, including, for example, starting infusions, knowing the proper vein placement, assessing patients during therapy, and knowing the advantages and disadvantages of different delivery methods. After researching the problem, they discovered that not all programs preparing students for registered nurse licensure included this competency in their undergraduate curricula. They decided to take collective action by writing a resolution to encourage all schools of nursing to incorporate or increase levels of instruction on the concepts of intravenous insertion and therapy in their curricula. As members of the National Student Nurses Association, they first brought the **resolution** to their state association convention, where it was presented to the voting members. The resolution passed and was then brought to the National Student Nurses Association House of Delegates to be presented to over 500 voting **delegates** (Fig. 4–1). During the debate, delegates expressed concerns about insufficient safety devices, fear of becoming infected with blood-borne pathogens, and lack of worker's compensation coverage if infection did occur. Following a lively debate, the resolution was adopted by the House of Delegates and is now part of the NSNA's policies. As a result of this policy, the NSNA will work with other organizations, such as the National League for Nursing, to encourage nursing schools to prepare

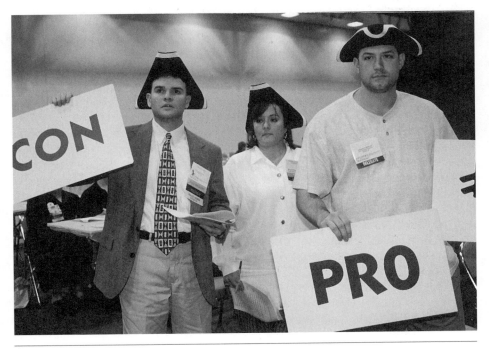

Figure 4–1
Students serving as delegates to the National Student Nurses Association House of Delegates learn leadership and political skills while having fun and meeting others from around the United States, Puerto Rico, and Guam. In this photo, students voice their views about resolutions being considered by the delegates (Courtesy of National Student Nurses Association).

students with basic intravenous insertion and maintenance skills. In addition, the NSNA will use its communication tools and educational programs to raise awareness about this issue.

By participating in collaborative decision making, students can take important actions on issues critical to them as students and to their future as professional nurses. A powerful synergy results when students from different nursing programs and cultural backgrounds and perspectives get together and share ideas, analyze issues, make informed decisions, and take collective action.

Example B
Nurses working in a hospital are concerned about inadequate staffing and fear for the well-being of patients. Caring for older, more acutely ill patients with shortened hospital stays is complicated by fewer staff registered nurses, many of whom are working mandatory overtime, and utilization of **unlicensed assistive personnel** whose skill level is inadequate to meet patient care needs. When registered nurses try to work within the hospital chain of command to solve staffing problems and to address concerns about quality of care, they

find their issues go unresolved. In some cases, those registered nurses raising concerns suddenly become targeted as troublemakers. Many nurses want to report unsafe staffing to the appropriate state agency, or the Joint Commission on Accreditation of Healthcare Organizations (JCAHO), but fear reprisal if their employer were to find out.

Nurses need abundant support, strategies, and resources to tackle issues that obstruct their ability to meet a primary professional imperative: ensuring that patients receive safe and appropriate care. For some, **contracts** are in place that include provisions giving staff nurses control over staffing and that additionally may prohibit or limit mandatory overtime. The majority of nurses, however, do not have contracts. All nurses need to know their rights and responsibilities and to understand the potential consequences of actions and recourse available. In addition, they need an organization that can provide this type of information and support.

Working through a state nurses association (SNA), together with other nurses, registered nurses can shape legislative and regulatory strategies and can create public education and communication campaigns to ensure that quality of care is monitored and reported in a standardized manner and that nurses advocating for patient well-being are protected in the process. Additional resources come from the ANA to support and augment the work of state nurses associations and to share strategies and accomplishments with the membership. The ANA and the SNAs also are working on protections for nurses who speak out against unsafe patient care practices. Several states have secured **whistleblower** protections through legislation, and many more are seeking similar protections. At the federal level, the ANA has advocated for inclusion of whistleblower protections in the Patient Safety Act, which the ANA helped draft, and the Patients' Bill of Rights, both under consideration by the 106th Congress.

Example C

While caring for others, registered nurses face the risk of needlesticks every day, exposing themselves to potentially lethal blood-borne pathogens such as human immunodeficiency virus (HIV) and hepatitis C. Registered nurses and other health care workers sustain between 600,000 and 1 million needlestick and sharps injuries every year, resulting in at least 1,000 new cases of HIV infection, hepatitis C, or hepatitis B. The technology exists to protect health care workers from needlesticks, yet less than 15 percent of U.S. hospitals use safe needle devices, such as retractable needles. The ANA is fighting this situation through its Safe Needles Save Lives Campaign, by educating the public about this issue, and by empowering nurses to take individual and collective action.

The Safe Needles Save Lives Campaign encompasses all of the ANA's work on this issue. The ANA worked with members of Congress to craft the Health Care Workers Needlestick Prevention Act of 1999, which was introduced in the U.S. Senate and House of Representatives in May 1999. Also, ANA is working with its state nurses associations to introduce needlestick prevention legislation at the state level. Some states have already passed legislation mandating the use of safe needle devices, while similar legislation is moving forward in other states. Due to the ANA's efforts, the Occupational Safety and Health Administration (OSHA) is considering measures to mandate use of safe needle devices.

Example D

Technologies, such as ventilators, keep comatose people alive even though their quality of life is no longer what they would have desired. Lifetime savings of families may be wiped out by maintaining a family member in a persistent vegetative state.

Nurses frequently face situations in which patients or their families no longer want to continue this kind of existence, yet in the health care system there are not adequate legal and decision mechanisms to deal with end of life issues. In response to the need for guidance on ethical issues, a special task force of the ANA (1985) created a document entitled the **Code for Nurses** to help nurses clarify their responsibilities. Appendix A contains an abbreviated form of the *Code*.

Although the *Code for Nurses* provides broad direction, the ANA also provides specific guidance on particular ethical issues and has published a number of position statements, including one on assisted suicide (Box 4–1) (American Nurses Association, 1994).

These examples of the range of activities and issues addressed by professional associations demonstrate how associations work on behalf of the profession and ultimately benefit the public by helping nurses to provide high quality nursing care.

Joining and Using Professional Associations in Nursing

Nurses have a responsibility to belong to one or more nursing associations, both as an extension of their interest in nursing and to support their fellow nurses. A strong professional organization is a characteristic of mature pro-

---

BOX 4–1

Summary of the American Nurses Association's Position Statement on Assisted Suicide

Nurses, individually and collectively, have an obligation to provide comprehensive and compassionate end-of-life care, which includes the promotion of comfort and the relief of pain, and at times, foregoing life-sustaining treatments. The American Nurses Association (ANA) believes that the nurse should not participate in assisted suicide. Such an act is in violation of the *Code for Nurses with Interpretive Statements* (*Code for Nurses*) and the ethical traditions of the profession.

Reprinted with permission of the American Nurses Association (1994). Position statement on assisted suicide. Washington, D. C.: American Nurses Association.

fessions (see Chapter 6). Following is a discussion of how nurses can make effective decisions about which nursing associations to join and how they can learn to use these groups to meet their needs for professional growth and to stimulate activities on behalf of members of the group (otherwise known as collective action).

Types of Associations

A list (not comprehensive) of nursing associations in the United States appears in Box 4–2. This list dramatically demonstrates the number and variety of associations that nurses can join. Understandably, individual nurses often express confusion about which associations to join. In general, associations can be classified as one of three main types:

1. Broad purpose professional associations.
2. Specialty practice associations.
3. Special interest associations.

The ANA is the broad-purpose association in nursing. Individual nurses belong to state nurses associations, and SNAs constitute the ANA, which is a federation made up of 53 state and territorial nurses associations. Its purposes are threefold:

1. To work for the improvement of health standards and the availability of health care services for all people.
2. To foster high standards for nursing.
3. To stimulate and promote the professional development of nurses and advance their economic and general welfare.

As the nursing profession grew and diversified, many nurses limited their practices to specialty areas, such as maternal/infant, school, or community health, critical care, or perioperative or emergency/trauma nursing. Members of specialty nursing associations frequently choose also to belong to an SNA because specialty associations focus only on standards of practice or professional needs of the specific specialty or group.

Examples of special purpose organizations include Sigma Theta Tau International, Honor Society of Nursing, which one must be invited to join, and the American Association for the History of Nursing, which focuses on a particular area of study in nursing. A comprehensive updated list of nursing organizations is available on the World Wide Web (www.nsna.org/resources/weblinks/associate.html and www.nursingworld.org/affil/index.htm) (see also Web Resources at the end of the chapter).

Nurses are also connected internationally through the International Council of Nurses (ICN). The ICN is a federation of national nurses associations (NNAs), representing nurses in 118 countries (The ANA represents U.S. registered nurses in the ICN, and the NSNA represents U.S. nursing students in the ICN.). Founded in 1899, the ICN is the world's first and widest reaching

BOX 4–2
A Selection of Nursing Organizations in the United States*

- American Nurses Association
- American Academy of Ambulatory Nursing Administration
- American Academy of Nurse Practitioners
- American Assembly for Men in Nursing
- American Association for Continuity of Care
- American Association for the History of Nursing
- American Association of Colleges of Nursing
- American Association of Critical-Care Nurses
- American Association of Diabetes Educators
- American Association of Neuroscience Nurses
- American Association of Nurse Anesthetists
- American Association of Nurse Attorneys
- American Association of Occupational Health Nurses
- American Association of Office Nurses
- American Association of Spinal Cord Injury Nurses
- American College of Nurse-Midwives
- American Holistic Nurses' Association
- American Nephrology Nurses' Association
- American Organization of Nurse Executives
- American Psychiatric Nurses' Association
- American Radiological Nurses Association
- American Society of Plastic and Reconstructive Surgical Nurses
- American Society of PeriAnesthesia Nurses
- Association of Black Nursing Faculty in Higher Education
- Association of Community Health Nursing Educators
- Association of Nurses in AIDS Care
- Association of periOperative Registered Nurses
- Association of Pediatric Oncology Nurses
- Association of Rehabilitation Nurses
- Association of Women's Health, Obstetric and Neonatal Nurses
- Chi Eta Phi
- Dermatology Nurses Association
- Drug and Alcohol Nursing Association
- Emergency Nurses Association
- Hospice Nurses Association
- Intravenous Nurses Society
- National Alliance of Nurse Practitioners
- National Association of Hispanic Nurses
- National Association of Neonatal Nurses
- National Association of Orthopaedic Nurses
- National Association of Pediatric Nurse Practitioners and Associates
- National Association of School Nurses
- National Black Nurses Association
- National Flight Nurses Association
- National Gerontological Nurses Association
- National League for Nursing
- National Nurses Society on Addictions
- National Organization for the Advancement of Associate Degree Nursing
- National Student Nurses Association
- Nurses Organization of the Veterans Administration
- Oncology Nursing Society
- Sigma Theta Tau International
- Society for Peripheral Vascular Nursing
- Transcultural Nursing Society

* World Wide Web access to many of these associations is available online at http://www.nsna.org/resources/weblinks/associate.html and www.nursingworld.org/affil/index.htm

international organization for health professionals. Operated by nurses for nurses, the ICN works to ensure quality nursing care for all, sound health policies globally, the advancement of nursing knowledge, the presence worldwide of a respected nursing profession, and a competent and satisfied nursing workforce. For additional details about the ICN's activities in professional nursing practice, nursing regulation, and the socioeconomic welfare of nurses, visit the ICN home page at http://www.icn.ch.

Benefits of Belonging to Professional Associations

A variety of benefits result from membership in professional associations. Most nurses were drawn to their profession because it exemplifies caring for others, it makes a difference in others' lives, and it demands full use of their intellectual, interpersonal, and emotional talents. Once in nursing, however, both students and practicing nurses have many needs.

Developing Leadership Skills

Students have opportunities to learn from and socialize with their peers in school and at the state and national levels of the National Student Nurses Association. As NSNA members, they benefit from developing leadership and organizational skills to help them in many phases of their professional and personal lives. They need to learn how associations function and how to participate as active, effective members. The NSNA, which has local and state chapters in addition to the national organization, provides all of these opportunities and more. The mission of the NSNA (1995) is to:

- Organize, represent, and mentor students preparing for initial licensure as registered nurses (in associate degree, diploma, baccalaureate, and generic master's and doctoral programs) as well as those nurses enrolled in baccalaureate completion programs.
- Promote development of the skills that students will need as responsible and accountable members of the nursing profession.
- Advocate for high-quality health care.

Through a new program, the NSNA Leadership U, the NSNA recognizes students for their leadership and management competencies with a certificate presented at the annual NSNA convention. For complete details about all of the NSNA's programs, visit their web site at www.nsna.org.

Earning Recognition through Certification

Practicing nurses want to be recognized, through both compensation and position, for their level of professional expertise. They may do this through **certification** in a specialty area, which is granted by professional associations. Certification is a formal but voluntary process of demonstrating expertise in a particular area of nursing. Certified nurses often receive salary supplements and special opportunities. For information about credentials in nursing, visit the ANA's web site at www.nursingworld.org and web sites of specialty nursing organizations www.nsna.org/resources/weblinks/associate.html.

Legislative Lobbying Power

As their careers develop, nurses may obtain master's-level preparation or become nurse practitioners and practice independently outside an institution. These nurses desire and deserve direct reimbursement for their work. They need state laws that mandate direct reimbursement of nurses. Others work in nursing homes and may be concerned that there are not enough registered nurses available to provide the quality of care the residents need. They need laws that regulate nurse-to-patient ratios and control educational requirements for unlicensed assistive personnel.

Some nurses work in settings in which they have little voice in the quality of care, are inadequately compensated for their level of education and responsibility, and are required to "float" to cover specialized units for which they have not been trained. These nurses may wish to be represented for purposes of **collective bargaining** so they can negotiate for improved salary and work conditions.

In each of these instances, nursing's general purpose association, the ANA, is involved in vital work supporting nurses as they fulfill their roles as professionals. State nurses associations **lobby** state representatives to support laws affecting nursing, such as those mandating insurance companies to reimburse nurse practitioners for the services they provide. State associations also influence debate on laws determining how many registered nurses are required to staff nursing homes and educational requirements for unlicensed assistive personnel, for whom nurses are legally responsible. If invited to do so, many state nurses associations assist nurses in dealing with workplace issues, such as salaries, working conditions, and staffing ratios.

Other Benefits

These examples—developing leadership skills, achieving recognition through certification, and banding together for legislative lobbying—represent major benefits of association membership. There are many others, such as publications, eligibility for group health and life insurance, networking with peers, continuing education, and discounts on products and services.

Deciding on Which Associations to Join

Once you have decided to belong to an association, visit the group's web site to find out more. Then ask yourself the following questions:

1. What are the purposes of this association?
2. Are the association's purposes compatible with my own?
3. How many members are there nationally, statewide, and locally?
4. What activities does the association undertake?
5. How active is the local chapter?
6. What opportunities does the association offer for involvement and leadership development?
7. What are the benefits of membership?
8. Does this organization lobby for improved health care legislation? How successful is it?

9. Is membership in this association cost-effective?
10. Even if I am not active, what benefit will I derive from the legislative agenda and other activities that the association undertakes to advocate for nurses and patients?

Answering these questions and speaking with current association members should provide nurses with adequate information to make reasoned decisions.

Becoming a Productive Association Member

Members get involved with a nursing association by attending meetings, volunteering for leadership and committee opportunities, and participating in the association's activities. Members directly influence the association's priorities and, in the absence of association staff, provide the volunteer labor that makes the association function. By becoming active participants in professional associations, nurses become part of something larger than their personal work situation, an organization central to their professional role, and a way through which they can make a difference throughout their professional lives. By adding their voices to those of other nurses, nursing concerns are heard, with a difference in the lives of patients and nurses resulting.

Perspectives of Nursing Leaders About Professional Associations

To present readers with a personal view of what organizations do and mean to nurses, the presidents of four major nursing organizations were asked to describe the benefits members receive and what they personally have attained through involvement with their own organizations.

National Student Nurses Association, Kristen Liane Hiscox, President*

The mission of the NSNA is to promote the development of skills that students will need as responsible and accountable members of the nursing profession. This is accomplished through interaction between students and faculty, as well as through networking with the many outstanding leaders of the nursing profession. As a nursing student, I readily recognize the value of participating in professional organizations. In today's rapidly changing health care environment, nursing organizations must continue to safeguard the delivery of high quality nursing and health care. Nursing students depend on nursing educators and leaders to strengthen the foundation of nursing so that we may inherit a structure that enables us to serve the needs of society and

---

* At the time of this communication, Hiscox was a senior nursing student in a baccalaureate program at the Medical College of Georgia School of Nursing in Athens, Georgia.

to advance the profession of nursing. There are many opportunities for nursing organizations to work together to empower and enlighten the next generation of nurse leaders. Just as our nursing ancestors link the past to the present, nursing students link the profession of nursing from the present to the future.

The NSNA seeks to promote professional growth through leadership development opportunities and career development workshops as well as through participation in community health projects, legislative activities, recruitment into the nursing profession programs (Breakthrough to Nursing), and fund-raising activities. The NSNA has produced a Bill of Rights and Responsibilities for Students of Nursing and a Code of Academic and Clinical Professional Conduct. These important documents provide a guideline for ethical conduct and grievance procedures for nursing students. Students gain many valuable skills when they serve in school, state, and national NSNA leadership positions. For example, they learn about developing and directing public policy by writing and debating resolutions. During the process of presenting and defending resolutions in the House of Delegates, they learn about Robert's Rules of Order and Parliamentary Procedure.

Furthermore, the NSNA offers members many tangible benefits such as discounts on products and services used by students. All NSNA members receive *Imprint,* the only magazine published by nursing students for nursing students. Members have many opportunities to enhance their education and plan their careers at the midyear career planning conferences and annual conventions.

The NSNA is the voice of nursing students. As the NSNA president, I serve as the spokesperson for nursing students at professional nursing organizations such as the ANA, the NLN, the National Federation for Specialty Nursing Organizations, the National Organization Liaison Forum, and the International Council of Nurses. I invite all nursing students to become members of the NSNA and to have their voices heard throughout the country and around the world. With unlimited opportunities, "the sky's the limit" when you belong to the NSNA. Visit our web site at http://www.nsna.org for more information (Hiscox, 1999).

American Nurses Association, Dr. Beverly L. Malone, President

For more than 100 years, the American Nurses Association has represented the nation's registered nurses as the only professional organization that addresses ethics, clinical standards, public policy, and the **economic and general welfare** of nurses. Through the ANA's constituent state nurses associations, nurses unite their voices for a common cause: to protect patients, support individual nurses, and advance the nursing profession. The ANA has made unprecedented strides at securing a seat for nursing in the national health care policy arena (Fig. 4–2). On the international level, the ANA represents U.S. nurses in the International Council of Nurses.

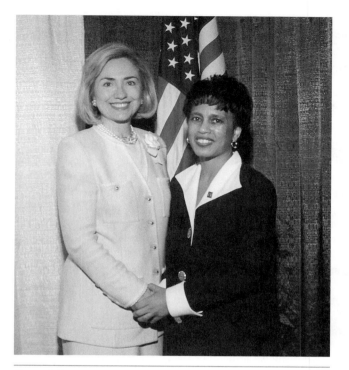

Figure 4–2
Hillary Rodham Clinton and Dr. Beverly L. Malone, President, American
Nurses Association (Courtesy of American Nurses Association).

On the eve of the new millennium, the ANA built on its strong foundation
by reshaping itself into a house for all nurses. At the 1999 House of Delegates,
the delegates voted to modify ANA's organizational structure. The new structure includes a national labor entity for nurses who use collective bargaining
as a tool, a **workplace advocacy** component for nurses who use other strategies to advocate in the workplace, one congress to strengthen its policy making, and a federal nurses association to be inclusive of active duty military
nurses and uniformed Public Health Service nurses.

As rich old traditions are blended with the exciting potential of the new,
nurses have much to gain from SNA/ANA membership. *The American Nurse,*
the *American Journal of Nursing,* and the ANA's Nursing World website
(www.nursingworld.org) give members unparalleled access to crucial information. Through local and state meetings, publications, and vigorous advocacy efforts, the state nurses associations enhance collegiality and enable
members to influence state legislation and policy and address workplace concerns.

The ANA, as the voice and advocate for the profession, needs the membership, support, and commitment of each nurse. Membership in your SNA

and the ANA is a demonstration of professionalism for it is the means to ultimately create a strong, vibrant, and valued profession influencing positive patient outcomes and a health care system sensitive to all who are in need (Malone, 1999).

National League for Nursing, Dr. Nancy Langston, President

The National League for Nursing was established in 1893 at the Chicago World's Fair as the Association of School Superintendents of the United States and Canada. As such it is the oldest organization for nursing in this country. The mission of the NLN is: "The National League for Nursing advances quality nursing education that prepares the nursing work force to meet the needs of diverse populations in an ever-changing health care environment."

The National League for Nursing is the national organization concerned with quality nursing for all types of nursing education programs, from licensed practical nurse through master's degree programs; until 1998 it was the only organization that accredited schools of nursing as one of the mechanisms for ensuring quality. In 1997 the NLN created a separate and independent unit named the National League for Nursing Accrediting Commission to fulfill the function of accreditation.

In addition to the very visible activity of accreditation, the NLN is concerned with activities and programs related more broadly to quality education; for example, the NLN is a leader in curriculum development, serves as a resource for cutting-edge knowledge of teaching/learning strategies, particularly relevant for nursing education, and provides a testing service that schools of nursing use to assist them in assessing student knowledge comprehensively and in various subject areas.

The membership of the National League for Nursing is both unique and visionary. The membership consist of individuals and organizations, such as schools of nursing and other organizations with an interest in nursing education. Individual members include nurses from nursing education and practice settings. Furthermore, there are nonnurse members. This category of membership positions NLN as unique among professional associations, in that the NLN is the only professional association that has individuals other than members of the profession within its organization. The public members make clear and visible the perspective that definitions of quality for a profession must include the ideas of people beyond the profession. This inclusivity of membership is the reason that the name of the organization is the National League FOR Nursing rather than the National League OF Nursing.

My advice to students is to be active in the NSNA and the day you graduate become a member of the ANA and a specialty organization. Then, within a few years, as you begin to see and understand more fully the benefits and responsibilities of a professional to support our collective vision and voice and begin to reflect on your education and think about what it should be to prepare nurses for the future, add the NLN to your membership commitments. These three memberships will keep you connected to the state of science in your practice and to the profession, including its future. For more information about the NLN visit our web site at http://www.nln.org (Langston, 1999).

Sigma Theta Tau International, Dr. Eleanor Sullivan, President

Sigma Theta Tau International, Honor Society of Nursing, provides leadership and scholarship in practice, education, and research to enhance the health of all people. We support the learning and professional development of our members, who strive to improve nursing care worldwide.

The vision of Sigma Theta Tau International is to create a global community of nurses who lead by using scholarship, technology, and knowledge to improve the health of the world's people.

The honor society is organized into chapters within accredited schools of nursing that grant baccalaureate and higher degrees. Currently, 383 chapters in over 400 college and university campuses provide professional activities and opportunities for approximately 115,000 members residing in 70 different countries and territories. As members of Sigma Theta Tau International, inductees connect with a global community of leaders and scholars who use their knowledge to influence practice. Participation in the society provides members with opportunities and resources for individualized career development, mentoring, education, publishing, leadership skill development, research, and knowledge building and use.

The society nurtures the leadership and scholarship skills of members through four primary initiatives: 1) research, 2) leadership, 3) electronic knowledge generation and sharing (through the Virginia Henderson International Nursing Library), and 4) programming, publication, and public relations. Research opportunities include funding, paper and poster presentations at international assemblies, and sponsorship for attendance at local, regional, and international research conferences. Leadership opportunities include individually designed mentoring, skills workshops in clinical leadership, health care policy and management, publishing, grant writing, entrepreneurism, and organizational leadership. The Virginia Henderson International Nursing Library provides members with the services of the Registry of Nursing Research, an individualized literature and book review service, clinical knowledge base indexes, and the *Online Journal of Knowledge Synthesis,* a clinically focused, evidence based, peer reviewed journal. Programming opportunities on critical, timely clinical issues are available through local, regional, international, and online offerings. The society's research journal, *Journal of Nursing Scholarship* and news magazine, *Reflections*, provide opportunities for publishing and showcase nursing research and clinical scholarship and leadership. The public relations opportunities include media training and conferences linking media, nursing, and public information officers.

Membership in Sigma Theta Tau International is an honor that creates new beginnings for professional development in scholarship and leadership. It is a springboard for placing members in the forefront of the profession and is highly regarded by employers and other leaders in the profession and health care. In summary, Sigma Theta Tau International provides many avenues globally to connect, develop, and showcase nursing excellence. Please visit our web site at http://www.nursingsociety.org for more information about our programs (Sullivan, 1999).

Analysis of Selected Issues Nursing Associations Address

Through the work of associations practicing nurses and nurse educators can address issues of critical importance to themselves, their students, their patients, and the future of the profession. The National League for Nursing, for example, strives to maintain high quality nursing education programs at all levels of nursing education (associate degree, diploma, baccalaureate, and advanced degree). In another example, the ANA works to unify nurses through its state nurses associations to benefit nurses and patients through professional practice advocacy. The ANA also manages a comprehensive federal legislative agenda. Each of these issues will be described briefly.

Nursing Education

High quality nursing education is important to nursing students, nursing educators, registered nurses, and the recipients of nursing care. The NLN helps to advance the quality of nursing education that prepares the nursing workforce to meet the needs of diverse populations in an everchanging health care environment. For more than 100 years, the NLN has helped to shape the development of nursing curricula and educational models that anticipate, reflect, and respond to the everchanging health care needs of diverse student and patient populations. The dynamic nature of nursing education and the need to examine priorities continually is reflected in the NLN's Blue Ribbon Panel on Priorities for Nursing Education Research. The Blue Ribbon Panel report identified three areas of research that should be established as priorities in nursing education. These priorities are important to nursing students and include:

1. A need to understand the changing role of the student in learning. New learning structures will demand that the nursing student take a more active role in the education process. This new model will focus more on the participation of the student, as opposed to the student simply attending lectures.
2. Nursing students should understand the coming changes in nursing education that focus on bridging the gap between education and practice.
3. Nursing students should expect not only to be engaged in the health care of their communities for educational purposes but also to play an integral role in the delivery of the health care in that community.

By encouraging member schools to address these priorities, the NLN ensures that nursing education remains relevant to our changing health care system and society.

Professional Practice Advocacy

In an effort to address the needs of all registered nurses, the American Nurses Association's 1999 House of Delegates passed historic bylaw changes to streamline and revitalize the organization as it moves into the next millennium. These bylaw changes reinforced ANA's overarching commitment to **professional practice advocacy** for the nation's 2.6 million registered nurses. Professional practice advocacy embraces activities including education, lobbying, and individual and collective advocacy in order to advance nursing's agenda. Professional practice advocacy uses the tools of collective bargaining or workplace advocacy to achieve its objectives.

Strengthening the voice of nurses in collective bargaining units nationwide, the ANA has created a national labor entity, the United American Nurses (UAN). The United American Nurses is a separate entity within the ANA that focuses on ongoing labor activities and supports state nurses associations in organizing and collective bargaining efforts. The UAN focuses on existing problem areas with offers to organize and represent groups of registered nurses who want support through collective bargaining to deal with issues such as staffing levels and workplace safety. The ANA also strengthened its role in workplace advocacy by creating a Workplace Advocacy Task Force to develop strategies and recommendations to ensure that nurses who are not represented by collective bargaining have access to meaningful workplace advocacy.

Federal Lobbying Efforts

The American Nurses Association has achieved many important and historic advances at the federal level in recent years. Its strength on Capitol Hill is a direct result of the collaboration and coordination of three critical components of its federal legislative program: lobbying, grassroots activities, and political action. The backbone of nursing's power in the U.S. Congress is the political and **grassroots activism** of thousands of nurses across the country. As that participation continues to increase, so will the voices and victories of nursing in the federal legislative arena.

Legislative agendas are constantly changing as new congressional sessions occur. Some examples of the ANA's legislative agenda for the first session of the 106th Congress (1999) were:

- The Patients' Bill of Rights. The ANA is working to make sure that this legislation covers all patients, no matter what type of insurance they have or where they live, and that it holds health plans accountable for their decisions. The ANA is also lobbying vigorously to protect nurses who advocate for their patients by blowing the whistle on unsafe conditions or practice.

- The Health Care Worker Needlestick Prevention Act. The ANA supports legislation that would require health care facilities to use safe devices. This will reduce the risk of contacting blood-borne disease from accidental needlestick injuries, which are currently sustained by thousands of health care workers each year. Introduced in the House of Representatives by Representatives Pete Stark (D-Calif.) and Marge Roukema (R-NJ), this bill has more than 100 bipartisan cosponsors. An identical bill was introduced in the Senate by Senator Barbara Boxer (D-Calif.).

- Medicaid reimbursement. The ANA is advocating for direct Medicaid reimbursement for all nurse practitioners and clinical nurse specialists. Under current law, state Medicaid programs are required to provide direct reimbursement to pediatric and family nurse practitioners and certified nurse midwives. Legislation has been introduced in both the House of Representatives and the Senate to provide Medicaid reimbursement to all nurse practitioners and clinical nurse specialists. These bills emphasize that better utilization of nurse practitioners and clinical nurse specialists will help to increase access to quality care for the nation's underserved populations.

- Nurse Education Act. In the 105th Congress, ANA worked successfully to ensure passage of a bill that would provide federal government support for nurses to return to school for their bachelor of science degree in nursing or advanced practice nursing degree. In the 106th Congress, ANA worked to ensure that Congress provided adequate funding for these Nurse Education Act programs during the fiscal year 2000 appropriations process. The ANA also worked to achieve adequate funding for the National Institute for Nursing Research and the Occupational Safety and Health Administration.

- Medicare. The ANA was deeply involved in discussions on Capitol Hill to find ways to modify many of the Medicare provisions of the Balanced Budget Act of 1997. For instance, drastic cuts in reimbursement for home health agencies created a crisis for patient care, and ANA worked to find both short-term and long-term solutions to this problem.

- Health care records privacy. The ANA worked for passage of legislation to guarantee the confidentiality of patients' health information that, at the same time, promoted access to high quality care and the continued viability of health research.

- Community Nursing Organization Demonstration Project. The ANA worked to achieve an extension of the Community Nursing Organization Demonstration Project, based on the positive experiences of the four pioneer projects, which are nurse-operated programs serving Medicare beneficiaries in home and community-based settings. The initial demonstration project was scheduled to expire on January 1, 2000.

- Patient Safety Act. The ANA continued to advocate for the provisions contained in the Patient Safety Act that were addressed during the 105th

Congress. These included reporting of institutional staffing and outcomes information, protection from retaliation for nurses who advocate for their patients, and community accountability for hospital mergers and acquisitions.

The American Nurses Association has also proposed to reform the ailing Medicare program, reaffirming a long-standing commitment to strengthening the program. Recommending that much of Medicare's framework remain the same, the ANA also advocates strong measures to simplify and improve the program to better meet the diverse health care needs of the growing population of older Americans. A fundamental underpinning of the ANA's proposal is the transformation of the Medicare program to a "beneficiary-focused coordinated model of care" that focuses on primary health care services, prevention, wellness, and early intervention. This is in contrast to the current "medical model of care" in which the emphasis is on treatment of disease and in which coordination of care among health care providers is negligible. The ANA was the first health professional association to support Medicare when it was introduced as legislation and has been an ardent supporter of the Medicare program since its inception in 1966. In September 1998, the ANA delivered testimony before the National Bipartisan Commission on the Future of Medicare regarding its support for the program. Recognizing its significance, the ANA will remain actively involved in the public policy debate surrounding Medicare reform.

For the latest ANA legislative initiatives, visit their website at http://www.nursingworld.org.

Summary of Key Points

- Professional associations are the vehicle through which nursing takes collective action to improve health care and nursing.
- There are many nursing associations from which to choose, and they offer a variety of benefits to the public, to the nursing profession as a whole, and to individual members.
- Membership in professional associations is considered essential for true professionals, but selecting which associations to join can be a challenge. Prospective members can ask several key questions to help them select wisely.
- The ANA, which represents all nurses, is at the forefront in addressing issues of importance to all nurses, including nurse staffing, occupational health, and safety and the enactment of legislative proposals that address protections for nurses in the workplace and patients' rights.
- The NSNA develops leaders whose future membership in their state nurses associations will strengthen the profession.
- The NLN ensures quality of nursing education through accreditation of schools of nursing, consultation in curriculum construction and teaching-learning strategies, and standardized aptitude and achievement testing.

- Sigma Theta Tau International is the Honor Society for Nursing. Membership is by invitation. It encourages scholarship, research, practice, and leadership skills in its members.

Critical Thinking Questions

1. Look in the local newspaper for articles about legislation that supports nursing's concerns, that is, the Patient's Bill of Rights or the Health Care Worker Needlestick Prevention Act. Then write a letter to the editor of your local paper about these bills. Sample letters on various nursing topics are available at the ANA's Nursing World website, www.nursingworld.org. On the Nursing World homepage, click on "RN=Real News." Once you've entered the RN=Real News area, click on the "Nurses Toolkit" button, then on "Letters to the Editor."

2. Find out if there is a student nurses association on your campus. If there is, learn all you can about it and consider joining. If there isn't one, consider establishing one (resources: www.nsna.org; click on "Get Involved").

3. As a student, attend local or state nurses association meetings to gain a better sense of the issues in the profession, so that you can be prepared for what lies ahead when you graduate. How is the association addressing these issues? Do they interest you? How can you get involved?

4. You read in local newspapers that students at the university where you attend nursing school have a high rate of drug and alcohol use. The following week another story appears about a senior university student who died following a car crash. The student was driving under the influence of alcohol. How can nursing students address the need for education about drug and alcohol use? What collective action can you initiate to address this or another issue of importance to your college or university community (resources: www.nsna.org; click on "Publications" to download *Guidelines for Planning Community Health Projects*)?

5. Enrollments in the nursing program that you attend have dropped 20 percent over the past two years. This year, there are over 35 unfilled places for nursing students. The faculty is concerned about a nursing shortage in the community and the decline in enrollments. The student nurses association chapter has formed a recruitment committee to address this issue. Why are students not considering nursing as a career? Why are students considering nursing as a career? How many registered nurses will be needed in the future? Plan a collective action project that can be implemented by the student nurses association to increase interest in the nursing profession (resources: www.nsna.org; click on "Publications" to download *Guidelines for Planning Breakthrough to Nursing Projects*).

6. Students at your school have to struggle to pay tuition. Many students work part-time while attending school full-time. They have taken out student loans and have applied for scholarships to help pay tuition and school-related expenses. A faculty member announces in class that the Nurse Education Act in going before Congress for reauthorization. What collective actions can the student nurses association take to ask Congress to increase funding for undergraduate nursing education (resources: www.nsna.org;

click on "Publications" to download *Guidelines for Planning Legislative Activities;* Mason, D. and Leavitt, J. (1998). *Policy and Politics in Nursing and Health Care,* 3rd ed. Philadelphia, WB Saunders)?

7. Nursing students are not immune to the pressures of university life such as competition for good grades. A classmate asks you to share a paper you prepared for a leadership course she is now taking so that she can see how you handled the assignment. You willingly give her a copy of your A+ paper. At the end of the semester, the faculty member who teaches the leadership course calls you into her office. She shows you the paper you wrote for her course last semester, but it now has your classmate's name on it instead of yours! What collective action can the student nurses association take to prevent plagiarism and cheating (resources: www.nsna.org; click on "Publications" to download the NSNA *Bill of Rights and Responsibilities for Students of Nursing* and the NSNA *Code of Academic and Clinical Professional Conduct*)?

Web Resources

American Nurses Association, http://www.nursingworld.org

International Council of Nurses, http://www.icn.ch

National League for Nursing, http://www.nln.org

National Student Nurses Association, http://www.nsna.org

Sigma Theta Tau International, http://www.nursingsociety.org

References

American Nurses Association (1994). *Position statement on assisted suicide.* Washington, D. C.: American Nurses Association.

American Nurses Association (1985). *Code for nurses with interpretive statements.* Kansas City, Mo.: American Nurses Association.

Aydelotte, M. K. (1990). The evolving profession: The role of the professional organization. In N. L. Chaska (Ed.), *The nursing profession: Turning points.* St. Louis: Mosby.

Hiscox, K. L. (1999). Personal communication.

Langston, N. (1999). Personal communication.

Malone, B. L. (1999). Personal communication.

Merton, R. K. (1958). The functions of the professional association. *American Journal of Nursing,* 58(1), 50–54.

National Student Nurses Association (1995). *Mission statement.* New York: National Student Nurses Association.

Sullivan, E. (1999). Personal communication.

Nursing Today

Kay K. Chitty and Cathy Campbell

5

Key Terms

Advanced Practice Nurse (APN)
Ambulatory Care
Autonomy
Case Management
Certified Nurse-midwife (CNM)
Certified Registered Nurse
    Anesthetist (CRNA)
Clinical Coordinator
Clinical Ladder
Clinical Nurse Specialist (CNS)
Community Health Nursing
Critical Path
Entrepreneur
Extended Care
Flexible Staffing
Informatics Nurse

Nurse Manager
Nurse Practitioner (NP)
Occupational Health Nurse

Parish Nurse
Private Practice
School Nurse

Learning Outcomes

After studying this chapter, students will be able to:

- Describe the "average" registered nurse of today.
- Identify the broad range of settings in which today's registered nurses practice.
- Discuss emerging practice opportunities for nurses.
- Cite similarities and differences in nursing roles in various practice settings.
- Explain the roles of advanced practice nurses and the preparation required to assume them.

F ar-reaching economic and social changes in the United States have profoundly changed the way health care is provided. Many of the changes outlined in Chapter 3 have opened avenues to new and exciting employment opportunities for nurses. This chapter provides an overview of the registered nurse (RN) population in the United States and briefly presents a selection of employment options available to nurses today in both hospital and community settings. Integrated into this chapter are interviews with several nurses who describe their work and the rewards and challenges of their positions.

Current Status of Nursing in the United States

What is the profile of nurses today? Is there an "average" registered nurse? Where do nurses work? What incomes do they earn in today's market? Are there enough opportunities to provide employment for all nurses? As health care changes and nursing evolves to meet new challenges, the answers to these questions also change.

Characteristics of Registered Nurses

In order to provide current information about practicing nurses, the federal government conducts a national survey of registered nurses in the United States every four years. The most recent survey was conducted in March 1996. Data from this survey were published in 1997 by the U. S. Department of Health and Human Services, Division of Nursing, in a document entitled *The Registered Nurse Population: March 1996*. This document and others published by the American Nurses Association (ANA) and the National League for Nursing (NLN) provide a comprehensive look at the characteristics of registered nurses today.

Numbers

Registered nurses represent the largest group of health care providers in the United States. More than 2.5 million individuals held licenses as registered nurses in 1996, with over 2.1 million (82.7 percent) of that number actively working in nursing. The remainder of the registered nurse population (17.3 percent) was either not working at all or working in fields other than nursing. These figures indicate that 59 percent of employed registered nurses worked full-time.

Gender

Not surprisingly, the Division of Nursing's 1996 survey also showed that most registered nurses were women. Among those employed, only 5.4 percent were men, up from 4.3 percent in 1992 and 3.3 percent in 1988. The number of men is growing at a rate faster than that for the total registered nurse population, however, with an average annual growth rate between 1992 and 1996 of 8.9 percent. The historic status of nursing as a female-dominated profession is gradually changing as the number of male graduates of basic nursing programs increases (See Chapter 3, Fig. 3–2).

Race and Ethnicity

As of 1996, the total registered nurse population was overwhelmingly composed of white, non-Hispanic individuals (89.7 percent). The 1996 survey showed that distribution by ethnic/racial backgrounds of the 10.3 percent employed nonwhite registered nurses included African-American, 4.2 percent; Asian/Pacific Islander, 3.4 percent; Hispanic, 1.6 percent; and Native American/Alaskan Native, 0.5 percent. There were over 18,000 registered nurses whose racial/ethnic background was unknown, accounting for 0.7 percent of the total.

Although the number of nonwhites in the registered nurse population is growing at a rate higher than that of the total population, the need exists both to recruit and to retain nonwhite members in the practice of nursing. Nursing has a long way to go before the racial/ethnic composition of the profession more accurately reflects that of American society, which the 1996 survey found was 72 percent white and 28 percent nonwhite.

Age

In respect to age, the registered nurse population is similar to the rest of American society: It is getting older. This "graying" of the work force can be illustrated by comparing 1980 statistics with those from 1996. In 1980, the average age of all registered nurses was 40.3 years. This figure had risen to 44.3 years by 1996. With large numbers of new nurses entering practice each year, the average age might be expected to remain the same or decline. Many new nurses are beginning second careers, however, and are significantly older than the typical college graduate.

Education

Nursing has more levels of preparation than most professional groups, due to the variety of educational pathways that one can take to become a registered nurse. In 1996, of the 2,115,815 employed registered nurses, 23.7 percent had diplomas as their highest nursing-related educational preparation; 34.6 percent held associate degrees; 31.8 percent had baccalaureate degrees; 9.1 percent held master's degrees in nursing; and 0.6 percent were doctorally prepared (U. S. Department of Health and Human Services, 1997). Figure 5–1 illustrates the educational preparation of registered nurses in the United States in 1996.

Employment Opportunities for Nurses

As members of the largest health care profession in the United States, nurses serve in diverse settings such as hospitals, clinics, offices, homes, schools, workplaces, community centers, nursing homes, children's camps, and homeless shelters, among others. Increasingly, as state nurse practice acts are revised to cover advanced practice roles, registered nurses work in private prac-

Figure 5–1
Educational preparation of registered nurses in the United States, 1996 (Data from The Registered Nurse Population, March 1996, Division of Nursing, U. S. Department of Health and Human Services, 1997, p. 40).

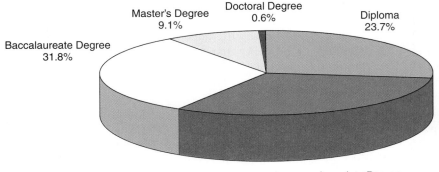

tice. Nurses in private practice must have advanced degrees or specialized education, training, and certification.

In 1996, hospitals were the primary work site for registered nurses (reported by 60 percent of those employed). Community settings showed the largest increase in employment from 1992 to 1996, with 8.5 percent of registered nurses working in **ambulatory care** settings such as physicians' offices, nurse-managed practices, or health maintenance organizations. Community or public health settings such as health departments or visiting nurse services employed another 17 percent of nurses, whereas 8.1 percent of nurses worked in nursing homes or **extended care** facilities based in and out of hospitals. The remainder of the registered nurses worked in settings such as schools of nursing, nursing organizations, governmental offices, or insurance companies (U. S. Department of Health and Human Services, 1997).

Not all nurses provide direct patient care as the primary part of their roles. A small but important group of nurses spend the majority of their time conducting research, teaching undergraduate and graduate students, managing companies as chief executives, and consulting with health care organizations. Nurses who have advanced levels of education, such as master's and doctoral degrees, are prepared to become researchers, educators, administrators, and advanced practice nurses, including nurse practitioners, clinical nurse specialists, certified nurse-midwives, and certified registered nurse anesthetists. These advanced-practice roles are discussed in greater detail later in this chapter.

In deciding which of the many available practice options to select, nurses should consider several salient points: educational preparation required; their special talents, likes, and dislikes; and whether their preparation, talents, and preferences are a good match with the employment opportunity under consideration. Although a majority of nurses are employed in hospitals, many others are pursuing challenges elsewhere. Numerous new opportunities and roles are being developed that use nurses' skills in different and exciting ways. What follows are descriptions of a sampling of the broad range of settings in which nurses now practice. In some instances, nurses are interviewed. It must be stressed that these areas represent only a sampling of the growing number of opportunities available.

Hospital Nursing

Nursing care originated in home and community settings and moved into hospitals only within the last century, with 60 percent of employed registered nurses working in hospitals in 1996. Hospitals vary widely in size, services offered, and geographic location. In general, nurses in hospitals work with patients who have medical or surgical conditions, with children, with women and their newborns, with cancer patients, and with people who have had severe traumas or burns. Nurses work in various units, such as operating rooms or emergency departments, and in many other capacities. In addition to providing direct patient care, they serve as educators, managers, and administrators who teach or supervise others and establish the direction of nursing hospitalwide. A number of generalist and specialist certification opportunities are appropriate for hospital-based nurses, including medical-surgical nurse, pediatric nurse, perinatal nurse, acute care nurse practitioner, gerontological nurse, psychiatric and mental health nurse, nursing administration, nursing administration advanced, nursing continuing education and staff development nurse, and informatics nurse. There is perhaps no other setting that offers so much variety as the hospital.

The educational credentials required of registered nurses practicing in hospitals can range from associate degrees and diplomas to doctoral degrees. Generally, entry-level positions require only a license. Many hospitals require nurses to hold baccalaureate degrees to advance up the clinical ladder or to assume management positions. **Clinical coordinators,** who are responsible for the management of more than one unit, are generally expected to have a master's degree.

Most new nurses choose to work in acute care hospitals initially to gain experience in organizing and delivering patient care. For some, staff nursing is extremely gratifying, and they continue in this role for their entire careers. Others pursue additional education, often provided by the hospital, and staff specialty units such as coronary care. Although specialty units usually require experience and advanced training, some hospitals do allow exceptional new graduates to work in these units.

Some nurses find that management is their strength. **Nurse managers,** formerly called head nurses, are in charge of all activities on their units, including patient care, continuous quality improvement, personnel selection and evaluation, and resource management. Being a nurse manager in a hospital today is somewhat like running a business, and nurses need an entrepreneurial spirit and some business background to be most effective in this role.

Most nurses in hospitals provide direct patient care. In the past, it was necessary for nurses to assume administrative or management roles to be promoted or receive salary increases. Such positions removed them from bedside care. Today, clinical ladder programs allow nurses to progress while staying in direct patient care roles.

A **clinical ladder** is a multiple-step program that begins with entry-level staff nurse positions. As nurses gain experience, participate in continuing education, demonstrate clinical competence, pursue formal education, and become certified, they are eligible to move up the rungs of the ladder.

At the top of most clinical ladders are clinical nurse specialists, who are nurses with master's degrees in specialized areas of nursing, such as oncology. The role varies but generally includes responsibility for serving as a clinical mentor and role model for other nurses as well as setting standards for nursing care on one or more particular units. The oncology clinical specialist, for example, works with the nursing staff on the oncology unit to help them stay informed of the latest research in the care of cancer patients. The clinical specialist is a resource person for the unit and often provides direct care to patients or families with particularly difficult or complex problems, establishes nursing protocols, and is responsible for seeing that nurses adhere to high standards of care.

Salaries and responsibilities increase at the higher levels of clinical ladders. The clinical ladder concept benefits nurses by allowing them to advance while still working directly with patients. Hospitals also benefit by retaining experienced clinical nurses in direct patient care, thus improving the quality of nursing care throughout the hospital.

One of the greatest drawbacks to hospital nursing in the past was the necessity for nurses to work rigid schedules, which usually included evenings, nights, and weekends. Although hospital nurses still must work a fair share of undesirable times, **flexible staffing** is becoming the norm. Sometimes nurses on a particular unit negotiate with each other and establish their own schedules that meet personal needs while ensuring that appropriate patient care is provided.

Each hospital nursing role has its own unique characteristics. In the following profile, a registered nurse discusses his role as a bedside nurse in a burn unit:

> A burn nurse has to be gentle, strong, and patient enough to go slow. You must be confident enough to work alone; you must believe that what you're doing is in the patient's best interest because some of the procedures hurt far worse than anyone can imagine. Every burn is unique and a challenge. Fifteen years ago, the prognosis for surviving an extensive burn was not good, but with today's techniques for fluid replacement and the development of effective antibiotics, many patients are surviving the first few critical days. During the long hours of one-on-one care you really get to know your patient. There is nothing more rewarding.

When the "fit" between nurses and their role requirements is good, nursing is a gratifying profession, as an oncology nurse demonstrated as she discussed her role:

> Being an oncology nurse and working with people with potentially terminal illnesses brings you close to patients and their families. The family room for our patients and their families is very homelike. Families bring food in and have dinner with their loved one right here. Working with dying patients is a tall order. You must be able to support the family and the patient through many stages of the dying process, including anger and depression. Experiencing cancer is always traumatic, with the diagnosis, the treatment, and the struggle to cope. But today's statistics show that more people experience cancer and live. Because of research and early detection, being diagnosed with cancer is no longer the automatic death sentence it used to be. I love getting involved with patients and their families and feel that I can contribute to their positive mental attitude, which can impact their disease process, or hold their hand and help them to die with dignity. They cry, I cry—it is part of my nursing, and I would have it no other way.

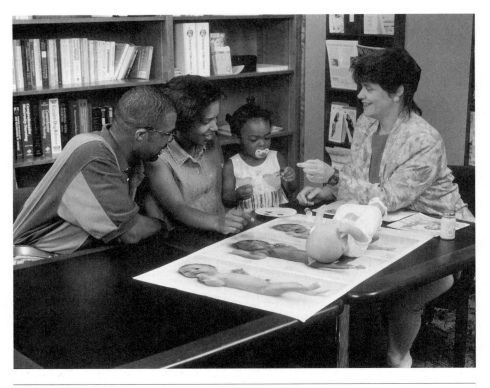

Figure 5–2
Hospital nurses work closely with the families of patients as well as with the patients themselves (Courtesy of Memorial Hospital, Chattanooga, Tennessee).

These are only two of the many possible roles nurses in hospital settings may choose. Although brief, these descriptions convey a flavor of the responsibility, complexity, and fulfillment to be found in hospital-based nursing (Fig. 5–2).

Community Health Nursing

Lillian Wald is credited with initiating **community health nursing** when she established the Henry Street Settlement in New York City. Community health nursing today is a broad field encompassing what were formerly known as public health nursing and home health nursing. Community health nurses work in ambulatory clinics, health departments, hospices, and a variety of other community-based settings, including homes, where they provide nursing care to home-bound patients.

Community health nurses may work for either government or private agencies. Those working for public health departments provide care in clinics, schools, retirement communities, and other community settings. They focus on improving the overall health of communities by planning and implementing health programs as well as delivering care. They provide educational programs in health maintenance, disease prevention, nutrition, and child care. They conduct immunization clinics and health screenings and work with teachers, parents, physicians, and community leaders toward a healthier community. Many health departments also have a home health component.

Since 1980, there has been a tremendous increase in the number of private agencies providing home health services, a form of community health nursing. In fact, home health care is a fast-growing segment of the health care industry (Fig. 5–3). Many home health nurses predict that most health care services in the future will be provided in the home. This is especially true as patients are being discharged earlier from the hospital to control costs.

Home health care has traditionally been, and will continue to be, nursing's "turf." Home health nurses across the United States provide quality care in the most cost-effective and, for patients, comfortable setting possible—the home. Patients cared for at home today are sicker than ever. Therefore, more high-technology equipment is being used in the home. Equipment and procedures formerly unheard of outside of hospital settings, such as ventilators, intravenous pumps and, chemotherapy set ups, are routinely encountered in home care today.

Home health nurses must possess up-to-date nursing knowledge and be secure in their own nursing skills. They do not have the backup of physicians

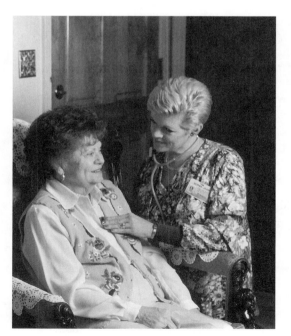

Figure 5–3
Home health nursing is a fast-growing segment of the health care industry (Courtesy of Memorial Hospital, Chattanooga, Tennessee).

or more experienced nurses as they might in a hospital. They must have good assessment skills, make independent judgments, recognize patients' and families' teaching needs, and have good communication skills. They must also know what their limits are and seek help when the patient's needs are beyond the scope of their abilities. A registered nurse working in home health relates her experience:

> I have always found a tremendous reward in working with the terminally ill and the elderly, and I get a great deal of contact with this particular population working in home health. One patient I cared for developed a pressure ulcer while at home. I was able to assess the patient's physiological needs as well as teach the family how to care for their loved one to prevent future skin breakdown. Within a few weeks the skin looked good, and the family felt important and involved. To me this is real nursing.

Community health nursing is growing as more and more nursing care is delivered outside the walls of hospitals. The American Nurses Credentialing Center offers certification in both community health and home health nursing at the generalist and clinical specialist levels. The increase in demand for nurses to work in a variety of community settings is expected to increase for the foreseeable future.

Nurse Entrepreneurs

A nurse **entrepreneur** identifies a need and creates a service to meet the identified need. Some nurses are creative and energetic people who like the idea of new forms of expression. They are challenged by the risks of starting a new enterprise and make good candidates for entrepreneurship.

Nurse entrepreneurs enjoy the **autonomy** that is derived from owning and operating their own health-related businesses. Groups of nurses, some of whom are faculty in schools of nursing, have opened nurse-managed centers to provide direct care to clients. Nurse entrepreneurs are self-employed as consultants to hospitals, nursing homes, and schools of nursing. Others have started **private practices** and carry their own caseloads of patients with physical or emotional needs. They are sometimes involved in presenting educational workshops and seminars. Some nurses establish their own creative apparel businesses, which provide articles of clothing for premature babies or physically challenged individuals. Others own and operate their own health equipment companies and home health agencies. In today's burgeoning health care environment, there is no limit to the opportunities available to nurses with the entrepreneurial spirit. Here are a few comments from one such entrepreneur, the chief executive officer of a privately owned home health agency:

> I enjoy working for myself. I know that my success or failure in my business is up to me. Having your own home health agency is a lot of work. You have

to be very organized and have excellent communication skills. You cannot be afraid to say no to the people. There is nothing better than the feeling you get from a family calling to say our nurses have made a difference in their loved one's life, but I also have to take the calls of complaint about my agency. Those are tough.

Increasingly, nurses are taking the business of health care into their own hands. They seem to agree that the opportunity to create their own companies has never been better. One such company offers nursing care for mothers, babies, and children. The emphasis is the care of women whose pregnancies may be complicated by diabetes, hypertension, or multiple births. "Our main specialty is managing high-risk pregnancies and high-risk newborns," reports the registered nurse founder. She continued:

> Home care for these individuals is a boon not only to the patients themselves, but also to hospitals, insurance companies, and doctors. With the trend toward shorter hospital stays, risks are minimized if skilled maternity nurses are on hand to provide patients with specialty care in their homes.

As with almost any endeavor, there are disadvantages that come with owning a small business. There is the risk of losing your investment if the business is unsuccessful. Fluctuations in income are common, especially in the early months, and regular paychecks may become a memory, at least at first. A certain amount of pressure is created because of the total responsibility for meeting deadlines and paying bills, salaries, and taxes. But there is great opportunity, too. Aspiring entrepreneurs can eliminate much of the risk involved in small business ownership by completing four preliminary steps:

1. Conduct a thorough needs assessment to determine whether the service or product is needed and wanted by consumers.
2. Develop a detailed business plan complete with short-term and long-term goals, marketing plans, and schedules for business development.
3. Have enough capital to carry the business for at least a year, even if there is no profit, and keep overhead low.
4. Prepare appropriately by learning about effective business practices, for example, budgeting, accounting, personnel policies, and legal aspects of small business.

In addition to financial incentives, there are also intangible rewards in entrepreneurship. For some people, the autonomy and freedom to control their own practice are more than enough to compensate them for increased pressure and initial uncertainty.

With rapid changes occurring daily in the health care system, there are always new and exciting possibilities. Alert nurses who possess creativity, initiative, and business savvy have tremendous opportunities as entrepreneurs. The accompanying Research Note describes the work of one such nurse.

Kathleen Vollman is a critical care nurse practicing in Detroit. She has a master's degree. In the early 1980s she observed that about 60 to 70 percent of her patients with acute respiratory distress syndrome (ARDS) died of lack of oxygen. Attempts to oxygenate them with ventilators often further injured their lungs. Inspired by an article on animal research left in the break room by a pulmonologist, Kathleen began to think about positioning patients for maximum oxygenation.

First she tried turning her patients with ARDS from side to back to side every 30 minutes, as had been done in the animal study. She took blood gas readings in each position and developed a schedule for each patient based on that person's unique responses. Patients seemed to do better when she used this noninvasive independent nursing function of positioning.

Encouraged by her patients' responses, she read more research studies and found two articles dealing with the beneficial effect of prone (face down) positioning on gas exchange. She tried this with positive results but encountered problems turning very sick patients into the prone position. Solving this problem became the subject of her master's research.

Kathleen and a relative who is a mechanical engineer developed a turning frame and tested it first on healthy people in a simulated critical care environment. After testing, the device was modified twice and then tested with ARDS patients. Data were collected for over 10 months and showed the usefulness of the frame in improving oxygenation of these critically ill patients. Kathleen has since won several research awards and has patented her device. She licensed it to a major maker of hospital beds and now the Voll-

man Prone Positioner is marketed internationally. The device costs $2,000 and can be reused after disinfecting. Kathleen serves as a consultant to the company on the marketing of the device and the education of those who will use it.

This is an example of how a practicing nurse, making an observation and thinking creatively through possible solutions, became a researcher, inventer, and, ultimately, entrepreneur. This is not an overnight success story, however; it has been over 15 years since Kathleen made her initial observations. She continues her research into prone positioning science today.

From Vollman, K. M. (1999). My search to help patients breathe. *Reflections,* 25(2), 16–18, and Vollman, K. M., and Bander, J. L. (1996). Improved oxygenation utilizing a prone positioner in patients with acute respiratory distress syndrome. *Intensive Care Medicine,* 22, 1105–1111.

Office Nursing

Nurses who are employed in medical office settings work directly with physicians and their patients. Nursing activities include performing health assessments, drawing blood, giving immunizations, administering medications, and providing health teaching. Nurses in office settings also act as liaisons between patients and physicians. They amplify and clarify orders for patients as well as provide emotional support to anxious patients. They may visit hospitalized patients, and some assist the employing physician in surgery. Often, they supervise other office workers, such as practical nurses, nurse aides, scheduling clerks, and record clerks. Educational requirements, hours of work, and specific responsibilities vary, depending on the preferences of the employer.

A registered nurse who works for a group of three nephrologists describes a typical day:

> I first make rounds independently on patients in the dialysis center, making sure that they are tolerating the dialysis procedure and answering questions

regarding their treatments and diets. I then make rounds with one of the physicians in the hospital as he visits patients and orders new treatments. The afternoon is spent in the office assessing patients as they come for their physician's visit. I may draw blood for a diagnostic test on one patient and do patient teaching regarding diet to another. No two days are alike, and that is what I love about this position. I have a sense of independence but still have daily patient contact.

Registered nurses considering employment in office settings need good communication skills because a large part of their responsibilities includes communicating with patients, families, physicians, pharmacists, and hospital admitting clerks. They should inquire about the specifics of the position because office nursing roles range from performing only routine tasks to the challenging, multifaceted functions described by the nurse interviewed.

Occupational Health Nursing

Many large companies today employ **occupational health nurses** to provide basic health care services, health education, screenings, and emergency treatment to company employees. Corporate executives have long known that good employee health reduces absenteeism, insurance costs, and worker errors, thereby improving company profitability. Occupational health nurses represent an important investment by companies. They are often asked to serve as consultants on health matters within the company. They may participate in health-related policy development, such as policies governing employee smoking or family leaves (formerly known as maternity leaves). Depending on the size of the company, the nurse may be the only health professional employed and therefore may have a good deal of autonomy.

The usual educational requirement for nurses in occupational health roles is licensure. Some positions call for a baccalaureate degree in nursing. These nurses must possess knowledge and skills that enable them to perform routine physical assessments, including vision and hearing screenings for all employees. Good interpersonal skills to provide counseling and referrals for lifestyle problems, such as stress or substance abuse, are a plus for these nurses. They must also know first aid and cardiopulmonary resuscitation (CPR). If employed in a heavy manufacturing setting where burns or traumas are a risk, they must have special training in those medical emergencies.

Occupational health nurses also have responsibilities for identifying health risks in the entire work environment. They must be able to assess the environment for potential safety hazards and work with management to eliminate or reduce them. They need a working knowledge of governmental regulations, such as the requirements of the Occupational Safety and Health Administration (OSHA), and must ensure that the company is complying with them. They also need to understand worker's compensation regulations and coordinate the care of injured workers with the treating physician.

Nurses in occupational settings have to be confident in their nursing skills, be effective communicators with both employees and managers, motivate employees to adopt healthier habits, and be able to function independently in providing care. Certification for occupational health nurses is available through the American Board for Occupational Health Nurses (ABOHN).

School Nursing

Nurses choosing **school nursing** must love to work with children, their families, and teachers. The purpose of school nursing is to enhance the educational process by improving the well-being of the target population, children and adolescents. Although many states have well-developed school nurse programs, others do not. Very few states have the recommended minimum number of school nurses of 1 nurse per 750 students. Other states have up to 10,000 students per school nurse (Carey and Mullins, 1995). With such high ratios, it is difficult to imagine how children in these states can be deriving substantial health benefits from the school nurse program.

Health care futurists believe that school nursing is the wave of the future (Moccia, 1992). The role of school nurse has expanded to include members of the school child's immediate family. It will require many more school nurses as well as a willingness by states and local school boards to pay them for the nation's children to enjoy the full potential of school nurse programs.

Most school systems require nurses to have a minimum of a baccalaureate degree in nursing, whereas some school districts have higher educational requirements. Prior experience working with children is also usually required. School health has become a specialty in its own right, and in states where school health is a priority, graduate programs in school health nursing have been established. The American Nurses Credentialing Center offers certification as a school nurse at two levels, generalist and nurse practitioner.

School nurses need a working knowledge of human growth and development to detect developmental problems early. Counseling skills are important because many children turn to the school nurse as counselor. School nurses keep records of children's required immunizations and are responsible for seeing that immunizations are current. When an outbreak of a childhood communicable disease occurs, school nurses educate parents, teachers, and students about treatment and prevention of transmission.

Although the essentially well child is the focus of the school nurse's work, the practice of mainstreaming has brought many chronically ill, injured, developmentally delayed, and physically challenged students into regular school classrooms. School nurses must work closely with families, teachers, and the community to provide these children with the special care they need while at school.

School nurses work closely with teachers to incorporate health concepts into the curriculum. They conduct vision and hearing screenings. Parents may expect school nurses to make referrals to qualified physicians and other health care providers when routine screenings identify problems outside the nurses' scope of practice.

School nurses must be prepared to handle both routine illnesses of children and adolescents and emergencies. One of their major concerns is safety. Accidents are the leading cause of death in children of all ages, yet accidents are preventable. First aid for minor injuries and emergency care for more severe ones are additional skills school nurses use.

Preventive aspects of child health are a major focus of school health nurses. In terms of safety, prevention requires both protection from obvious hazards and education of teachers, parents, and students about how to avoid accidents. School nurses practice safety, are alert to safety needs in the school and surrounding environment, and recognize the need for safety education in contributing to accident reduction.

School nursing is a complex and multifaceted field that is constantly expanding. It represents a challenge for those nurses who choose it as a career.

Case Management Nursing

Case management is a dynamic, challenging, and relatively new field in nursing. It involves systematic collaboration with patients, their significant others, and their health care providers to coordinate high quality health care services in a cost-effective manner with positive patient outcomes. The case manager is the person responsible for this process, and while registered nurses are not the only professionals who act as case managers, they are uniquely prepared for this role. Due to their broad educational backgrounds, skill in arranging and providing patient education and referrals, orientation toward holistic care and health promotion, and communication and interpersonal skills, nurses are particularly well suited for case management.

Depending on the case management model being followed, the nursing case manager may follow the patient from the diagnostic phase through hospitalization, rehabilitation, and back to home care. Through careful planning, every step of the patient's care can be coordinated in a timely manner.

One key to making case management work is the use of critical paths that include specific time lines and standard treatment protocols. A **critical path** is an abbreviated version of the case management plan that is used for daily decision making about patient care. It lists key nursing and medical interventions that should occur within a certain time line to ensure positive patient outcomes. Case management is considered successful if the patient is well enough for discharge within the Diagnostic-Related Grouping–directed length of stay. Appendix B shows a sample critical path such as those being used for case management in many institutions across the United States.

Both patient and nurse satisfaction are high with the one-on-one relationship fostered with case management. Patients like the security of having one familiar person coordinating their care, and a nursing case manager has the satisfaction of coordinating a patient's care from beginning to end (McKenzie,

Torkelson, and Holt, 1989). Certification in nursing case management is offered by the American Nurses Credentialing Center. You may hear case management nursing referred to as "care management nursing," a name more consistent with nursing's values.

Parish Nursing

The resurgence of interest in spirituality and its relation to wellness and healing has prompted an emerging practice area known as **parish nursing.** It includes a holistic approach to healing that involves partnerships between churches and healthcare providers. Since it was developed in the Chicago area in the mid-1980s by a hospital chaplain, Dr. Granger E. Westberg, parish nursing has spread rapidly and now includes more than 5,000 nurses in paid and volunteer positions across the country (Abuelouf, 1998). According to the American Nurses Association definition,

> Parish nursing is a unique, specialized practice of professional nursing that focuses on the promotion of health within the context of the values, beliefs, and practices of a faith community, such as a church, synagogue, or mosque, and its mission and ministry to its members (families and individuals), and the community it serves (American Nurses Association, 1998, p. 1).

Parish nurses serve as members of the ministry staff or clergy of a faith community. They practice independently, within the legal scope of the state's nurse practice act. In a unique partnership, the American Nurses Association and the Health Ministries Association, Inc., an interfaith organization supporting wellness within places of worship, jointly published the *Scope and Standards of Parish Nursing Practice* in 1998. This document sets forth the responsibilities for which parish nurses are accountable and reflects the values and priorities of the specialty. Interview 5–1 contains an interview with a parish nurse.

Informatics Nurse

Another new and exciting specialty area within nursing is nursing informatics (NI). The **informatics nurse** combines nursing science with information management science and computer science to manage information nurses need and to make it accessible. This field encompasses "the full range of activities that focus on information handling in nursing" (American Nurses Association, 1994, p. 4) and assists nurses to do the work of nursing efficiently and effectively.

In contrast to computer science systems analysts, informatics nurses must understand the information they handle and how other nurses will use it. Nursing knowledge is specialized and must be accessible by nurse users or

Interview with a Parish Nurse

Interviewer: Describe a typical day in your practice.

Parish Nurse: There is no "typical" day. Every day is different, which is what I love about parish nursing. There are many aspects of my work, a number of which are not usually thought of as nursing. I help the congregation understand the interaction and connection between body, mind, and spirit. This is important because unhealthy behaviors or emotions often affect us physically in harmful ways.

Interviewer: What is the focus of your practice?

Parish Nurse: One aspect is health maintenance, such as teaching nutrition and diet, dental health, medication management, blood pressure screenings, and the like. I also visit parishioners in their homes, mostly older adults. Recently I visited a lady with a stasis ulcer on her leg. After my assessment and much discussion, she agreed to let me make a referral to a wound specialist. I don't do invasive procedures like a home health nurse might do. My focus is in the role of teaching, counseling, supporting, and often just encouraging people about how to improve their lives physically, mentally, and spiritually both within the congregation and the community.

Interviewer: What has surprised you about parish nursing?

Parish Nurse: It surprised me how much writing I do. I am frequently asked to write an article for a newsletter or a small local paper about my current programs or about what I do as a parish nurse. I also make a lot of presentations, which takes some research. I sure didn't appreciate writing all of those papers in school, but now I'm glad because it gave me confidence in my writing and research skills.

Interviewer: How did you prepare yourself to be a parish nurse?

Parish Nurse: By searching and establishing my own spiritual foundation and having an open mind and heart, in order to hear God's calling. Parish nursing is a calling by God. I do not believe you can be totally effective in assisting others in discovering and improving their spirituality for better health unless you have achieved a certain amount of spiritual awareness within your own life. Education wise, I have a BSN and a master's degree in gerontological nursing. I have primarily worked in the areas of rehabilitation nursing and longterm care, which has prepared me well for what I do.

Interviewer: What is the most challenging part of your work?

Parish Nurse: The most challenging part of my work is learning about the philosophy of health ministry and parish nursing and applying it to my practice. Although parish nursing has been around for 12 to 15 years, it is still a relatively new field. I am the first parish nurse for my congregation and there are fewer than a dozen other parish nurses in our community, although that number is growing. This is an exciting time for our congregation as we explore the role of health ministry and parish nursing together.

Amy L. Corder, RN, MSN, CRRN

it is useless in improving patient care. Complex information systems are "more likely to fail when end-users are not consulted during the design phase" (American Nurses Association, 1994, p. 6). Because they are nurses themselves, informatics nurses are best able to understand the needs of nurses who use the systems and can design them with the needs, skills, and time constraints of those nurses in mind.

Informatics nurses may work in clinical areas, ensuring that the caregiver nurse is provided with complete and accurate information about patients' health needs and nursing care requirements. They may also practice in nonclinical areas such as nursing education or administration, where they design ways to make information needed by teachers, students, and managers easily accessible. In addition to practicing in hospitals and universities, informatics nurses also work in the military, health maintenance organizations, and research settings.

Information technology can help nurses deliver more effective care in a number of ways. Some examples of the practice of nursing informatics include computerizing a nursing document or system; writing a program to support nursing care of patients; developing an interactive video disc system for educational purposes; helping nurse managers develop systems to use nursing resources effectively (people, money, supplies); or designing systems to collect and aggregate clinical data so they can be analyzed to assess the cost and outcomes of nursing care.

As a minimum, informatics nurses should have a bachelor's degree in nursing and additional knowledge and experience in the field of informatics. "Advanced practice in nursing informatics requires preparation at the graduate level in nursing" (American Nurses Association, 1994, p. 10). Certification for informatics nurses is available through the American Nurses Credentialing Center.

Nursing Opportunities Requiring Higher Degrees

Many registered nurses choose to pursue roles that require a master's degree, doctoral degree, or specialized education in a specific area. They include clinical nurse specialists, nurse managers, nurse executives in hospital settings, nurse educators, whether in clinical or academic settings, and other advanced practice nurses.

Nurse Educators

About 2 percent of registered nurses work in nursing education. Nurse educators in accredited schools of nursing must hold a minimum of master's degree in nursing, and in 1998, 48 percent had doctoral degrees in nursing or other fields (American Association of Colleges of Nursing, 1999). That is a significant increase from 1992, when 21.4 percent of nursing faculty were doctorally prepared, and even more favorable when compared with only 10.6 percent in 1984 and 3 percent in 1972 (Anderson, 1994).

Most (96.7 percent) nursing faculty are women, 8.5 percent are members of minority groups, and 37 percent of faculty teaching in colleges and universities hold tenure (American Association of Colleges of Nursing, 1999). In 1995, only 8.3 percent of graduate students chose nursing education and prepared for a teaching role. This trend seems to be continuing and contributes to anxiety about a shortage of nursing faculty in the future, since current faculty are aging, and many will retire in the next decade.

Advanced Practice Nursing

Advanced practice nursing is growing rapidly, with approximately 161,712 registered nurses in 1996 reporting having the education and credentials to work as advanced practice nurses, up from 140,000 in 1992. This growth is spurred

Total Advanced Practice Nurses: 161,712

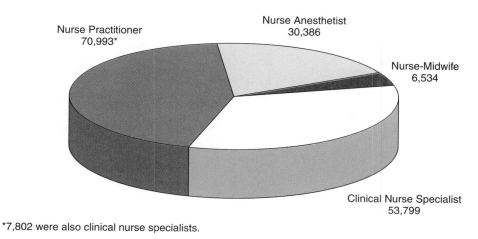

*7,802 were also clinical nurse specialists.

Figure 5–4

Numbers of advanced practice nurses by areas of specialty (Data from the Registered Nurse Population March 1996, Division of Nursing, U. S. Department of Health and Human Services, 1997, p. 18).

by several factors, including increased demand for primary care coupled with increased specialization of physicians and heightened demand for efficient and cost effective treatment. **Advanced practice nurse (APN)** is an umbrella term applied to a registered nurse who has met advanced educational and clinical practice requirements beyond the two to four years of basic nursing education demanded of all registered nurses. There are four categories of advanced practice nurses: nurse practitioner, clinical nurse specialist, certified nurse-midwife, and certified registered nurse anesthetist (Fig. 5–4). Patient acceptance of advanced practice nurses is high. A growing body of evidence is accumulating that confirms that advanced practice nurses deliver high quality care, exceeding that delivered by physicians on several measures. It is estimated that 60 to 80 percent of primary and preventive care traditionally performed by physicians can be done by advanced practices nurses for less money (American Nurses Association, 1997).

Nurse Practitioner

Nurse practitioners (NPs) work in clinics, nursing homes, their own offices, or physicians' offices. Other work for hospitals, health maintenance organizations (HMOs), or private industry. Most nurse practitioners choose a specialty area such as adult, family, or pediatric health care. They are qualified to handle a wide range of basic health problems. These nurses can perform physical examinations, take medical histories, diagnose and treat common acute and chronic illnesses and injuries, order and interpret laboratory tests and x-ray films, and counsel and educate clients (Fig. 5–5).

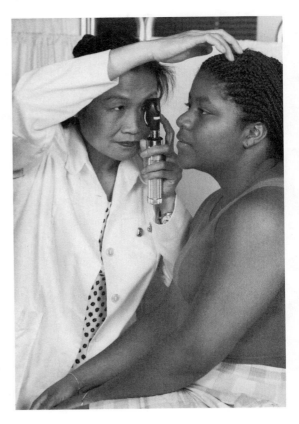

Figure 5–5
A nurse practitioner examines her patient
(Photo by Fielding Freed).

In 1999, nurse practitioners could legally write prescriptions in 40 states with some physician supervision, whereas in 17 states and the District of Columbia, nurse practitioners could prescribe independent of physician involvement (Pearson, 1999). Some nurse practitioners are independent practitioners and can be reimbursed by Medicare or Medicaid for their work.

Opportunities for nurses in expanded roles in health care has created a boom in nurse practitioner education. There were 150 nurse practitioner education programs in 1992. By 1999, this number had increased to 313. These programs grant master's degrees or postmaster's certificates and prepare nurses to sit for national certification examinations. Approximately 36 states have nurse practice acts requiring nurse practitioners to be nationally certified by the ANA or other nursing specialty organizations. By 1996, approximately 76 percent of the 70,993 nurse practitioners in the United States were nationally certified or had state recognition as advanced practice nurses or nurse practitioners (U. S. Department of Health and Human Services, 1997).

Clinical Nurse Specialist
Similar to nurse practitioners, **clinical nurse specialists (CNS)** work in a variety of settings, including hospitals, clinics, nursing homes, their own offices,

private industry, home care, and health maintenance organizations. They hold advanced nursing degrees—master's or doctoral—and are qualified to handle a wide range of physical and mental health problems. They are experts in a particular field of clinical practice, such as mental health, gerontology, cardiac care, cancer care, community health, or neonatal health, and perform health assessments, make diagnoses, deliver treatment, and develop quality control methods. Additionally, clinical nurse specialists work in consultation, research, education, and administration. Direct reimbursement to some clinical nurse specialists is possible through Medicare, Medicaid, Champus, and private insurers. In 1996, there were 53,799 clinical nurse specialists in the United States (American Nurses Association, 1996).

Certified Nurse-Midwife

There were an estimated 6,700 certified nurse-midwives in the United States in 1999 (American College of Nurse-Midwives, 1999). A **certified nurse-midwife (CNM)** provides well-woman care and attends to or assists in childbirth in various settings, including hospitals, birthing centers, and homes. According to the National Center for Health Statistics, in 1997, certified nurse-midwives attended 258,227 births. This represented about 8.47 percent of all U.S. births that year (American College of Nurse-Midwives, 1999). Births attended by nurse-midwives had fewer episiotomies, fewer forceps deliveries, and fewer low-birth-weight and premature infants, according to an ANA study (American Nurses Association, 1993). Certified-nurse midwives are able to prescribe medication in 50 states and jurisdictions (American College of Nurse-Midwives, 1999). Most of the 47 American College of Nurse-Midwives–accredited nurse-midwife programs offer a master's degree, accounting for an average of 1.5 years of specialized education beyond basic nursing school.

Because of patient acceptance and a good safety record, nurse-midwives are expected to increase in the future. The accompanying News Note summarizes a report by Ralph Nader, the consumer advocate, describing the value of certified nurse-midwives in a reformed health care system.

Certified Registered Nurse Anesthetist

There are over 30,000 **certified registered nurse anesthetists (CRNAs)** in the United States. Nurse anesthetists administer more than 65 percent of all anesthetics given to patients each year and are the only anesthesia providers in nearly one-third of U.S. hospitals. In rural hospitals, they provide 85 percent of anesthetics. Working with physician anesthesiologists or frequently independently, they are found in a variety of settings—operating rooms, dentist's offices, and ambulatory surgical settings.

Two to three years of specialized education in a master's program is required beyond the required four-year bachelor's degree. Nurse anesthetists must also meet national certification and recertification requirements. There were 30,386 nurse anesthetists in 1996, nearly all of whom were nationally certified (U. S. Department of Health and Human Services, 1997).

"Nader Group Sees CNMS Replacing OBS in 'Majority of American Births'"

Washington, D.C.—If Ralph Nader and his Public Citizen advocacy group have anything to say about it, the majority of American births, "not too long from now," will be attended by *certified nurse-midwives* (CNMs).

Releasing his Health Research Group's latest findings, Nader called the press to his Washington headquarters in November to explain why CNMs are a "better alternative" for birthing and maternity care and why they should outnumber obstetricians in a rational health care system. The research group is publishing a survey supporting that argument together with a national *Consumer's Guide to Nurse-Midwifery,* a 252-page directory that the researchers compiled with detailed descriptions of the services offered by 414 hospital-based practices and 41 freestanding birth centers.

"The 4000-plus CNMs in the U.S. offer . . . sensible, woman-oriented, old-fashioned care along with the latest medical and scientific expertise," said Public Citizen's head health researcher, physician Sidney Wolfe.

A group of new mothers told reporters about their contrasting experiences with OBs and CNMs. Johns Hopkins CNM Lisa Summers pointed out that healthy women are most in need of providers who don't answer questions "with our hand on the doorknob." Ruth Watson Lubic, founder of New York's Maternity Center Association, called on insurers to pay for prenatal and follow-up care, "rather than another 24 hours in an institution."

"Get the Message Out"

The powerful consumer group announced that it's pushing state and federal officials to loosen restrictive laws and to fund expanded education programs. It's urging consumers to choose a CNM as a primary care provider and spread the message: "Talk to your friends . . . Write to your legislators . . . Ask your insurance company to cover nurse-midwifery . . . Let the administrator of your local hospital know that you would like to see nurse-midwives given admitting privileges."

Wolfe stressed that CNMs should play a major role in cutting health care costs and curbing infant mortality rates. Assistant Secretary for Health Philip Lee endorsed the campaign and pledged continued federal support.

The $3,000-plus cost of cesarean births was spotlighted as an example of what's wrong with the current delivery system. While nearly one in four U.S. babies are now born by cesarean section, Public Citizen's data on 127,000 births showed a rate of only 11.6% for hospital births attended by CNMs. At freestanding birth centers, the rate dropped to 6.7%.

The CNMs who were surveyed also averaged a 68.9% rate of vaginal birth after cesarean—2.8 times higher (better) than the national average. The rates can't be explained away by risk profiles; most of the CNMs surveyed care for moderate- and high-risk as well as low-risk women.

Resurgence Seen in U. S.

As recently as 1975, fewer than 1% of American births in-hospital were attended by CNMs. By contrast, midwives supply much of the prenatal and labor and delivery care in many countries with better mortality records. But the past two decades have seen a steady rise that in 1993 reached 178,537—4.4% of U.S. hospital births.

(continued)

NEWS NOTE (Continued)

The 460 practices that answered Public Citizen's questions are responsible for an estimated 50% to 60% of CNMs' childbirth activity.

"Nurse-midwifery is not assembly-line care," the survey found. Over 90% of the practices reported that they offer 11 of 14 "options" in care, from oral fluids, room to ambulate, and use of a bath, shower, or hot tub to encouragement of alternative positions.

Besides comparable outcomes and control over their childbirth experience, CNMs' clients "can look forward to longer prenatal visits, greater emphasis on education and birth preparation, and greater emotional support," the Nader group concluded.

Yet the responses showed CNMs still struggling for acceptance. Over 60% were coping with some kind of restriction: limits on prescribing and reimbursement, refusal of admitting privileges, and hospital policies that assume a medical model of care.

Reprinted with permission of *American Journal of Nursing* (1996). Nader group sees CNMs replacing OBs in "majority of American births." 96(1), 62, 65. Used with permission of Lippincott-Raven Publishers, Philadelphia, Pa.

Issues in Advanced Practice Nursing

Beginning in the early 1990s, some nursing leaders (Jones, 1994; Sparacino, 1993) began to express the belief that the boundaries between the roles of clinical nurse specialists and nurse practitioners were increasingly blurred. They wondered if nursing might benefit from having a common educational base and common title for these two advanced practice roles. This continues to be debated at the national level.

Linda Pearson (1995), editor-in-chief of the journal *The Nurse Practitioner* claimed that it is clear to insurance companies what physicians, hospitals, and dentists do, but that it is often not as clear what advanced practice nurses do. This impedes progress toward direct reimbursement for services for these highly qualified professionals. Nurses were challenged to be clear to the public about the services they are qualified to provide.

Pearson addressed another challenge, in 1995, when she asserted that although there had been some progress in state legislation to improve the scope of practice of advanced practice nurses, there was little to celebrate regarding national legislation (Pearson, 1995). By 1998, she sounded more optimistic, stating, "APNs and many other professionals have worked very hard with their state and national legislators to obtain the most autonomous practice possible. The success is showing!" (Pearson, 1998).

At the turn of the century, both the public and legislators at state and national levels had begun to appreciate the role advanced practice nurses played in increasing the efficiency of primary health care delivery while reducing costs. But until the U. S. Congress approves legislation to provide primary health care for all citizens and makes provisions for advanced practice nurses to share fully in the provision of that care, the practice parameters of advanced practice nurses are at the mercy of the various state legislatures.

There are substantial practice barriers because of the overlap between traditional medical and nursing functions. "The independent practice of nurses is a politically charged arena, with organized medicine firmly against all efforts of nurses to be recognized as independent health care providers who receive direct reimbursement for their services" (Stafford and Appleyard, 1994, p. 24). Nurses, through their professional associations, are continuing the efforts to change laws that limit the scope of nursing practice.

Employment Outlook in Nursing

In spite of some concerns about an oversupply of registered nurses as hospitals downsize (Pew Health Professionals Commission, 1995), the Bureau of Labor Statistics, a division of the U. S. Department of Labor, is confident about nursing's overall employment prospects. According to the Bureau, nurses can expect their employment opportunities to grow faster than the average in other occupations through the year 2006 (U. S. Department of Labor, 1998). Several factors are fueling this growth, including technological advances and the increasing emphasis on primary care. The aging of the nation's population also has an impact, since older people are more likely to require medical care. And as aging nurses retire, many additional job openings will result.

Opportunities in hospitals, traditionally the largest employers of nurses, will grow more slowly than those in community-based sectors. The most rapid hospital-based growth is projected to occur in outpatient facilities, such as same-day surgery departments, rehabilitation programs, and outpatient cancer centers.

Home health care positions are expected to increase the fastest of all. This is in response to the expanding elderly population's needs and preference for home care. Technological advances also are making it possible to bring increasingly complex treatments into the home.

Another expected area of high growth is nursing homes, which is a response to the larger number of frail elderly in their eighties and nineties requiring long-term care. As hospitals come under greater pressure to decrease the average patient length of stay, nursing home admissions will increase, as will growth in long-term rehabilitation units.

Another factor influencing employment patterns for registered nurses is the tendency for sophisticated medical procedures to be performed in physicians' offices, clinics, ambulatory surgical centers, and other outpatient settings. Registered nurses' expertise will be needed to care for patients undergoing procedures formerly performed only in hospital settings (U. S. Department of Labor, 1998).

Nurse practitioners can expect to find themselves in demand for the foreseeable future. The evolution of integrated health care networks focusing on primary care and health maintenance are ideal settings for advanced nursing practice.

Nursing Salaries

Salaries vary widely according to practice setting, level of preparation and credentials, and region of the country. The latest survey of *The Registered Nurse Population: 1996* (U. S. Department of Health and Human Services, 1997) shows positive signs in terms of salaries for registered nurses. The 1996 average annual salary of a full-time registered nurse in a staff position was $38,567, up from $35,212 in 1992. This represents an increase of 9.5 percent in four years (U. S. Department of Health and Human Services, 1997). While salaries are up nationwide, discussing salaries from a national perspective is often misleading. Salaries in urban areas are much higher than those in rural communities. Readers should bear this in mind when reviewing these figures. Regional salaries are more realistic measures. Figure 5–6 shows the average annual salaries of staff nurses in each geographical area of the United States. Regional variations are apparent.

The salaries of doctorally prepared nursing professors (the highest ranking faculty members) in the nation's colleges and universities averaged $66,132 in the 1998–99 academic year (American Association of Colleges of Nursing, 1999). Associate and assistant professors earned less, as did instructors. Nondoctorally prepared faculty also earned less at all ranks.

Nationwide, the average salary of nurse practitioners and certified nurse-midwives in 1996 was $54,182, but this varies widely according to specialty and geographic area. The average salary of clinical nurse specialists was $47,160, whereas certified registered nurse anesthetists averaged $86,319 (American Nurses Association, 1997). Clearly, additional preparation increases earning potential.

Figure 5–6

Average annual salaries of full-time registered nurses in staff positions by geographic region, March 1996 (Data from The Registered Nurse Population March 1996, Division of Nursing, U. S. Department of Health and Human Services, 1997).

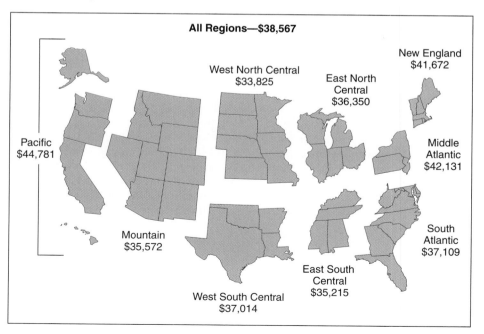

Summary of Key Points

- There are more than 2.5 million registered nurses in the United States, and over 2.1 million are actively practicing.
- Sixty percent of working nurses are employed in hospitals, a traditional setting for nursing practice, but one that will see dramatic changes as health care in the United States continues to become more community based.
- An exciting trend is the establishment of practice settings in home health, school nursing, and small health-related businesses.
- Increased use of advanced practice nurses can be part of the solution to the U. S. health care crisis brought on by the aging of the baby boom generation, technological advances, and cost-containment measures in the health care industry.
- Advanced practice nurses are capable of delivering high-quality care to many segments of the population not currently receiving health care or receiving substandard care.
- If the nation is to benefit from the services of advanced practice nurses, legal barriers to their practice must be removed through political action of organized nursing and politically active nurses.
- Although opinions are mixed, government projections are for the demand for nurses, particularly advanced practice nurses, to increase through the year 2005 and beyond.

Critical Thinking Questions

1. What characteristics do nurses of today have in common, and how do they differ?
2. Think of the areas of nursing that interest you most. How do your personal and professional qualifications compare with the characteristics needed in the roles discussed in this chapter?
3. Interview nurses in various practice settings, especially those not covered in this chapter. Find out how they prepared for their positions, what their daily activities are, and what they find most challenging and rewarding about their work.
4. Call the nurse recruiter or personnel office of a nearby hospital and inquire about salaries and other benefits for entry-level and advanced nursing practice positions. How do they compare with those listed in this chapter?
5. Interview an advanced practice nurse working in your community. What does he or she see as the major impediments to practice? Find out what legislative initiatives are being undertaken to remove these barriers in your state.

Web Resources

American Academy of Nurse Practitioners, http://www.aanp.org

American Association of Colleges of Nursing, http://www.aacn.nche.edu

American Association of Nurse Anesthetists, http://www.aana.org

American Association of Occupational Health Nurses, http://www.aaohn.org

American Board of Occupational Health Nurses, http://www.abohn.org

American College of Nurse-Midwives, http://www.acnm.org

American College of Nurse Practitioners, http://www.nurse.org/acnp

American Nurses Credentialing Center, http://www.ancc.org

Home Health Care Nurses Association, HHNA @puetzamc.com

International Parish Nurse Resource Center, http://www.advocatehealth.com/sites/pnursctr.html

National Association of School Nurses, http://www.nasn.org

(The) Nurse Practitioner (journal), http://www.springnet.com/np

Nursing Informatics, http://www.fitne.net

U. S. Department of Health and Human Services, Division of Nursing, http://158.72.83.3/bhpr/dn/dn.htm

References

Abuelouf, A. (1998). Community health ministry: Meeting many needs. *Tennessee Nurse,* 61(6), 22, 31.

American Association of Colleges of Nursing (1999). *1997–1998 salaries of instructional and administrative faculty in baccalaureate and graduate programs in nursing,* Washington, D. C.: American Association of Colleges of Nursing.

American College of Nurse-Midwives (1999). Basic facts about certified nurse-midwives. Available from http://www.acnm.org/press/basicfac.htm.

American Journal of Nursing (1996). Nader group sees CNMs replacing OBs in "majority of American births." 96(1), 62, 65.

American Nurses Association (1993). *Advanced practice nursing: A new age in health care.* Kansas City, Mo.: American Nurses Association.

American Nurses Association (1994). *The scope of practice for nursing informatics.* Washington, D. C.: American Nurses Association.

American Nurses Association (1997). *Workforce trends among U. S. registered nurses.* Available from http://www.nursingworld.org/readroom/usworker.htm.

American Nurses Association and Health Ministries Association (1998). *Scope and standards of parish nursing practice.* Washington, D. C.: American Nurses Association and Health Ministries Association.

Anderson, C. A. (1994). Nursing faculty: Who are they, what do they do, and what challenges do they face? In J. C. McCloskey and H. K. Grace (Eds.), *Current issues in nursing* (pp. 32–37). St. Louis: Mosby.

Carey, A. R., and Mullins, M. E. (1995). Schools lack enough nurses. *USA Today* (Source: Asthma Zero Mortality Coalition).

Jones, D. A. (1994). Advanced practice: Merging the roles of the nurse practitioner and clinical specialist. In O. L. Strickland and D. J. Fishman (Eds.), *Nursing issues in the 1990's* (pp. 126–132). Albany: Delmar.

McKenzie, C. B., Torkelson, N. G., and Holt, M. A. (1989). Care and cost: Nursing case management improves both. *Nursing management,* 20(10), 30–34.

Moccia, P. (1992). In 1992: A nurse in every school. *Nursing & Health Care,* 13(1), 14–18.

National League for Nursing (1997). *Nursing data review 1997.* New York: National League for Nursing.

Pearson, L. J. (1995). Annual update of how each state stands on legislative issues affecting advanced nursing practice. *The Nurse Practitioner,* 20(1), 13–63.

Pearson, L. J. (1999). Annual update of how each state stands on legislative issues affecting advanced nursing practice. *The Nurse Practitioner,* 24(1), 16–83.

Pew Health Professions Commission (1995). *Critical challenges: Revitalizing the health professions for the twenty-first century* (Third Report). San Francisco: University of California, Center for the Health Professions.

Sparacino, P. S. A. (1993). The advanced practice nurse: Is the time right for a singular title? *Clinical Nurse Specialist,* 7(1), 3.

Stafford, M., and Appleyard, J. (1994). Clinical nurse specialists and nurse practitioners: Who are they, what do they do, and what challenges do they face? In J. C. McCloskey and H. K. Grace (Eds.), *Current issues in nursing* (pp. 32–37). St. Louis: Mosby.

U. S. Department of Health and Human Services, Division of Nursing, (1997). *The registered nurse population: March 1996.* Washington, D. C.: Government Printing Office.

U. S. Department of Labor, Bureau of Labor Statistics (1998). *Occupational outlook handbook, 1998–99 edition.* Washington, D. C.: Government Printing Office.

U. S. Department of Labor, Bureau of Labor Statistics (1992). *Occupational wage survey: Hospitals.* Washington, D. C.: Government Printing Office.

Vollman, K. M. (1999). My search to help patients breathe. *Reflections,* 25(2), 16–18.

Defining Profession

Kay K. Chitty

Key Terms

Accountability
Altruism
Autonomy
Code of Ethics
Cognitive
Collegiality
Flexner Report
Helping Profession
Nursing Process
Occupation
Profession
Professional
Professionalism

Learning Outcomes

After studying this chapter, students will be able to:

- Identify the characteristics of a profession.
- Distinguish between the characteristics of professions and occupations.
- Describe how professions evolve.
- Evaluate nursing's current status as a profession.
- Explain the elements of nursing's contract with society.
- Recognize characteristic behaviors of professional nurses.

What is a **profession,** and who can be called a professional? These terms are used loosely in everyday conversation. Historically, only medicine, law, and the ministry were accepted as professions. Today, however, **professional** is a term commonly used to identify many types of people, ranging from wrestlers and rock stars to college professors and archaeologists. Are all these individuals professionals? The answer to that question depends on how profession is defined.

In sports, a professional is distinguished from an amateur by being paid. Amateur golfers, for example, are not supposed to accept money; professional golfers compete for it. So in sports, making money is one characteristic of being a professional. Professionals are generally better at what they do than are others. Therefore, in most fields, expertise is also a part of being a professional. As you will see, however, there are many other criteria to be examined in a discussion of what makes a true profession.

Characteristics of a Profession

Over the years, many thoughtful people have grappled with the meaning of **professionalism.** In the early 1900s, the Carnegie Foundation issued a series of papers about professional schools. The first of these reports was based on sociologist Abraham Flexner's 1910 study of medical education (Flexner, 1910). The **Flexner Report,** as it became known, is a classic piece of educational literature that provided the impetus for the much-needed reform of medical education.

Flexner went on to study other disciplines and later, in a paper about social work, published a list of criteria that he believed were characteristic of all true professions (Flexner, 1915). Since Flexner's original criteria were published, they have been widely used as a benchmark for determining the status of various occupations in terms of professionalism and have had a profound influence on professional education in several disciplines, including nursing.

In recent years there has been concern that traditional definitions of profession, such as Flexner's, are incomplete because they embody only the masculine worldview. Some believe that adhering to traditional criteria for professions has had the effect of relegating nursing, teaching, social work, and other female-dominated fields to the status of "semiprofessions."

Flexner's Criteria

With contemporary feminist concerns in mind, let us examine Flexner's criteria of a profession. He believed that professional work:

1. Is basically intellectual (as opposed to physical) and is accompanied by a high degree of individual responsibility.
2. Is based on a body of knowledge that can be learned and is refreshed and refined through research.
3. Is practical, in addition to being theoretical.
4. Can be taught through a process of highly specialized professional education.
5. Has a strong internal organization of members and a well-developed group consciousness.
6. Has practitioners who are motivated by altruism (the desire to help others) and who are responsive to public interests (Fig. 6–1).

Since 1915, a number of other authorities have also identified criteria for professions, which built on and vary slightly from Flexner's.

Bixler's and Bixler's Criteria

Genevieve and Roy Bixler, a husband and wife team of nonnurses who were nevertheless advocates and supporters of nursing, first wrote about the status of nursing as a profession in 1945. In 1959, they again appraised nursing according to their original seven criteria, noting the progress made (Bixler and Bixler, 1959). Their criteria included the following:

1. "A profession utilizes in its practice a well-defined and well-organized body of specialized knowledge which is on the intellectual level of the higher learning" (p. 1142).

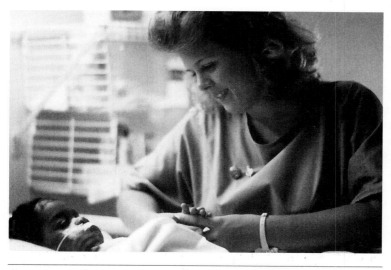

Figure 6-1
According to Flexner, professionals are motivated by altruism, a desire to help others (Courtesy of Medical University of South Carolina).

2. "A profession constantly enlarges the body of knowledge it uses and improves its techniques of education and service by the use of the scientific method" (p. 1143).
3. "A profession entrusts the education of its practitioners to institutions of higher education" (p. 1144).
4. "A profession applies its body of knowledge in practical services which are vital to human and social welfare" (p. 1145).
5. "A profession functions autonomously in the formulation of professional policy and in the control of professional activity thereby" (p. 1145).
6. "A profession attracts individuals of intellectual and personal qualities who exalt service above personal gain and who recognize their chosen occupation as a life work" (p. 1146).
7. "A profession strives to compensate its practitioners by providing freedom of action, opportunity for continuous professional growth, and economic security" (p. 1146).

A comparison of Flexner's and Bixler's and Bixler's criteria reveals many similarities. General agreement exists about what constitutes a profession, but not all people agree about which occupations are professional. How contemporary nursing stacks up as a profession is discussed later.

The Evolution from Occupation to Profession

Professions usually evolve from occupations that originally consisted of tasks but developed more specialized educational pathways and publicly legitimized status. The established professions, such as law, medicine, and the ministry, generally followed a typical developmental pattern of stages that occurred sequentially. First, practitioners performed full-time work in the discipline. They then determined work standards, identified a body of knowledge, and established educational programs in institutions of higher learning. Next, they promoted organizing into effective occupational associations. Then they worked toward legal protection that limited practice of their unique skills by outsiders. Finally, they established codes of ethics (Carr-Saunders and Wilson, 1933).

Occupation is often used interchangeably with *profession,* but their definitions differ. Webster defines *occupation* as "what occupies, or engages, one's time; business; employment." *Profession* is defined as "a vocation requiring advanced training . . . , and usually involving mental rather than manual work, as teaching, engineering, etc.; especially, medicine, law, or theology (formerly called the learned professions)" (*Webster's,* 1996). There is widespread overall agreement that a profession is different from an occupation in at least two major ways—preparation and commitment.

Preparation

Professional preparation usually takes place in a college or university setting. Preparation is prolonged to include instruction in the specialized body of knowledge and techniques of the profession. Professional preparation includes more than knowledge and skills, however. It also includes orientation to the beliefs, values, and attitudes expected of the members of the profession. Standards of practice and ethical considerations are also included. These components of professional education are part of the process of socialization into a profession and are discussed in Chapter 8. According to Miller (1985), preparation enables professional practitioners to act in a logical, rational manner rather than relying on intuition and speculation. Notice that this gives no credence to intuition, long considered a feminine attribute, as an important consequence of preparation.

Commitment

Professionals' commitment to their profession is strong. They derive much of their personal identification from their work and consider it an integral part of their lives. People engaging in a profession often consider it their "calling." Professionals' commitment to their profession historically has transcended their expectation of material reward. Although people may readily change occupations, it is less common for people to change professions. Several critical differences between occupations and professions are summarized in Table 6–1.

Helping Professions

Historically, nursing has been considered one of the helping professions. Groups in this category include, among others, social workers, teachers, counselors, probation officers, and youth workers. A **helping profession** is pri-

TABLE 6-1
Comparison of Characteristics of Occupations and Professions

Occupation	Profession
Training may occur on the job.	Education takes place in a college or university.
Length of training varies.	Education is prolonged.
Work is largely manual.	Work involves mental creativity.
Relies largely on experience or trial and error to guide decision making.	Relies largely on science or theoretical constructs to guide decision making.
Values, beliefs, and ethics are not prominent features of preparation.	Values, beliefs, and ethics are an integral part of preparation.
Commitment and personal identification vary.	Commitment and personal identification are strong.
Workers are supervised.	Workers are autonomous.
People often change jobs.	People unlikely to change professions.
Material reward is main motivation.	Commitment transcends material reward.
Accountability rests with employer.	Accountability rests with individual.

marily committed to assisting clients. Personalized care of clients is central to a helping profession's practice, and their needs take precedence above all else. There is a selfless dedication to duty and putting the needs of others first. Making a substantial salary is not usually the most important factor to those in the helping professions. The helping professions are imbued with a service ideology and a sense of vocation. Helping professionals often see their role as the regulation and control of problematical areas of social life.

The concept of caring is a central part of the helping professions. Helping professionals demonstrate their particular type of caring through their professional expertise. A challenge for nursing and the other helping professions is attempting to care in a society that, by and large, does not value caring but instead values material goods and profits as measures of success.

Nursing as a Profession

An ongoing subject for discussion in nursing circles has been the question: "Is nursing a profession?" Much has been written on both sides of this issue over the years. Nursing sociologists do not all agree that nursing is a profession. Some believe that it is, at best, an *emerging profession*. Others cite the progress nursing has made toward meeting the commonly accepted criteria for full-fledged professional status. Still others believe that nursing leaders, by embracing the masculine orientation to professionalism embodied in the work of Flexner and others, supported the existing patriarchal order, thereby prolonging the subordination of nursing to male-dominated professions such as medicine.

Kelly's Criteria

Kelly (1981, p. 157), for example, reiterated and expanded Flexner's criteria in her 1981 listing of characteristics of a profession:

1. The services provided are vital to humanity and the welfare of society.
2. There is a special body of knowledge that is continually enlarged through research.
3. The services involve intellectual activities; individual responsibility (**accountability**) is a strong feature.
4. Practitioners are educated in institutions of higher learning.
5. Practitioners are relatively independent and control their own policies and activities (**autonomy**).
6. Practitioners are motivated by service (**altruism**) and consider their work an important component of their lives.
7. There is a **code of ethics** to guide the decisions and conduct of practitioners.
8. There is an organization (association) that encourages and supports high standards of practice.

Recognizing that feminine strengths, such as informed intuition, are not included in traditional lists of criteria for a profession, let us examine how well contemporary nursing fulfills them.

"The Services Provided Are Vital to Humanity and the Welfare of Society"

If any group of students were asked why they chose nursing, most would reply, "To help people." Certainly nursing is a service that is essential to the well-being of people and to society as a whole. Nursing promotes the maintenance and restoration of health of individuals, groups, and communities. Assisting others to attain the highest level of wellness of which they are capable is the goal of nursing. Caring, meaning nurturing and helping others, is a basic component of professional nursing.

"There Is a Special Body of Knowledge That Is Continually Enlarged through Research"

In the past, nursing was based on principles borrowed from the physical and social sciences and other disciplines. Today, however, there is a body of knowledge that is uniquely nursing's. Although this was not always so, the amount of investigation and analysis of nursing care has expanded rapidly in the past 30 years. Nursing theory development is also proceeding swiftly. Nursing is no longer based on trial and error but increasingly relies on theory and research as a basis for practice. Several theoretical models of nursing are discussed in Chapter 11, and issues in research are discussed in Chapter 12.

"The Services Involve Intellectual Activities; Individual Responsibility (Accountability) Is a Strong Feature"

Nursing has developed and refined its own unique approach to practice, called the **nursing process**. The nursing process is essentially a **cognitive** (mental) activity that requires both critical and creative thinking and serves as the basis for providing nursing care. There is more about the nursing process in Chapter 15.

Individual accountability in nursing has become the hallmark of practice. Accountability, according to the American Nurses Association's (ANA) *Code for Nurses* (1985, p. 8), is "being answerable to someone for something one has done. It means providing an explanation to self, to the client, to the employing agency, to the nursing profession, and to society." Through legal opinions and court cases, society has demonstrated that it, too, holds nurses individually responsible for their actions as well as for those of unlicensed personnel under their supervision.

"Practitioners are Educated in Institutions of Higher Learning"

As presented in Chapter 2, the first university-based nursing program began in 1909 at the University of Minnesota. Several studies, including Esther Lucille Brown's 1948 report, *Nursing for the Future,* called for nursing education to be based in universities and colleges. Recall that another milestone was the 1965 position paper of the ANA, which called for all nursing education to take place in institutions of higher education (American Nurses Association, 1965).

The majority of programs offering basic nursing education are now associate degree and baccalaureate programs located in colleges and universities. There are growing numbers of master's and doctoral programs in nursing, although the number of graduates is small compared with other health professions. Because professional status and power increase with postgraduate education, a legitimate question is "How can nursing take its place as a peer among the professions when most nurses currently in practice hold less than a baccalaureate degree?" The differentiation between professional nursing and technical nursing is a challenging issue that nursing has not yet resolved. Educational diversity within nursing has slowed the progress toward acceptance of the baccalaureate or higher degree as the prerequisite for professional practice. Lack of resolution of these differences threatens to undermine nursing's continued steady development as a profession (Christman, 1998).

"Practitioners Are Relatively Independent and Control Their Own Policies and Activities (Autonomy)"

Autonomy, or control over one's practice, is another controversial area for nursing. Although many nursing actions are independent, most nurses are employed in hospitals, where authority resides in one's position. One's place in the hierarchy, rather than expertise, confers or denies power and status. Physicians are widely regarded as gatekeepers, and their authorization or supervision is required before many activities can occur. Nurse practice acts in most states reinforce nursing's arguable self-determination by requiring that nurses perform certain actions only when authorized by supervising physicians or hospital protocols.

There are at least three groups that have historically attempted to control nursing practice: organized medicine, health service administration, and organized nursing. Both the medical profession and health service administration have historically attempted to maintain control of nursing because they believe it is in their best interest to keep nurses dependent on them. Both are well organized and have powerful lobbies at state and national levels.

Organized nursing promotes independence and autonomy, but its power is fragmented by subgroups and dissension. Rivalry among diploma-educated, associate degree-educated, and baccalaureate-educated nurses saps the vitality of the profession. The proliferation of nursing organizations (see Box 4–2 for a partial list) and competition among them for members also diminish nursing's potential. Only 8 percent of the 2.5 million registered nurses in the United States are members of the ANA (American Nurses Association, 1999). The fact that most nurses are not members of any professional organization impairs nursing's ability to lobby effectively. These are major challenges for nursing if it is to realize its potential collective professional power and autonomy.

"Practitioners Are Motivated by Service (Altruism) and Consider Their Work an Important Component of Their Lives"

As a group, nurses are dedicated to the ideal of service to others, which is also known as altruism. This ideal has sometimes become intertwined with economic issues and historically has been exploited by employers of nurses. No one questions the right of other professionals to charge reasonable fees for the services they render; when nurses want higher salaries, however, others sometimes call their altruism into question. Nurses must take responsibility for their own financial well-being and for the health of the profession. This will, in turn, ensure its continued attractiveness to those who might choose nursing as a career. If there are to be adequate numbers of nurses to meet society's needs, salaries must be comparable with those in competing disciplines. Being concerned with salary issues does nothing to diminish a nurse's altruism or professionalism.

Another issue, consideration of work as a primary component of life, has been a thornier problem for nurses. Commitment to a career is not a value equally shared by all nurses. Some still regard nursing as a job and drop in and out of practice depending on economic and family needs. This approach, although appealing to many female nurses and conducive to traditional family management, has retarded the development of professional attitudes and behaviors for the profession as a whole.

BOX 6–1
The Florence Nightingale Pledge

I solemnly pledge myself before God and in the presence of this assembly to pass my life in purity and to practice my profession faithfully.

I will abstain from whatever is deleterious and mischievous, and will not take or knowingly administer any harmful drug. I will do all in my power to maintain and elevate the standard of my profession, and will hold in confidence all personal matters committed to my keeping and all family affairs coming to my knowledge in the practice of my calling.

With loyalty will I endeavor to aid the physician in his work and devote myself to the welfare of those committed to my care.

Reprinted with permission of Pillitteri, A. (1991). Documenting Lystra Gretter's student experiences in nursing. *Nursing Outlook*, 39(6), 273–279.

"There Is a Code of Ethics to Guide the Decisions and Conduct of Practitioners"

An ethical code does not stipulate how an individual should act in a specific situation; rather, it provides professional standards and a framework for decision making. The trust placed in the nursing profession by the public requires that nurses act with integrity. To aid them in doing so, both the International Council of Nurses (ICN) and the ANA have established codes of nursing ethics through which standards of practice are established, promoted, and refined. Appendix A contains the ANA's Code for Nurses.

In 1893, long before these codes were written, "The Florence Nightingale Pledge" (Box 6–1) was created by a committee headed by Lystra Eggert Gretter and presented to the Farrand Training School for Nurses located at Harper Hospital in Detroit, Michigan (Pillitteri, 1991). The Nightingale pledge can be considered nursing's first code of ethics.

"There Is an Organization (Association) That Encourages and Supports High Standards of Practice"

As shown in Chapter 4, nursing has a number of professional associations that were formed to promote the improvement of the profession. Foremost among these is the ANA, the purposes of which are to foster high standards of nursing practice, promote professional and educational advancement of nurses, and promote the welfare of nurses to the end that all people have better nursing care (Fig. 6–2) (American Nurses Association, 1970). The ANA is also the official voice of nursing and therefore is the primary advocate for nursing interests in general. Unfortunately, fewer than 1 out of 10 nurses belongs to this official professional organization. The political power that could be derived from the unified efforts of 2.5 million registered nurses nationwide would be impressive; that goal has not yet been realized.

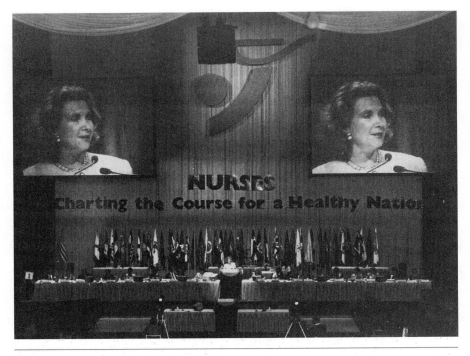

Figure 6-2
Professionals belong to associations that encourage and support ethical standards of practice (Courtesy of American Nurses Association).

Nursing's Social Policy Statement: A Contract with Society

Although criteria for professions vary, all professions have one criterion in common: an obligation to the recipients of their services. Nursing, therefore, has an obligation to those who receive nursing care. The nature of the social contract between the members of the nursing profession and society is summarized in *Nursing's Social Policy Statement*. This document, the result of several years of work by literally hundreds of nurses, serves "as a framework for understanding nursing's relationship with society and nursing's obligation to those who receive nursing care" (p. 1). A careful reading of this brief document will provide the reader with the essence of nursing's professionalism. It is available from the publications department of the American Nurses Association.

Collegiality as an Attribute of the Professional Nurse

An often overlooked but increasingly important aspect of professionalism in nursing is **collegiality.** The promotion of collaboration, cooperation, and recognition of interdependence among members of the nursing profession is the essence of collegiality. Professional nurses demonstrate collegiality by sharing with, supporting, assisting, and counseling other nurses and nursing students. These behaviors can be seen when nurses, for example, take part in professional organizations, mentor less experienced nurses, willingly serve as role models for nursing students, welcome learners and their instructors in the practice setting, assist researchers with data gathering, publish in professional literature, and support peer-assistance programs for impaired nurses. The value placed on collegiality as a professional attribute can be seen in the ANA's 1998 (p. 15) publication, *Standards of Clinical Nursing Practice,* 2nd edition, which includes collegiality as one of only eight standards of professional performance. The practice of nursing would be enhanced if the commitment nurses feel toward their clients was equalled by their commitment to one another and to the next generation of professional nurses.

Characteristic Behaviors of Professional Nurses

If being a professional nurse is different from practicing the occupation of nursing, there must be certain behaviors that differentiate the two. As students develop their ideas of how they want to function as nursing professionals, it may help to have an ideal in mind. Many students already know a nurse they consider to be a role model of professionalism. If not, there may be interest in hearing about Joan, the subject of the following case study.

Joan: A Case Study in Professionalism	Professional Behaviors Demonstrated
Joan is a 32-year-old married mother of two. She graduated from River City College of Nursing at the age of 26 and has been practicing since her graduation. Her first position was as a staff nurse at Providence Hospital, a 300-bed private hospital. Nursing administration at Providence encourages nurses to provide individualized nursing care while protecting the dignity and autonomy of each patient and family. She chose Providence because the philosophy of nursing there paralleled her own. Another reason for selecting this hospital was that Joan wanted to practice oncology (cancer) nursing, and there is an oncology unit at Providence.	Has developed own philosophy of nursing
Each day Joan uses the nursing process in caring for her patients and in dealing with their families. That means she assesses their condition, plans and implements their care, and evaluates the care she has given. Then she enters what she has done in each patient's database in the accepted format. She communicates clearly to the other members of the nursing staff and to the other health care professionals involved in the care of the patients on her unit.	Self-determination Uses critical thinking Collaborates and communicates with other health professionals; demonstrates collegiality
After two years as a staff nurse, Joan accepted a position as a team leader. This means that now she takes responsibility not only for	

Demonstrates self-regulation and accountability for self and others

Committed to lifelong learning

Active in professional organization

Mentors aspiring professionals

Recognizes own limits; seeks help when needed

Contributes to expansion of nursing's body of knowledge

Provides leadership

Uses principles of time management

Delegates responsibility wisely

Represents profession to the public

Models altruism

Is self-aware

her own practice but also for that of licensed practical nurses and nursing assistants on her team. To do this effectively, she stays abreast of changes in her state's nursing practice act and Providence Hospital's policies and procedures. In addition, she updates her knowledge by reading current journals and research periodicals. She makes it a policy to attend at least two nursing conferences each year to stay on top of trends. She belongs to her professional organization and participates as an active member. She finds that this is another source of the latest information on professional issues.

Joan looks forward to working with the nursing students at Providence Hospital. She remembers when she was a student and how a word from a practicing nurse could make or break her day. Of course, students do mean extra work, but she sees this as a part of her role and patiently provides the guidance they need, even when she is busy.

In the course of her daily work, Joan sometimes has a question about certain procedures. She is not embarrassed to seek help from more experienced nurses, from textbooks, or from other health professionals. Sometimes she offers suggestions to the head nurse and the oncology clinical nurse specialist about possible research questions and participates in gathering data when the unit takes on a research study.

Providence Hospital uses a shared governance model, which means nurses serve on committees that develop and interpret nursing policies and procedures. Joan serves on two committees and chairs another. Right now the hospital is preparing a self-study for an upcoming accreditation, so the meetings are frequent. Instead of complaining about the meetings, Joan prepares and organizes her portion of the meeting so that everyone's time is used most effectively. She has to delegate some of her patient care responsibilities to others while she is attending meetings. Because she has taken the time to know the other workers' skills and abilities, she does not worry about what happens while she is gone.

At the end of the day when Joan goes home, she occasionally gets a call from a friend with a health-related question or a request to give a neighbor's child an allergy injection. Although she is tired, she recognizes that in the eyes of others, she represents the nursing profession. She is proud to be trusted and respected for her knowledge, skills, and dedication. Helping others through nursing care is something Joan has wanted to do since she was small, and she finds it very fulfilling.

Lately, Joan has recognized in herself some troubling signs: She has been irritable and impatient with family and co-workers and generally out of sorts. She has gained weight and is exercising less than usual. She wonders if working with terminally ill patients and their families is the source of her stress. Joan's husband suggested that she take "a break" from nursing and stay home with the children, but after talking it over with her nurse manager, she decided to ask for assignment to different nursing responsibilities for a while. She knows that she needs to be her own advocate and take care of herself. Next week she will begin a three-month stint in outpatient surgery, where she believes the emotional intensity will be a bit lower.

Demonstrates commitment to nursing as a career

Models healthy coping behaviors

This brief description illustrates more than 18 characteristic behaviors exhibited by professional nurses. Nursing is clearly much more than an occupation to Joan and to many others like her. The accompanying Research Note (Holl, 1994) describes several factors that are related to the development of professionalism in nurses.

Summary of Key Points

- Commitment to a profession is different from commitment to a job or an occupation.
- Flexner, Bixler and Bixler, and Kelly, all of whom have studied professions, agree that there are several characteristics that all true professions have in common.
- A body of knowledge, specialized education, service to society, accountability, autonomy, and ethical standards are a few of the hallmarks of professions.
- The feminist perspective includes the belief that the emphasis on professionalism has not helped nursing and has prevented nurses from appreciating, valuing, exploring, and refining the feminine caring experience (Wuest, 1994).
- Although nursing has a briefer history than some traditional professions and is still dealing with autonomy, preparation, and commitment issues,

RESEARCH NOTE

Research Note

Rita M. Holl conducted a study of registered nurses to determine which characteristics influenced professional beliefs and decision making. The characteristics she was interested in included age, years of practice, area of practice, level of education, certification, and membership in professional organizations.

She developed a survey instrument and asked 133 registered nurse subjects how they would deal with real-life nurse-patient situations. Results were analyzed according to the degree of independence required, the degree to which they met the patient's needs, and their professional standards.

Holl found that professional beliefs and decision making were related to level of education, membership in professional organizations, and certification. Critical care nurses demonstrated higher levels of independent decision making than did nurses in other areas of practice. The results of this study supported, in general, the notion that nurses who continue their education and belong to professional organizations are more likely to be independent thinkers and to participate in creative problem solving.

Adapted with permission of Holl, R. M. (1994). Characteristics of the registered nurse and professional beliefs and decision making. *Critical Care Nursing Quarterly*, 17(3), 60–66.

great progress has been made in moving nursing toward full professional status.

- An awareness of the characteristics of professions and professional behavior helps nurses assume leadership in continuing progress toward professionalism.
- *Nursing's Social Policy Statement* can be thought of as nursing's contract with society.
- Being a professional is a dynamic process, not a condition or state of being.
- Professional growth evolves throughout the different stages of nurses' careers.

Critical Thinking Questions

1. How might nursing be different today if all its practitioners viewed it as their profession rather than a job?
2. What impact might the traditional male orientation to work as a lifelong career commitment have on the potential for success of men in nursing?
3. What is the relationship between training and education?
4. On a scale of 1 to 10, rate nursing on each of Flexner's, Bixler's, and Bixler's, and Kelly's criteria for professions.
5. Identify at least two concerns about traditional views of professionalism expressed by nurses with a feminist perspective.
6. Describe at least five characteristic behaviors of professional nurses.
7. Discuss the Nightingale Pledge (Box 6–1) as a historical document, as an ethical statement, and as a reflection of Florence Nightingale's social and cultural environment. What value does this document have for today's nurse?

Web Resources

Characteristics of a profession, http://www.ship.edu/ ~ library/instruction/professions.htm

List of professional characteristics in nurses, http://www.jan.ucc.nau.edu/ ~ erw/nur301/profession/characteristics/assign1-2-2.html

References

American Nurses Association (1965). *Educational preparation for nurse practitioners and assistants to nurses: A position paper.* Kansas City, Mo.: American Nurses Association.

American Nurses Association (1970). *Association bylaws.* Kansas City, Mo.: American Nurses Association.

American Nurses Association (1985). *Code for nurses with interpretive statements.* Washington, D. C.: American Nurses Association.

American Nurses Association (1995). *Nursing's social policy statement.* Washington, D. C.: American Nurses Association.

American Nurses Association (1998). *Standards of clinical nursing practice* (2nd ed.), Washington, D. C.: American Nurses Association.

American Nurses Association (1999). Personal communication via MEMBERINFO @ana.org.

Bixler, G. K., and Bixler, R. W. (1959). The professional status of nursing. *American Journal of Nursing,* 59(8), 1142–1147.

Brown, E. L. (1948). *Nursing for the future.* New York: Russell Sage Foundation.

Carr-Saunders, A. M., and Wilson, P. A. (1933). *The professions.* Oxford: Clarendon Press.

Christman, L. (1998). Who is a nurse? *Image: Journal of Nursing Scholarship,* 30(3), 211–214.

Flexner, A. (1910). *Medical education in the United States and Canada: A report to the Carnegie Foundation for the advancement of teaching.* Bethesda, Md.: Science & Health Publications.

Flexner, A. (1915). Is social work a profession? *School Society,* 1(26), 901.

Holl, R. M. (1994). Characteristics of the registered nurse and professional beliefs and decision making. *Critical Care Nursing Quarterly,* 17(3), 60–66.

Kelly, L. (1981). *Dimensions of professional nursing* (4th ed.). New York: Macmillan.

Miller, B. K. (1985). Just what is a professional? *Nursing Success Today,* 2(4), 21–27.

Pillitteri, A. (1991). Documenting Lystra Gretter's student experiences in nursing. *Nursing Outlook,* 39(6), 273–279.

Webster's new world dictionary. (1996). New York: Simon and Schuster.

Wuest, J. (1994). Professionalism and the evolution of nursing as a discipline: A feminist perspective. *Journal of Professional Nursing,* 19(6), 357–367.

Defining Nursing

Kay K. Chitty

7

Learning Outcomes

After studying this chapter, students will be able to:

- Recognize the evolutionary nature of definitions.
- Compare early definitions of nursing with contemporary ones.
- Recognize the impact of historical, social, economic, and political events on definitions of nursing.
- Identify commonalities in existing definitions of nursing.
- Develop personal definitions of nursing.

Definitions of nursing seek to describe who nurses are and what they do. It may be surprising to learn that finding a universally acceptable definition of nursing has been a long sought after but elusive goal. It seems that even nurses themselves have been unable to agree on one definition. For more than 150 years individuals, including the venerable Florence Nightingale, and organizations, such as the International Council of Nurses (ICN) and the American Nurses Association (ANA), have made attempts to achieve a consensus on a definition of nursing. Some efforts have been more successful than others. Despite the inability of those in the profession to agree on one definition, most of the definitions reviewed in this chapter have commonalities. Considering the variations in knowledge and technology during the different points in history when these definitions were written, the similarities are remarkable. All the definitions were rooted in history, affected by significant political, economic, and social events that shaped the form of nursing as it is now known.

Why Define Nursing?

Why is it important for people to spend time trying to define nursing? Having an accepted definition of nursing is helpful in a variety of ways and provides a framework for nursing practice. It establishes the parameters, or boundaries, of the profession; identifies the purposes and functions of the work; and guides the educational preparation of aspiring practitioners. Definitions of nursing are often included in laws, such as nurse practice acts.

Definitions Identify Purposes and Functions

To illustrate the benefits of defining human activity, suppose a person was told that he had been selected to play on a major league baseball team, but he did not know how to play. So he asked the team owner, "What is important for me to know about baseball?" And she said, "Just win games!" Then he went to a pitcher, who showed him a fast ball, a curve ball, and a slider. From there he went to a batting coach, who showed him how to hit fast balls, slow balls, and sliders. When he went to a fielding coach, he was told how to cover the bases and catch balls. Next, he consulted a trainer who showed him how to condition his body to avoid injuries. He has spent a great deal of time and still does not have an overall picture of baseball. Now, suppose he had been told initially, "Baseball is a game played with a ball and a bat on a large field on which there are three bases and a home plate. There are two nine-member teams, one at bat and one in the field. The object of the game is for a member of the batting team to hit a pitched ball and to run around the bases to home plate without being called out. The team with the most runs at the end of nine turns at bat wins."

Although this description leaves out a lot of detail, it succinctly states the boundaries of the game and the purpose of the game and gives guidance on how to play the game. Therefore, this overview would be more useful as a first step in an attempt to master baseball than the unorganized approach of talking to owners, players, and coaches and coming up with a piecemeal appreciation of the game.

So it is with definitions. They are a good place to begin in attempting to understand any complex enterprise such as nursing.

Definitions Differentiate Nursing from Other Health Occupations

The proliferation of various types of health care workers in the past two decades has led to the development of over 200 different allied health occupations (Jacox, 1997). Each new advance in technology bred a new "technician" who needed to be educated, hired, oriented, and paid with health care dollars. The resulting cost led to significant redesign of the health care system during the 1990s, accompanied by a period of redefining roles within the system. Defining the essence of nursing care has become even more important in light of these changes in order to manage the overlap of nursing with other fields without losing the core identify of nursing.

Definitions Are Needed in Legislation Regulating Practice

Another very practical reason to define nursing is that nursing practice is regulated by the states. Nurse practice acts need to reflect the increasing expertise and autonomy of nurses today so that the lay public and legislators who pass laws regulating nursing practice understand what nurses do. Otherwise, nurse practice acts will remain restrictive and inhibit professional growth (Dracup and Bryan-Brown, 1997).

Evolution of Definitions of Nursing

In the last century and a half since nursing became a progressively formal area of study and practice, many have attempted to distill into one definition the essence of nursing. This section reviews a number of definitions that evolved over the years.

Nightingale Defines Nursing

Florence Nightingale was the first person to recognize that the complex and multifaceted nature of nursing led to difficulty in defining it. Considering how relatively undeveloped nursing was during her time, Nightingale's definitions contain surprisingly contemporary concepts. Remember that during Nightingale's day, formal schooling in nursing was just beginning. In writing *Notes on Nursing: What It Is and What It Is Not* in 1859, she became the first person to attempt a written definition of nursing. She wrote, "And what nursing has to do . . . is put the patient in the best condition for nature to act upon him" (Nightingale, [1859] 1946, p. 75). She also wrote:

> I use the word nursing for want of a better. It has been limited to signify little more than the administration of medicines and the application of poultices. It ought to signify the proper use of fresh air, light, warmth, cleanliness, quiet, and the proper selection and administration of diet—all at the least expense of vital power to the patient (Nightingale, [1859] 1946, p. 6).

Although Nightingale lived in a time when little was known about disease processes and available treatments were extremely limited, these definitions foreshadowed contemporary nursing's focus on the therapeutic **milieu** (environment) as well as the modern emphasis on **health promotion** and **health maintenance.** She accurately observed that while possessing observational skills does not make a good nurse, without these skills a nurse is ineffective. Indeed, observation has always been an integral part of the process of nursing. Nightingale was also the first person to differentiate between nursing provided by a professional nurse using a unique body of knowledge and nursing care such as a mother would perform for an ill child.

Early Twentieth-Century Definitions

Fifty years after Nightingale wrote *Notes on Nursing,* the search for a definition began in earnest. Following the English model, many schools of nursing had been established in the United States, and numbers of "trained nurses" were in practice. They sought to develop a professional identity for their rapidly expanding discipline. Shaw's *Textbook of Nursing* (1907, pp. 1–2) defined nursing as an art: "It properly includes as well as the execution of specific orders, the administration of food and medicine, the personal care of the patient." Harmer's *Textbook of the Principles and Practice of Nursing* (1922) elaborated on Shaw's bare-bones definition: "The object of nursing is not only to cure the sick . . . but to bring health and ease, rest and comfort to mind and body. Its object is to prevent disease and to preserve health" (p. 3). The fourth edition of the Harmer text, which showed the influence of coauthor and nursing notable Virginia Henderson, redefined nursing: "Nursing may be defined as that service to an individual that helps him to attain or maintain a healthy state of mind or body" (Harmer and Henderson 1939, p. 2). Henderson's perceptions represented the emergence of contemporary nursing and were so inclusive that they remained useful for many years.

Post–World War II Definitions

World War II, similar to all wars, helped advance the technologies available to treat people, which, in turn, influenced nursing. The war also made nurses aware of the influential role emotions play in health, illness, and nursing care. Hildegard Peplau (1952), widely regarded as a pioneer among contemporary nursing theorists and herself a psychiatric nurse, defined nursing in interpersonal terms: "Nursing is a significant, therapeutic, interpersonal process . . . . Nursing is an **educative instrument** . . . that aims to promote forward movement of personality in the direction of creative, constructive, productive, personal and community living" (p. 16). She reinforced the idea of the patient as an **active collaborator** in his own care.

During the late 1950s and early 1960s, the number of master's programs in nursing increased. As more nurses were educated at the graduate level and learned about the research process, they were anxious to test new ideas about nursing. Nursing theory was born (See Chapter 11 for an indepth discussion of nursing theory).

One of the theorists who began work during this period was Dorothea Orem. Her 1959 definition of nursing captures the flavor of her later, more completely elaborated self-care theory of nursing: "Nursing is perhaps best described as the giving of direct assistance to a person, as required, because of the person's specific inabilities in self-care resulting from a situation of personal health" (Orem, 1959, p. 5). Orem's belief, that nurses should do for a person only those things the person cannot do without assistance, also emphasized the patient's active role.

By 1960, Henderson's earlier definition had evolved into a statement that had such universal appeal that it was adopted by the ICN:

> The unique function of the nurse is to assist the individual, sick or well, in the performance of those activities contributing to health or its recovery (or to a peaceful death) that he would perform unaided if he had the necessary

strength, will or knowledge. And to do this in such a way as to help him gain independence as rapidly as possible (Henderson, 1960, p. 3).

Never before or since has one definition of nursing been so widely accepted both in the United States and throughout the world. Many believe it is still the most comprehensive and appropriate definition of nursing in existence.

Another pioneer nursing theorist, Martha Rogers, included the concept of the nursing process in her definition: "Nursing aims to assist people in achieving their **maximum health potential.** Maintenance and promotion of health, prevention of disease, nursing diagnosis, intervention, and rehabilitation encompass the scope of nursing's goals" (Rogers, 1961, p. 86).

A Controversial Definition

Definitions are not usually considered controversial, but in 1980, the ANA issued a statement of beliefs called *Nursing: A Social Policy Statement* that contained perhaps the most controversial definition of nursing to date. It stated: "Nursing is the diagnosis and treatment of human responses to actual and potential health problems" (p. 9). This definition was criticized for a number of reasons, a chief one being that it failed to identify health as a goal of nursing. The emphasis on diagnosis and treatment of health problems seemingly ignored the health promotion and maintenance aspects that other theorists have defined as the essence of nursing.

Terming the ANA definition "incomplete and in part illogical," prominent nurse educator Rozella Schlotfeldt (1987) went so far as to assert that the definition, by its incompleteness, could "delay or deter progress in theory development" (p. 6). She suggested that a more accurate and appropriate definition, and one that could inform and guide current and future practitioners, would be: "Nursing is the appraisal and the enhancement of the health status, health assets, and health potentials of human beings" (p. 67).

The ANA responded to the criticisms, and the 1995 revision of what is now titled *Nursing's Social Policy Statement* defined nursing much more comprehensively. The new definition included four essential features of contemporary nursing practice (American Nurses Association, 1995, p. 6):

- Attention to the full range of human experiences and responses to health and illness without restriction to a problem-focused orientation.
- Integration of objective data with knowledge gained from an understanding of the patient or group's subjective experience.
- Application of scientific knowledge to the processes of diagnosis and treatment.
- Provision of a caring relationship that facilitates health and healing.

A Focus on Caring, Humanism, and Holism

After a period of intense interest in **high-tech nursing** during the late 1960s and 1970s, modern nursing returned to its **high-touch** roots, so to speak, in the late 1970s with a renewed interest and public recognition as the health discipline that "cares." That movement has continued to the present.

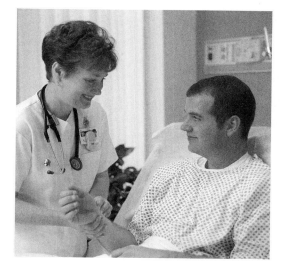

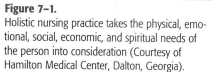

Figure 7–1.
Holistic nursing practice takes the physical, emotional, social, economic, and spiritual needs of the person into consideration (Courtesy of Hamilton Medical Center, Dalton, Georgia).

A **caring** professional is one who watches over, attends to, and provides for the needs of others. Contemporary nursing stresses **humanistic nursing care,** that is, viewing professional relationships as human to human rather than nurse to patient. The meaning of the patient's experience is an important aspect of humanistic nursing. **Holism** is also receiving emphasis in modern definitions of nursing. Holism is a system of comprehensive care that takes the physical, emotional, social, economic, and spiritual needs of the person into consideration (Fig. 7–1).

Jean Watson, a nursing theorist, illustrated the return to caring and humanism in 1979 when she wrote "Nursing is both scientific and artistic. I seek to combine science with humanism . . . . Nursing is a therapeutic interpersonal process . . . . Nursing is a **scientific discipline** that derives . . . its practice base from scientific research" (p. xvii).

Other theorists have included the concept of caring in their definitions of nursing. Orem (1991) defined the focus of caring as the return of the patient to his own (self-) care rather than formation of a caring relationship with the nurse. Leininger (1991) identified caring factors as "comfort measures." They included compassion; empathy; helping and coping behaviors; stress-alleviating measures; touching; nurturance; succorance; protective, restorative, and stimulative behaviors; health maintenance; instruction; and consultation. Nurses can expect to hear more about the caring aspects of nursing as a counterbalance to the dizzying array of technologies anticipated in the future.

This brief review of selected definitions of nursing generated during the past 150 years is summarized in Box 7–1.

BOX 7-1
Themes in the Evolution of Definitions of Nursing, 1859–1995

Nightingale, [1859] (1946)

"I use the word nursing for want of a better. . . . It ought to signify the proper use of fresh air, light, warmth, cleanliness, quiet, and the proper selection and administration of diet—all at the least expense of vital power to the patient.

"It has been said and written scores of times, that every woman makes a good nurse. I believe, on the contrary, that the very elements of nursing are all but unknown" (p. 6).

"And what nursing has to do . . . is put the patient in the best condition for nature to act upon him" (p. 75).

- The nurse's center of concern is the patient.
- Nature and a healthful, restful environment are the nurse's allies.
- Health maintenance and restoration are the nurse's goals.

Shaw, 1907

"Nursing is an art. . . . It properly includes as well as the execution of specific orders, the administration of food and medicine, the personal care of the patient. . . . To fill such a position requires certain physical and mental attributes as well as special training" (pp. 1–2).

- More than knowledge and skills are needed by nurses. The attribute of personal caring is also required.

Harmer, 1922

"Nursing is rooted in the needs of humanity. . . . Its object is not only to cure the sick . . . but to bring health and ease, rest and comfort to mind and body. Its object is to prevent disease and to preserve health" (p. 3).

- Disease prevention and health promotion are the focus.
- Nursing is based on human needs.

Harmer and Henderson, 1939

"Nursing may be defined as that service to an individual that helps him to attain or maintain a healthy state of mind or body" (p. 2).

- Nursing deals with the health of both psyche (mind) and soma (body).

Peplau, 1952

"Nursing is a significant, therapeutic, interpersonal process. . . . Nursing is an educative instrument . . . that aims to promote forward movement of personality in the direction of creative, constructive, productive, personal and community living" (p. 16).

- Effective nursing results from a therapeutic relationship between nurse and patient.

Orem, 1959

"Nursing is . . . described as the giving of direct assistance to a person, as required, because of the person's specific inabilities in self-care resulting from a situation of personal health" (p. 5).

- Nursing is doing for a person what he cannot do at this time because of health-related limitations. Return to self-care is the goal.

Henderson, 1960

"The unique function of the nurse is to assist the individual, sick or well, in the performance of those activities contributing to health or its recovery (or to a peaceful death) that he would perform unaided if he had the necessary strength, will or knowledge. And to do this in such a way as to help him gain independence as rapidly as possible" (p. 3).

- Both well and ill people are the focus of nursing.
- Responsibility for care is shared by nurse and patient.
- The goal is independence of the patient.

Rogers, 1961

"Nursing aims to assist people in achieving their maximum health potential. Maintenance and promotion of health, prevention of disease, nursing diagnosis, intervention, and rehabilitation encompass the scope of nursing's goals" (p. 86).

- Each person has a personal maximum health potential. Nursing seeks to strengthen each human being's capacity to achieve that potential.

Watson, 1979

"Nursing is both scientific and artistic. I seek to combine science with humanism. . . . Nursing is a therapeutic interpersonal process. . . . Nursing is a scientific discipline that derives . . . its practice base from scientific research" (p. xvii).

- Nursing represents a balance between science and humanism.
- The interpersonal features of nursing are paramount.
- Nurses care for people with a holistic approach even while using the scientific approach.

American Nurses Association, 1980

"Nursing is the diagnosis and treatment of human responses to actual and potential health problems" (p. 9).

- Nursing focuses on human responses to illness or the threat of illness.

Schlotfeldt, 1987

"Nursing is the appraisal and the enhancement of the health status, health assets, and health potentials of human beings" (p. 67).

- Regardless of where a person is on the continuum of wellness to illness, nursing focuses on enhancing that person's health care status.

(continued)

BOX 7–1
Themes in the Evolution of Definitions of Nursing, 1859–1995 (*Continued*)

American Nurses Association, 1995
"Attention to the full range of human experiences and responses to health and illness without restriction to a problem-focused orientation; integration of objective data with knowledge gained from an understanding of the patient or group's subjective experience; application of scientific knowledge to the processes of diagnosis and treatment; and provision of a caring relationship that facilitates health and healing" (p. 6).

- Reflects the multifaceted, complex nature of nursing.
- Integrates the science of caring with traditional knowledge.
- Retains the commitment to care of both healthy and ill people, individually or in groups and communities.
- Reflects a commitment to holism.

Developing Definitions of Nursing

Since the profession of nursing is ever evolving and is influenced by changing social, economic, and political forces, so too will definitions of nursing continue to evolve. Faculties of schools of nursing, leaders in agencies and institutions providing nursing care, individuals, and state legislatures all, from time to time, attempt to define nursing.

Definitions Developed by Schools of Nursing

Students may not realize that faculties of accredited schools of nursing are encouraged to develop definitions of nursing as part of the school's statement of philosophy. Some of the most spirited discussions during faculty meetings center around what one or another faculty member believes nursing really is. A description of nursing that combines humanistic and holistic values can be found in the University of Rochester School of Nursing's comprehensive philosophy statement:

> We believe that the profession of nursing has as its essence, assisting people to attain and maintain optimal health and to cope with illness and disability. Nursing derives its rights and responsibilities from society and is, therefore, accountable to society as well as to the individuals who comprise it. The nurse functions as a caring professional in both autonomous and collaborative professional roles, using critical thinking, ethical principles, effective communication, and deliberative action to render holistic care, facilitate access to health care, and aid consumers in making decisions about their health (Radke et al., 1991, p. 12).

Another thoughtful and somewhat more specific definition comes from the University of Akron (Ohio) College of Nursing faculty, who wrote:

> Nursing is an art and a science. The discipline of nursing is concerned with individual, family, and community, and their responses to health within the context of the changing health care environment. Professional nursing includes the appraisal and the enhancement of health. Personal meanings of health are understood in the nursing situation within the context of familial, societal, and cultural meanings. The professional nurse uses knowledge from theories and research in nursing and other disciplines in providing nursing care. The role of the nurse involves the exercise of social, cultural, and political responsibilities, including accountability for professional actions, provision of quality nursing care, and community involvement (University of Akron College of Nursing, 1999, p. 4).

Although these two definitions are quite different, commonalities are evident.

Definitions Developed by Hospitals

Most hospitals have developed definitions of nursing to guide practice in that institution. Accreditation guidelines for hospitals require that much consideration be given to defining the nursing care provided. The following definition was developed by the Division of Nursing at St. Vincent's Medical Center in Jacksonville, Florida:

> The practice of nursing is the caring and competent application of a specialized body of knowledge and judgment within the framework of the nursing process. This process encompasses the assessment, planning, intervention, and evaluation of actual and potential health care needs. Nursing Practice is further based on the core values of Baptist St. Vincent's, the philosophy of the Division of Nursing, and the Nurse Practice Act of the State of Florida (St. Vincent's Medical Center Division of Nursing, 1999, p. 1).

Most hospital definitions of nursing make reference to the **nurse practice act** of the state in which the hospital is located, and many simply adopt the practice act's definition as their own. This prevents any conflict between the legal scope of practice and practices sanctioned by the institution. Approximately two-thirds of the hospitals surveyed for this chapter used nurse practice act definitions as their own. For example, Hamilton Medical Center in Dalton, Georgia, simply recognizes the definition of nursing as defined by the Georgia Board of Nursing:

> [Nursing is] . . . the performance for compensation of any act in the care and counsel of the ill, injured, or infirm, and in the promotion and maintenance of health with individuals, groups, or both throughout the life span. It requires substantial specialized knowledge of the humanities, natural sciences, social sciences and nursing theory as a basis for assessment, nursing diagnosis, planning, intervention, and evaluation. It includes, but is not limited to, provision of nursing care; administration, supervision, evaluation, or any combi-

nation thereof, of nursing practice; teaching; counseling; the administration of medications and treatments as prescribed by a physician practicing medicine in accordance with Article 2 of Chapter 34 of this title, or a dentist practicing dentistry in accordance with Chapter 11 of this title, or a podiatrist practicing podiatry in accordance with Chapter 35 of this title (Hamilton Medical Center, 1999).

Definitions Developed by State Legislatures

It is important to keep in mind that the most significant definition of nursing for every nurse is contained in the nurse practice act of the state in which a nurse practices. Regardless of how restrictive or permissive it may be, this definition constitutes the legal definition of nursing in a particular state, and the wise nurse maintains familiarity with the latest version of the act. Ohio's nurse practice act contains wording typical of many states' acts:

> "Practice of nursing as a registered nurse" means providing to individuals and groups nursing care requiring specialized knowledge, judgment, and skill derived from the principles of biological, physical, behavioral, social, and nursing sciences. Such nursing care includes:
>
> 1. Identifying patterns of human responses to actual or potential health problems amenable to a nursing regimen;
> 2. Executing a nursing regimen through the selection, performance, management, and evaluation of nursing actions;
> 3. Assessing health status for the purpose of providing nursing care;
> 4. Providing health counseling and health teaching;
> 5. Administering medications, treatments, and executing regimens prescribed by licensed physicians, dentists, optometrists, and podiatrists; or until January 1, 2010, advanced practice nurses authorized to prescribe under section 4723.56 of the Revised Code;
> 6. Teaching, administering, supervising, delegating, and evaluating nursing practice (Akron General Medical Center Department of Nursing, 1999).

If the language in this nurse practice act sounds like familiar nursing language, that is not accidental. State nurses associations and boards of nursing are actively involved with legislators to assist them in drafting laws that accurately reflect the nature and scope of nursing. The current nurse practice act in each state can be obtained by calling or writing the state board of nursing. The addresses of the boards of nursing are found in Appendix C.

Developing Your Own Definition of Nursing

All nursing students and practicing nurses, whether or not they realize it, are in the process of developing and refining their own definitions of nursing. From time to time, it is helpful to write down just what your personal definition is and compare it with those developed by nursing scholars over the years. It can also be informative to compare your own early definitions with ones you develop later as you mature in the profession.

Summary of Key Points

- Although attempting to define nursing has been an interesting activity since the days of Nightingale, all attempts have fallen short of capturing the scope, diversity, and richness that constitutes nursing.
- Storlie struck a chord of timeless truth in 1970 when she wrote "The glorious thing about nursing is that it cannot be defined. The irony is that we never give up trying. . . . Nursing will resist being reduced to so-called facts no matter how precise the researcher" (Storlie, 1970, pp. 254–255).
- Definitions reviewed in this chapter have more commonalities than differences.
- Definitions have evolved over time even though many themes are constant.
- It may be possible to find definitions by some of the same authors that are different from the ones given in this chapter because definitions change over time as both society and nursing change and as each individual's perceptions about, and experiences in, nursing change.
- Although nursing may wish for one, succinct definition, the dynamic nature of the nursing profession, society, and health care will likely prevent us from ever developing one eternal, universally accepted definition of nursing.

Critical Thinking Questions

1. Obtain your school's definition of nursing. How is it similar to or different from definitions in this chapter?
2. From the definitions of nursing presented in this chapter, select the one you most prefer and explain your choice.
3. Using your thoughts as well as elements of others' definitions, write your own definition of nursing. Explain it to a classmate, giving your rationale for what you included and excluded. Keep it among your professional papers to refer to in later years.
4. How might new technologies, economic factors, social trends, and new practice options for nurses affect future definitions of nursing?
5. How has your personal definition of nursing changed over time?
6. Using the appropriate address from Appendix C, obtain a copy of the nurse practice act for your state. Find the legal definition of nursing and compare it with other definitions found in this chapter. How are they alike, and how are they different?

Web Resources

American Nurses Association *Nursing's Social Policy Statement* ordering information, http://www.nursingworld.org/anp/pdescr.cfm?Cnum=6.#NP-107

International Council of Nursing, http://www.icn.ch

References

Akron General Medical Center Department of Nursing (1999). *Definition of nursing.* Akron, Ohio: Akron General Medical Center Department of Nursing.

American Nurses Association (1980). *Nursing: A social policy statement.* Kansas City, Mo.: American Nurses Association.

American Nurses Association (1995). *Nursing's social policy statement.* Washington, D. C.: American Nurses Association.

Dracup, K., and Bryan-Brown, C. W. (1997). Making a profession visible: Three nurses' stories. *American Journal of Critical Care,* 6(4), 256–258.

Hamilton Medical Center (1999). *Definition of nursing.* Dalton, Georgia: Hamilton Medical Center.

Harmer, B. (1922). *Textbook of the principles and practice of nursing.* New York: Macmillan.

Harmer, B., and Henderson, V. (1939). *Textbook of the principles and practice of nursing* (4th ed.). New York: Macmillan.

Henderson, V. (1960). *Basic principles of nursing care.* London: International Council of Nurses.

Jacox, A. (1997). Determinants of who does what in health care. *Online Journal of Issues in Nursing.* Available from http://www.nursingworld.org/ojin/tpc5/tpc5_1.htm.

Leininger, M. M. (Ed.). (1991). *Culture care diversity and universality: A theory of nursing.* New York: National League for Nursing.

Nightingale, F. [1859] (1946). 1859 ed. *Notes on nursing: What it is and what it is not.* Reprint, Philadelphia: J. B. Lippincott.

Orem, D. (1959). *Guidelines for developing curricula for the education of practical nurses.* Washington, D. C.: Government Printing Office.

Orem, D. (1991). *Nursing: Concepts of practice* (4th ed.). St. Louis: Mosby.

Peplau, H. (1952). *Interpersonal relations in nursing: A conceptual frame of reference for psychodynamic nursing.* New York: G. P. Putnam's Sons.

Radke, K. J. et al. (1991). Curriculum blueprints for the future: The process of blending beliefs. *Nurse Educator,* 16(2), 9–13.

Rogers, M. (1961). Educational revolution in nursing. New York: Macmillan.

St. Vincent's Medical Center Division of Nursing (1999). *Definition of nursing.* Jacksonville, Fla.: St. Vincent's Medical Center Division of Nursing.

Schlotfeldt, R. M. (1987). Defining nursing: A historic controversy. *Nursing Research,* 36(1), 64–67.

Shaw, C. W. (1907). *Textbook of nursing* (3rd ed.). New York: Appleton.

Storlie, F. (1970). Nursing need never be defined. *International Nursing Review,* 70(17), 255–258.

University of Akron College of Nursing (1999). *Philosophy of the College of Nursing.* Akron, Ohio: University of Akron College of Nursing.

Watson, J. (1979). *The philosophy and science of caring.* Boston: Little, Brown.

Professional Socialization

Kay K. Chitty

Learning Outcomes

After studying this chapter, students will be able to:

- Discuss how students' initial images of nursing are modified by professional education.
- Differentiate between formal and informal socialization.
- Identify internal and external factors that influence an individual's professional socialization.
- Describe developmental models of professional socialization and how they can be used.
- Differentiate between the elements of professional socialization that are the responsibility of nursing programs and those that are the individual's responsibility.
- Discuss Kramer's model for minimizing reality shock.
- Describe practical steps to ease the transition from student to professional nurse.
- Discuss employer expectations.

In Chapter 3, societal influences that have affected the development of nursing were discussed, and the media's impact on nursing's image was explored. It is clear that the image of nursing held by the public over the years has been influenced in large measure by books, television, and motion pictures. Nursing students, too, are affected by the images portrayed by these media as well as by contact with nurses they know. They bring an outsider's view of the nursing profession to school with them.

During formal schooling, the complex process of exchanging an outsider's perception for an insider's understanding of nursing begins. This process requires that students **internalize,** or take in, the knowledge, skills, attitudes, beliefs, norms, culture, values, and ethical standards of nursing and make these a part of their own self-image and behavior (Jacox, 1973).

The process of internalization and development of an occupational identity is known as **professional socialization.** Put another way, "Socialization brings nurses into *existence*" (Colucciello, 1990, p. 17). Professional socialization in nursing is believed to occur largely, but not entirely, during the period students are in basic nursing programs. It continues after graduation when they enter nursing practice. In this chapter, the effects of both school and work settings on nurses' professional socialization are examined.

Education and Professional Socialization

What kinds of educational experiences are needed to make the transition from student to professional nurse? How does a student make the transition from novice to initiate, a person who thinks and feels like a nurse? Learning any new role is derived from a mixture of formal and informal socialization. Little boys, for example, learn how to assume the father role by what their own fathers purposely teach them (formal socialization) and by observing their own and other fathers' behavior (informal socialization). In nursing, **formal socialization** includes lessons the faculty intends to teach, such as how to plan nursing care, write a paper on professional ethics, perform a physical examination on a healthy child, or practice communication with a psychiatric patient (Fig. 8–1). **Informal socialization** includes lessons that occur incidentally, such as the unplanned observation of a nurse teaching a young mother how to care for her premature infant, participating in a student nurse association, or hearing nurses discuss patient care in the nurses' lounge. Part of professional socialization is simply absorbing the **culture of nursing,** that is, the rites, rituals, and valued behaviors of the profession. This requires that students spend enough time with nurses in work settings for adequate exposure to the nursing culture to occur. Most nurses agree that informal socialization was often more powerful and memorable than formal socialization in their own development.

Learning a new vocabulary is also part of professional socialization. Each profession has its own jargon, which is not generally understood by outsiders. Professional students usually enjoy acquiring the new vocabulary and practicing it among themselves.

Learning any new role creates some degree of anxiety (Wooley, 1978). Disappointment and frustration sometimes occur when students' learning expectations come into conflict with educational realities. Students' ideas of what they need to learn, when they need to learn it, and what might be the best way to learn it may differ from how their education actually unfolds. They sometimes become disillusioned when they observe nurses behaving in ways that are in contrast to their ideas about how nurses *should* behave. Knowing in advance that these things may happen can help students accurately assess the sources of their anxiety and manage it more effectively.

Internal Influencing Factors

As students progress through nursing programs, a variety of internal and external factors challenge their customary ways of thinking. **Internal factors** include personal feelings and beliefs. Some of these may conflict with profes-

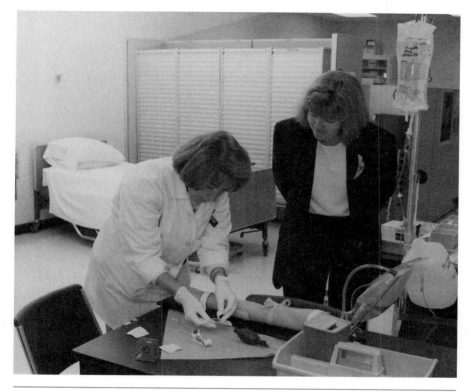

Figure 8–1
During formal schooling, students internalize the knowledge, skills, and beliefs of nursing (Courtesy of University of Akron).

sional values. For example, if students believe in a higher power, they may be uncomfortable working with patients who have no such belief. Yet nursing's *Code for Nurses* (American Nurses Association, 1985) requires that nurses work with all patients regardless of their beliefs. Other areas that sometimes challenge students' thinking are substance abuse; self-destructive behaviors; abortion; issues related to sexuality, such as sexual preference; genetic manipulation; and end-of-life issues.

External Influencing Factors

External factors also influence professional development. Growing children are first influenced by the values, beliefs, and behaviors of the significant adults around them and later by peers. Ideas about health, health care, and nursing are also shaped through this process. If a nurse's family valued fitness, for example, it may be difficult for that nurse to empathize with an overweight patient who refuses to exercise. In this example, a family value (fitness) comes into conflict with a professional value (empathy toward all patients without judging them).

Nurses need to be aware of their biases and discuss them with peers, instructors, and professional role models. Failure to do so may adversely affect the nursing care provided to certain patients. Professional nurses make every effort to avoid imposing their personal beliefs on others (See Chapter 18 for further discussion of self-awareness and nonjudgmentalism as necessary attributes of professional nurses.).

As seen from this brief discussion, socialization is much more than the transmission of knowledge and skills. It serves to develop a common nursing consciousness and is the key to keeping the profession vital and dynamic. It is not surprising, therefore, that a good deal of attention has been paid to this important process.

Models of Professional Socialization

In thinking about professional socialization, it is helpful to have theoretical models to consider. Cohen (1981) and Hinshaw (1976) described developmental models appropriate for beginning nursing students. Bandura (1977) described an informal type of socialization he called **modeling,** which is useful when learning any new behavior. Benner (1984) identified five stages nurses pass through in the transition from "novice to expert." Throwe and Fought (1987) described a developmental model of professional socialization specifically designed to meet the needs of registered nurse (RN) students. Each of these models is considered briefly.

Cohen's Model

Cohen (1981) proposed a model of professional socialization consisting of four stages. Basing her work on developmental theories and studies of students' attitudes toward nursing, she asserted, "Students must experience each stage in sequence to feel comfortable in the professional role" (p. 16). She believed that a positive outcome in all of the four stages is necessary for satisfactory socialization to occur.

Cohen called the first stage in her model *stage I, unilateral dependence.* Owing to inexperience and lack of knowledge, students at this stage rely on external limits and controls established by authority figures such as teachers. During stage I, students are unlikely to question or analyze critically the concepts teachers present because they lack the necessary background to do so.

In *stage II, negativity/independence,* students' critical thinking abilities and knowledge bases expand. They begin to question authority figures. Cohen called this **cognitive rebellion.** Much as a young child learns that he can say no, students at this level begin to free themselves from external controls and to rely more on their own judgment. They think critically about what they are being taught.

In *stage III, dependence/mutuality,* Cohen described students' more reasoned evaluation of other's ideas. They develop an increasingly realistic appraisal process and learn to test concepts, facts, ideas, and models objectively. Students at this stage are more impartial; they accept some ideas and reject others.

In *stage IV, interdependence,* students' needs for both independence and **mutuality** (sharing jointly with others) come together. They develop the capacity to make decisions in collaboration with others. The successfully socialized student completes stage IV with a self-concept that includes a professional role identity that is personally and professionally acceptable and compatible with other life roles. Table 8–1 summarizes the key behaviors associated with each of Cohen's stages.

Readers may wish to compare themselves and nursing classmates to these four stages. A word of caution, however: Although it is interesting and useful, this is a model that has not been scientifically tested and validated (confirmed). At least one researcher, McCain (1985), concluded that her study "did not support the Cohen model. . . ." because students in McCain's sample of 422 bachelor of science in nursing (BSN) student volunteers in a large southern state university did not show evidence of progression through Cohen's developmental stages (p. 185). McCain recommended further testing of Cohen's model.

Hinshaw's Model

Another potentially useful model describing the educational aspects of professional socialization was proposed by Hinshaw in a 1976 publication for the National League for Nursing.

TABLE 8–1
Cohen's Stages of Professional Socialization*

Stage	Key Behaviors
I: Unilateral dependence	Reliant on external authority; limited questioning or critical analysis
II: Negativity/independence	Cognitive rebellion; diminished reliance on external authority
III: Dependence/mutuality	Reasoned appraisal; begins integration of facts and opinions following objective testing
IV: Interdependence	Collaborative decision making; commitment to professional role; self-concept now includes professional role identity

*Data from Cohen, H. A. (1981). *The nurse's quest for professional identity.* Menlo Park, Calif.: Addison-Wesley.

In this model, *stage I, initial innocence,* is characterized by idealized images and expectations of nursing. Students have gained these images from the media and from their own experiences with nurses. For example, they may expect that as nursing students they will immediately begin to work with sick patients, or that nurses are always treated with respect by other health care workers, or that they will always be able to make things better for their patients.

In *stage II, incongruities,* students realize that their innocent images of nursing differ from the real structure and challenges of a nursing program. For example, they discover that they must complete anatomy, physiology, nutrition, and a host of other courses before working with patients, or they discover that students are expected to defer to more experienced nurses and instructors, or they encounter patients with chronic, intractable pain. This **dissonance** (lack of harmony) between their expectations and the real situation produces tension and frustration. During the dissonant stage, differences are sufficiently well formulated to discuss with others. Students at this stage may overtly question whether or not they should continue in the program and may choose not to do so.

In *stage III, identification,* students select and carefully observe role models. Role models may be particularly admired instructors or nurses seen in clinical settings. This stage is closely followed by *stage IV, role simulation,* in which they practice the role behaviors they observed. At first, the new behaviors may feel strange or phony, which sometimes causes confusion and self-doubt. Students learning therapeutic communication techniques, for example, often feel awkward and obvious when they first try out these techniques in conversation.

In *stage V, vacillation,* there is a desire to cling to the old ideas and images about nursing while recognizing that new ideas and images are based on life experiences. Evidence of this stage can be seen in new graduates who feel guilty when they are unable to provide intense, individualized care for every patient because of patient load and time constraints.

The last stage, *internalization,* occurs when there is stable and reliable use of the internalized professional model. This can be seen in nurses who, after practicing for some time, have developed a balance between their expectations of themselves as professionals, employers' expectations, and their other life role expectations. Table 8–2 contains the stages of socialization described in the Hinshaw model.

Bandura's Concept of Modeling

Another method of professional socialization is modeling, as discussed by Bandura (1977). In modeling, students learn by observing role models. Bandura believed that there are two requirements for successful modeling: Models must be seen as competent, and students must have an opportunity to practice the behaviors they see modeled. This is different from the informal socialization process described earlier because modeling involves a con-

---

TABLE 8-2
Hinshaw's Stages of Professional Socialization

Stage	Key Behaviors
I: Initial innocence	Initial image of nursing unaffected by reality
II: Incongruities	Initial expectations and reality collide; questions career choice; may drop out
III: Identification	Observes behaviors of experienced nurses
IV: Role simulation	Practices observed behaviors; may feel unnatural in role
V: Vacillation	Old images emerge and conflict with new professional image
VI: Internalization	Acceptance and comfort with new role

Data from Hinshaw, A. S. (1976). Socialization and resocialization of nurses for professional nursing practice. New York: National League for Nursing.

---

scious decision on the part of learners to model themselves after the selected role model.

Students who wish to try modeling should identify nurses or instructors who share their values and attitudes and observe them closely. The next step is to "try out" the behaviors they most admire. Because people are not equally talented in all areas, students may choose to observe several models, each of whom excels in a different area. The basis of modeling as a method of professional socialization is careful observation and intentional simulation of the admired behaviors or characteristics. This is a legitimate method of acquiring desirable professional behaviors that can be useful to students interested in being more active in their own socialization.

Benner's Stages of Nursing Proficiency

Benner wondered how nurses made the transition from inexpert beginners to highly expert practitioners. She described a stepwise process of five stages of nursing practice, upon which she based her 1984 book, *From Novice to Expert.* The stages are "novice," "advanced beginner," "competent practitioner," "proficient practitioner," and "expert practitioner." Advancing from stage to stage occurs gradually as nurses have more experience in patient care. Clinical judgment is stimulated when the nurse's "preconceived notions and expectations" (p. 3) collide with or are confirmed by the realities of everyday practice.

Benner's *novice,* or *stage I,* begins with students entering nursing school. Because they generally have little background upon which to base their clinical behavior, they must depend rather rigidly on rules and expectations established for them. Their practical skills are limited.

By the time learners enter the *advanced beginner,* or *stage II,* period, they have discerned that a particular order exists in clinical settings (Benner,

Tanner, and Chesla, 1996). Their performance is marginally competent. They can base their actions on both theory and principles but tend to experience difficulty formulating priorities, viewing many nursing actions as equally important.

Competent practitioners, or *Stage III,* learners usually have two to three years experience in a setting. As a result, they feel competent, organized, and efficient most of the time. These feelings of mastery are due to planning and goal-setting skills and the ability to think abstractly and analytically. They can coordinate several complex demands simultaneously.

It generally takes three to five years of practice to reach the level of *proficient practitioner,* represented by *Stage IV.* These nurses are able to see patient situations holistically rather than in parts, to recognize and interpret subtleties of meaning, and to recognize easily priorities for care. They can focus on long-term goals and desired outcomes.

Expert practitioner, or *Stage V,* status is reached only after extensive practice experience. These nurses perform without conscious thought, intuitively, automatically grasping the significance of the patient's complete experience. They move fluidly through nursing interventions, acting on the basis of their feeling of "rightness" of nursing action. They may find it difficult to express verbally why they selected certain actions, so integrated are their responses. Their expertise seems, both to themselves and to observers, to "come naturally." Table 8–3 summarizes Benner's stages from novice to expert.

TABLE 8-3
Benner's Stages of Nursing Proficiency

Stages	*Nurse Behaviors*
I: Novice	Has little background and limited practical skills; relies on rules and expectations of others for direction
II: Advanced beginner	Has marginally competent skills; uses theory and principles much of the time; experiences difficulty establishing priorities
III: Competent practitioner	Feels competent, organized; plans and sets goals; thinks abstractly and analytically; coordinates several tasks simultaneously
IV: Proficient practitioner	Views patients holistically; recognizes subtle changes; sets priorities with ease; focuses on long-term goals
V: Expert practitioner	Performs fluidly; grasps patient needs automatically; responses are integrated; expertise comes naturally

Data from Benner, P. (1984). *From novice to expert: Excellence and power in clinical nursing practice.* Menlo Park, Calif.: Addison-Wesley.

Throwe's and Fought's Model for Socialization of Registered Nurse Students

When registered nurses return to school for their baccalaureate degrees, their needs are different from those of basic nursing students. They may experience feelings of frustration and anger caused by returning to the student role. Often, these nurses have practiced for years and wonder what anyone can teach them about nursing. It may seem almost insulting when they are placed in classes with students who are just beginning in nursing education. What needs to be recognized is that these registered nurses are not being socialized into nursing; they are in the process of **resocialization,** a process that often creates uncomfortable tension.

Throwe and Fought (1987) believed that the stages registered nurses must master during resocialization could be assessed using Erikson's theory. Erikson (1950) described eight developmental stages individuals master as they progress from infancy to old age. Throwe and Fought designed a framework for registered nurses in BSN programs to assess their own growth as they progress through school. The framework can also be used by faculty and non-RN students to help them appreciate and support registered nurses' experiences. Table 8–4 contains Throwe's and Fought's assessment tool.

TABLE 8–4
Assessment Tool for Socialization to the Professional Nurse Role

Developmental Task	Role-Resisting Behaviors Observed	Role-Accepting Behaviors Observed
Trust/mistrust: Learns to trust the worlds of education and work through consistency and repetitive experiences	Physically isolated from peers both in class and clinicals; does not initiate interactions with others; responds only if called on	Involved with classmates; readily and quickly forms/joins groups when directed; initiates discussions with others; asks for clarification
Autonomy/doubt: Begins to develop independence while under supervision	Delays joining groups for unstructured activities; does not contribute equally; forgets or suppresses assignment dates; does not meet target dates; self-conscious about being evaluated by others	Joins groups for unstructured activities (study groups); shares information with group; prepares for activities; meets target dates; able to interact in the teaching/learning environment; begins to develop independence with guidance
Initiative/guilt: Can independently identity, plan, and implement skills/ assignments	Perceives objectives and assignments as not worthwhile; stress-related symptoms increase; has difficulty setting priorities; waits for instructor to initiate priority setting; lacks initiative to deal with conflicts; unaware of available resources	Objectives and assignments take on meaning; applies new skills, content to other work settings; effective in time management; renegotiates deadline extensions when appropriate; takes initiative in resolving conflict situations; aware of and uses available resources

(continued)

TABLE 8-4
Assessment Tool for Socialization to the Professional Nurse Role (*Continued*)

Developmental Task	Role-Resisting Behaviors Observed	Role-Accepting Behaviors Observed
Industry/inferiority: Behavior is dominated by performance of tasks and curiosity—individuals need encouragement to attempt and master skills	Elicits performance rewards and feedback from others; needs direct encouragement, especially when performing affective and cognitive skills; last to volunteer to demonstrate new behaviors; seeks rewards by performing old familiar skills rather than those in new dimensions; demonstrates disengaging behaviors (late, uninterested, resistive to learning opportunities)	Able to reward self; confidence thrives; eager to try out new skills; takes risks; volunteers to demonstrate new behaviors; profits from guidance and direction of others; applies self beyond family/work settings; curiosity channeled through educational system
Identity/role confusion: Individual searches for continuity and structure; is concerned with how he or she is accepted by others; is concerned how he or she is accepted by self; each individual struggles to shape or formulate own identity	Needs a structured clinical setting to develop ego identity further; sees old job as ideal and denies need for change; serious about learning (content and clinical practice); frustrated with nursing as a career choice; too ideological or overly critical of others	Searches for continuity and structure but can adapt to unstructured clinical settings; identifies role models in clinical setting; articulates need for change or for modification of job-related roles and procedures; appears to enjoy learning and performing in clinical settings; realistic about own achievements and progress in educational system
Intimacy/isolation: Seeks to combine identity with other self-selected individuals	Participates as a member, but resists group leader role; does not participate in professional meetings; unsupportive of others' educational advancement; feels no increased esteem in performing new role behaviors; meets minimal requirements and sees instructor only in evaluative role; resists using newly developed skills, more comfortable with previous level of performance; avoids giving feedback to agency personnel	Volunteers to lead work/study groups; participates in professional organizations; recruits others and represents school; demonstrates pride in new role behaviors and shares with others in work settings; seeks out instructor for additional learning, information, and professional growth opportunities; values symbols of profession (using assessment tools, RN name tags); evaluates ability of clinical agencies to facilitate meeting learner objectives; provides feedback to agency personnel

TABLE 8-4
Assessment Tool for Socialization to the Professional Nurse Role (*Continued*)

Developmental Task	Role-Resisting Behaviors Observed	Role-Accepting Behaviors Observed
Generativity/stagnation: Efforts are made to guide and direct incoming students; assists others	Avoids social interaction and information sharing with incoming students; provides minimal care, unconcerned about continuity of patient care; selects patients with common, familiar clinical disorders; no increased ease of learning or improved test-taking abilities; does not elect to test out of course requirements; stagnates in same job setting	Guides and directs incoming students; provides quality nursing care to patient, family, and community; takes calculated risks (questions level of care, seeks multiple learning opportunities, shares level of expertise, elects to test out of required/elective courses); demonstrates critical problem-solving skills; attains mastery of test-taking skills; self-directed learner; demonstrates clinical problem solving in own work setting; uses holistic approach to delivery of health care
Ego integrity/despair: Acceptance of one's own progress, achievement, and goals through realistic self-appraisal	Frustrated with progress and achievement, stagnated in developing new goals; crisis prone when changing roles; self-appraisal unrealistic; does not participate in structured educational opportunities; returns to old job and does not modify role performance; sees no reward in risk taking; high risk for dissatisfaction with profession	Accepts progress, achievement, and goal attainment; realistic in self-appraisal; resets professional goals (graduate school, participation in continuing education, certification); joins new perspectives on old job by use of critical thinking; takes risks (new jobs, different clinical setting, and leadership roles)

Reprinted with permission of Throwe, A. N., and Fought, S. G. (1987). Landmarks in the socialization process from RN to BSN. *Nurse Educator,* 12(6), 15–18.

Actively Participating in One's Own Professional Socialization

So far in this discussion, professional socialization has sounded like something that happens *to* students. Although much is out of their control, students do not have to be passive recipients of socialization. As active participants, they can influence the socialization process. For some ideas about how to become an active participant in the socialization process, use the checklist in Box 8–1.

BOX 8–1

A Do-It-Yourself Guide to Professional Socialization

Listed are 20 possible behaviors demonstrated by students who take responsibility for their own professional socialization. Place a check next to the behaviors you regularly exhibit. Be honest with yourself.

1. I interact with other students in and out of class.
2. I participate in class by asking intelligent questions and initiating discussion occasionally.
3. I have formed or joined a study group.
4. I use the library, labs, and teachers as resources.
5. I organize my work so I can meet deadlines.
6. If I have a conflict with another student or a teacher, I take the initiative to resolve it.
7. I don't let minor personality problems distract me from my goals.
8. I seek out new learning experiences and sometimes volunteer to demonstrate new skills to others.
9. I have chosen professional role models.
10. I am realistic about my performance.
11. I try to accept constructive criticism undefensively.
12. I recognize that trying to do good work is not the same as doing good work.
13. I recognize that each teacher has different expectations, and it is my responsibility to learn what is expected by each.
14. I demonstrate respect for my teachers' time by making appointments whenever possible.
15. I demonstrate respect for my classmates and patients by never coming to class or clinical unprepared.
16. I recognize my responsibility to help create a dynamic learning environment and am not satisfied to be merely an academic spectator.
17. I participate in the student nurse association and encourage others to do the same.
18. I represent my school with pride.
19. I project a professional appearance.
20. One of my goals is to become a self-directed, lifelong learner.

Scoring: 1 to 10 checks: You need to examine your behavior and think about taking more responsibility for your own socialization; 11 to 15 checks: You are active in your own behalf. See if you can begin using some of the remaining behaviors on the list or come up with your own; more than 15 checks: You are a role model of positive action in your own professional socialization process.

As consumers of educational services, students need to know what to expect of their nursing programs in terms of professional socialization. Schools are responsible for some activities, whereas the individual is responsible for others. The checklist in Box 8–2 provides ideas about what takes place in nurs-

BOX 8-2
A Consumer's Guide to Professional Socialization

The following statements indicate some positive socialization attitudes and behaviors students should expect in their nursing programs. Check the ones that apply to your program.

1. My teachers are interested in students' learning.
2. My teachers can tolerate ideas that are different from their own.
3. My program offers me the opportunity to explore different values.
4. Considering the size of the community, my program offers me rich clinical opportunities.
5. My program emphasizes knowledge and techniques as well as values, ethics, and social behaviors of the nursing profession.
6. My teachers provide regular, direct, constructive feedback on my performance.
7. The program's philosophy and curriculum have been explained to me.
8. The faculty members take pride in the school and actively work to improve it.
9. Faculty members model healthy personal behaviors.
10. Faculty members model professional behavior and project a positive nursing image on campus and in the community.
11. My teachers model respect for each other and for nurses in agencies where we have clinical experiences.
12. Faculty members respect students and avoid authoritarianism (big me/little you).
13. My program makes every effort to accept students who have the potential to succeed.
14. My teachers maintain school standards.
15. My teachers help students cope with anxiety.
16. My program encourages students to participate in extracurricular activities available in the institution.
17. My teachers avoid favoritism.
18. My teachers keep on top of new developments in nursing and health care and are clinically competent.
19. My teachers value teaching as much as they value their other academic interests.
20. My teachers view me as a consumer of educational services.

Scoring: Compare your responses to other students' scores and identify commonly agreed-on areas of strength and weakness. Discuss both strengths and weaknesses in class. With your teacher as a resource, decide how to use the information in a positive way.

ing programs around the United States to enhance students' professional socialization. Students can compare their experiences with those in this guide. The Research Note in this chapter describes the findings of a study of the socialization of students in nursing education programs.

Postgraduate Resocialization to the Work Setting

When nurses graduate, is their professional socialization over? Most authorities believe that socialization, similar to learning, is a lifelong activity. The transition from student to professional is just another of life's challenges and, similar to most challenges, is one that helps people grow. Most new nursing graduates feel somewhat unprepared and overwhelmed with the responsibilities of their first positions. Although agencies that employ new graduates realize that the orientation period will take time, graduates may have unrealistic expectations of themselves and others.

During the early days of practice, most graduate nurses quickly realize that the ideals taught in school are not always possible to achieve in everyday practice. This is largely owing to time constraints and produces feelings of conflict and even guilt. In school, students are taught to spend time with patients and to consider their emotional as well as their physical needs. In practice, the emphasis seems to be on finishing tasks, completing checklists and flowsheets, and the like. Talking with patients, engaging in patient teaching, or counseling family members may be viewed as an unproductive use of time. In the early days of professional practice, having time to do comprehensive,

RESEARCH NOTE

Because she believed that "the primary purpose of socialization is to transmit and transform our culture" (p. 17), Margaret L. Colucciello designed a study to examine the degree of professional socialization of 216 midwestern university nursing students at sophomore, senior, and graduate levels. The student volunteers each completed a 25-item inventory developed by Richard Hall that measures degree of professionalism on five attitudinal dimensions: the use of professional organizations as a major reference, a belief in service to the public, a belief in self-regulation, a sense of calling to the field, and autonomy.

The study findings were surprising and dismaying: The degree of professionalism for each attribute was actually lower as the students progressed academically. According to Colucciello, this finding "is antithetical to nursing education's curriculum goals. It appears that socialization into the profession of nursing creates nurses who exhibit average or minimal commitment to the field" (p. 24). She cited other studies that showed that as nurses become "more socialized they begin to face the realities of their role expectations and responsibilities. The idealistic view of nursing is replaced by an awareness of the actuality" (p. 25).

Colucciello called for curricular changes in nursing education to improve role socialization, a rethinking of the role of the nurse educator, use of nontraditional scheduling and adult learning strategies to promote autonomy, and fostering students' identification and internalization of nursing's role by increasing clinical practicum experiences to learn the work culture of nursing. She encouraged the use of debates, simulations, role reversals, and realistic, autonomous clinical experiences and research with instructor guidance and collaboration with nursing administration in clinical settings to make students feel more a part of the system.

Adapted with permission of Colucciello, M. L. (1990). Socialization into nursing: A developmental approach. *NursingConnections,* 3(2), 17–27.

individualized nursing care planning, such a staple of life for nursing students, may seem like an unrealistic luxury.

New nurses also must adapt to collaborating with other nursing care personnel, such as nursing assistants, patient care technicians, and other unlicensed assistive personnel who assist them in caring for patients. This is a difficult adjustment for some nurses who are unaccustomed to delegating, are unsure of the abilities of others, or believe only they can provide quality care.

Kramer's Reality Shock

Kramer (1974) termed the feelings of powerlessness and ineffectiveness experienced by new graduates **reality shock.** Although Kramer's initial observations were published more than 25 years ago, they remain relevant. She observed that psychological stresses generated by reality shock decrease the ability of individuals to cope effectively with the demands of the new role. Unfortunately, some new nurses drop out at this point before they take steps to resolve reality shock.

Kramer identified several ways to drop out: disengaging mentally and becoming part of the problem; driving self and others to the breaking point by trying to do it all; "**job hopping**" (looking for the perfect, nonstressful job that is completely compatible with professional values); or prematurely returning to school. Sadly, both for themselves and the nursing profession, some individuals even sacrifice all the years of education they have invested in nursing and decide not to work in nursing at all. This is a loss neither nursing nor society can afford.

Being aware that there are stages most new graduates go through before settling comfortably into their professional roles can help reduce anxiety and increase coping. Kramer identified a model for resolving reality shock that consists of four stages.

1. *Mastery of skills and routines.* In busy acute care settings, which most new nurses choose for their first jobs, certain activities must be accomplished each day, and specific behaviors are required to accomplish them. During this stage, nurses focus on the mastery of essential skills and routines. They may temporarily lose sight of the bigger picture and may have to be reminded not to focus so much on the technical aspects of care that they fail to see patients' emotional needs.
2. *Social integration.* In this stage, which overlaps with the first stage, new nurses face the challenge of fitting into the work group. Issues of getting along and being accepted surface. Most people have a desire for peer recognition and approval. It is sometimes a challenge to retain the goodwill of co-workers while keeping high ideals and standards. Learning that they may have to sacrifice the esteem of some workers to maintain their professional values can be a painful, but necessary, lesson for nurses in this stage.
3. *Moral outrage.* Once they realize that they cannot do it all because their commitments to the needs of the organization, to the profession, and to patients often conflict, frustration and anger result. Is it more important

to attend a staff meeting or to talk to Mr. Jameson's daughter, who needs to discuss home care versus nursing home placement for her father? Managing these sorts of priorities is a challenge even for experienced nurses.

4. *Conflict resolution.* Kramer identified several possible resolutions of these problems:
   a. Change behavior while retaining values. For example, find a new work setting that is more compatible with beliefs or, if that is impossible, leave nursing altogether.
   b. Give up professional values (attending to patients' emotional needs) and accept the values of the work organization (get work done quickly) and just try to fit into the employer's existing system.
   c. Give up both sets of values; for example, adopt a "go-with-the-flow" attitude; survival becomes the goal.
   d. Become a "bicultural nurse" (p. 162), who learns to use the values of both the nursing profession and the work organization to influence positive change in the employment setting.

According to Kramer, adopting **biculturalism** is the most effective of these options.

Biculturalism

Biculturalism is a term used to describe nurses who learn to balance both cultures—the ideal nursing culture they learned about in school and the real one they experience in practice—and use the best of both.

How do bicultural nurses behave? First, they are realists. They recognize that there is no perfect work situation. They also recognize that if they are able to establish credibility and gain respect, they can later be leaders in making improvements.

Next, they accept the fact that newcomers have to demonstrate competence before they can become leaders. They know that people follow only those whom they respect. So they invest time in proving themselves before they start trying to make changes in the system. During this time, they demonstrate, through their own work, the approach to nursing care they value. They do this quietly and without fanfare, however, seeking support from like-minded peers.

Bicultural nurses observe the political system around them. Who are the real opinion makers? Who are the formal and informal leaders? Are they the same? When changes are made, who is involved, and how is it done? Who can be counted on to react to new ideas positively, and who is always negative and complaining? Is there anything that "turns on" the complainers? Are there some people who are so chronically underfunctioning that they just cannot or will not change? Answering these questions provides an appraisal of some of the political realities in the system.

Bicultural nurses willingly serve on committees to demonstrate their ability to address institution-wide issues and to meet others within the system who may share their values. They limit their committee service, however, to those committees that they believe are useful and constructive.

Bicultural nurses work at having rewarding personal lives. They realize that when people meet most of their emotional needs at work, they are vulnerable. They want to fit in so badly that they tend to sacrifice their professional values if they conflict with those of the work system or with the values of others.

Bicultural nurses take care of themselves. They negotiate for a position, not just accept what is offered. They expect reasonable compensation and work hours most of the time, although they work their fair share of undesirable shifts. They do not routinely allow their employer to take advantage of them and set them up for physical and emotional exhaustion, or burnout. They are cooperative. They demonstrate commitment and loyalty to the organization and show that nursing is more than just a job to them.

Bicultural nurses demonstrate many of the professional behaviors discussed in Chapter 6. In the final analysis, biculturalism and professionalism have many of the same attributes.

Minimizing Reality Shock

Much can be done to reduce reality shock in the transition from student to professional. Students must recognize that schools cannot provide enough clinical experience to make graduates comfortable on their first day as new nurses. They can take responsibility for obtaining as much practical experience as possible outside of school. Working in a health care setting during summers, on school breaks, and on weekends is helpful. They should avoid work during the school week, if at all possible, or keep it to an absolute minimum because academic responsibilities take priority during that time, and exhausted students make poor learners.

Some schools offer programs in which students are paired with practicing nurses (**preceptors**) and work closely with them to experience life as registered nurses do. If your school offers such a program, take advantage of it. If not, seek out information about similar programs at area hospitals. Many agencies, including hospitals and the military, are now providing excellent opportunities for students nearing graduation to function in expanded roles.

Knowing Employers' Expectations

New nurses approaching graduation should realistically appraise their strengths, weaknesses, and preferences. To reduce reality shock, it is important to ensure that there is a good "match" between one's abilities and employers' expectations. Ellis and Hartley (1998, pp. 399–401) suggest that nurses examine themselves in seven areas in which employers of new graduates have expectations.

1. *Theoretical knowledge* should be adequate to provide basic patient care and to make clinical judgments. Employers expect new nurses to be able to recognize the early signs and symptoms of patient problems, such as an allergic reaction to a blood transfusion, and take the appropriate nursing action, that is, turn off the transfusion. They are expected to

know potential problems related to various patient conditions, such as postoperative status, and what nursing actions to take to prevent complications.

2. The ability to *use the nursing process* systematically as a means of planning nursing care is important. Employers evaluate nurses' understanding of the phases of the process: assessment, analysis, nursing diagnosis/outcome identification, planning, intervention, and evaluation. They expect nurses to ensure that all elements of a nursing care plan are used in delivering nursing care and that there is documentation in the patient's record to that effect. The ability to follow critical paths or other already-developed plans of care is also expected.

3. *Self-awareness* is critically important. Employers ask prospective employees to identify their own strengths and weaknesses. They need to know that new nurses are willing to ask for help and recognize their limitations. New graduates who are unable or unwilling to request help pose a risk to patients that employers are unwilling to accept.

4. *Documentation ability* is an increasingly important skill that employers value. Although patient documentation systems differ from facility to facility, employers expect new graduates to know what patient data should be charted and that all nursing care should be entered in patient records. Accuracy, legibility, spelling, and use of correct grammar and approved abbreviations are all minimal expectations. The increasing use of bedside computers for patient record keeping places another demand on new graduates. Employers increasingly expect graduates to adapt computer skills to the agency's systems in a reasonable time.

5. *Work ethic* is another area in which employers are vitally interested. **Work ethic** means that prospective employees understand what is expected of them and are committed to providing it. Nursing is not, and never has been, a nine-to-five profession. Although work schedules are more flexible today than ever before, patient care still goes on around the clock, on weekends, and on holidays. Employers expect new graduates to recognize that the most desirable positions and work hours do not usually go to entry-level workers in any field. Nursing is no different in this respect from accounting, broadcasting, or investment banking. In nursing, others cannot leave work until they turn patient care responsibilities over to a qualified replacement; therefore, being late to work or "calling in sick" when not genuinely incapacitated are luxuries professional nurses cannot afford. Tardy nurses quickly lose credibility with their peers. Employers expect new nurses to recognize and accept that employment means some sacrifices in personal convenience—as in every other profession.

6. *Skill proficiency* of new graduates varies widely, and employers are aware of this. Most large facilities now provide fairly lengthy orientation periods when each nurse's skills are appraised and opportunities are provided to practice new procedures. In general, smaller and rural facilities have less formalized orientation programs, and earlier independent functioning is expected. It is useful to keep a log of nursing procedures learned during

school. Many schools provide a skills checklist that is helpful in identifying areas in which students need more practice. Students can then be assertive in seeking specific types of patient assignments.

7. *Speed of functioning* is another area in which new nurses very widely. By the end of the orientation period, the new graduate should be able to manage the average patient load without too much difficulty. Time management is a skill that is closely related to speed of functioning. Managing time well means managing yourself well and requires self-discipline. The ability to organize and prioritize nursing care for a group of patients requires time management skills (See Box 8–3 to determine what can be done to keep poor time management from becoming a problem.).

8. Collaboration skills, including communication with patients, families, co-workers, and other health professionals, are increasingly important. The delivery of high quality nursing care is related to how well the care delivery team works together. Nurses are expected to take the lead in establishing a tone of mutual respect within the team. This requires the effective application of the communication and collaboration skills discussed in Chapter 17.

Other Measures to Reduce Reality Shock

Other measures to reduce reality shock include seeking an employment situation with an **internship** or long orientation period. Inquire about preceptor opportunities, that is, working alongside an experienced nurse, and assess the level of professional development activities offered in each facility under consideration.

Recognize that all large systems have a certain amount of **inertia** (disinclination to change), and as good as a new nurse's ideas are, they may not be welcomed. Learning how change is accomplished in the institution is an important first step in becoming a positive influence on its system of operation. Identifying which battles to fight and which to ignore is a learning process for all new professionals.

Talking with other new graduates about feelings is one of the best ways to combat reality shock. Take the initiative to form a group for mutual support—others need it too! Another interpersonal strategy is to seek a professional mentor. A **mentor** is an experienced nurse who is committed to nursing and to sharing knowledge with less experienced nurses to help advance their careers. A mentor can be a great source of all types of knowledge as well as another source of support. Mentoring involves forming a relationship through which ideas, experiences, and successful behavior patterns are transmitted.

Ask a nurse whose work you admire to be a mentor and identify what he or she can offer. Some inexperienced nurses are fearful of approaching potential mentors with this request. They should remember that this process is not a one-way street; it has benefits to both parties because it complements and validates the mentor's knowledge and self-esteem as well as providing important information and support to the nurse being mentored.

BOX 8-3
Time Management Self-Assessment

Good time management is a skill that can be developed. Listed are principles reflecting good time management. Circle the answer most characteristic of how you manage your time.

1. I spend some time each day planning how to accomplish school and other responsibilities.
   0. Rarely
   1. Sometimes
   2. Frequently

2. I set specific goals and dates for accomplishing tasks.
   0. Rarely
   1. Sometimes
   2. Frequently

3. Each day I make a "to do" list and prioritize it. I complete the most important tasks first.
   0. Rarely
   1. Sometimes
   2. Frequently

4. I plan time in my schedule for unexpected problems and unanticipated delays.
   0. Rarely
   1. Sometimes
   2. Frequently

5. I ask others for help when possible.
   0. Rarely
   1. Sometimes
   2. Frequently

6. I take advantage of short but regular breaks to refresh myself and stay alert.
   0. Rarely
   1. Sometimes
   2. Frequently

7. When I really need to concentrate, I work in a specific area that is free from distractions and interruptions.
   0. Rarely
   1. Sometimes
   2. Frequently

8. When working, I turn down other people's requests that interfere with completing my priority tasks.
   0. Rarely
   1. Sometimes
   2. Frequently

9. I avoid unproductive and prolonged socializing with fellow students or employees during my workday.
   0. Rarely
   1. Sometimes
   2. Frequently

10. I keep a calendar of important meetings, dates, and deadlines and carry it with me.
    0. Rarely
    1. Sometimes
    2. Frequently

Scoring: Give yourself 2 points for each "Frequently," 1 point for each "Sometimes," and 0 points for each "Rarely." If your score is 0–10, you need to improve your time management skills; 11–15, you are doing fine and can still improve; 16–18, you have very good time management skills; and 19–20, your time management skills are too good to be true!

In preparing for a relationship with a mentor, you must first:

1. Complete a self-assessment to identify your professional and personal needs and skills.
2. Select a mentor who seems to share your nursing values and beliefs.
3. Ask for an appointment to share your needs and values and determine the areas of mutual interest in the mentoring process.
4. Be prepared to communicate openly with your mentor. Be aware that to grow you must be willing to identify your vulnerabilities and needs (Hagenow and McCrea, 1994).

An exciting new opportunity to pair with a mentor is now possible through the World Wide Web. If you would like to establish a mentoring relationship online, log on to *www.nursingnet.org* and learn about NursingNet's mentoring project. This website was created and is maintained by practicing nurses who seek to improve professionalization in nursing.

Summary of Key Points

- Professional socialization is a critical process that turns novices into fully functioning professionals.
- The two major components of socialization to professional nursing are socialization through education and socialization in the workplace.
- There are several models of professional socialization that identify stages in the process and key behaviors occurring at each stage.
- Individuals have significant responsibility for active participation in their own professional socialization. They should identify needed learning experiences and seek opportunities that provide them.
- Reality shock has been identified as a stressful period new nurses may experience upon entering nursing practice. Understanding the stages and how to resolve them can assist new graduates through this transition.
- Knowing what employers expect can help students plan more effectively and help them be more assertive in seeking experiences they need.

Critical Thinking Questions

1. Describe how both formal and informal socialization experiences in school are modifying your image of nursing.
2. Select one model of socialization discussed in this chapter and place yourself in one of the stages. Give your rationale for that placement. If none of the models fits your experience, design one and share it with the class.
3. List five things you can do to take active responsibility for your own professional socialization.
4. Interview a new nurse and assess his or her reality shock experience. How is this individual handling the transition from student to practicing nurse? What can you learn from his or her experience?

5. Identify several personal and professional areas in which a mentor might be helpful to you. Select a potential mentor and talk with him or her about your needs. If possible, establish a relationship with a mentor using guidelines in this chapter.

Web Resources

National Student Nurses Association, http://www.nsna.org

Nursing Center, http://nursingcenter.com

NursingNet, http://www.nursingnet.com

References

American Nurses Association. (1985). *Code for nurses with interpretive statements.* Washington, D. C.: American Nurses Association.

Bandura, A. (1977). *Social learning theory.* Englewood Cliffs, NJ: Prentice-Hall.

Benner, P. (1984). *From novice to expert: Excellence and power in clinical nursing practice.* Menlo Park, Calif.: Addison-Wesley.

Benner, P., Tanner, C. A., and Chesla, C. A. (1996). *Expertise in nursing practice: Caring, clinical judgment, and ethics.* New York: Springer.

Cohen, H. A. (1981). *The nurse's quest for professional identity.* Menlo Park, Calif.: Addison-Wesley.

Colucciello, M. L. (1990). Socialization into nursing: A developmental approach. *NursingConnections, 3*(2), 17–27.

Ellis, J. R., and Hartley, C. L. (1998). *Nursing in today's world*: Challenges, issues, trends (6th ed.). Philadelphia: J. B. Lippincott.

Erikson, E. (1950). *Childhood and society.* New York: W. W. Norton.

Hagenow, N. R., and McCrea, M. A. (1994). A mentoring relationship: Two viewpoints. *Nursing Management, 25*(12), 42–43.

Hinshaw, A. S. (1976). *Socialization and resocialization of nurses for professional nursing practice.* New York: National League for Nursing.

Jacox, A. (1973). Professional socialization of nurses. *Journal of the New York State Nurses' Association, 4*(4), 6–15.

Kramer, M. (1974). *Reality shock: Why nurses leave nursing.* St. Louis, Mo.: Mosby.

McCain, N. L. (1985). A test of Cohen's developmental model for professional socialization with baccalaureate nursing students. *Journal of Nursing Education, 24*(5), 180–186.

Throwe, A. N., and Fought, S. G. (1987). Landmarks in the socialization process from RN to BSN. *Nurse Educator, 12*(6), 15–18.

Wooley, A. S. (1978). From RN to BSN: Faculty perceptions. *Nursing Outlook, 26*(2), 104–106.

Philosophies of Nursing

Kay K. Chitty

Key Terms

Aesthetics
Belief
Bioethics
Epistemology
Ethics
Logic
Metaphysics
Nonjudgmental
Philosophy
Politics
Values

Learning Outcomes

After studying this chapter, students will be able to:

- Define and give examples of beliefs.
- Define and give examples of values.
- Cite examples of nursing philosophies.
- Discuss the impact of beliefs and values on nurses' professional behaviors.
- Explain why nurses need a philosophy of nursing.
- Identify personal beliefs, values, and philosophies as they relate to nursing.

Up to now, this book has focused on describing and defining nursing from the outside. The historical milestones of the profession, how its practitioners are educated, the social context in which nursing has evolved, the organizations nurses belong to, how nursing measures up as a profession, how nurses define their profession, and how new nurses are socialized have all been examined. Now we will begin to examine what nurses themselves think, believe, and value, and how their care of patients is influenced by these thoughts, beliefs, and values. In other words, nursing will be explored from the inside.

Certain beliefs have evolved during the development of professional nursing. Specific statements of beliefs were generated by the members of the American Nurses Association (ANA) and published in the *Code for Nurses with Interpretive Statements* (see Appendix A). Statements such as the *Code* exist to affirm the beliefs of the profession and to guide the practice of nursing.

Beliefs about nursing and values pertaining to nursing are at the core of philosophies of nursing. This chapter examines the relationship of beliefs, values, and philosophies to the practice of nursing; reviews several philosophies of nursing that were developed by an individual, two hospitals, and two schools of nursing; and assists readers in beginning to develop their own philosophies of nursing.

Beliefs

A **belief** represents the intellectual acceptance of something as true or correct. Beliefs can also be described as convictions or creeds. Beliefs are opinions that may be, in reality, true or false. They are based on attitudes that have been acquired and verified by experience. Beliefs are generally transmitted from generation to generation.

Although all people have beliefs, relatively few have spent much time examining their beliefs. In nursing, it is important to know and understand one's beliefs because the practice of nursing frequently challenges nurses' beliefs. Although this conflict may create temporary discomfort, it is ultimately good because it forces nurses to consider their beliefs carefully. They have to answer the question: "Is this something I really believe, or have I accepted it because some influential person [such as a parent or teacher] said it?" Abortion, advance directives, the right to die, the right to refuse treatment, alternative lifestyles, and similar issues confront all members of contemporary society. Professional nurses must develop and refine their beliefs about these and many other issues. This is often difficult to do.

Beliefs are exhibited through attitudes and behaviors. Simply observing how nurses relate to patients, their families, and nursing peers reveals something about those nurses' beliefs. Every day nurses meet people whose beliefs are different from, or even diametrically opposed to, their own. Effective nurses recognize that they need to adopt **nonjudgmental** attitudes toward patients' beliefs. A nurse with a nonjudgmental attitude makes every effort to convey neither approval nor disapproval of patients' beliefs and respects each person's right to his or her beliefs (Fig. 9–1).

An example of differences in beliefs that directly affect nursing is the position taken by some religious groups that all healing should be left to a divine power. Seeking medical treatment, even lifesaving ones such as blood transfusions or chemotherapy for cancer, is not condoned. From time to time, there have been news reports of parents who are charged with criminal acts because they did not take a sick child to a physician. Typical of such incidents was the one reported in Pennsylvania when a 2-year-old boy developed a form of kidney cancer. His parents never took him to a physician because they believed that ". . . life rests in God's hands and that trust in medicine harms one's spiritual and eternal interests, which are more important than physical well-being. . . ." (Levine, 1989, p. 220). These parents were ultimately convicted of involuntary manslaughter and endangering the welfare of a child.

Because you are in a health profession, you clearly have beliefs about the value of modern medicine. Think about how your health care beliefs differ from those of this family. What feelings might you have if assigned to work with a family with these beliefs? From this brief exercise, it can be seen how difficult maintaining a nonjudgmental attitude toward the beliefs of patients can be. It is nevertheless essential.

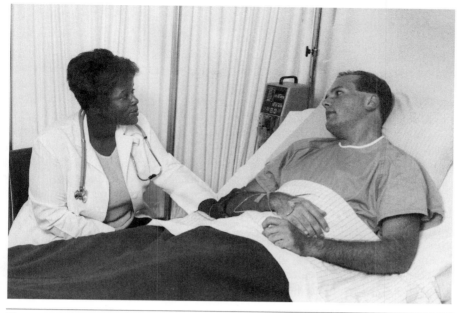

Figure 9–1
Professional nurses make every effort to maintain a nonjudgmental attitude toward patients. A nonjudgmental attitude is one of nursing's values (Photo by Fielding Freed).

Three Categories of Beliefs

People often use the terms *beliefs* and *values* interchangeably. Even experts disagree about whether they differ or are the same. Although they are related, beliefs and values are differentiated in this chapter and discussed separately.

Rokeach (1973, pp. 6–7) identified three main categories of beliefs:

1. *Descriptive* or *existential beliefs* are those that can be shown to be true or false. An example of a descriptive belief is "The sun will come up tomorrow morning."
2. *Evaluative beliefs* are those in which there is a judgment about good or bad. The belief "Dancing is immoral" is an example of an evaluative belief.
3. *Prescriptive* (encouraged) and *proscriptive* (prohibited) *beliefs* are those in which certain actions are judged to be desirable or undesirable. The belief "Every citizen of voting age should vote in every election" is a prescriptive belief, whereas the belief "People should not engage in sexual intercourse outside of marriage" is a proscriptive belief. Prescriptive and proscriptive beliefs are closely related to values.

Values

Values are the social principles, ideals, or standards held by an individual, class, or group that give meaning and direction to life. A value is an abstract representation of what is right, worthwhile, or desirable. Values reflect what people consider desirable and consist of the subjective assignment of worth to behavior. Although many people are unaware of it, values help them make both small, day-to-day choices and important life decisions. Just as beliefs influence nursing practice, values also influence how nurses practice their profession, often without their conscious awareness. Diann Uustal (1985), a contemporary nurse who has written and spoken extensively about values, said, "Everything we do, every decision we make and course of action we take is based on our consciously and unconsciously chosen beliefs, attitudes and values" (p. 100). Uustal asserts that "Nursing is a behavioral manifestation of the nurse's value system. It is not merely a career, a job, an assignment; it is a *ministry*" (1993, p. 10). She believes that nurses must give "caring attentiveness and presence" to their patients and to do otherwise "is equivalent to psychological and spiritual abandonment" (Uustal, 1993). Do you agree or disagree with these statements?

Nature of Human Values

Values evolve as people mature. An individual's values today are undoubtedly different from those of ten, or even five, years ago. Rokeach (1973, p. 3) made several assertions about the nature of human values:

1. Each person has a relatively small number of values.
2. All human beings, regardless of location or culture, possess basically the same values to differing degrees.
3. People organize their values into value systems.
4. People develop values in response to culture, society, and even individual personality traits.
5. Most observable human behaviors are manifestations or consequences of human values.

Authorities agree that values influence behavior and that people with unclear values lack direction, persistence, and decision-making skills (Raths, Harmin, and Simon, 1978). Because much of nursing involves having a clear sense of direction, the ability to persevere, and the ability to make sound decisions quickly and frequently, effective nurses must have a strong set of professional nursing values. A number of professional nursing values are listed in Box 9–1.

Process of Valuing

Valuing is the process by which values are determined. There are three identified steps in the process of valuing: choosing, prizing, and acting.

BOX 9-1
Professional Nursing Values

Accountability	Nonjudgmental attitude
Caring	Openness to learning
Collaboration	Partnerships with patients
Competence	Patient advocacy
Cooperative work relationships	Patient education
Dependability	Promotion of health
Dignity of the patient	Promotion of patient self-determi-
Empathy	nation
Ethical conduct	Providing care regardless of pa-
Flexibility	tient's ability to pay
Health promotion	Quality care (physical, emotional,
Holism	spiritual, social, intellectual)
Honesty	Respect for each person
Illness prevention	Sharing self through nursing inter-
Individualized patient care	ventions
Integrity	Support of fellow nurses
Involvement with families	Teamwork
Knowledge	Trust
Listening	

From Uustal, D. B. (1985). *Values and ethics in nursing: From theory to practice.* East Greenwich, R. I.: Educational Resources in Nursing and Wholistic Health.

Choosing is the cognitive (intellectual) aspect of valuing. Ideally, people choose their values freely from all alternatives after considering the possible consequences of their choices.

Prizing is the affective (emotional) aspect of valuing. People usually feel good about their values and cherish the choices they make.

Acting is the kinesthetic (behavioral) aspect of valuing. When people affirm their values publicly by acting on their choices, they make their values part of their behavior. A real value is acted upon consistently in behavior.

All three steps must be taken, or the process of valuing is incomplete. For example, a professional nurse might believe that learning is a lifelong process and that nurses have an obligation to keep up with new developments in the profession. This nurse would choose continued learning and appreciate the consequences of the choice. He or she might even publicly affirm this choice and feel good about it. If the nurse follows through consistently with behaviors such as reading journals, attending conferences, and seeking out other learning opportunities, continued learning can be seen as a true value in his or her life.

Values Clarification

Nurses as well as people in other helping professions need to understand their values. This is the first step in self-awareness, which is important in maintaining a nonjudgmental approach to patients.

A variety of values clarification exercises have been developed to help people understand their values. Considering your reactions to these statements can help in beginning to identify some nursing values you hold:

1. Patients should always be told the truth about their diagnoses.
2. Nurses, if asked, should assist terminally ill patients to die.
3. Severely impaired infants should be kept alive, regardless of their future quality of life.
4. Nurses should never accept gifts from patients.
5. A college professor should receive a heart transplant before a homeless person does.
6. Nurses should be role models of healthy behavior.

As you react both emotionally and intellectually to these statements, something about your personal and professional values is revealed. Determining where you stand on these and other nursing issues is an important step in clarifying your values. Box 9–2 contains a values clarification exercise you may want to complete to assist you further in understanding the valuing process.

Values Undergirding Nursing's Social Policy Statement

Professional groups, such as nursing, "have collective identities that are evidenced by their actions. These actions stem from a set of values and choices. . . . [B]y examining the actions of groups, . . . , their basic values can be logically inferred" (Mohr, 1995, p. 30).

Organized nursing, through the ANA, sets forth the values that undergird the profession. This is done in a document published from time to time that is designed to explain "nursing's relationship with society and nursing's obligation to those who receive nursing care" (American Nurses Association, 1995, p. 1). The most recent version, entitled *Nursing's Social Policy Statement,* was published in 1995. It set forth several underlying values and assumptions on which the *Statement* is based (American Nurses Association, 1995, pp. 3–4):

- Humans manifest an essential unity of mind/body/spirit.
- Human experience is contextually and culturally defined.
- Health and illness are human experiences.
- The presence of illness does not preclude health nor does optimal health preclude illness.

Another value inherent in this document is that "the relationship between a nurse and patient involves full and active participation of the patient and the nurse in the plan of care and occurs within the context of the values and beliefs

BOX 9–2
Clarifying Your Values

Once you have identified a value, it is important to assess its significance to you and to clarify your willingness to act on the value. The following clarifying questions are organized based on the steps of the valuing process and can help you answer questions about what you value. Identify a value (or values) that is (are) important to you. Write your value(s) in the space provided.

_____

_____

_____

_____

Next, use these questions to assess the importance of a belief or attitude and to determine if it is a value. Rephrase the questions to suit your own style of conversation.

Choosing Freely
1. Am I sure I've thought about this value and chosen to believe it myself?
2. Who first taught me this value?
3. How do I know I'm "right?"

Choosing from among Alternatives
4. What other alternatives are possible?
5. Which alternative has the most appeal for me and why?
6. Have I thought much about this value/alternative?

Choosing after Considering the Consequences
7. What consequences do I think might occur as a result of my holding this value?
8. What "price" will I pay for my position?
9. Is this value worth the "price" I might pay?

Complement to Other Values
10. Does this value "fit" with my other values, and is it consistent with them?
11. Am I sure this value doesn't conflict with other values I deem important to me?

Prize and Cherish
12. Am I proud of my position and value? Is this something I feel good about?
13. How important is this value to me?
14. If this were not my value, how different would my life be?

Public Affirmation
15. Am I willing to speak out for this value?

Action
16. Am I willing to put this value into action?
17. Do I act on this value? When? How consistently?
18. Is this a value that can guide me in other situations?
19. Would I want others who are important to me to follow this value?

(continued)

BOX 9–2
Clarifying Your Values (*Continued*)

20. Do I think I'll always believe this? How committed to this value am I?
21. Am I willing to do anything about this value?
22. How do I know this value is "right?" Are my values ethical?

Reprinted with permission of Uustal, D. B. (1993). *Clinical ethics and values: Issues and insights in a changing healthcare environment* (pp. 36–37). East Greenwich, R. I.: Educational Resources in Healthcare.

of the patient and the nurse" (American Nurses Association, 1995, p. 4). Chapter 19 contains more about values and their relationship to nursing practice.

Philosophies

Philosophy is defined as the study of the principles underlying conduct thought, and the nature of the universe (Webster's, 1996). A more literal translation, based on the Greek root words, means "the love of exercising one's curiosity and intelligence" (Edwards, 1967, p. 216). A simple explanation of philosophy is that it entails a search for meaning in the universe. Nursing students often learn about philosophers such as Plato, Socrates, Aristotle, Bacon, Kant, Hegel, Kierkegaard, Russell, de Chardin, Descartes, and others in nonnursing classes. These philosophers were searching for the underlying principles of reality and truth. Nursing philosophies and theories often derive from or build upon the ideas of these and other philosophers.

Philosophy begins when someone contemplates, or wonders, about something. If a group of friends sometimes sits and discusses the relationship between men and women and ponder the differences in men's and women's natures and approaches to life, one might say that they were developing a philosophy about male and female ways of being. It is important to remember that philosophy is not the exclusive domain of a few erudite individuals; everyone has a personal philosophy of life that is unique.

People develop personal philosophies as they mature. These philosophies serve as blueprints or guides and incorporate each individual's value and belief systems. Nurses' personal philosophies interact directly with their philosophies of nursing and influence professional behaviors.

Branches of Philosophy

Before examining professional philosophies, we briefly explore the discipline of philosophy itself. Philosophy has been divided into specific areas of study. This section reviews six branches: epistemology, logic, aesthetics, ethics, politics, and metaphysics.

1. **Epistemology** is the branch of philosophy dealing with the theory of knowledge. The epistemologist attempts to answer such questions as "What can be known?" and "What constitutes knowledge?" Epistemology attempts to determine how we can know whether our beliefs about the world are true.
2. **Logic** is the study of correct and incorrect reasoning. In logic, the nature of reasoning itself is the subject. It is logical behavior, for example, for fair-skinned individuals to stay out of the midday sun unless wearing protective clothing. Chapter 15 presents the method of logical thinking that nurses use to plan and implement effective patient care, called the nursing process.
3. **Aesthetics** is the study of what is beautiful. Painting, sculpture, music, dance, and literature are all associated with beauty. Judgments about what is beautiful, however, differ from individual to individual and culture to culture. For example, Eastern music may sound discordant to the Western ear and vice versa.
4. **Ethics** is the branch of philosophy that studies the propriety of certain courses of action. Moral principles and values make up a system of ethics. Behavior depends on moral principles and values. Ethics, therefore, underlie the standards of behavior that govern us as individuals and as nurses. **Bioethics** is a term describing the branch of ethics that deals with biological issues. Bioethics and nursing ethics are complex areas of study that are explored in Chapter 19.
5. **Politics,** in the context of a discussion of philosophy, means the area of philosophy that deals with the regulation and control of people living in society. Political philosophers study the conditions of society and suggest recommendations for improving them.
6. **Metaphysics** is the consideration of the ultimate nature of existence, reality, and experience. Metaphysicians believe that through contemplation we can come to a more complete understanding of reality than even science can provide.

This brief review of the branches of philosophy is presented as a backdrop for the discussion of philosophies of nursing.

Philosophies of Nursing

Philosophies of nursing are statements of beliefs about nursing and expressions of values in nursing that are used as bases for thinking and acting. Most philosophies of nursing are built on a foundation of beliefs about people, environment, health, and nursing. Each of these four foundational concepts of nursing is discussed in some detail in Chapter 10.

Individual Philosophies

If asked, most nurses could list their beliefs about nursing, but it is doubtful that many have written a formal philosophy of nursing. They are influenced on a day-to-day basis, however, by their unwritten, informal philosophies. It is

BOX 9-3
One Nurse's Philosophy

I believe that the essence of nursing is caring about and caring for human beings who are unable to care for themselves. I believe that the central core of nursing is the nurse-patient relationship and that through that relationship I can make a difference in the lives of others at a time when they are most vulnerable.

Human beings generally do the best they can. When they are uncooperative, critical, or otherwise unpleasant, it is usually because they are frightened; therefore, I will remain pleasant and nondefensive and try to understand the patient's perception of the situation. I pledge to be trustworthy and an advocate for my patients.

I realize that my cultural background affects how I deliver nursing care and that my patients' cultural backgrounds affect how they receive my care. I try to learn as much as I can about each individual's cultural beliefs and preferences and individualize care accordingly.

My vision for myself as a nurse is that I will provide the best care I can to all patients, regardless of their financial situation, social status, lifestyle choices, or spiritual beliefs. I will collaborate with my patients, their families, and my health care colleagues and work cooperatively with them, valuing and respecting what each brings to the situation.

I am individually accountable for the care I provide, for what I fail to do and to know. Therefore, I pledge to remain a learner all my life and actively seek opportunities to learn how to be a more effective nurse.

I will strive for a balance of personal and professional responsibilities. This means I will take care of myself physically, emotionally, socially, and spiritually so I can continue to be a productive caregiver.

useful to go through the process of writing down one's own professional philosophy and revising it from time to time. Comparing recent and earlier versions can reveal professional and personal growth over time. It is also helpful to read one's philosophy of nursing from time to time to make sure daily behaviors are consistent with deeply held beliefs. Box 9-3 contains one nurse's philosophy of nursing.

Collective Philosophies
Although few individuals write down their nursing philosophies, it is common for hospitals and schools of nursing to express their collective beliefs about nursing in written philosophies. In fact, both hospitals and schools of nursing are required by their accrediting bodies to develop statements of philosophy. Philosophical statements should be relevent to the setting. They are intended to guide the practice of nurses employed in that setting. Examining some of these statements clarifies what constitutes a collective philosophy of nursing.

Philosophies of Nursing in Two Hospital Settings. First look at the philosophy of the Division of Nursing at Beth Israel Hospital in Boston (Box 9–4). Notice that

BOX 9-4
Beth Israel Hospital Philosophy of Nursing

Introduction

This revised statement of philosophy and purpose has drawn on the seminal thinking of Benner, Henderson, Orlando, and Wiedenbach and on multiple documents developed by the Beth Israel Hospital nursing services and programs over a twenty-year period, including the Statement of Philosophy first issued in 1974.

Statements such as this are meaningless unless they are translated into action. Our philosophy and purpose are perhaps most succinctly expressed in the words of one of our patients: "My primary nurse was truly a gem in the profession of nursing. She combines not only the highest level of professionalism in nursing, but also the many personal qualities which go beyond that in assisting patients to make a full recovery. She had a knack for getting me to motivate myself. Her concern was genuine, her advice sound, and her willingness to assist in my long-range rehabilitation goals ever present."

Purpose

The purpose of the Beth Israel's nursing services and programs is to ensure that each patient receives professional nursing care that is patient-centered and goal-directed, and to support healthcare education and research in nursing and other disciplines. Beth Israel nurses and their associates in the division of nursing carry out their activities with one focus in mind—assisting the patient to achieve optimal health outcomes.

Philosophy

Nursing as a Professional Service

We agree with Virginia Henderson that professional nursing is a complex service that assists ". . . people (sick or well) in the performance of those activities contributing to health, or its recovery (or to a peaceful death) that they would perform unaided if they had the necessary strength, will, or knowledge. It is likewise the unique contribution of nursing to help people to be independent of such assistance as soon as possible." The activities that nurses help patients carry out (or those that nurses carry out for patients) include the therapeutic plans prescribed by physicians, by other health care providers, and by nurses themselves. In carrying out these activities, nurses practice an art through which technical, observational, analytical, and communication skills as well as scientific knowledge and clinical judgment are systematically applied to the health needs of others in a caring manner. Caring means being connected and having things matter. Thus by caring, the nurse creates possibilities for coping in the face of risk and vulnerability.

We believe that physical and emotional comfort is a universal health need, the provision of which is a historical and fundamental nursing responsibility. Nursing is further distinguished from other direct healthcare services by its tradition of continuity. For hospitalized patients, this includes 24-hour accountability for observing, recording, and reporting of the patient's condition, and for di-

(continued)

BOX 9-4
Beth Israel Hospital Philosophy of Nursing (*Continued*)

rect provision of care and comfort. For patients residing in the community, care is generally provided on an intermittent basis, incorporating the family and/or significant other in the plan to insure continuity. The nursing care in this setting includes identifying and facilitating access to community resources and supports, and encouraging patients to achieve their optimal level of functioning. Continuity of care across the spectrum of health and illness is valued and provided by all Beth Israel nurses whatever their area of practice.

We believe that for each patient, continuity, personalization, and excellence of care is best achieved when it is planned and evaluated by a collaborative patient care team whose individual members have continuous accountability for that care. We further believe that nursing care for each patient should be planned, coordinated, and delivered by a professional registered nurse, and that direct care should be provided by a primary nurse and any designated associates. The desired endpoint of all nursing activity is to maintain or improve the patient's health status and comfort.

The art and science of professional nursing is acquired through formal higher education. It becomes refined through continuing education and training, experience, self-evaluation, evaluation by a manager, and peer review.

The Beth Israel Nursing Services philosophy also contains statements about patients, families, professional nursing, and the environment for nursing care.

this philosophy includes statements of belief about nursing services, recipients of nursing care, and professional nurses themselves.

Box 9-5 contains the philosophy of nursing of Memorial Hospital in Chattanooga, Tennessee. It describes a commitment to excellence in nursing service, practice, and leadership.

Notice differences and similarities in the two philosophies as well as statements with which one might agree or disagree. Remember that these are both philosophies of departments of nursing in hospital settings. Before taking a position in a hospital or health care agency, it is a good idea to ask for a copy of the philosophy of nursing of that institution. Read it carefully and make sure you accept the beliefs and values it contains, for it will influence nursing care in that setting.

Philosophies of Two Schools of Nursing. Now examine philosophical statements of two schools of nursing. The philosophy of the faculty in the Department of Nursing at the University of North Florida is printed in Box 9-6. Box 9-7 contains the philosophy of the Department of Nursing at Central Missouri State University. After reading them, identify the similarities and differences between the philosophies of nursing in hospitals and the ones in these schools of nursing.

An important point about philosophies of nursing is that they are dynamic and change over time. When a collective philosophy is written, it reflects the

BOX 9–5
Memorial Health Care System Philosophy of Nursing

Philosophy of Nursing
Nursing Care throughout the Memorial Health Care System is committed to upholding the corporate values and the mission of Catholic Health Initiatives. We affirm that the corporate values of Reverence, Compassion, Integrity, and Excellence are in congruence with our professional values. Therefore, we believe that these principles must characterize nursing care.

Reverence
We believe . . .

- that each of our patients, regardless of circumstances, possesses intrinsic value from God and should be treated with dignity and respect.
- that meeting the needs of patients and other customers should always be our number one priority.
- that nurses should collaborate with other health care team members to meet the holistic needs of our patients, which include physical, psychosocial and spiritual aspects of care.
- that patient confidentiality and privacy should be preserved.
- that we should be sensitive to individual needs and give support, praise and recognition to encourage professional and personal development.

Compassion
We believe . . .

- that each encounter with patients and families should portray compassion and concern.
- that our profession is a science and an art, the essence of which is nurturing and caring.
- that our primary duty is to restore and maintain the health of our patients in a spirit of compassion and concern.
- that compassion should be characterized in our day to day personal interactions as well as being a motivating factor in management decisions.

Integrity
We believe . . .

- that the nursing process is an integral part of our practice as professional nurses.
- that we should aggressively promote patient and family education to allow each individual the opportunity to prevent illness and/or achieve optimal health.
- that we should encourage and support collaborative decision-making by those who are closest to the situation, even at the risk of failure.
- that we are accountable to our patients, patients' families, and to each other for our professional practice.
- that we should possess an energy level and personal style that empowers and inspires enthusiasm in others.
- that justice should be applied equitably in all employment practices and personnel policies.

(continued)

BOX 9-5
Memorial Health Care System Philosophy of Nursing
(*Continued*)

Excellence
We believe . . .

- that monitoring and evaluating nursing practice is our responsibility and is necessary to continuously improve care.
- that we should pursue professional growth and development through education, participating in professional organizations and support of research.
- that we should provide a progressive environment, utilizing current technology guided by responsible stewardship, to promote the highest quality patient care and employee satisfaction.
- that we should consider suggestions and criticisms as challenges for improvement and innovation.
- that each patient should receive quality care that is cost-effective, competitive and based on the latest technology.

Reprinted by permission of the Department of Nursing, Memorial Health Care System, a division of Catholic Health Initiatives. (1999). *Philosophy of nursing*. Chattanooga, Tenn.: Memorial Health Care System.

existing values and beliefs of particular group of people who wrote it. When the group members change, the philosophy may change. Therefore, once a collective philosophy is written, it should be "revisited" regularly and modified to reflect accurately the group's current beliefs about nursing practice (Cody, 1990).

Developing a Personal Philosophy of Nursing

Developing a philosophy of nursing is not merely an academic exercise required by accrediting bodies. Having a written philosophy can help guide nurses in the daily decisions they must make in nursing practice.

Writing a philosophy is not a complex, time-consuming task. It simply involves writing down one's beliefs and values about nursing. It answers the question: Why do you practice nursing the way you do? A philosophy should provide direction and promote effectiveness. If it does not, it is a time-wasting collection of words.

Box 9–8 is designed to help you develop your own personal philosophy of nursing. After you write a beginning philosophy, save it. As you progress through your educational program, take it out and revise it regularly, saving each version. After you graduate, look back at all the different versions and see how your values and beliefs about nursing have changed over time.

BOX 9-6

Philosophy of the Department of Nursing, University of North Florida

The philosophy of the Department of Nursing supports the mission of the University of North Florida and the College of Health and reflects the academic goals of the greater university community. The faculty have defined a philosophy of nursing that considers two domains: the patient who is the recipient of care, and the nurse who is the care-giver. The patient domain includes beliefs about persons, environment and health.

The faculty of the Department of Nursing view patients as biopsychosocial beings with inherent dignity and worth who strive to meet a hierarchy of human needs throughout the life span. When unable to satisfy these needs, patients are at risk for alterations in health status. As risks manifest themselves in health problems, patients seek relief in the form of health care from health professionals. Nursing responds to a need for care and support and, in some cases, the need for treatments and curing techniques. Patients of nursing may be individuals, families, groups, or communities.

Patients live in an environment with an internal and external dimension. The internal environment is an open system composed of four subsystems: physical, psychological, spiritual, and cultural. The external environment is composed of groups of individuals and families, each living within their unique sociocultural milieu. These groups function in a universe influenced by political and economic forces. The dynamic relationship between internal and external environments has a profound effect on health status and on how persons adapt to physical, psychological, social, and environmental changes.

Health is viewed as a dynamic state of being on a continuum from optimal wellness to illness. Changes on this continuum are influenced and, in some cases, caused by internal and external environmental stressors. A state of health exists when a person functions as an integrated whole, living and interacting with environments in a productive manner. Movement on the health-illness continuum depends on the severity of stressors, the adaptive mechanisms of the person and the accessibility to and quality of health care services available.

The nurse/care-giver domain includes beliefs about nursing, education, and professional practice and research. Nursing is a human service that assists patients to achieve optimal wellness and cope with periods of illness and disability. The nurse uses problem-solving skills and caring behaviors to facilitate the patient's adaptive responses in an effort to maintain, promote and/or restore an optimal state of health or facilitate a peaceful death. Specific caring behaviors are determined by the patient's individual needs and may be assistive, supportive, or facilitative in nature. The nurse assumes independent and interdependent roles at various times, based on mutually identified needs of the patient. Nurses fulfill their professional role as members of a health care team working together in the best interest of the patient.

(continued)

BOX 9–6

Philosophy of the Department of Nursing, University of North Florida (*Continued*)

Nursing education takes place through a planned teaching-learning process. Faculty are responsible for assisting students to achieve their full potential and are sensitive to the individual needs of students. Learning readiness, self-directed learning, recognition of the value of past experience and education, and the development of a problem-solving orientation to learning are important aspects of the teaching-learning process. Students and faculty cooperate in assuming a shared responsibility for planning and implementing learning activities within the context of the curriculum and through individual course offerings. Learning is facilitated when the educational environment provides an open, accepting atmosphere in which the faculty and students work together to achieve mutual goals. Higher education is a process through which the student is afforded opportunities to develop a liberal education as well as a rich knowledge base on which to build a professional career.

Baccalaureate nursing education is specifically concerned with preparation for the first professional degree in nursing. This education prepares the student for professional practice and leadership roles within an ever changing health care industry. It also serves as a foundation for graduate education and advanced nursing practice.

Professional nursing practice is based on concepts and theories from the discipline of nursing and from other fields, including the sciences and humanities. Professional nurses use the nursing process, which demands the ability to assess, analyze, plan, implement and evaluate nursing care. The nursing process is the basis of scientific nursing practice and requires nurses to analyze data from many sources. A strong foundation from the natural sciences and the humanities assists nurses in developing the critical thinking skills essential to the nursing process. The scientific base of practice continues to be developed throughout the nursing curriculum and provides the graduate with the knowledge and skills to practice nursing in a responsible manner.

Nursing is a discipline that uses research as a process to develop a distinct body of knowledge which will provide a basis for scientific practice. Research serves as the basis for changes that influence and improve nursing practice and patient care outcomes. The professional nurse prepared at the baccalaureate level should be an informed consumer of research findings and should be able to collaborate with others to study questions that arise from the practice of nursing and related issues.

Reprinted by permission of Department of Nursing, University of North Florida (1999). *Philosophy of the Department of Nursing*. Jacksonville, Fla.: University of North Florida.

BOX 9-7
Philosophy of the Department of Nursing, Central Missouri State University

The philosophy of the Department of Nursing is founded on the belief that the profession of nursing makes an essential contribution to society and that education for professional nursing and advanced practice nursing is best conducted in an institution of higher learning. For these purposes, we believe:

- Persons are the focus of nursing. Persons are moral beings endowed with individual qualities, but hold in common with others the basic need for dignity, respect, and recognition of their individual worth and uniqueness.
- Health is the actualization of inherent and acquired human potential, either as individual, aggregate, or collective humanity.
- Nursing is a human science and an art concerned with the diagnosis and treatment of human responses to actual or potential health changes (ANA).
- The professional nurse functions in an ethical manner as an independent practitioner or as a collaborator with other health team members.
- In the future the professional nurse will practice in expanded roles and, with additional formal education, will practice in advanced practice nursing roles in increasing numbers and in a variety of settings, many of which will be outside acute care institutions.
- Teaching is an interactive, interpersonal activity whereby the teacher is a learner, facilitator, and collaborator. The role of the teacher is to provide structure, climate, and dialogue so the student can explore and discover self.
- Learning is a process whereby the student begins to view wholes, develop insights into situations, find meanings, evaluate rules and values, project consequences, and predict from knowns to unknowns using both data and intuition.
- Communication, Critical Thinking, Nursing Process, Professionhood, Valuing, Environment, and Interpersonal Relationships are essential graduate outcomes.
- Formative and summative assessments are important to the development and achievement of graduate outcomes.

Through fulfillment of these beliefs, our baccalaureate degree students, upon graduation, will be prepared to practice nursing as generalists in rural and urban settings. Through their baccalaureate nursing education, our students will be provided with the foundation for further study and advancement. We feel our advanced nursing degree students, upon graduation, will be prepared to practice nursing as specialists in primarily rural areas. Through their master's level nursing education, students are provided with the foundation for advanced practice specialty practice, and advanced study at the doctoral level.

Reprinted by permission of the Department of Nursing, Central Missouri State University. (1999). *Philosophy of nursing.* Warrensburg, Mo.: Central Missouri State University.

BOX 9–8
Philosophy of Nursing Work Sheet

Purpose: To write a beginning philosophy of nursing that reflects the beliefs and values of _____ [Your Name].
Today's date is _____.
I chose nursing as my profession because nursing is _____.
I believe that the core of nursing is _____.
I believe that the focus of nursing is _____.
My vision for myself as a nurse is that I will _____.
To live out my philosophy of nursing, every day I must remember this about:

1. My patients _____.
2. My patients' families _____.
3. My fellow health care professionals _____.
4. My own health _____.

Summary of Key Points

- People develop beliefs and values that affect their attitudes and behaviors.
- Beliefs and values influence how nurses practice their profession.
- Nurses need to be aware of their beliefs and values to prevent the unintentional intrusion of personal values into nurse-patient relationships.
- A statement of beliefs can be called a philosophy.
- The purpose of developing a philosophy of nursing is to shape and guide nursing practice.
- There are numerous philosophical statements about nursing and nursing education.
- Philosophies can either express individual beliefs or beliefs of a group, such as a nursing faculty.
- As nurses progress professionally, they collect ideas about the practice of nursing that they agree with and support. From these, they develop their own personal philosophies of nursing.
- As nurses mature in the profession, they may find that their philosophies about nursing also change, even though underlying values may not.

Critical Thinking Questions

1. Name two of your health-related values. How did these become your values? Describe how you expect these values to influence your nursing practice.
2. After reading "One Nurse's Philosophy" in Box 9–3, identify at least 10 of that nurse's professional values that are listed in Box 9–1, "Professional Nursing Values."
3. Compare the nursing philosophies of Beth Israel and Memorial hospitals. What are three common elements and three differences? If you or a family

member needed to be hospitalized and you had to select a hospital based on the philosophy of nursing, which of these two hospitals would you choose? Why?

4. Obtain the philosophy statement of the faculty of your school of nursing. What concepts are included? Which beliefs do you agree with and disagree with? Why?

5. Using the work sheet in Box 9–8, write a beginning philosophy of nursing. Share your philosophy with one other person.

6. Discuss how having or not having a philosophy of nursing influences a nurse's practice.

7. Discuss how the current focus on "the bottom line" impacts your own and nursing's professional values.

Web Resources

Personal philosophy, http://www.orths.com/robert/nurse/nurse.html

Sample hospital philosophy, http://www.sw.org/jobs/nsg/f_philos.htm

Values clarification, http://www.astro.clpccd.cc.ca.us/Nursing70/values.html

References

American Nurses Association (1995). *Nursing's social policy statement.* Washington, D. C.: American Nurses Association.

Beth Israel Hospital Division of Nursing (1996). *Statement of philosophy and purpose.* Boston: Beth Israel Hospital.

Central Missouri State University, Department of Nursing (1999). *Philosophy of nursing.* Warrensburg, Mo.: Central Missouri State University.

Cody, B. (1990). Shaping the future through a philosophy of nursing. *Journal of Nursing Administration,* 20(10), 16–22.

Edwards, P. (Ed.) (1967). *Encyclopedia of philosophy.* New York: Macmillan.

Levine, C. (1989). God's will versus doctor's orders. *Parents' Magazine,* 64(3), 220, 222, 226–227.

Memorial Health Care System Department of Nursing. (1999). *Memorial Health Care System philosophy of nursing.* Chattanooga, Tenn.: Memorial Health Care System.

Mohr, W. K. (1995). Values, ideologies, and dilemmas: Professional and occupational contradictions. *Journal of Psychosocial Nursing,* 33(1), 29–34.

Raths, L., Harmin, M., and Simon, S. (1978). *Values and teaching* (2nd ed.). Columbus, Ohio: Charles Merrill.

Rokeach, M. (1973). *The nature of human values.* New York: Free Press.

University of North Florida, Department of Nursing (1999). *Philosophy of the department of Nursing.* Jacksonville, Fla.: University of North Florida.

Uustal, D. B. (1985). *Values and ethics in nursing: From theory to practice.* East Greenwich, R. I.: Educational Resources in Nursing and Wholistic Health.

Uustal, D. B. (1993). *Clinical ethics and values: Issues and insights in a changing healthcare environment.* East Greenwich, R. I.: Educational Resources in Healthcare.

Webster's New World Dictionary and Thesaurus. (1996). New York: Macmillan.

Major Concepts in Nursing

Kay K. Chitty

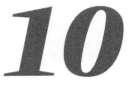

Key Terms

Adaptation
Closed System
Culture
Environment
Evaluation
Extended Family
Feedback
Health
Health Behaviors
Health Beliefs
High-Level Wellness
Holism
Homeostasis
Human Motivation
Input
Abraham Maslow
Nuclear Families
Nursing

Open System
Output
Person
Self-Actualization

Self-Efficacy
Subsystems
Suprasystem
System

Learning Outcomes

After studying this chapter, students will be able to:

- Summarize the concepts basic to professional nursing.
- Describe the components and processes of systems.
- Explain human needs.
- Recognize how environmental factors such as family, culture, social support, the Internet, and community influence health.
- Explain the significance of a holistic approach to nursing care.
- Apply Rosenstock's model of health beliefs and Bandura's theory of perceived self-efficacy to personal health behaviors and health behaviors of others.
- Devise a personal plan for achieving high-level wellness.

There are certain basic concepts, or ideas, that are essential to an understanding of professional nursing practice; they are the building blocks of nursing. These concepts are person, environment, and health. Everything professional nurses do is in some way related to one of these basic interrelated concepts. A general overview of systems will assist you in understanding how the concepts relate to each other and to nursing.

Systems

A **system** is a set of interrelated parts that come together to form a whole. Each part is a necessary or integral component required to make a complete, meaningful whole. These parts are input, output, evaluation, and feedback (von Bertalanffy, 1968).

Components of Systems

The first component of a system is **input,** which is the information, energy, or matter that enters a system. For a system to work well, input should contribute to achieving the purpose of the system.

A second component of a system is **output,** the end result or product of the system. Outputs vary widely, depending on the type and purpose of the system. **Evaluation** is the third component of a system. Evaluation means measuring the success or failure of the output and consequently the effectiveness of the system. For evaluation to be meaningful in any system, outcome criteria, against which performance or product quality is measured, must be identified.

The process of communicating what is found in evaluation of the system is called **feedback,** the final component of a system. Feedback is the information given back into the system to determine whether or not the purpose, or end result, of the system has been achieved. Figure 10–1 depicts the components of systems and how they relate to each other.

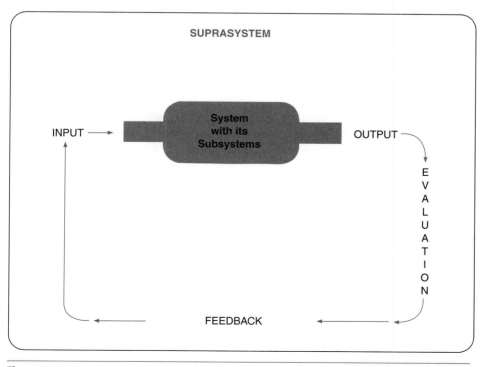

Figure 10–1
Major components of a general systems model.

Examples of Systems

It may be helpful to use a familiar example to clarify the components of systems. In a college system, *input* consists of students, faculty, ideas, the desire to learn, and knowledge. Because the purpose of the system is to educate, the students need to be ready to learn, the faculty should be prepared to teach, and the ideas and knowledge tramsmitted must be clear and understandable. The *output,* or product, of the system is educated graduates. For *evaluation* of the output, a standardized examination of reading comprehension, mathematics, and analytical skills may be used. Student scores on the comprehensive examination provide *feedback* to the faculty and administrators. If students score well, the system has achieved its purpose. If not, changes need to be made in the input or in the system itself, for example, to admit brighter students, hire more talented faculty, or design more rigorous courses and curricula.

Systems are usually complex and consist of several parts called **subsystems.** Let us examine a hospital as a system. Technically, it is a system for providing health care, but the success of the system depends on the functioning of many subsystems. The subsystems include the laboratory, radiology, housekeeping, laundry, central supply, medical records, dietetics, nursing, pharmacy, and medical staff. All these subsystems function collaboratively to make the health care provider system—the hospital—work.

Open and Closed Systems

The hospital and all its subsystems are **open systems.** An open system promotes the exchange of matter, energy, and information with other systems and the environment. The larger environment outside the hospital is called the **suprasystem.** A **closed system** does not interact with other systems or with the surrounding environment. Matter, energy, and information do not flow into or out of a closed system. There are few totally closed systems. A completely balanced aquarium approaches a closed system.

Two more points are essential to a beginning understanding of systems. First, the whole is different from and greater than the sum of its parts. Stated another way, the system is different from and greater than the sum of its subsystems. Anyone who has ever been in a hospital, for example, knows that what happens there is different from and more than the sum of the following equation: laundry + pharmacy + nurses + physicians = hospital. Something additional occurs when all the various subsystems and the people who make them up join forces to work with patients and their families.

Dynamic Nature of Systems

The final point to be made about systems is that change in one part of the system creates change in other parts. If the hospital admissions office, for example, decides to admit patients only between the hours of 8:00 A.M. and

10:00 A.M., that decision creates changes in the nursing units, housekeeping, the business office, surgery, the laboratory, and other hospital subsystems. If that change were implemented without prior communication to the other subsystems and coordinated planning, it could create chaos in the system.

The exchange of energy and information within open systems and between open systems and their suprasystems is continuous. The dynamic balance within and between the sybsystems, the system, and the suprasystems helps create and maintain **homeostasis,** or internal stability.

All living systems are open systems. The internal environment is in constant interaction with a changing environment external to the organism. As change occurs in one, the other is affected. For example, walking into a cold room (change in the external environment) affects a variety of physiological and psychological subsystems of the person's internal environment. These, in turn, affect a person's blood flow, ability to concentrate, feeling of comfort, and so on (changes in internal environment).

The openness of human systems makes nursing intervention possible. Understanding systems helps nurses assess relationships among all the factors that affect patients, including the influence of nurses themselves. Nurses who understand systems view patients holistically, including the subsystems (respiratory system, gastrointestinal system, and so on) and suprasystem (family, culture, and community). These nurses appreciate the influence of change in any part of the system. For instance, when a diabetic patient has pneumonia (change in subsystem), the infection increases the blood sugar and may result in hospitalization. Hospitalization may adversely affect the patient's role in the family and community (change in suprasystem). Key concepts of systems are summarized in Box 10–1. With this beginning understanding of systems as a foundation, the three basic concepts that are fundamental to the practice of professional nursing can now be examined.

BOX 10–1
Key Concepts about Systems

- A system is a set of interrelated parts.
- The parts form a meaningful whole.
- The whole is different from and greater than the sum of its parts.
- Systems may be open or closed.
- All living systems are open systems.
- Systems strive for homeostasis (internal stability).
- Systems are part of suprasystems.
- Systems have subsystems.

Person

The term **person** is used to describe each individual man, woman, or child. There are a number of different approaches to the study of person. This chapter briefly examines the concept of people as systems with human needs.

As mentioned previously, each individual has numerous subsystems that make up the whole person. There are circulatory, musculoskeletal, respiratory, and neurological subsystems that compose the physiological subsystem. There are also psychological, social, cultural, and spiritual subsystems that combine with the physiological subsystem to make up the whole person. Each person is unique and different from all others. This uniqueness is determined both genetically and environmentally.

Certain personal characteristics are determined before birth by the genes received from parents. Genetically determined characteristics include eye, skin, and hair color; height; gender; and a variety of other features. Other characteristics about persons are determined by the environment. The availability of loving parents or parent substitutes, level of sufficient nutritious foods, cultural beliefs, degree of educational opportunities, adequacy of housing, quality and quantity of parental supervision, and safety are all environmental factors that influence how a person develops.

Human Needs

In addition to having personal characteristics, people have *needs.* A human need is something that is a requirement for the person's well-being. In 1954, psychologist **Abraham Maslow** published *Motivation* and *Personality.* In this book, Maslow discussed **human motivation** and the relationship between motivation and needs, suggesting that human behavior is motivated by needs. He identified five levels of needs and organized them into a hierarchical order, as shown in Figure 10–2.

Basic Needs
The most basic level of needs consists of those necessary for physiological survival: food, oxygen, rest, activity, shelter, and sexual expression. These are needs all human beings, regardless of location or culture, have in common. Maslow identified the second level of needs as safety and security. These include physical as well as psychological safety and security needs. Psychological safety and security include having a fairly predictable environment with which one has some familiarity. The third level of needs consists of love and belonging. To a greater or lesser extent, each person needs close, intimate relationships, social relationships, and group affiliations. Next in Maslow's hierarchy is the need for self-esteem. This includes the need to feel self-worth, self-respect, and self-reliance. The highest level of needs was termed **self-actualization.** Self-actualized people have realized their maximum potential and use their capabilities to the fullest extent possible. People do not stay in a

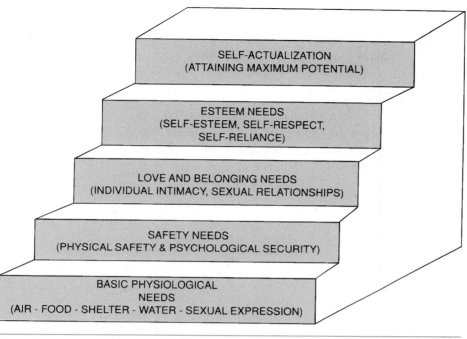

Figure 10–2
Maslow's hierarchy of needs.

state of self-actualization but may have "peak experiences" during which they realize self-actualization for some period of time. Maslow believed that many people strive for self-actualization, but few consistently reach that level.

Assumptions about Needs

Maslow's hierarchy rests on several basic assumptions about human needs. One assumption is that basic needs must be at least partially satisfied before higher-order needs can become relevant to the individual. For example, a starving person can hardly be concerned with self-esteem until a life-sustaining level of nutrition is established.

A second assumption about human needs is that individuals meet their needs in different ways. One person may need eight or nine hours of sleep to feel rested, whereas another may require only five or six hours. Each individual's sleep needs may vary at different stages of life. Older people usually require less sleep than younger people. Individuals also eat different diets in differing quantities and at differing intervals. Some prefer to eat only twice a day, whereas others may snack six or eight times a day to meet their nutritional needs. Sexual energy also varies widely from person to person. The frequency with which normal adults desire sexual activity is determined by a broad range of individual factors.

Even though sleep, food, and sex are considered basic human-needs, the manner in which these needs are met as well as the extent to which any one of them is considered a need varies according to each individual. It is therefore extremely important to determine a person's needs to be able to provide appropriate, individualized nursing care. If a patient is uncomfortable eating three large meals such as those served in most hospitals, nurses can help that person by saving parts of the large meals in the refrigerator on the nursing unit and serving them to the patient between regularly scheduled meals. This is a simple example of what is meant by the term *individualized nursing care.* Individualized nursing care recognizes each individual's unique needs and tailors the plan of nursing care to take that uniqueness into consideration.

Adaptation and Human Needs

Another aspect of human needs that must be considered is the nature of people to change, grow, and develop. Carl Rogers (1961), a well-known psychologist, built a theory of personhood based on the idea that people are constantly adapting and discovering themselves. His book *On Becoming a Person* is considered a classic in psychological literature. Roger's idea that a person's needs change as the person changes is important for nurses to remember. Nurses can tap into the human potential to grow and develop to assist patients to change unhealthy behaviors and to reach the highest level of wellness possible.

The concept of **adaptation** is also helpful in understanding that people admitted to hospitals and removed from their customary, familiar environments frequently become anxious. Even the most confident person can become fearful when in an uncertain, perhaps threatening, situation. Under these circumstances, nurses have learned to expect people to regress slightly and to become more concerned with basic needs and less focused on the higher needs in Maslow's hierarchy. A "take-charge" professional person, for example, may become somewhat demanding and self-absorbed when hospitalized. As you will see in Chapter 11, several nursing theorists based their models on adaptation.

Homeostasis

When a person's needs are not met, homeostasis is threatened. Remember that homeostasis is a dynamic balance achieved by effectively functioning open systems. It is a state of equilibrium, a tendency to maintain internal stability. In humans, homeostasis is attained by coordinated responses of organ systems that automatically compensate for environmental changes. When someone goes for a brisk walk, for example, heartbeat and respiratory rates automatically increase to keep vital organs supplied with oxygen. When the individual comes home and sits down to read the newspaper, heart rate and breathing slow down. No conscious decision to speed up or slow down these physiological functions has to be made. Adjustments occur automatically to maintain homeostasis.

Individuals, as open systems, also endeavor to maintain balance between external and internal forces. When that balance is achieved, the person is healthy, or at least is resistant to disease. When environmental factors affect the homeostasis of a person, the person attempts to adapt to the change. If adaptation is unsuccessful, disequilibrium may occur, setting the stage for the development of illness or disease. How individuals respond to stress is a major factor in the development of illness. Stress is discussed more fully in Chapter 17.

Environment

The second concept basic to professional nursing practice is **environment.** Environment includes all the circumstances, influences, and conditions that surround and affect individuals. The environment can be as small as a premature infant's isolette or as large as the universe. Included in environment are the social and cultural attitudes that profoundly shape human experience.

The environment can either promote or interfere with homeostasis and well-being of individuals. As seen in Maslow's hierarchy of needs, there is a dynamic interaction between a person's needs, which are internal, and the satisfaction of those needs, which is often environmentally determined.

Nurses have always been aware of the influence of environment on people, beginning with Florence Nightingale, who understood well the elements of a healthful environment in which restoration and preservation of health and prevention of disease and injury were possible. Concerns about the health of the public have led governmental entities at local, state, and national levels to promulgate standards and regulations that assure citizens of the safety of their food, water, air, cosmetics, medications, workplaces, and other areas where health hazards may occur. Environmental factors to be discussed in this section are family, culture, social support, and community.

Family Influences

The most direct environmental influence on people is the family. The quality and amount of parenting provided to infants and growing children constitute a major determinant of health. Children who are nurtured when young and vulnerable, who are allowed to grow in independence and self-determination, and who are taught the skills they need for social living are likely to grow into strong, productive, autonomous adults.

Influences on Extended and Nuclear Families

For most of the history of humankind, immediate and **extended families** were relatively intact units that lived together or lived within close proximity to each other. Children were nurtured by a variety of relatives as well as by their own parents. This closeness was profoundly affected by industrialization, which fostered urbanization. When families ceased farming, which was a family endeavor, and moved to cities where fathers worked in factories, the first dilution of family influence on children began. The **nuclear family** (mother and father and their children) moved away from former sources of nurturing, as older relatives such as grandparents, aunts, and uncles, often stayed in rural areas.

During World War II, more women began to work, taking them out of the home and away from young children for hours each day. The increased geographic mobility of families since World War II also had a destructive effect on the role of extended family in the lives of children, as nuclear families often live half a continent or more away from grandparents and other family members. The intense attention children traditionally received from adult relatives diminished, sometimes to the detriment of the child's well-being.

Single-Parent Families

Today, there are more single-parent families in the United States than ever before, most of which are headed by women. As of 1994, U. S. Census data revealed that there were nearly 10 million women with a total of 16 million children under age 21 and no father present. In addition to single mothers, there were also 1.6 million single custodial fathers in the United States in 1994 (U. S. Bureau of the Census, 1995).

Only 54 percent of the single and divorced mothers were receiving child support due from absent fathers, with the average yearly support ranging from $2,500 to $3,000. Custodial fathers fared even worse, with only 41 percent receiving child support averaging $2,300 annually. Louis Sullivan, former secretary of the Department of Health and Human Services, stated, "Many of this country's societal problems can be traced back to parents not supporting their children" (Half of single moms, 1991).

More than 35 percent of households with single female heads were below the poverty level (U. S. Bureau of the Census, 1995). Lack of money often means adequate nutrition and health care are not attainable, adversely affecting the health status of all family members. Life is challenging for single parents of both sexes who must perform traditional breadwinner roles as well as traditional nurturing roles in the family. The combination of bearing multiple roles alone over long periods of time can be extremely stressful, even exhausting, to single parents.

Long-term stress affects the mental and physical health of these adults, which, in turn, affects their parenting abilities. Although many single parents manage stress well and are able to provide excellent parenting, some children's needs are neglected. The impact of this neglect can be seen in the behavior and school performance of children who have not learned the skills they need to be successful. With 26 percent of all children in the United States being born to unmarried women (U. S. Bureau of the Census, 1995), the trend to single-parent households is likely to continue.

The examples given here represent only a few of the ways families influence the well-being of individuals. There are many others. Understanding a patient's family and home environment is part of a complete nursing assessment. Modification of the home environment may be needed, particularly when a person is returning home with a physical disability, or where there is neglect or abuse. Nurses, social workers, and others involved in discharge planning must collaborate to ensure that needed changes occur before patients return to homes and families.

Cultural Influences

Culture is an extremely important environmental influence affecting individuals. Culture consists of the attitudes, beliefs, and behaviors of social and ethnic groups that have been perpetuated through generations. Patterns of language, dress, eating habits, activities of daily living, attitudes toward those outside the culture, health beliefs and values, spiritual beliefs or religious orientation, and attitudes toward children, women, men, marriage, education, work, and recreation all are influenced by culture.

According to Census Bureau estimates, there were 25 million foreign-born Americans in 1998, a dramatic increase from under 20 million only eight years earlier. As mentioned in Chapter 3, the United States is fast becoming the first truly multicultural society. Because basic beliefs about health and illness vary widely from culture to culture, nurses need to develop *cultural competence* to meet the needs of culturally diverse patients. For example, "A traditional Vietnamese folk remedy, *ventouse* . . . , involves placing a heated cup on the skin. It's believed that as the cup cools, it draws away excess energy or 'wind' causing the illness" (Grossman, 1994, p. 58). This practice can cause bruising, which can be mistaken for a sign of abuse. This is just one indication that cultural beliefs of patients have great relevance to nurses. Most cultural differences are more subtle than this and can escape the notice of nurses who have not developed cultural competence.

Effective nurses learn to be aware of and to respect cultural influences on patients. Whenever possible, they pay attention to patients' cultural preferences. They recognize that some cultural groups attribute illness to bad fortune. Individuals from cultures with these beliefs do not see themselves as active participants in their own health status. This attitude is a challenge for nurses who value the collaboration of patients in their own health care planning.

These are only two examples of the influence of cultural beliefs on the nurse-patient interaction. Wise nurses realize that integration of a patient's cultural health beliefs into the individualized treatment plan can make a strong impact on that patient's desire and ability to get well.

Understanding the relationship between culture and health is the basis for "transcultural nursing," a field of nursing practice initiated by nurse-anthropologist Madeline Leininger. Additional discussion of the influence of culture is included in Chapter 17.

Influence of the Social Environment

In addition to families and cultural groups, individuals are also influenced by the social environment in which they live. Social institutions such as families, neighborhoods, schools, churches, professional associations, civic groups, and recreational groups may constitute a form of social support. Social support also includes such factors as presence in the home of a spouse; proximity to neighbors, children, and other supportive individuals; access to medical care; coping abilities; educational level; and so on.

Holmes and Rahe (1967) published a study of the relationship of social change to the subsequent development of illness. People with many social changes that disrupt social support, such as death of a loved one, divorce, job changes, moving, or unemployment, were much more likely to experience illness in the following 12 months than people with few social changes. Both positive and negative changes created the need for social readjustment. In 1995 this study was updated and the Recent Life Changes Questionnaire (Box 10–2) was devised to reflect more accurately contemporary concerns (Miller and Rahe, 1997). Numerous other researchers have found additional evidence that social support has a direct relationship to health.

In assessing patients, nurses need to remember that the adequcy of social support is determined by the patient, not the nurse. Individuals vary in their need and desire for social support. When it is determined that strengthening social support is desirable, nurses can encourage patients to use interest groups, parenting classes, marriage enrichment groups, religious groups, formal and informal educational groups, and self-help groups to develop stronger support from the social environment.

Increasingly, people receive support online, in chat rooms and other forums. People with new insulin pumps, for example, can "talk" with over 700 others who have similar pumps, ask questions, and get helpful tips to assist them. There are literally hundreds of online support groups, ranging from those for Alzheimer's caregivers to weight loss groups.

Community, National, and World Influences

Community environment also influences the health status of people. The types and availability of jobs, housing, schools, and health care as well as the overall economic well-being profoundly affect the citizens in a community. Although nurses may not think they have an obvious role, they can be instrumental in improving the community environment. Identifying health needs and bringing these to the attention of community planners, offering screening programs, serving on health-related committees and advisory boards, and lobbying political leaders can bring about positive change in a community. Nurses have also become politically active by running for elected offices at local, state, and national levels. They can energetically support political candidates who have sound environmental platforms. More information about political activism in nursing is found in Chapter 21.

On a broader perspective, environment also includes the nation, the world, and the universe. A seemingly isolated incident such as an earthquake in Turkey may have worldwide health repercussions as disease epidemics occur in its aftermath. Although nothing can be done to prevent natural disas-

BOX 10–2
Recent Life Changes Questionnaire, Revised 1995

The following 74 potential life changes inquire about recent events in a person's life. Six-month totals equal to or greater than 300 LCU, or one-year totals equal to or greater than 500 LCU, are considered indicative of high recent life stress.

Life Change Event	*Life Change Units*
Health	
An injury or illness which:	
kept you in bed a week or more or sent you to the hospital	74
was less serious than above	44
Major dental work	26
Major change in eating habits	27
Major change in sleeping habits	26
Major change in your usual type and/or amount of recreation	28
Work	
Change to a new type of work	51
Change in your work hours or conditions	35
Change in your responsibilities at work:	
more responsibilities	29
fewer responsibilities	21
promotion	31
demotion	42
transfer	32
Troubles at work:	
with your boss	29
with coworkers	35
with persons under your supervision	35
other work troubles	28
Major business adjustment	60
Retirement	52
Loss of job:	
laid off from work	68
fired from work	79
Correspondence course to help you in your work	18
Home and family	
Major change in living conditions	42
Change in residence:	
move within the same town or city	25
move to a different town, city, or state	47
Change in family get-togethers	25
Major change in health or behavior of family member	55
Marriage	50
Pregnancy	67
Miscarriage or abortion	65

(continued)

BOX 10-2
Recent Life Changes Questionnaire, Revised 1995
(*Continued*)

Gain of a new family member:	
birth of a child	66
adoption of a child	65
a relative moving in with you	59
Spouse beginning or ending work	46
Child leaving home:	
to attend college	41
due to marriage	41
for other reason	45
Change in arguments with spouse	50
In-law problems	38
Change in the marital status of your parents:	
divorce	59
remarriage	50
Separation from spouse:	
due to work	53
due to marital problems	76
Divorce	96
Birth of grandchild	43
Death of spouse	119
Death of the family member:	
child	123
brother or sister	102
parent	100

Personal and social

Change in personal habits	26
Beginning or ending school or college	38
Change of school or college	35
Change in political beliefs	24
Change in religious beliefs	29
Change in social activities	27
Vacation	24
New, close, personal relationship	37
Engagement to marry	45
Girlfriend or boyfriend problems	39
Sexual difficulties	44
"Falling out" of a close personal relationship	47
An accident	48
Minor violation of the law	20
Being held in jail	75
Death of a close friend	70
Major decision regarding your immediate future	51
Major personal achievement	36

Financial

Major change in finances:
increased income	38
decreased income	60
investment and/or credit difficulties	56
Loss or damage of personal property	43
Moderate purchase	20
Major purchase	37
Foreclosure on a mortgage or loan	58

Reprinted with permission of Miller, M. A., and Rahe, R. H. (1997). Life changes scaling for the 1990s. *Journal of Psychosomatic Research, 43*(3), 279–292.

ters, nurses can contribute to a healthier world environment by promoting or participating in humanitarian responses to international disasters.

Nurses' Potential Impact on the Environment

Individual nurses, in the interest of world health, may choose to engage in a variety of environmentally sound practices in their personal lives and encourage others to do the same. These include recycling of household trash and hazardous materials such as batteries and paint, using pump rather than aerosol sprayers, avoiding insecticides and unnecessary use of gardening chemicals, buying energy-efficient appliances and automobiles, walking when possible instead of driving, and refusing to buy from or invest in companies that engage in environmentally unsound practices such as polluting air and water.

Professionally, nurses need to be aware that hospitals are among the highest producers of waste, including biohazardous waste. For example, hospitals are a major source of mercury pollution. This highly toxic substance, used in thermometers, blood pressure measuring devices, and other medical devices, ultimately flows into the environment where it contaminates water. It then is concentrated in the bodies of predator fish such as tuna and swordfish, which are eventually consumed by humans. Mercury, even in small doses, poses serious health risks to pregnant women and young children. Nurses can be instrumental in encouraging their employers to avoid purchasing and using mercury-containing devices and to dispose of them properly when they are discarded.

In an effort to reduce environmental pollution, some health care facilities have committees dedicated to identifying and recommending environmentally sound products. Nurses can volunteer to serve on these committees or recommend the purchase of fewer disposable products and products with wasteful packaging. The accompanying News Note discusses the initiatives of a health-related group, Health Care Without Harm, to reduce hazardous waste emanating from health care facilities.

NEWS NOTE

Study Shows Mercury in Tuna Threatens Developing Babies and Young Children: Hospitals Will Reduce Threat by Eliminating Mercury from Health Care

According to a report released today, some of the most commonly eaten fish contains levels of mercury that pose a risk to pregnant women and young children. In response to the problem of mercury pollution, healthcare providers like Kaiser Permanente, Dartmouth-Hitchcock Medical Center in Lebanon, New Hampshire, and New York's Beth Israel Medical Centers are creating model programs for mercury elimination. By phasing out the purchase and use of mercury-containing products and devices, hospitals will eventually decrease the amount of mercury moving up the food chain until it reaches its highest concentrations in top predator fish like tuna, swordfish and shark.

These findings are included in the report *Protecting by Degrees*, written by the Environmental Working Group for Health Care Without Harm, a coalition of more than 170 groups dedicated to environmentally responsible health care.

Test results reported in *Protecting By Degrees* are consistent with studies done by the U. S. Food and Drug Administration (FDA) in 1993. In both instances, chunk light tuna contained levels of mercury that create serious health risks:

- A 140-pound pregnant woman risks subtle but permanent brain damage to her fetus by eating less than half of a six-ounce can of tuna per day.
- An average four-year-old exceeds the EPA's "safe" dose if he or she eats one six-ounce can per week.

"Tuna fish has too much mercury to be eaten regularly by pregnant women and young children. But that's not the fault of the tuna or the people who caught or canned it," explained Charlotte Brody, RN, Co-Coordinator of Health Care Without Harm. "Industries that use mercury and the governments that regulate them must take responsibility for getting mercury out of our fish and out of our children's developing brains."

"Health care groups like Kaiser Permanente, Dartmouth-Hitchcock and New York's Beth Israel Medical Center are leaders in developing a cure for the mercury problem," said Todd Hettenbach, EWG policy analyst and primary author of the report. "These hospitals are voluntarily eliminating mercury because of the threat to public health and showing other health care providers and other industries that it can be done."

Safe, cost-comparable alternatives exist for most of the mercury use in hospitals. Thermometers and blood pressure-measuring devices are two of the most commonly used mercury-containing devices. A mercury fever thermometer, like those used in the home, contains enough mercury to potentially contaminate 9,000 cans of tuna fish. A desk-mounted sphygmomanometer (used for measuring blood pressure) contains enough mercury to potentially contaminate 492,000 six-ounce cans of chunk light tuna.

"As we learned with mercury instruments, some of the weapons we use to fight disease can also be weapons that compromise a healthy environment," said David Lawrence, M. D., chairman and Chief Executive Officer of Kaiser Foundation Health Plan and Kaiser Foundation Hospitals. "We need to address the long-term consequences of treatment options and challenge ourselves to devise effective alternatives that do less environmental harm."

Health Care Without Harm is an international campaign made up of health care professionals, hospitals, environmental advocates, organizations of health-impacted individuals, religious organizations and labor unions. The campaign's mission is to transform the health care industry so it is no longer a source of environmental harm by eliminating the pollution in health care practices without compromising safety or care. The Environmental Working Group, a member organization of Health Care Without Harm, is an environmental research organization based in Washington, D. C.

HCWH press release issued Thursday, May 6, 1999. Available from http://www.noharm.org.

Health

Health is the third major concept fundamental to the practice of professional nursing. Health can be viewed as a continuum rather than as an absolute state. Each individual's health status varies from day to day, depending on a variety of factors, such as rest, nutrition, and stressors. Illness is also not an absolute state. People can have chronic illnesses such as diabetes or seizure disorders and still work, take part in recreational activities, and maintain acceptably healthy lives. Figure 10–3 depicts the health-illness continuum.

Defining Health

There are numerous definitions of health. The World Health Organization (WHO) defined health as "a state of complete physical, mental and social well-being and not merely the absence of disease or infirmity" (1947, p. 29). This definition was the first modern recognition of health as multidimensional. The WHO definition presented a holistic view of health that reflected the interplay between the psychological, social, spiritual, and physical aspects of human life.

A holistic view of health focuses on the interrelationship of all the parts that make up a whole person. Jan Christian Smuts (1926) first introduced the concept of **holism** in modern Western thought by emphasizing the harmony between people and nature. When viewing health holistically, individual health practices must be taken into account. Health practices are culturally determined and include nutritional habits, type and amount of exercise and rest, how one copes with stress, quality of interpersonal relationships, expression of spirituality, and numerous other lifestyle factors. As a profession, nurses value a holistic view of health.

Parsons (1959) defined health as "the state of optimum capacity of an individual for the effective performance of his roles and tasks." This definition focused on the roles individuals assume in life and the impact health or illness has on the fulfillment of those roles. A few examples of roles that are familiar may include the student role, the parent role, the breadwinner role, and the friend role. Given the activities inherent in each of these roles, it is easily seen that the state of health profoundly influences how people carry out their roles in life.

Figure 10–3
The health-illness continuum—a holistic health model.

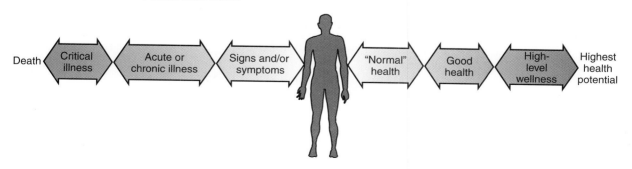

Yet another description of health is the opposite of illness (Dunn, 1959). Dunn, in his classic text, *High Level Wellness* (1961), described health as a continuum with high-level wellness at one end and death at the other. He described **high-level wellness** as functioning at maximum potential in an integrated way within the environment. A prisoner of war kept in solitary confinement and given a diet of rice for many months certainly would have difficulty maintaining health. If he keeps active, both physically and mentally, and retains a positive outlook, however, he is likely to be healthier than the prisoner who does none of these things. Using Dunn's definition and taking his environment into consideration, the prisoner may even be said to have attained high-level wellness.

Nurse-theorist Nola Pender (1987) described health promotion as "approach behavior," whereas prevention is "avoidance behavior" (p. 5). This may be a useful concept for nurses to keep in mind when seeking to help patients expand their positive potential for health.

A National Health Initiative: Healthy People 2000/2010

On September 6, 1990, then U. S. Secretary of Health and Human Services Louis W. Sullivan released a report to the United States entitled *Healthy People 2000*. Heralded as an unprecedented cooperative effort, the preparation of the report involved over 200 people representing government, private businesses, voluntary and professional associations, and concerned individual citizens. *Healthy People 2000* was designed to stimulate initiatives to improve significantly the health of all Americans in the last decade of the century.

Goals of Healthy People 2000
Three broad goals for health of the public in the 1990s were identified (U. S. Department of Health and Human Services, 1990, p. 1):

1. Increase the span of healthy life for Americans.
2. Reduce health disparities among Americans.
3. Achieve access to preventive services for all Americans.

To meet these goals, 300 measurable objectives were identified in 22 different priority areas under the broad categories of health promotion, health protection, and preventive services. The report challenged American citizens, organizations, and communities to change behaviors and environments to support good health for all. United States public health agencies were charged with the responsibility for overseeing the initiatives in each of the 22 priority areas.

It was the hope of those involved in preparing the plan that it would stimulate sustained support from a diverse base of individuals, groups, communities, associations, and governmental agencies to improve health outcomes. Particular emphasis was placed on improving access to health care by the poor, minorities, and rural populations, all of whom have borne "a disproportionate burden of suffering compared to the total population" (p. 1).

Tracking Progress toward Healthy People 2000 Goals: 1995 Report
Although the *Healthy People 2000* initiative stimulated much discussion and activity among those concerned about health, as of 1995, progress with respect to the health of U. S. citizens was mixed. According to McGinnis and Lee (1995), a preliminary examination of trends showed mixed results. In the area of health promotion, 10 of the 17 priority areas were

> proceeding in the right direction, four are proceeding in the wrong direction, one is without change, and two have no data available on which to make comments. Particularly good progress continued for reductions in adult use of tobacco products and in alcohol-related automobile deaths. Positive but less striking gains are recorded for the proportion of adults exercising regularly, eating less fatty diets, and reporting stress-related problems (pp. 1124–1125).

They attributed some of the gains to the fact that more workplaces had health promotion programs for their workers. On the downside, the number of people with sedentary lifestyles was unchanged and a higher proportion of the population was overweight in 1995 than in 1990. The trends for youth were also mixed, with improvements in tobacco, alcohol, and marijuana use but alarming increases in the areas of homocides, other violence, and pregnancies.

Reporting on the 10 *Healthy People 2000* priorities in the area of health protection, McGinnis and Lee reported that 8 of the 10 were "proceeding in the right direction while one is progressing in the wrong direction and one has insufficient data available on which to base a conclusion" (p. 1125). There were fewer motor vehicle deaths, owing to reductions in drunk driving, increased use of child safety devices, increased seat belt use, speed limit enforcement, and the introduction of air bags in new cars. Air quality had improved, and reductions were noted in blood lead levels in children. Indoor air quality remained a challenge, as did the incidence of work-related injuries. Food safety had improved. Fewer old people had complete tooth loss, although children's oral health was not documented.

The mid-decade report also pointed out progress in reducing cholesterol levels and controlling hypertension, reductions in coronary heart disease and stroke deaths, and increasing use of recommended cancer screening services. Prenatal care during the first trimester had also improved, as had the number of children receiving childhood immunizations. They noted that problems remained for vulnerable populations, such as ethnic minorities and the chronically ill. As a result of the mixed progress, a number of midcourse corrections were recommended (McGinnis and Lee, 1995).

Tracking Progress toward Healthy People 2000 Goals: 1999 Report
By 1999, U. S. Secretary of Health and Human Services Donna Shalala issued a more encouraging report. She reported that 15 percent of the objectives had met their targets. "As the century draws to a close, we can be proud that we have made significant strides in improving the health of Americans. *Healthy People 2000* lets us measure the overall progress we have achieved in preventing disease and promoting health during this decade," said Secretary Shalala (U. S. Department of Health and Human Services, 1999a). Upon closer inspection, how-

ever, the report also showed that one fifth of the original objectives were moving away from their targets, particularly in the areas of reducing obesity and increasing physical activity. A related finding was that the incidence, prevalence, complications, and mortality from diabetes were all on the rise.

Infant mortality had declined throughout the 1990s with the death rate for children between 1 and 14 years of age down by 26 percent, surpassing the objective. Severe childhood asthma was rising and was a major cause of hospitalizations.

Death rates in young people ages 15 to 24 declined substantially and met the year 2000 target of 85 deaths per 100,000. Alcohol-related vehicular deaths and suicides were lower, while heavy drinking among high school and college students had increased.

Mortality was also down in the 25 to 64 age group and was close to the year 2000 target. Cancer deaths were below the target, with breast and colorectal cancer deaths both down. Lung cancer deaths continued to rise but at a slower rate.

Older Americans also showed improvements in life expectancy rates, reflecting the continuing decline in heart disease and stroke-related deaths. Suicide rates for elderly white males, considered a high-risk group, were lower, but deaths from falls and vehicular accidents increased (U. S. Department of Health and Human Services, 1999b).

From the results of this report, it can be seen that when federal, state, and local health entities combine their efforts, improvements in the health of citizens can be made. Convincing individual Americans to change their lifestyles, however, even when to do so would result in improved health, remains a challenge. The next phase of the project, called *Healthy People 2010,* was launched in January 2000. Box 10–3 lists the *Healthy People 2010* focus areas, some of which are different from the *Healthy People 2000* priorities (U. S. Department of Health and Human Services, 1999b).

BOX 10–3
Healthy People 2010 Focus Areas

- Physical activity and fitness
- Nutrition
- Tobacco use
- Educational and community-based programs
- Environmental health
- Food safety
- Injury/violence prevention
- Occupational safety and health
- Oral health
- Access to quality health services
- Family planning
- Maternal, infant, and child health
- Medical product safety
- Public health infrastructure
- Health communication prevention and health promotion
- Disability and secondary conditions
- Heart disease and stroke
- Kidney disease
- Mental health and mental disorders
- Respiratory diseases
- Sexually transmitted diseases
- Substance abuse

From *Healthy People 2010 Factsheet.* Available from http://www.health.gov/healthypeople.

Health Beliefs and Health Behaviors

Health is affected by **health beliefs** and **health behaviors.** Health behaviors include those choices and habitual actions that promote or diminish health, such as eating habits, frequency of exercise, use of tobacco products and alcohol, sexual practices, and adequacy of rest and sleep (Fig. 10–4).

Rosenstock (1966) was interested in determining why some people change their health behaviors while others do not. For example, when the surgeon general's report on smoking first came out in 1960, some people immediately quit smoking. Over the years, evidence condemning smoking has accumulated and been widely communicated, yet many intelligent people still smoke. Rosenstock wondered why. He formulated a model of health beliefs

Figure 10–4

More Americans are engaging in health behaviors such as regular exercise, yet obesity is still on the rise (Photo by Fielding Freed).

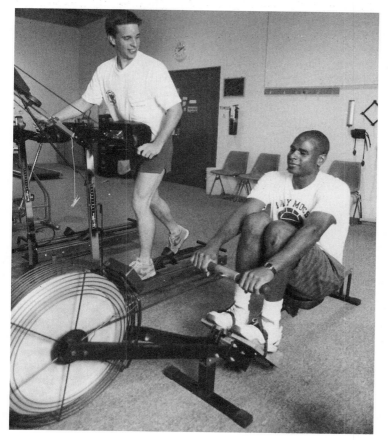

that illustrates how people behave in relationship to health maintenance activities. His model included three components:

1. An evaluation of one's vulnerability to a condition and the seriousness of that condition.
2. An evaluation of how effective the health maintenance behavior might be.
3. The presence of a trigger event that precipitates the health maintenance behavior.

Using Rosenstock's model, a man chooses to participate in a stop-smoking program depending on his perception of smoking-related heart disease and his personal susceptibility to it. If because of family history he believes he is susceptible to heart disease and that it may cause his death prematurely and if he believes that not smoking will substantially reduce his risk, he is likely to participate in the program. If, however, the stop-smoking program is at an inconvenient location, scheduled at an inconvenient time, or not affordable, he is less likely to participate. If his sibling, who smokes, has a massive heart attack, he may be motivated to attend the stop-smoking program despite the inconvenience and cost. The illness of his sibling is what Rosenstock termed "a cue to action," or trigger event. A trigger event propels a previously unmotivated individual into changing health behaviors.

Albert Bandura (1992), a cognitive psychologist, developed an approach designed to assist people to exercise influence over their own health-related behaviors. He observed that whether or not people considered altering detrimental health habits depended upon their belief in themselves as having the ability to modify their own behavior. He called this belief in their own abilities perceived **self-efficacy.** High belief in one's self-efficacy leads to efforts to change, whereas low perceived self-efficacy leads to a fatalistic lack of change.

Bandura identified four components needed for an effective program of lifestyle change: information, skill development, skill enhancement through guided practice and feedback, and creating social supports for change (Bandura, 1992). Using Bandura's model, a man wishing to stop smoking needs knowledge of the potential dangers of smoking, guidance on how to translate concern into action, extensive practice and opportunities to perfect skills, and strong involvement in a social network supportive of nonsmoking.

According to nurse-writer Patricia Butterfield (1995), most health belief models place "the burden of action exclusively on the client and assume that only clients who have distorted or negative perceptions will fail to act" (p. 74). She suggested that nurses familiarize themselves with the work of Nancy Milio (1976) and focus their attention "upstream" at the causes of poor health of the entire population. Milio recommended intervening at the population level rather than attempting to change individual behaviors. She advocated making health-promoting choices more readily available and cheaper than health-damaging options and using national-level policy making to affect society's health. This is precisely what the *Healthy People 2000* initiative is attempting to do, with some success.

Using the Milio/Butterfield model of health behaviors, a man wishing to stop smoking would be supported by population-based interventions such as "mobilizing comprehensive smoking cessation programs in schools and workplaces and encouraging politicians to end federal subsidization of the tobacco industry" (Butterfield, 1995, p. 76). There is little question that had population-based interventions been put into place soon after the 1960 surgeon general's report, smoking would be all but eliminated today.

No one definition or theory of behavior can fully explain the complex state called health. It is important for nurses to recognize that health is relative, ever changing, and affected by both genetics and environment. It affects the entire person physically, socially, psychologically, and spiritually.

Influence of the Internet on Health

With more than 100 million Americans estimated to be online, the Internet has had an impact on every aspect of life. People shop; make travel reservations; check out the latest movies, plays, and books; and meet potential spouses online. Is it any wonder, then, that they also seek information about health online? The World Wide Web, with its ready availability of information, ranging from the latest clinical trials and research studies to the most popular herbal remedies and diet fads, has changed the way we learn about health. Even Dr. Koop has his own website offering news and advice on a wide variety of health topics (www.drkoop.com).

With the proliferation of health information sites, Americans are now armed with more information than has ever before been available to consumers. They are demanding to be equal partners in making health care decisions once decided only by the professionals they consulted. Health care practitioners encounter numerous patients each day who enter examining rooms with printouts of the latest research and advice, culled from the mountains of data available.

Support groups are available by the score. There is no need to dress, drive across town, or even leave the comforts of home to be in touch with dozens of people who share similar concerns or health problems. Cyberspace support groups have another advantage not shared by face-to-face groups: anonymity.

Some people are concerned about the validity of information available on the Web (Chase, 1999). In fact, there is a lot of misinformation transmitted along with well-founded information from respected sources. The difficulty for the average citizen is telling the difference. Box 10–4 contains some helpful hints to improve the likelihood of obtaining valid health information from the Web.

The increased reliance on the Web for health information is expected to continue. It is also understandable, since the Web is readily available, day or night, while getting an appointment with a primary care provider can take days or weeks.

Nurses have an obligation to adapt to this new influence on health by helping their patients obtain sound advice from the Web. Sharing legitimate sites and guidelines for assessing the quality of information are ways to help patients become better consumers of online health data. This means that nurses themselves must be knowledgeable and stay up-to-date on both helpful and unhelpful web sites. Nurses also should be nondefensive when pa-

BOX 10-4
Assessing Health-Related Sites on the World Wide Web

- Consult books that list health-related web sites. Sites listed usually must meet standards set by the book's author or editor.
- Use the Department of Health and Human Services' Healthfinder site to find online support groups (www.healthfinder.gov).
- Go online and "lurk" before getting involved. Monitor conversations or read postings to determine if you want to participate.
- Determine who runs the web site. University-based sites may prove objective and less commercial that those run by companies or individuals wishing to profit from the site.
- Find out if the group has a moderator who can control monopolizers, commercial pitches, and inappropriate behavior.
- Ask for supporting data about cures, particularly "miracle" cures. Rumors and unsupported claims are rampant on the Web and cause untold harm.
- Until you are confident about the quality of data, cross-check it with other print and electronic sources.

From Chase, M. (1999). Health journal: A guide for patients who turn to the Web for solace and support. *Wall Street Journal*, September 17, 1999, B1.

tients question traditional advice, citing the Web as their source. Use these exchanges as opportunities to correct misinformation, if needed. Perhaps you will learn something new yourself.

Devising a Personal Plan for High-Level Wellness

Each individual nurse has a personal definition of health, certain health beliefs, and individual health behaviors. How nurses view health behaviors in their own lives has both direct and indirect impacts on nursing practice. Sedentary nurses, for example, are less likely to encourage patients to become fit. This directly affects their effectiveness as nurses. Not exercising, most would agree, disqualifies a person from being a healthy role model. In case of nurses, being unfit also has an indirect effect of portraying a poor image of nursing.

Nurses have a professional responsibility to model positive health behaviors in their own lives, but nurses are individuals, too. Being or becoming a healthy role model may require some effort. If you are not the positive role model for health you would like to be, Box 10–5 will help you get started.

Putting It All Together: Nursing

Nursing integrates concepts from person, environment, and health to form a meaningful whole. Nursing is an example of an open system that freely interacts with, influences, and is influenced by external and internal forces.

BOX 10-5

**Self-Assessment: Developing a Personal Plan
for High-Level Wellness**

Nurses' personal health behaviors send a powerful message to consumers of
nursing care. Are you in a position to demonstrate that you practice what you
preach? In answering the following questions, you can assess how well you are
meeting your responsibilities in this area of nursing.

1. I weigh no more than 10 pounds over or under my ideal weight.
   T   F
2. I eat a balanced diet, including breakfast, each day.
   T   F
3. Of the total calories in my diet, less than 30 percent come from fat.
   T   F
4. I exercise aerobically at least three times each week.
   T   F
5. I get at least seven hours of sleep each night.
   T   F
6. I do not smoke or use any other form of tobacco.
   T   F
7. I use alcohol in moderation and take mood-altering medication only when
   prescribed by my physician.
   T   F
8. I identify and control the sources of stress in my life.
   T   F
9. I have a balanced lifestyle, with work and diversional activities both playing an important role.
   T   F
10. I have friends, neighbors, or family members who are sources of social
    support for me.
    T   F
11. I practice safe sex.
    T   F

Directions for scoring: If you could not honestly answer "true" to all 11 questions,
you need to set goals to enable you to do so.

1. On a piece of paper, begin your personal plan for high-level wellness.
   Write down at least two things you can do to address each "false" answer
   you gave to the self-assessment questions.
2. Share your health goals with one other person in your class. Make a contract with that person to serve as your "health coach."
3. Review your progress with your health coach at least once per week for
   the remainder of the term.
4. Begin your quest for high-level wellness today!

Nursing is the provision of health care services that focus on maintaining,
promoting, and restoring health. Nursing involves collaborating with patients
and their families to help them cope and adapt to situations of disequilibrium
in an effort to regain homeostasis. Nursing is also health and wellness pro-

motion, including patient teaching to maximize rehabilitation and restoration of high-level wellness.

Nursing is integrally involved with people at points along the health-illness continuum. The purpose of nursing is to assist people in maintaining health, avoiding or minimizing disease and disability, restoring them to wellness, or assisting them to achieve a peaceful death.

Nursing care is provided regardless of diagnosis, individual differences, age, beliefs, gender, sexual preference, or other factors. As a profession, nursing supports the value, dignity, and uniqueness of every person.

Nurses require advanced knowledge and skills; they also must care about their patients. Nursing requires concern, compassion, respect, and warmth as well as comprehensive, individualized planning of care to facilitate patients' growth toward wellness. Nursing links theory and research in an effort to answer difficult questions generated during nursing practice. Nursing's role is to assist patients to achieve health at the highest possible level. Figure 10–5 depicts the relationships among nursing's major concepts.

Figure 10–5
Concepts and subconcepts basic to professional nursing.

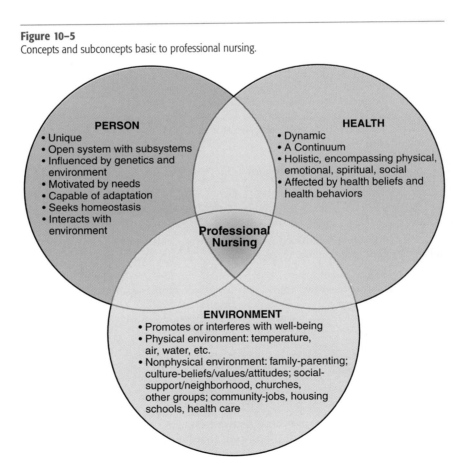

Summary of Key Points

- Nursing integrates three basic components—person, environment, and health—to form its focus.
- Knowledge of systems and human needs can be used to understand nursing's major concepts.
- Persons are viewed as unique open systems who are motivated by needs.
- Maslow organized human needs into a hierarchy consisting of five levels that range from basic physiological needs, which are common to all people, to self-actualization, which is attained by few.
- Environment consists of all the circumstances, influences, and conditions that affect an individual. The physical environment and family, cultural, social, and community environments all have an impact.
- Health is dynamic and viewed as a continuum.
- There are numerous definitions of health.
- Nurses view health holistically, including its effect on an individual's physical, emotional, social, and spiritual functioning as well as its effect on the family.
- Health is affected by health beliefs and health behaviors.
- As an open system nursing integrates person, environment, and health into a meaningful whole.
- Nursing assists people to achieve health at the highest possible level, given their environmental and genetic constraints.

Critical Thinking Questions

1. Discuss systems in relation to your family. What are the family equivalents of inputs, subsystems, suprasystems, outputs, evaluation, and feedback? Does your family tend to be an open or closed system?
2. Describe Maslow's hierarchy of needs and place yourself on the hierarchy today, one week ago, and when you were a senior in high school.
3. Write your own personal definition of health and share it with one other person. Evaluate your definition in terms of holism.
4. What are factors that influence an individual's personal health behaviors? Make a list of your health behaviors, including those that promote health and those that diminish health. Analyze why you continue both the healthy and the nonhealthy behaviors. Identify population-based initiatives that could influence you to make more health-generating choices.
5. Using a search engine, assess the array of support groups online. Enter the discussion group of one that interests you and simply observe. How would you evaluate the quality of the support and information being shared?
6. Look through the yellow pages of your local telephone book under "social services" and "organizations." What types of social support do you find that might be useful to patients? Compare these with the online choices. Which type of support—face-to-face or online—is more appealing to you?
7. Conduct an assessment of your community in terms of one of the following: availability of jobs, quality of public education, availability of health ser-

vices, environmental hazards, and quality of air and water. What is the impact of the factor you selected on the health of the community's citizens? What can you do to strengthen the environmental health of your community?

Web Resources

American Nurses Association's environmental web page, http://www.nursingworld.org/rnnoharm

General medical information, http://www.reutershealth.com

Health Care Without Harm, http://www.noharm.org

Healthy People 2000, http://www.health.gov/healthypeople

U. S. Bureau of the Census, http://www.census.gov

U. S. Department of Health and Human Services' Health Finder, http://www.healthfinder.gov

World Health Organization, http://www.who.int

References

Bandura, A. (1992). A social cognitive approach to the exercise of control over AIDS infection. In R. J. DiClemente (Ed.), *Adolescents and AIDS: A generation in jeopardy.* Newbury Park, Calif.: Sage Publications.

Butterfield, P. G. (1995). Thinking upstream: Conceptualizing health from a population perspective. In J. M. Swanson and M. Albrecht (Eds.), *Community health nursing.* Philadelphia: W. B. Saunders.

Chase, M. (1999). Health journal: A guide for patients who turn to the Web for solace and support. *Wall Street Journal,* September 17, 1999, B1.

Dunn, H. L. (1959). High-level wellness for man and society. *American Journal of Public Health,* 49(6), 786–792.

Dunn, H. L. (1961). *High-level wellness.* Thorofare, N. J.: Slack.

Flynn, J., and Heffron, P. (1984). *Nursing: From concept to practice.* East Norwalk, Conn.: Appleton & Lange.

Grossman, D. (1994). Enhancing your cultural competence. *American Journal of Nursing,* 94(7), 58–62.

Half of single moms get support. (1991). *Citizen-News* (Dalton, Ga.), October 14, 1991, 4A.

Holmes, T. H., and Rahe, R. H. (1967). The social readjustment rating scale. *Journal of Psychosomatic Research,* 11(2), 213–218.

Maslow, A. (1954). *Motivation and personality.* New York: Harper & Row.

McGinnis, J. M., and Lee, P. R. (1995). *Healthy People 2000* at mid-decade. *JAMA,* 273(14), 1123–1129.

Milio, N. (1976). A framework for prevention: Changing health-damaging to health-generating life patterns. *American Journal of Public Health,* 66, 435–439.

Miller, M. A. and Rahe, R. H. (1997). Life changes scaling for the 1990s. *Journal of Psychosomatic Research,* 43(3), 279–292.

Parsons, T. (1959). Definitions of health and illness in light of American values and social structure. In E. G. Jaco (Ed.), *Patients, physicians and illness* (pp. 165–187). New York: Free Press.

Pender, N. J. (1987). *Health promotion in nursing practice* (2nd ed.). Norwalk, Conn.: Appleton & Lange.

Rogers, C. (1961). *On becoming a person.* Boston: Houghton Mifflin.

Rosenstock, I. M. (1966). Why people use health services, part II. *Milbank Memorial Fund Quarterly,* 44(3), 94–124.

Smuts, J. C. (1926). *Holism and evolution.* New York: Macmillan.

U. S. Bureau of the Census. (1990). *Statistical abstract of the United States: 1990.* Washington, D. C.: Government Printing Office.

U. S. Bureau of the Census. (1995). *Population profile of the United States: 1995.* Washington, D. C.: Government Printing Office.

U. S. Department of Health and Human Services. (1990). *Healthy people 2000: Fact sheet.* Washington, D. C.: Government Printing Office.

U. S. Department of Health and Human Services. (1999a). *Healthy people 2000 review 1998–1999.* Washington, D. C.: Government Printing Office.

U. S. Department of Health and Human Services. (1999b). *Healthy people 2010: Fact sheet.* Washington, D. C.: Government Printing Office.

von Bertalanffy, L. (1968). *General systems theory: Foundations, development, applications.* New York: George Braziller.

World Health Organization. (1947). *Constitution.* Geneva: World Health Organization.

Nursing Theory: The Basis for Professional Nursing

Martha Raile Alligood

11

Key Terms

Abstract
Adaptation
Patricia Benner
Concept
Conceptual Model/Framework
Criteria
Virginia Henderson
Dorothy Johnson
Imogene King
Knowledge
Madeleine Leininger
Metaparadigm
Middle-range Theory
Myra Levine
Florence Nightingale
Betty Neuman
Margaret Newman
Dorothea Orem
Ida Orlando
Rosemarie Parse

Phenomena
Philosophy
Martha Rogers
Callista Roy
Structure of Knowledge

Systems
Theory
Jean Watson

Learning Outcomes

After studying this chapter, students will be able to:

- Explore elements of selected nursing philosophies, nursing conceptual models, and theories of nursing.
- Consider how selected nursing theoretical works guide nursing practice.
- Delineate the role of nursing theory for different levels of nursing education.
- Describe the function of nursing theory in research and theory-based practice.
- Relate the role of nursing theory in education, research, and practice to the development of the profession.

What is Theory?

The purpose of this chapter is to introduce you to nursing's major theoretical works. Some of you may be asking, "What is theory and why is it important for us to study nursing theory?" **Theory** has many definitions, but generally it is a group of related concepts, definitions, and statements that propose a view of nursing **phenomena** from which to describe, explain, or predict outcomes (Chinn and Kramer, 1998; Powers and Knapp, 1995). More simply, it is "a group of related concepts that propose actions to guide practice" (Alligood and Marriner-Tomey, 1997, p. 225). Theories represent **abstract** ideas rather than concrete facts. As such, theories are tentative and when new knowledge becomes available, theories that are no longer useful are modified or discarded. Therefore, theories are considered propositions that suggest new understandings, and although some may serve us for centuries, new theories are always being generated.

Professional nurses are conscious of the need for both nursing theory development and theory-based practice to be complementary activities. As nursing develops as a professional practice and a scholarly discipline, there is increasing interest in the theoretical basis of nursing. Some scholars believe that continued theory development and the expansion of theory-based practice are the most crucial challenges facing nursing today (Alligood, 1997a, Chinn and Kramer, 1998; Fawcett, 1997; Holder and Chitty, 1997; Meleis, 1997).

There are many reasons to be interested in theory, and three primary ones will be discussed (Holder and Chitty, 1997). First, as seen in Chapter 6, one criterion for a profession is a distinct body of **knowledge** as the basis for practice. Nursing's interest in developing a body of substantive nursing knowledge has been noted as a major driving force within the profession throughout the twentieth century (Alligood, 1997a). Theory testing and the development of new theory in theory-based research is a means of building that knowledge and establishing nursing as a profession.

Second, commitment to theory-based practice using sound, reliable knowledge is intrinsically valuable to nursing; that is to say, by its very nature, knowledge is desirable. The evolving development of knowledge in and of itself is an important activity for nurse scholars to pursue. For nursing to be recognized and respected as a scholarly discipline contributing to society is helpful to the development of the profession.

Third, theory is a useful nursing practice tool for reasoning, critical thinking, and decision making (Alligood, 1997c; Alligood and Marriner-Tomey, 1997; Marriner-Tomey and Alligood, 1998). Nursing practice settings are complex, and the amount of data (information) confronting nurses is virtually endless. Nurses must analyze a vast amount of information about each patient and decide what to do. A theoretical approach helps practicing nurses not to be overwhelmed by the mass of information and to progress through the nursing process in an orderly manner. Theory enables them to organize and understand what happens in practice, to analyze critically patient situations for clinical decision making; to plan care and propose appropriate nursing interventions; and to predict patient outcomes from that care and evaluate its effectiveness. Box 11–1 summarizes the ways in which theory helps practicing nurses.

BOX 11–1
Nursing Theory and the Practicing Nurse

Theory assists the practicing nurse to:

- Organize patient data
- Understand patient data
- Analyze patient data
- Make decisions about nursing interventions
- Plan patient care
- Predict outcomes of care
- Evaluate patient outcomes

Because theory is abstract, it is useful to consider theoretical works in the context of a **structure of knowledge.** Figure 11–1 illustrates the structure of nursing knowledge as conceptualized by Fawcett (1995). This structure is useful in that it specifies a metaparadigm consisting of the major concepts of the discipline: person, environment, health, and nursing. It also differentiates types of theoretical works based on the nature of the work itself (philosophies, models, and theories) and levels of abstraction. Although nursing theory dates back to Florence Nightingale, most nursing theory was developed in the latter half of the twentieth century (Alligood, 1997a; Alligood and Choi, 1998).

There are a number of nursing theory textbooks that provide an overview and critique of developments in nursing theory (see Chinn and Kramer, 1998; Fawcett, 1993, 1995; Fitzpatrick and Whall, 1996; George, 1995; Marriner-Tomey and Alligood, 1998). Although these texts may differ in their approach, each addresses person, environment, health, and nursing as major concepts. Together, they compose the most abstract aspect of the structure of nursing knowledge, which is known as a metaparadigm (Fawcett, 1993, 1995).

A **metaparadigm** is defined as "the global concepts which identify the phenomena of interest for a discipline" (Alligood and Marriner-Tomey, 1997, p. 224). Whereas the best source for indepth understanding of theoretical works is the primary source (actual writing) of the theorist, explanatory texts are helpful to introduce novices to the theoretical basis of the discipline of nursing. Explanatory texts trace the historical development of various theories and specify **criteria** to analyze, critique, and evaluate each work. These texts, which began to be published in the early 1980s, contribute to the general understanding of nursing theory and theoretical developments in nursing among undergraduate and graduate students and faculty.

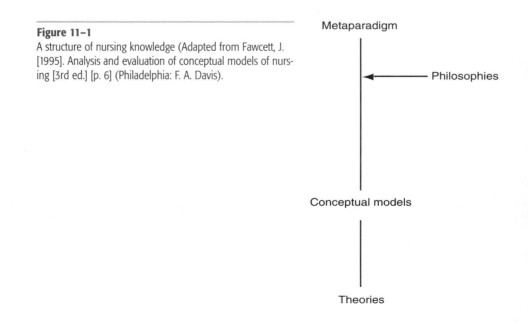

Figure 11–1
A structure of nursing knowledge (Adapted from Fawcett, J. [1995]. Analysis and evaluation of conceptual models of nursing [3rd ed.] [p. 6] (Philadelphia: F. A. Davis).

In this chapter, nursing theoretical works will be considered according to three general types: nursing philosophies, nursing models, and theories of nursing (Marriner-Tomey and Alligood, 1998). Selected works from each of the three provide a broad overview of theory within the discipline of nursing. This introduction is designed to help you develop a basic understanding of nursing theory on which you can build as you pursue your nursing education.

Nursing Philosophies

Chapter 9 introduced nursing philosophies and discussed their functions in nursing practice and educational institutions. **Philosophies** provide broad, general views of nursing that clarify values and answer broad disciplinary questions such as "What is nursing?" "What is the profession of nursing?" "What do nurses do?" "What is the nature of human caring?" and "What is the nature of nursing practice and the development of practice expertise?" Four philosophies have been selected because they represent different positions in the development of nursing theory.

Nightingale's Philosophy

Florence Nightingale's work represents the beginning of professional nursing, as noted in Chapter 1. In her often cited work, *Nursing: What It Is and What It Is Not* ([1859] 1969), Nightingale answered the philosophical question "What is nursing?" She envisioned nursing as different from the work of household servants, which were common in her day. She developed a logical distinction between medicine and nursing by clarifying that nursing is concerned with health rather than illness.

Though we draw many ideas from the writings of Nightingale, her unique perspective for nursing practice focused on the relationship of patients to their surroundings. She set forth nursing principles that were foundational to nursing and remain relevant to nursing practice today. Her description of the importance of observation of the patient and accurate recording of information and her principles of cleanliness, which clarified clean areas from dirty ones, are examples. Both can be seen in hospital-based nursing practice today.

Using Nightingale's Philosophy in Practice
Nightingale believed that the health of patients was related to their surroundings. She discussed the need for pure air and water, efficient drainage, cleanliness, and light. She emphasized the necessity of ventilation and sunlight and encouraged moving patients' beds to change their view and give them access to direct sunlight. Her discussion of diet spoke not only to the necessity of a balanced diet but also to the nurse's responsibility to observe and record what was eaten. She emphasized cleanliness of the patient, the bed linens, and the room itself. Her discussion of noise was especially interesting in light of at-

tention to noise pollution in recent years. She recognized the problem of noise in the room or in the hall for patients confined to bed. She emphasized the importance of rest and discouraged sudden disruption of sleep.

Nightingale gave nurses the responsibility for protection of patients from possible harm from visitors who mean well but may provide false hope, discuss upsetting news, or idly chatter, thereby tiring them. She focused on the nurse's responsibility for her patients even when the nurse was off duty. Finally, she suggested that patients might benefit from visits by small pets, yet another idea that speaks to the timeless relevance of her work.

The nurse whose practice is guided by Nightingale's philosophy is keenly aware of the importance of surroundings to health or recovery from illness. Her work presented an implicit theory that proposed changing patients' surroundings (environment) to bring about changes in patients. She held nurses responsible for patients and their surroundings.

Henderson's Philosophy

Virginia Henderson was another early philosopher of nursing. Henderson's work appeared at a time when efforts to clarify nursing as a profession emphasized defining nursing. As mentioned in Chapter 7, she provided a comprehensive definition: the "unique function of the nurse . . . is to assist the individual, sick or well in the performance of those activities contributing to health or its recovery (or a peaceful death) that he would perform unaided if he had the necessary strength, will or knowledge" (Henderson, 1966, p. 15). Although Henderson was recognized for many contributions to nursing throughout her career, this early work, which defined nursing and specified the role of the nurse in relation to the patient, remains noteworthy and relevant.

Henderson's philosophy of nursing linked her definition of nursing, which emphasized the functions of the nurse and the assistive aspects of nursing, with a list of basic patient needs, which are the focus of nursing care. Her work proposed an answer to the question "What is the nursing profession and what do nurses do?" She described the nurse's role as that of a substitute for the patient, a helper to the patient, or partner with the patient.

Henderson's 14 basic needs provided a general focus for patient care. She proposed that these needs clarified the elements of nursing care. The function of nurses was to assist patients if they were unable to perform these 14 functions themselves. Box 11-2 lists Henderson's 14 Basic Needs of the Patient.

Henderson's work has been used by nurses all over the world for direction in nursing education and practice. The needs she included might at first be viewed as physical, psychological, emotional, sociological, spiritual, and developmental areas. However, a more careful analysis reveals a holistic view of human development and health.

The first nine needs on Henderson's list stress the importance of breathing, eating and drinking, elimination, movement and positioning, sleep and rest, suitable clothing, maintenance of suitable environment for the body tem-

BOX 11-2
Henderson's 14 Basic Needs of the Patient

1. Breathe normally.
2. Eat and drink adequately.
3. Eliminate body wastes.
4. Move and maintain desirable position.
5. Sleep and rest.
6. Select suitable clothes—dress and undress.
7. Maintain body temperature within normal range by adjusting clothing and modifying the environment.
8. Keep the body clean and well groomed and protect the integument (skin).
9. Avoid dangers in the environment and avoid injuring others.
10. Communicate with others in expressing emotions, needs, fears, or opinions.
11. Worship according to one's faith.
12. Work in such a way that there is a sense of accomplishment.
13. Play or participate in various forms of recreation.
14. Learn, discover, or satisfy the curiosity that leads to normal development and health and use the available health facilities.

Reprinted with permission of Henderson, V. (1966). The nature of nursing: A definition and its implications for practice, research, and education. New York: Macmillan.

perature, cleanliness, and avoidance of danger or harm. Next, she included the psychological or sociological need to communicate and the spiritual need for worship and faith. She concluded with three needs that might be viewed as developmental: the need for work and the sense of accomplishment, the need for play and recreation, and the need to learn, discover, and satisfy curiosity.

Using Henderson's Philosophy in Practice
Nursing practice based on Henderson's work focuses on nursing care that is consistent with her definition of nursing. The nurse approaches patients from the perspective of the 14 basic needs. Henderson's clarity about the role and function of the nurse is a strength of her work. She utilized her definition of nursing and the basic needs approach in her well-known case study of a young patient who had undergone a leg amputation. Using this case, she demonstrated how the nurse's role changes on a day-to-day, week-to-week, and month-to-month basis in relation to the patient's changing needs and the contributions of other members of the health care delivery team (Henderson, 1966).

Watson's Philosophy

Jean Watson's initial philosophical work, *The Philosophy and Science of Caring,* was published in 1979. In it, she issued a call for a return to the earlier values of nursing and emphasized the caring aspects of nursing. Her work is recognized as a human science. Themes of caring can also be noted in her other professional accomplishments. For example, she established the Center for Human Caring at the University of Colorado in Denver, where nurses can incorporate knowledge of human caring as the basis of nursing practice and scholarship. Watson proposed 10 factors, which she labeled *carative* factors, a term she contrasted with *curative* to differentiate nursing from medicine. Watson's 10 carative factors are found in Box 11–3.

Watson's work (1979, 1988) addressed the philosophical question of the nature of nursing when viewed as a human-to-human relationship. She focused on the relationship of the nurse and the patient, drawing on philosophical sources for a new approach that emphasized how the nurse and patient change together through *transpersonal caring*. She proposed that nursing be concerned with spiritual matters and the inner knowledge of nurse and patient as they participate together in the transpersonal caring process. She equated health with harmony, resulting from unity of body, mind, and soul, for which the patient is primarily responsible. Illness or disease was equated with lack of harmony within the mind, body, and soul experienced in internal or external environments (Watson, 1979). According to Watson, nursing, based on human values and interest in the welfare of others, is concerned with health promotion, health restoration, and illness prevention.

Using Watson's Philosophy in Practice

Watson's carative factors guide nurses who use transpersonal caring in practice. Carative factors specify the meaning of the relationship of nurse and patient as human beings. Nurses are encouraged to share their genuine selves

---

BOX 11–3
Watson's Ten Carative Factors

1. The formation of a humanistic-altruistic system of values.
2. The instillation of faith-hope.
3. The cultivation of sensitivity to one's self and others.
4. The development of a helping-trust relationship.
5. The promotion and acceptance of the expression of positive and negative feelings.
6. The systematic use of the scientific problem-solving method for decision making.
7. The promotion of interpersonal teaching-learning.
8. The provision for a supportive, protective, and/or corrective mental, physical, sociocultural, and spiritual environment.
9. Assistance with the gratification of human needs.
10. The allowance for existential-phenomenological forces.

Reprinted with permission of Marriner-Tomey, A., and Alligood, M. R. (1998). Nursing theorists and their work (pp. 147). St. Louis: Mosby.

with patients. Patients' spiritual strength is recognized, supported, and encouraged for its contribution to health. In the process of transpersonal relationships, nurses develop and encourage an openness to understanding of self and others. This leads to the development of trusting, accepting relationships in which feelings are shared freely and confidence is inspired.

Watson recognized the scientific method as a tool for systematic solutions to problems and a guide for decision making. She suggested that teaching-learning, a vital aspect of nursing practice, also be carried out in an interpersonal manner true to the philosophy and nature of the caring relationship.

The nurse guided by Watson's work has responsibility for creating and maintaining an environment supporting human caring while recognizing and providing for patients' primary human requirements. In the end, this human-to-human caring approach leads the nurse to respect the overall meaning of life from the perspective of the patient. Watson's 1988 work formalized the theory of human caring from this philosophy.

Benner's Philosophy

Patricia Benner's work (1984) centered on the nature of nurses' personal knowledge of nursing practice. It emerged from research studies aimed toward understanding nurses' knowledge more completely. She sought personal and practical knowledge from nurses themselves about how they acquired nursing expertise. As a result, the focus of Benner's work is nursing practice.

Using Benner's Philosophy in Practice

Benner proposed seven domains of nursing practice that identify the role of the nurse in relation to the patient. They include *helping, teaching-coaching, diagnosing and monitoring, managing changes, administering and monitoring therapeutic interventions, monitoring for quality care,* and *organizing to enact the work role.* From her study of nurses within these domains she proposed five stages in the development of expertise. They are *novice, advanced beginner, competent, proficient,* and *expert.* These stages were summarized in Table 8–3, Chapter 8.

Benners' work is useful to practicing nurses. It provides descriptions of nursing practice from the perspectives of nurses at different levels of proficiency. Benner's work also has been useful as the profession moves toward differentiating levels of practice. Formerly, these levels were described mainly by educational preparation, however, Benner's work assists by describing specific behaviors at different levels of expertness.

Nursing Conceptual Models

Conceptual models (or conceptual frameworks) are the second type of theoretical work in the structure of nursing knowledge (Fawcett, 1995). They are broad conceptual structures providing comprehensive, holistic perspectives of nursing through the interrelationship of delineated concepts. They provide organizational frameworks for critical thinking about the processes of nursing (Alligood, 1997; Fawcett, 1995). As seen in Figure 11–1, models are less abstract and more formalized than the philosophies just discussed in this chapter; they are more abstract, however, than theories of nursing, which will be discussed later. It is important to note that nursing conceptual models are structures from which nursing theory can be derived. To illustrate, Box 11–4 contains a list of seven nursing conceptual models with an example of a theory derived from each. The name of the nursing conceptual model usually includes the name of the theorist who developed the model, for example, Rogers' Science of Unitary Human Beings (Alligood, 1997c). Each conceptual model addresses nursing's four major concepts—person, environment, health, and nursing—but defines those concepts in a unique way.

The conceptual models reviewed in the following sections were developed by Johnson, King, Levine, Neuman, Orem, Rogers, and Roy. The focus and perspective of each model is discussed, followed by a brief overview of how each model guides nursing practice.

Johnson's Behavioral System Model

Dorothy Johnson's work (1968, 1980) focused on human behavior. She proposed a system of nursing based on observation of patient behavior. The *behavioral phenomena of persons* was presented as a single system with seven

---

BOX 11–4

Conceptual Models of Nursing with a Theory Example from Each

Conceptual Models of Nursing	Theory Example
Johnson's Behavioral System	Theory of the person as a behavioral system
King's Interacting Systems	Theory of goal attainment
Levine's Conservation Model	Theory of therapeutic intention
Neuman's Systems Model	Theory of optimal client stability
Orem's Conceptual Model	Orem's self-care deficit theory
Rogers' Science of Unitary Human Beings	Theory of accelerating change
Roy's Adaptation Model	Theory of the person as an adaptive system

From Alligood, M. R. (1997). Models and theories: Critical thinking structures. In M. R. Alligood and A. Marriner-Tomey (Eds.). *Nursing theory: Utilization and application* (pp. 31–45). St. Louis: Mosby.

subsystems: *achievement behavior, affiliative behavior, aggressive/protective behavior, dependency behavior, eliminative behavior, ingestive behavior,* and *sexual behavior.* An eighth subsystem, *restorative behavior,* was added later (Holaday, 1997). Johnson contrasted the behavioral system approach for nursing with the physiological system approach of medicine or the social system approach of sociology.

Using Johnson's Model in Practice

When using Johnson's work as a guide for nursing practice, nurses view patients' behaviors in a systematic way according to the subsystems outlined above. Observation of patient behavior is paramount in this model. Each subsystem has its own structure, which assists nurses in considering what may be contributing to a patient's actual behaviors. Subsystem structures include a goal, which is based on *universal drive,* a *set,* a *choice,* and an *action.* An example of a "universal drive" is to maintain health; "set" is the usual behaviors of the patient that might help maintain health; "choice" is the range of behaviors the person considers to maintain health; and "action" is the observable healthy behavior (Holaday, 1997).

The nurse identifies the subsystem involved by observing a patient's behavior, then assesses the patient's set (usual behavior) in relation to the goal of the system. If the goal of the subsystem is not being met, the behavioral choices are reviewed in relation to action or the patient's actual behavior. An environmental assessment (internal and external) is also carried out to understand the impact of environment on a patient's behavior and to discover behavioral alternatives. A diagnostic analysis determines whether the behavior of the subsystem is *dominant, incompatible, discrepant,* or *insufficient.* Based on the diagnosis within the subsystem, nurse and patient select mutual goals and develop a plan for intervention.

If you wish to read more about the use of Johnson's model in practice, Holaday (1997) and Alligood (1997b) are suggested resources.

King's Interacting Systems Framework and Theory of Goal Attainment

Imogene King's work (1981) focused on persons, their interpersonal relationships, and social contexts with three interacting **systems:** *personal, interpersonal,* and *social.* Within each of these three systems King identified concepts that provide a conceptual structure describing the processes in each system. The three systems and their concepts are presented in Box 11–5.

King's interacting systems form a framework to view whole persons in their family and social contexts: the *personal system* identifies concepts that provide an understanding of individuals, personally and intrapersonally; the *interpersonal system* deals with interactions and transactions between two or more persons; and the *social system* presents concepts that consider social

---

BOX 11-5
King's Three Systems and Their Concepts

Personal System	*Interpersonal System*	*Social System*
Perception	Role	Organization
Self	Interaction	Power
Body image	Communication	Authority
Growth and development	Transaction	Status
Time	Stress	Decision making
Space		

From King, I. M. (1981). *A theory for nursing: Systems, concepts, process.* New York: John Wiley and Sons.

---

contacts, such as those at school, at work, or in social settings. King's work is unique as it provides a view of persons from the perspective of their interactions (or communications, both verbal and nonverbal) with other people at three interacting systems levels.

Using King's Model in Practice

When using King's work, nurses are guided by several aspects of the framework and her theory of goal attainment. First, the traditional steps of the nursing process—assessment, planning, goal setting, intervention, and evaluation—are augmented in several ways. It is difficult to describe a linear progression through these steps because there are many things occurring simultaneously.

Second, the focus of the process is guided by concepts at each of the system levels. For example, the personal system leads the nurse to pay close attention to a patient's perceptions, the interpersonal system steers the nurse to notice patients' roles and stresses in each role, and the social system cues the nurse to consider what seems to influence the patient's decision making.

A third aspect of the process focuses on interactions with the patient. Nurses are aware of their communication with patients, identifying steps from the first encounter to the attainment of the specified goal. King called these steps *perception, judgment, action, reaction, interaction,* and *transaction* (King, 1981).

King emphasized the importance of joint goal setting by nurse and patient, reminding nurses that this relationship involves mutuality. King's process provided a structure for the nurse to monitor the relationship's progress.

King specified the goal of nursing to be health. Examples of applications of King's work in nursing practice are available in the nursing literature (see

Alligood, 1995; Alligood and Marriner-Tomey, 1997; Frey and Norris, 1997; Frey and Sieloff, 1995). There is an organization of King scholars called, King International Nursing Group (KING).

Levine's Conservation Model

Myra Levine (1973, 1991) developed a model based on three major concepts: *wholeness, adaptation,* and *conservation.* The framework, which was first used to organize nursing school curricula, set forth a set of conservation principles as a comprehensive guide for nursing. Simply stated, Levine viewed human life as a process of maintaining wholeness through **adaptation,** which is facilitated by conservation. She believed that wholeness, meaning "keeping together," continues throughout life. According to Levine, the integrity of wholeness is sustained by the process of adaptation, or change, as humans interact with their environments. Wholeness is defined as health or well-being of persons, which is the outcome of properly functioning adaptive change. Illness and disease interrupt the normal process of adaptation and produce the need for nursing.

Levine asserted that nursing is a human interaction designed to promote human adaptation until wholeness is regained or the person can adapt without assistance. Nurses promote adaptation through conservation, which is guided by four principles: *conservation of energy, structure, personal integrity,* and *social integrity.* She proposed two theories from her model, the theory of redundancy and the theory of therapeutic intention. Both are testable in nursing practice and research (Schaefer, 1997).

Using Levine's Model in Practice

When using Levine's model to guide nursing practice, nurses use the four conservation principles in assessing patients. With information from this assessment, they make nursing judgments and propose hypotheses for interventions that promote adaptation. These hypotheses are tested by using them to guide nursing interventions and then evaluating patients' responses. Interventions are designed with Levine's theory of redundancy in mind. This means that nurses involve patients in choosing interventions to avoid conflicts with the patient's own conservation efforts (Schaefer, 1997). Schaefer and Pond (1991) Schaefer (1997) and Alligood (1997b) are resources for more information about the use of Levine's model in nursing practice.

Neuman's Systems Model

Betty Neuman (1995) designed a systems model in response to student requests for an organizing **framework** for the mass of information they encountered in nursing practice. The Neuman model, now in its third revision, viewed persons from the perspective of actual and potential stressors and associated health risk factors. Strengths and weaknesses were identified in relation to those stressors, and stress reduction goals were set as nursing outcomes. According to Neuman, the client, referred to as the *core* and *source of basic energy,* possesses unique survival capabilities in five areas: physiological, psychological, sociological, developmental, and spiritual. The client system includes the core as well as its system of *resistance* and *defenses.* The client is continuously exposed to internal and external factors, which are met by the lines of defense and/resistance.

Nursing interventions build on client strengths to shore up defenses and strengthen weaknesses. To this end, nursing interventions are based on the strengths and weaknesses in three possible levels of prevention. *Primary prevention* is for the promotion of health or wellness retention, *secondary prevention* is for treatment of symtoms while also conserving energy and strengthening the lines of resistance, and *tertiary prevention* is similar to what we sometimes call "recuperation," wherein strengths are supported while the client returns to health or wellness. This comprehensive model may be applied in all practice areas and is especially useful when working with families and communities.

Using Neuman's Model in Practice

Nurses practicing with Neuman's model interact with clients to identify actual and potential stressors. Next, the nurse and client identify client strengths and weaknesses in relation to the stressors. The approach is holistic and systematic. Based on the client's level of stress and health goals, a plan is developed. Nursing care provides primary, secondary, and tertiary prevention. Throughout the process the client is supported and assessed according to the many facets of the model. The emphasis is on maintaining client system balance, or *stability,* which is seen as the goal of nursing.

Applications of Neuman's work in nursing practice are available in the nursing literature (Alligood, 1997b; Sohier, 1997) as well as in her own text, *The Neuman Systems Model* (1995). Betty Neuman is still active writing and speaking about the model; however, she has appointed a Neuman Systems Model Trustee Group to continue refining the model in the new century.

Orem's Self-Care Model

An early nurse theorist, Dorothea Orem, published *Concepts of Nursing* in 1971. It is now in its fifth edition (1995). Over the years she formalized three interrelated theories: *theory of self-care, theory of self-care deficit,* and *theory of nursing system.* The model focuses on the patient's *self-care capacities* and the process of designing nursing actions to meet the patient's *self-care needs.* In this model, the nurse prescribes and regulates the nursing system for self-care.

Orem's (1995) work is widely used in nursing education and practice. It sets forth a comprehensive system for nursing practice in a variety of clinical settings.

Orem and Nursing Practice

When using Orem's work as a guide, the nurse carries out a systematic series of four operations: *diagnosis, prescription, regulation,* and *control.* Each of these specifies activities for the patient and the nurse.

Diagnostic operations begin with the establishment of the nurse-patient relationship and include contracting with the patient to explore current and potential self-care demands. *Diagnosis* is accomplished by examining *basic conditioning factors* in relation to the *universal, developmental,* and *health care deviation requisites* and related *self-care actions* of the patient. For example, recognizing a patient's inability to carry out self-care (called *deficits*) is a diagnostic operation. *Prescriptive operations* occur when therapeutic self-care requisites (based on deficits) are determined and the nurse reviews various methods, actions, and priorities with the patient. In *regulatory* operations the nurse designs, plans, and produces a system for care (Berbiglia, 1997).

This model has wide practical application. Numerous case examples of nursing care using Orem's model are available in the nursing literature (Alligood, 1997b; Berbiglia, 1997).

Rogers' Science of Unitary Human Beings

Another early theorist, Martha Rogers, first published her model in 1970. She believed that if nurses needed only knowledge from other disciplines to practice nursing, there was no need for higher education in nursing. So she set about identifying nursing's unique body of knowledge.

Rogers clarified "nursing" as a noun and defined it as a body of knowledge necessary for practice. She called this organized body of abstract knowledge *nursing science* and specified *nursing art* as the imaginative and creative use of knowledge in practice. She believed that nursing was both science and art and described nursing as a learned profession that focuses on the nature and direction of human development and human betterment.

Rogers' work focused on the process of humans and their environments. Her model has four main concepts: *energy fields, openness, pattern,* and *pandimensionality,* which Rogers used to describe the human developmental process in life.

Many theories have been derived from Rogers' conceptual system, a number by Rogers herself and numerous others by Rogerian scholars. Two theories derived from Rogers' work will be addressed in the theory section of this chapter, which follows.

The Society of Rogerian Scholars was formed in the late 1980s. It is an organization for nurses who practice and conduct research in Rogerian science and who wish to promote its development in the future. The organization sponsors annual meetings, biennial conferences, a newsletter, and a journal, *Visions: The Journal of Rogerian Science,* which is devoted to the development and dissemination of Rogerian science.

Using Rogers' Model in Practice

Rogers' model (1970, 1992) provides a very different view of nursing practice compared with other nursing models. Not only was hers an abstract model but it was also *acausal.* This means life events are viewed as emerging from the simultaneous actions of persons and the environment rather than from actions and reactions, or causes and effects, which are traditional views. This perspective allows nurses and patients to join in their life processes, participating in one another's patterns, while the nurse provides care and information. Nurses participate knowingly with patients toward increased understanding of patterns. Nursing care must be pertinent to the patient's life process.

Rogers' framework leads the nurse to respect the patient's preferences in all matters. The nurse and patient progress toward an outcome of well-being specified by the patient. Box 11–6 provides observations of a nurse who is a Rogerian practitioner. There are many examples of the use of Rogers' work in the nursing literature. Case applications may be found in Bultemeier (1997), Alligood (1997b), Barrett (1990), and Madrid (1994).

BOX 11–6
Using Nursing Science in Practice: Observations of a Rogerian Practitioner

Practice within the Rogerian model (framework) is ever dynamic and centers on continual pattern appraisal. The Rogerian framework is an abstract guide to nursing practice as it encompasses the simultaneous process of the human-environmental field. This dynamic emergent conceptual framework provides guidance for my practice toward systematic, innovative, and individualized care.

My practice is conceptually centered on the Rogerian concepts of resonancy, helicy, and integrality. These concepts guide my practice in selection of tools which facilitate pattern appraisal, mutual patterning, and evaluation of the human-environmental field. Pattern appraisal tools are based on mutual participation (of the patient and the nurse) and observation of emergent patterns. These patterns are often evident through perceived colors, smells, descriptive words, physical symptoms, and overt physical manifestations. The emergent pattern guides the patterning process always remembering the pandimensionality of the human-environment process. Patterning modalities frequently used in my practice include meditation, contemplation, reflection, journaling, therapeutic touch, massage, humor, music, metaphors, color, light, sleep, vitamins, and exercise. Evaluation is ongoing, integral, and centers on perceptions emerging via the mutual patterning of the patient and the nurse.

My professional practice is working with women at Women's Health Associates in Oak Ridge, Tennessee. I am an adjunct faculty member at the University of Tennessee, College of Nursing, in Knoxville and precept graduate students in my practice. In addition, I provide massage therapy to individuals in their homes. Nursing practice within the Rogerian model is ever evolving and rewarding . . .

Courtesy of Kaye Bultemeier, PhD, RNCS, Oak Ridge, Tennessee, 1999.

Roy's Adaptation Model

Sister Callista Roy first presented her adaptation model as a conceptual framework for a nursing curriculum in 1970 and updated all of her writing in a comprehensive text published in 1991 (Roy and Andrews, 1991). Her model is widely used for education, research, and nursing practice today. She focused on the individual as a *biopsychosocial adaptive system* and described nursing as a *humanistic discipline* that emphasizes the person's adaptive or coping abilities. Roy's work is based on adaptation and adaptive behavior, which is produced by altering the environment.

According to Roy, the individual and the environment are sources of stimuli that require modification to promote adaptation in the patient. Roy viewed the person as an adaptive system with *physiological, self-concept, role function,* and *interdependent* modes. These modes are manifestations of *cognator* and *regulator* coping responses to stimuli.

Roy's model provides a comprehensive understanding of nursing from the perspective of adaptation. When the demands of environmental stimuli are too high or the person's adaptive mechanisms are too low, the person's behavioral responses are ineffective for coping. Effective adaptive responses promote the integrity of the individual by conserving energy and promoting the survival, growth, reproduction, and mastery of the human system. Nursing promotes the patients' adaptation and coping, with progress toward *integration* as the goal (Phillips, 1997).

Using Roy's Model in Practice

The nurse using Roy's model focuses on the adaptation of the patient and on the environment. Adaptation is assessed and facilitated. Roy specified two assessments: of patients' adaptation behavior and of stimuli in the internal and external environments. Based on these assessments, the nurse develops nursing diagnoses to guide goal setting and interventions aimed at promoting adaptation. Simply stated, the nurse modifies the environment to facilitate patient adaptation.

Observable behavior is recognized and understood in the context of Roy's physiological, self-concept, role function, and interdependent modes. Descriptions of the behaviors included in each mode provide the nurse with a means of making evaluative judgments about the patient's progress toward the goal of adaptation (Phillips, 1997). Case applications are presented in Phillips (1997). Roy's model is very widely used in nursing practice and comprehensively described in the literature (Alligood, 1997b; Phillips, 1997; Roy, 1991).

Theories of Nursing

Nursing theories are the third and final type of theoretical work in the structure of nursing knowledge to be reviewed in this chapter. Theories are composed of sets of **concepts** which are related in statements or propositions.

King's theory of goal attainment is an example that was mentioned earlier. Theories are less abstract than nursing conceptual models, and they are more *prescriptive;* that is, they propose an explicit outcome that is testable in practice and research (Alligood, 1997c). Fawcett (1993) classified theories according to their breadth and depth. For example, *grand theories* are very broad, *theories* are less broad, and **middle-range theories** are the most specific. Theories are usually named for the outcome they propose or for specific characteristics of their content, for example Parse's theory of human becoming or Newman's theory of health as expanding consciousness (Alligood, 1997c).

Orlando's Nursing Process Theory

Ida Orlando first proposed her theory of effective nursing practice in 1961. She later revised it as a nursing process theory (1990). Her work actually proposed both: it is a theory about how nurses process their observations of patient behavior and about how they react to the patients based on inferences from their behavior, including what they say. Her early research revealed that processing observations as specified in the theory led to effective nursing practice and good outcomes.

This theory is specific to nurse-patient interactions. The goal of the nurse is to determine and meet patients' immediate needs and to improve their situation by relieving distress or discomfort. Orlando emphasized deliberate action (rather than automatic action) based on observation of the patients' verbal and nonverbal behavior, which leads to *inferences.* Inferences are confirmed or discomfirmed by the patient, leading the nurse to identify the patients' needs and provide effective nursing care.

Using Orlando's Theory in Practice

As a nursing practice theory, Orlando's theory specified how patients are involved in nurses' decision making. When used in practice, Orlando's theory guides interactions to predictable outcomes, which are different from outcomes that occur when the theory is not used. Nurses individualize care for each patient by attending to behavior, confirming with the patient ideas and inferences the nurse draws from interactions, and by identifying pressing needs.

Use of Orlando's theory improves the effectiveness of the nurse. It might be said that the nurse gets to the bottom line more quickly when *observing, listening,* and *confirming* with patients. Therefore, use of this theory saves time and energy for both the patient and nurse.

Leininger's Theory of Culture Care Diversity and Universality

Madeleine Leininger's (1978; 1991) work in cultural care grew out of her early nursing experiences. She observed that children of different cultures had widely varying behaviors and needs. After discussing the parallels between nursing and anthropology with the famed anthropologist Margaret Mead, Leininger pursued doctoral study in cultural anthropology. Through her doctoral work she became more convinced about the relationship of cultural differences and health practices. This led her to begin developing a theory of cultural care for nursing.

Leininger's work is formalized as a theory rather than as a conceptual model. It has stimulated the formation of the Transcultural Nursing Society, transcultural nursing conferences, newsletters, the *Journal of Transpersonal Caring,* and the awarding of master's degrees in the specialty area known as transcultural nursing.

Transcultural nursing's goal involves more than simply being aware of different cultures. It involves planning nursing care based on knowledge that is defined culturally, classified, and tested and then used to provide care that is *culturally congruent* (Leininger, 1978).

Leininger described theory as a creative and systematic way of discovering new knowledge or accounting for phenomena in a more complete way (Leininger, 1991). She encouraged nurses to use creativity to discover cultural aspects of human needs and use these findings to make culturally congruent therapeutic decisions. Her theory is broad, since it considers the impact of culture on all aspects of human life, with particular attention to health and caring practices.

As global migration continues and all societies become more diverse, Leininger's theory is more relevant than ever before.

Using Leininger's Theory in Practice

Leininger specified caring as the essence of nursing, and nurses who use Leininger's theory of cultural care in their practice view patients in the context of their cultures. Practice from a cultural perspective begins by respecting the culture of the patient and recognizing the importance of its relationship to nursing care. Use of the "sunrise model" (Fig. 11–2), which she created to guide the assessment of cultural data and its influence in the patient's life (Leininger, 1991), facilitates applying Leininger's theory. The nurse plans nursing care recognizing the health beliefs and folk practices of the patient's culture as well as the culture of traditional health services. To this end, care may be focused on *culture care preservation, accommodations,* or *repatterning* according to the patient's need. The nursing outcome of culturally congruent nursing care is health and well-being.

Newman's Theory of Health as Expanding Consciousness

Margaret Newman developed a theory of health derived from Rogers' Science of Unitary Human Beings. She focused on *pattern* and the *life process* to understand health and illness in a new way. Newman proposed a redefinition of health based on the original concept of wholeness. She saw health not as something apart from the person, as in "How is your health?" or to be gotten over, like an illness, but as a manifestation of the person's pattern of wholeness. As such, she saw health as a part of each person's wholeness: something to be gradually understood. She sought to design a means of recognizing the pattern of whole persons and their expanding conciousness throughout the process of life.

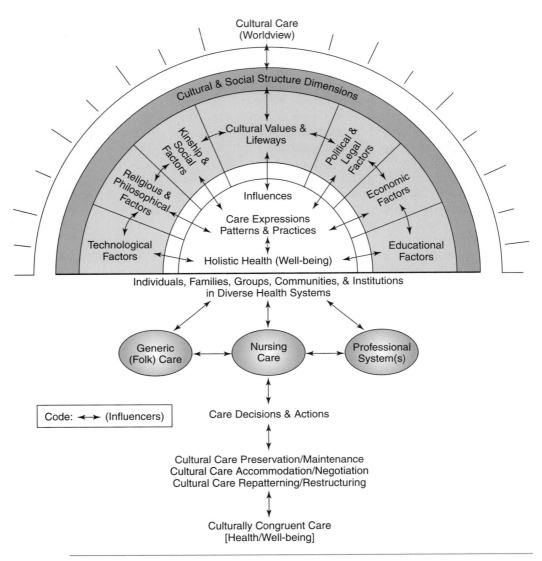

Figure 11–2
Leininger's sunrise model, created to facilitate the application in practice of the Theory of Culture Care Diversity and Universality (Courtesy Dr. Madeleine Leininger).

Using Newman's Theory in Practice

When using Newman's theory in nursing practice, the nurse's goal is to form meaningful relationships with patients and participate in their use of inner strengths as they move through higher and higher levels of consciousness (Fawcett, 1993; Newman 1986, 1994). Newman (1994) emphasized viewing patients in the context of their holistic patterns, or "pattern of the whole." Patients' perceptions of time are assessed in relation to their movement in space and time.

Newman's inclusive view incorporates all aspects of the person's process of living. Illness and disease are best understood as they exist in the patient's pattern. The nurse participates with patients with this goal: to establish relationships to facilitate their discovery of their inner strength as consciousness of their pattern unfolds. Health emerges from the patient's improved consciousness of life processes.

Parse's Theory of Human Becoming

Parse's work was first published as "theory of man-living-health" (1981) and later renamed "theory of human becoming" (1992). Parse derived her theory from two main sources: Martha Rogers' Science of Unitary Human Beings and existential phenomenology. Therefore, like Rogers, Parse viewed nursing as participation with the patient. Her work focused on the importance of health throughout life. She emphasized the nursing profession's history of focusing on health and contrasted that with the medical profession's history of treating illness and disease.

According to Parse, health is a cocreation with the universe as patients experience the being and becoming of life. Parse described this process, which like Rogers' model is acausal, in three existential phenomenological principles: The first principle proposed human meaning as a developing structure of *valuing* and *imaging* from which reality emerges through *languaging*; the second principle proposed a *patterned unity* of person and universe in rhythm of human behavioral patterns of *revealing-concealing, enabling-limiting,* and *connecting-separating*; the third principle proposed *co-transcendence* as the human capacity to grow (become) in process with the universe. She described transcendence as a rhythmical process originating from the intents and purposes of one's activity as possibilities become realities (Parse, 1981).

Using Parse's Theory in Practice

Nursing practice with Parse's theory involves participation with the patient. Within the relationship the nurse gains a perspective of the patient in the universe, being and becoming. This theory does not view nursing practice as an adjunct to medicine. Rather, nursing is seen as a profession in its own right focused on human becoming and health. The three principles help the nurse to recognize patient patterns and participate with patients in their becoming.

Theoretical Challenges for Nursing Education, Practice, and Research

These examples of nursing theoretical works illustrate that nursing theory has a vital role in nursing education, practice, and research. To move nursing forward and to improve the quality of nursing care, theory-based practice and theory testing and theory-generating research are required. Sound curricula based on nursing knowledge are also required. The relationship of theory to education and practice is illustrated in Figure 11–3.

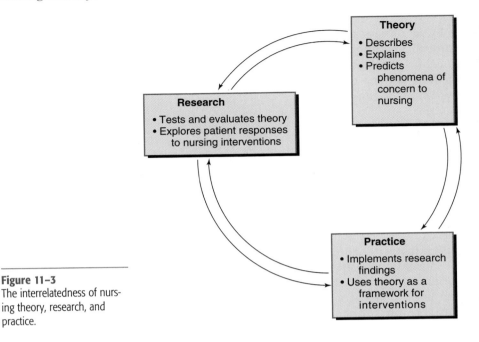

Figure 11–3
The interrelatedness of nursing theory, research, and practice.

Theory-Based Education

The nursing profession has grown phenomenally throughout the period of theory development. Schools of nursing have proliferated, preparing nurses from the associate degree level to the PhD level. Nurses prepared at each level of nursing are involved in nursing theory, as noted in Box 11–7.

BOX 11-7
Levels of Education and Use of Nursing Theory

Level of Nursing Education	*Use of Nursing Theory*
PhD in nursing	Conducts theory testing and theory development research for nursing science development; frames practice, administration, or research in nursing works
Master of science in nursing	Frames advanced practice with a nursing model or theory; uses theory to guide research with practice questions
Bachelor of science in nursing	Learns the nursing perspective in a nursing model or theory-based curriculum or courses. Uses models, theories, and middle-range theories to guide nursing practice
Associate degree in nursing	May have a nursing model or theory-guided curriculum or courses; is introduced to middle-range theories for nursing practice

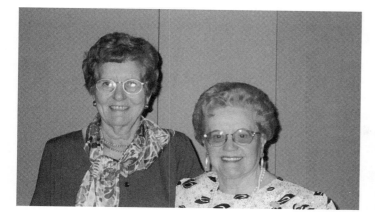

Figure 11–4
Madeleine Leininger, RN, PhD, FAAN (right) and Mary T. Boynton at the 1999 nursing theorist lecture at the College of Nursing, The University of Tennessee, Knoxville (Photo by Sally Helton, Courtesy of the College of Nursing, University of Tennessee, Knoxville).

The nursing profession has evolved from an applied vocation dependent on knowledge from other disciplines to the current stage of developing its own knowledge base. Efforts to develop nursing's knowledge base have stimulated—and been stimulated by—the development of the nursing PhD, a research degree that requires the generation of new, discipline-specific knowledge.

At the doctoral level nurses are concerned with the philosophy of science, that is, the nature of knowledge and how it is known; the generation of nursing knowledge; theory testing; and the development of new theory through research. The master's level nurse is concerned with advanced practice, which goes beyond the generic nursing process. Master's-level nurses use theoretical perspectives that focus on the patient and predict specific nursing outcomes. Many nurses conduct their first research studies as master's students. These studies usually focus on nursing practice and test nursing interventions with specific patient groups.

The baccalaureate nurse is introduced to the research process and the use of theory to guide it. The research emphasis for baccalaureate-level students is on learning to critique nursing research, thereby becoming informed consumers of research relevant to practice. Some curricula of bachelor of science in nursing programs are based on a selected nursing theoretical perspective; others introduce students to a variety of perspectives. Whether the curriculum is built around one or many nursing theoretical works, the focus at the baccalaureate level is utilization of nursing theory to guide practice.

The associate degree level of nursing education may also use nursing theoretical works to teach nursings' unique perspectives. Nurses with associate degrees often find middle-range theories, which are specific to patient care, particularly useful.

Basing nursing education on nursing theory benefits schools and colleges of nursing. Holding scholarly discussions about how to apply nursing theory in education, research, and practice establishes an environment of critical thinking, questioning, and learning. Hosting theorists as guest lecturers helps faculty and students see the theorists in a realistic light, as persons with information pertinent to nursing. A number of colleges of nursing have endowed distinguished lecturer programs. These programs often include annual events, drawing audiences from the campus and surrounding nursing community that look forward to the opportunity to hear nursing theorists discuss their work. Figure 11–4 shows Dr. Madeleine Leininger, the 1999 Mary T. Boynton Distinguished Lecturer at the University of Tennessee at Knoxville, pictured with Mary T. Boynton, for whom the lecture series was named.

Theory-based Practice

How is theory translated into practice? The answer to that question lies with theory-based practice. Theory-based practice occurs when nurses intentionally structure their practices around a particular nursing theory and use it to help them assess, plan, diagnose, intervene, and evaluate nursing care. Theory enables nurses to challenge conventional views of patients, the health-illness continuum, and traditional nursing interventions.

It is hoped that the introductions to various nursing theoretical works in this chapter will lead you to select works that resonate with your values to study more deeply. With increased understanding you may begin to develop the use of nursing theories in your practice.

There are many benefits to be gained from theory-based practice. You can explain your practice to others. That is, nursing theory provides the language for you to explain what you do, how you do it, and why. This facilitates the transmission of nursing knowledge to students who are new to the profession as well as contributes to the understanding of nursing by other health-related professionals. Furthermore, theory contributes to professional autonomy by providing a nursing guide for practice, education, and research. The study of theory will help you develop analytical skills, challenge your thinking, and clarify your values and assumptions (Holder and Chitty, 1997).

Many nurses have developed their ideas about nursing and continue to develop nursing assumptions based on education, experience, observation, and reading. Most nurses do not formally develop their own personal theories, although their ideas certainly influence the way they practice nursing. According to Wardle and Mandle (1989), who studied this practice in their research, personal theories tend to be incomplete and inconsistent as a basis for nursing practice. Relying on your personal theory as a basis for practice is usually ineffective and therefore not suggested. They recommend using a theory that has been tested or developed through nursing research and critiqued, analyzed, and evaluated for usefulness in nursing practice. There are many practice areas and client populations that remain to be addressed in formalized middle-range theories (Alligood, 1997 d).

As you engage in theory-based practice, remember to provide feedback to nurse researchers and theorists concerning your findings and experiences. You can do this through the World Wide Web, where you can find groups of nurses using, discussing, and refining all the theoretical works mentioned in this chapter. You can assist these scholars as they continue to advance the science of nursing and ultimately may join them in this quest.

Theory-based Research

Great strides have been made in the last 25 years in nursing research. The expansion of graduate nursing education at the master's level and the proliferation of nursing doctoral programs played a major role as more nurses than ever before were equipped with the knowledge and skills to conduct research. Nursing research tests and refines nursing's developing knowledge base. Ultimately, research findings enable nurses to predict reliably how nursing actions influence patient outcomes.

Research is vital to the future of nursing, and theory has an integral role in research. Unfortunately, nurse researchers still are publishing studies without including any discussion of the theory or theories that guided the study. Others continue to use theories from disciplines outside nursing that do not view persons holistically or from a nursing perspective. For these reasons, utilization of nursing theory to structure nursing research remains a challenge for nurse researchers.

Chapter 12 is devoted to understanding the research process. It is important for nurses to understand that theory, nursing practice, and research are interrelated. Each stimulates, improves, and advances the other. An example of how nurses use theory as a framework for research that contributes knowledge to nursing practice is presented in the study summarized in Box 11–8.

BOX 11–8

A Study Illustrating the Interrelationship of Theory, Research, and Practice

Even though breast cancer is the leading cause of cancer mortality in African-American women, fewer than half of these women who are older than 50 years report ever having had a mammogram and breast examination. Two-thirds report not practicing regular breast self-examination. Puzzled by these findings, Brown and Williams used Leininger's Culture Care Theory and the Health Belief Model to explore factors that prevented these women from using screening services.

According to Leininger's work, African-Americans value extended family networks, religious values, interdependence with other African-Americans, daily survival, folk foods, and folk-healing modes. The five variables of the Health Belief Model are susceptibility, seriousness, benefits, barriers, and health motivation.

After an extensive literature review, the researchers determined that some barriers to breast screening programs experienced by older African-American women were unique to their culture, whereas others were shared with all older women. Some barriers they identified that were unique to the African-American culture included heightened fear of cancer, underestimating its incidence, pessimism about cure, lack of awareness of screening tests, and use of a lay referral system that may delay treatment. In common with other older women, they attributed breast changes to age, were embarrassed, lacked knowledge about mammogram and breast self-examination, and believed that screening programs were too much trouble, inconvenient, or unnecessary. In addition, African-American individuals thought that health care providers were insensitive to their cultural and social needs.

(continued)

BOX 11-8

A Study Illustrating the Interrelationship of Theory, Research, and Practice (Continued)

Several guidelines for practice were identified as a result of this literature review. Nurses may

- Encourage the use of screening methods daily in their interactions with older African-American women.
- Reduce expenses by planning reduced-cost services.
- Increase the availability and accessibility of screening programs by using mobile units and community sites during evening and weekend hours.
- Plan and implement breast health educational programs using culturally sensitive materials.
- Work with African-American community leaders to promote breast cancer screening.

Adapted with permission of Brown, L. W., and Williams, R. D. (1994). Culturally sensitive breast cancer screening programs for older Black women. Used with permission from *Nurse Practitioner 19(3):21*, 26–6, 31 passim, © Springhouse Corporation/*www.springnet.com.*

Summary of Key Points

- Theory development is not a mysterious activity restricted to a few nursing scholars. It is, however, an activity that combines education, knowledge, and skill in a sustained effort.
- Nursing philosophies, models, and theories offer many perspectives on nursing, varying in their level of abstraction and their definitions of four major concepts: person, environment, health, and nursing.
- As nurses devise theories of nursing, present them for review by their colleagues in a peer review process, and publish them in the nursing literature, the discipline moves forward in the development of its unique knowledge base.
- There are scholarly contributions to be made by nurses at every level of educational preparation. To the extent that nurses question, read, study, and write about nursing practice, they contribute to the development of nursing knowledge.
- Nurses in practice settings contribute invaluable insights and observations, thereby building the knowledge base for nursing. Nursing theorists also rely on practicing nurses to test clinical interventions and explore the usefulness of their theories.
- Clinical research requires support by practicing nurses who recognize the importance of theory-based practice and research. Nurses contribute to the development of the profession by participating in research studies when possible and supporting research in practice settings.

- The nurse theorists whose works were reviewed in this chapter, as well as others too numerous to include, have made significant contributions to the development of nursing's unique body of knowledge.
- Many nurse theorists continue to develop and refine their work, whereas some are deceased or have retired from their work in theory development. However, each theoretical work has a community of scholars (Kuhn, 1970) who use the work in their own nursing research and practice and continue to expand, clarify, and refine these original works (Alligood and Marriner-Tomey, 1997; Fawcett, 1993, 1995; Marriner-Tomey and Alligood, 1998).

Critical Thinking Questions

1. Recognizing that your understanding of nursings' theoretical works is only beginning, which works introduced in this chapter appeal to you the most?
2. After exploring the features of the works you identified in question 1, which ones describe nursing in the way you think about it? What other feature(s) of the works intrigue you?
3. Which of the theoretical works would be useful to help you organize your thoughts for critical thinking and decision making in nursing practice?
4. Interview practicing nurses and ask them which nursing philosophies, models, or theories influence their thinking and practice of nursing.
5. Describe the use of nursing theory for nurses at your current level of nursing education.
6. Explain why theory development is important to the profession of nursing.

Web Resources

Center for Human Caring (Watson), http://uchsc.edu:80/ctrsinst/chc

Florence Nightingale Site, http://www.cfcsc.dnd.ca/links/bio/night.html

Levine's Conservation Model, http://www4.allencol.edu/~seyo/levine.html

Margaret Newman Web Site, http://www.tc.umn.edu/~hoym0003

Neuman Systems Model, http://www.lemmus.demon.co.uk/neuman1.htm

Nursing Theory Link Page, http://www.healthsci.clayton.edu/eichelberger/nursing.htm

Orlando Web Site, http://www.uri.edu/nursing/orlando/theory

Parse's Theory of Human Becoming, http://www.utoronto.ca/icps

Rogers Web Site, http://www.uwcm.ac.uk.uwcm/ns/mantha/homepage.html

Self-Care Deficit Nursing Theory, http://www.hsc.missouri.edu/~son/scdnt/scdnt.html

Sr. Callista Roy, http://www.bc.edu/bc-org/avp/son/theorist/nurse-theorist.html

The Nursing Theory, Page http://www.ualberta.ca/~jrnorris/nt/theory.html

Transcultural Nursing Society, http://www.tcns.org

References

Alligood, M. R. (1995). Theory of goal attainment: Application to adult orthopedic nursing. In M. A. Frey and C. Sieloff (Eds.). *Advancing King's systems framework and theory* (pp. 209–222). Thousand Oaks, Calif.: Sage Publications.

Alligood, M. R. (1997a). The nature of knowledge needed for nursing practice. In M. R. Alligood and A. Marriner-Tomey (Eds.). *Nursing theory: Utilization and application* (pp. 3–13). St. Louis: Mosby.

Alligood, M. R. (1997b). Models and theories in nursing practice. In M. R. Alligood and A. Marriner-Tomey (Eds.). *Nursing theory: Utilization and application* (pp. 15–30). St. Louis: Mosby.

Alligood, M. R. (1997c). Models and theories: Critical thinking structures. In M. R. Alligood and A. Marriner-Tomey (Eds.). *Nursing theory: Utilization and application* (pp. 31–45). St. Louis: Mosby.

Alligood, M. R. (1997d). Areas for further development of theory based nursing practice. In M. R. Alligood and A. Marriner-Tomey (Eds.). *Nursing theory: Utilization and application* (pp. 203–210). St. Louis: Mosby.

Alligood, M. R., and Choi, E. C. (1998). Evolution of nursing theory development. In A. Marriner Tomey and M. R. Alligood (Eds.). *Nursing theorists and their work* (pp. 55–66). St. Louis: Mosby

Alligood, M. R., and Marriner-Tomey, A. (1997). *Nursing theory: Utilization and application*. St. Louis: Mosby.

Barrett, E. (1990). *Visions of Rogers' science-based nursing*. New York: National League for Nursing.

Benner, P. (1984). *From novice to expert: Excellence and power in clinical nursing practice*. Menlo Park, Calif.: Addison-Wesley.

Berbiglia, V. (1997). Orem's self-care deficit theory in nursing practice. In M. R. Alligood and A. Marriner-Tomey (Eds.). *Nursing theory: Utilization and application* (pp. 129–152). St. Louis: Mosby.

Brown, L. W., and Williams, R. D. (1994). Culturally sensitive breast cancer screening programs for older black women. *Nurse Practitioner, 19*(3), 21, 25–26, 31, 35.

Bultemeier, K. (1997). Rogers' science of unitary human beings in nursing practice. In M. R. Alligood and A. Marriner-Tomey (Eds.). *Nursing theory: Utilization and application* (pp. 153–174). St. Louis: Mosby.

Chinn, P., and Kramer, M. (1998). *Theory and nursing: A systematic approach* (5th ed.). St. Louis: Mosby.

Fawcett, J. (1993). *Analysis and evaluation of nursing theories*. Philadelphia: F. A. Davis.

Fawcett, J. (1995). *Analysis and evaluation of conceptual models of nursing* (3rd ed.). Philadelphia: F. A. Davis.

Fawcett, J. (1997). Conceptual models of nursing, nursing theories, and nursing practice: Focus on the future. In R. A. Martha and A. Marriner-Tomey (Eds.). *Nursing theory: Utilization and application* (pp. 211–221). St. Louis: Mosby.

Fitzpatrick, J. and Whall, A. (1996). *Conceptual models of nursing: Analysis and application* (3rd ed.). Norwalk, Conn.: Appleton & Lange.

Frey, M. A., and Norris, D. (1997). King's systems framework and theory in nursing practice. In M. R. Alligood and A. Marriner-Tomey (Eds.). *Nursing theory: Utilization and application* (pp. 71–88). St. Louis: Mosby.

Frey, M. A., and Sieloff, C. L. (1995). *Advancing King's systems framework and theory for nursing*. Thousand Oaks, Calif.: Sage Publications.

George, J. B. (Ed.). (1995). *Nursing theories: The base for professional nursing practice* (4th ed.). Norwalk, Conn.: Appleton & Lange.

Henderson, V. (1996). *The nature of nursing: A definition and its implications for practice, research, and education.* New York: Macmillan.

Holaday, B. (1997). Johnson's behavioral system model in nursing practice. In M. R. Alligood and A. Marriner-Tomey (Eds.). *Nursing theory: Utilization and application* (pp. 49–70). St. Louis: Mosby.

Holder, P. J., and Chitty, K. K. (1997). Theory as a basis for professional nursing. In Kay Kittrell Chitty (Ed.). *Professional nursing: Concepts and challenges* (2nd ed.). Philadelphia: WB Saunders.

Johnson, D. (1968). One conceptual model for nursing. Paper presented at Vanderbilt University, Nashville, Tenn.

Johnson, D. (1980). The behavioral systems model for nursing. In J. Riehl and C. Roy (Eds.). *Conceptual models for nursing practice* (2nd ed.) (pp. 207–216). New York: Appleton-Century-Croft.

King, I. M. (1981). *A theory for nursing: Systems, concepts, process.* New York: John Wiley & Sons.

Kuhn, T. S. (1970). *The structure of scientific revolutions* (2nd ed.). Chicago: University of Chicago Press.

Leininger, M. (1978). *Transcultural nursing: Concepts, theories, and practices.* New York: John Wiley & Sons.

Leininger, M. (1991). *Culture care diversity and universality: A theory of nursing.* New York: National League for Nursing.

Levine, M. (1973). *Introduction to clinical nursing* (2nd ed.). Philadelphia: F. A. Davis.

Levine, M. (1991). The conservation model: A model for health. In K. M. Schaefer and J. B. Pond (Eds.). *The conservation model: A framework for nursing practice* (pp. 1–11). Philadelphia: F. A. Davis.

Madrid, M., and Barrett, E. A. M. (1994). *Rogers' scientific art of nursing practice.* New York: National League for Nursing.

Marriner-Tomey, A., and Alligood, M. R. (1998). *Nursing theorists and their work* (4th ed.). St. Louis: Mosby.

Meleis, A. (1997). *Theoretical nursing: Development and progress* (3rd ed.). Philadelphia: J. B. Lippincott.

Neuman, B. (1995). *The Neuman systems model* (3rd ed.). Norwalk, Conn.: Appleton & Lange.

Newman, M. (1986). *Health as expanding consciousness.* St. Louis: Mosby.

Newman, M. (1994). *Health as expanding consciousness* (2nd ed.). New York: National League for Nursing.

Nightingale, F. (1969). *Notes on nursing: What it is and what it is not.* 1859. Reprint, New York: Dover Publications.

Orem, D. (1995). *Nursing: Concepts of practice* (5th ed.). New York: McGraw-Hill.

Orlando, I. (1961). *The dynamic nurse-patient relationship: Function, process, and principles.* New York: G. P. Putnam's Sons.

Orlando, I. (1990). *The dynamic nurse-patient relationship: Function, process and principles* (reprint). New York: National League for Nursing.

Parse, R. R. (1981). *Man-living-health: A theory for nursing.* New York: John Wiley & Sons.

Parse, R. R. (1992). Human becoming: Parse's theory of nursing. *Nursing Science Quarterly,* 5(1), 35–42.

Phillips, K. D. (1997). Roy's adaptation model in nursing practice. In M. R. Alligood and A. Marriner-Tomey (Eds.). *Nursing theory: Utilization and application* (pp. 175–200). St. Louis: Mosby.

Powers, B. A., and Knapp, T. R. (1995). *A dictionary of nursing theory and research* (2nd ed.). Thousand Oaks, Calif.: Sage.

Rogers, M. (1970). *An introduction to the theoretical basis of nursing.* Philadelphia: F. A. Davis.

Rogers, M. (1992). Nursing science and the space age. *Nursing Science Quarterly,* 5(1), 27–34.

Roy, Sr. C. (1970, March). Adaptation: A conceptual framework for nursing. *Nursing Outlook,* 18(3), 42–45.

Roy, Sr. C., and Andrews, H. A. (1991). *The Roy adaptation model: The definitive statement.* Norwalk, Conn.: Appleton & Lange.

Schaefer, K. M. (1997). Levine's conservation model in nursing practice. In M. R. Alligood and A. Marriner-Tomey (Eds.). *Nursing theory: Utilization and application* (pp. 89–107). St. Louis: Mosby.

Schaefer, K. M., and Pond, J. B. (1991). *The conservation model: A framework for practice.* Philadelphia: F. A. Davis.

Sohier, R. (1997). Neuman's systems model in nursing practice. In M. R. Alligood and A. Marriner-Tomey (Eds.). *Nursing theory: Utilization and application* (pp. 109–127). St. Louis: Mosby.

Wardle, M. G., and Mandle, C. L. (1989). Conceptual models used in clinical practice. *Western Journal of Nursing Research,* 11(1), 108–114.

Watson, J. (1988). *Nursing: Human science and human care.* New York: National League for Nursing.

Watson, J. (1979). *Nursing: The philosophy and science of caring.* Boston: Little, Brown.

Understanding the Scientific Method and Nursing Research

Carol T. Bush

12

Key Terms

Applied Science
Conceptual Framework
Confidentiality
Data
Deductive Reasoning
Disseminate
Evidence-based Practice
Experimental Design
Galileo
Generalizable
Hypothesis
Inductive Reasoning
Informed Consent
Institutional Review Board
Newton
Nonexperimental Design
Nursing Research
Peer Review
Phenomena
Phenomenological Research
Population
Problem Solving
Protocol
Pure Science

Qualitative Research
Quantitative Research
Reliable
Replicate
Research Process

Research Question
Sample
Scientific Method
Subjects
Valid

Learning Outcomes

After studying this chapter, students will be able to:

- Differentiate between pure and applied science.
- Describe the historical development of the scientific method.
- Give examples of inductive and deductive reasoning.
- Discuss the limitations of the scientific method when applied to nursing.
- Differentiate between problem solving and research.
- List the steps in the research process.
- Describe the phases in the design of a qualitative study.
- Discuss contributions nursing research has made to nursing practice and to health care.
- Describe the relationship of nursing research to nursing theory and practice.
- Identify sources of support for nursing research.
- Discuss the roles of nurses in research.

In the 1960s, the nursing profession was poised on the threshold of a higher level of development. There was recognition that mature professions had strong scientific bases, which were lacking in nursing. Nursing scholars realized that nursing could achieve its potential and desired professional status only to the extent that the discipline was based on a scientifically derived body of knowledge unique to nursing. As a result of that recognition, nursing researchers set about developing knowledge, and nursing theorists began developing theories and testing them.

About the same time, nurses realized that a similar professionalization of patient care practices was needed. Using traditional methods to deal with familiar patient problems and trial and error or intuition to deal with unfamiliar ones was no longer seen as an acceptable way to care for patients and move the profession toward evidence-based practice. Practitioners of nursing, therefore, also developed a more scientific approach to patient care that is an adaptation of the classic scientific method. This problem-solving approach is called the nursing process and is presented in more depth in Chapter 15. An understanding of the scientific method is helpful in appreciating both nursing research and the nursing process.

Science and the Scientific Method

The study of any subject by using the **scientific method** or other methods of reasoning can be considered science. The scientific method is an orderly, systematic way of thinking about and solving problems. It has been used by scientists for centuries to discover and test facts and principles. When used under carefully planned and controlled conditions, the scientific method becomes research. The scientific method is the same, regardless of the discipline using it.

Pure and Applied Science and Research

Scientists divide scientific knowledge into two categories: pure and applied. **Pure science** or pure research, sometimes called basic science or basic research, summarizes and explains the universe without regard for whether the information is immediately useful. When Joseph Priestly discovered oxygen in 1774, he did not have an immediate use for that information. Therefore, that discovery could be classified as pure science, that is, information gathered solely for the sake of obtaining new knowledge. **Applied science** or applied research seeks to use scientific theory and laws in some practical way. The use of oxygen with premature infants is an example of applied science. The testing of this method to refine treatment guidelines is applied research. From this example, it can be seen that today's pure science can become tomorrow's applied science. Nursing makes use of applied scientific principles and is most effective in conducting applied research to improve patient outcomes through nursing care.

History of the Scientific Method

Until the time of Hippocrates (ca. 460–377 B.C.), in Western cultures illness was believed to be caused by evil spirits. Gradually, over the years and through the efforts of many scientists, humankind has learned a great deal about the human body, health, and illness. Most of this knowledge was developed after the scientific method came into widespread use.

A period of great intellectual activity, known as the Age of Reason, began in the 1600s and lasted until the late 1700s. During that time, scientists made unparalleled advances in understanding the laws by which nature operates by using reason and experimentation. **Galileo** (1564–1642), the Italian physicist and astronomer, and Sir Isaac **Newton** (1642–1727), the English philosopher and mathematician, are usually credited with developing and refining the scientific method. A scientific revolution and technological explosion resulted from the use of the scientific method. In the area of health care alone, profound and far-reaching scientific discoveries have changed human life dramatically. Selected important scientific discoveries related to health are listed in Box 12–1.

Each era has been characterized by scientific advances. For example, the 1990s was called the "Decade of the Brain," with impressive findings such as brain scans illustrating differences between the brains of persons with mental illness and substance abuse addictions and those of so-called normal persons. The future looks bright for continuation of brain-related research, which may someday unlock the secrets of human behavior. The National Institute of Nursing Research (NINR) is a member of the Council of Federal Liaisons. This group has endorsed the initiative "Decade of Behavior: 2000–2010," which highlights contributions already made by the behavioral and social sciences in addressing national challenges in health, education, and safety and potential future advances. You can learn more about the NINR's activities in this important area of research at http://www.nih.gov/ninr/decade_behavior.htm.

Inductive and Deductive Reasoning

The scientific method requires the use of two types of logic: inductive and deductive reasoning. In **inductive reasoning,** the process begins with a particular experience and proceeds to generalizations. Repeated observations of an experiment or event enable the observer to draw general conclusions. For example, the statement "All the St. Bernard dogs I have encountered are gentle; therefore, St. Bernards are gentle" is an example of inductive reasoning. It is obvious from this example that this type of logic leads to probabilities—not certainties—unless the world's entire population of St. Bernard dogs is observed.

Scientists also use **deductive reasoning,** a process through which conclusions are drawn by logical inference from given premises. It proceeds from the general case to the specific. For example, if the premises "All school children like chocolate" and "Missie is a schoolchild" are accepted, the conclusion "Missie likes chocolate" can be drawn. It may be entirely possible, however, that Missie, although a schoolchild, does not like chocolate at all. In deductive reasoning, the premises used must be correct or the conclusions will not be. Conclusions drawn through deductive processes are called valid rather than true. **Valid** is a term meaning "soundly founded," whereas true means "in accordance with the fact or reality" (Flexner, Stein, and Su, 1980). It is possible for a conclusion to be solidly founded without its being true. There is a subtle but real difference in the two terms.

As seen by these examples, neither inductive nor deductive processes alone are adequate. If scientists used only deductive logic, experience would

BOX 12-1
Important Health-related Events in the Evolution of Science

ca. 400 B.C.	Hippocrates taught that diseases have natural, not supernatural, causes.
A.D. 100	Galen laid the foundation for the study of anatomy and physiology.
ca. 1500	Leonardo da Vinci recognized the importance of observation and experimentation in learning.
1543	Andreas Vesalius published a book on human anatomy, based on observation.
1628	William Harvey published his theory on the circulation of blood.
1774	Joseph Priestly discovered oxygen.
ca. 1796	Edward Jenner discovered a method of smallpox vaccination.
1839	Matthias Schleiden and Theodor Schwann developed the theory that all living things are composed of cells.
1866	Gregor Mendel demonstrated the laws of heredity.
ca. 1876	Louis Pasteur demonstrated that microorganisms cause fermentation and disease.
1882	Robert Koch isolated the bacterium that causes tuberculosis.
1895	Wilhelm K. Roentgen discovered x-rays.
1898	Marie and Pierre Curie isolated the element radium.
ca. 1900	Paul Ehrlich originated chemotherapy, the treatment of diseases with chemicals (drugs).
1928	Alexander Fleming discovered penicillin.
1953	Jonas Salk developed the first effective polio vaccine.
1957	Arthur Karnberg grew deoxyribonucleic acid (DNA), the basic chemical of genes, in a test tube.
1978	The world's first test tube baby was delivered.
1982	William DeVries implanted the world's first artificial heart.
1989	The first authorized use of genetic engineering injecting genetically altered cells into patients with malignant melanoma was undertaken.
1992	A team of international scientists reported the discovery of the gene that causes fragile X syndrome, a common inherited form of mental retardation.
1998	A team of Scottish scientists, led by Dr. Ian Wilmut, reported the first successful cloning of an adult mammal, resulting in Dolly, the world's most famous sheep.

From Kuhn, T. S. (1970). The structure of scientific revolutions. In O. Neurath, (Ed.). *International encyclopedia of unified science* (2nd ed., vol 2). Chicago: University of Chicago Press; Ware, C. F., and Panikkar, K. M. (1966). *The twentieth century: History of mankind, cultural and scientific development* (vol. 6). New York: Harper & Row; and Time Magazine, available from, http://www.pathfinder.com/TIME/cloning/cloningl.html.

be ignored. If they used only inductive logic, relationships between facts and principles would be ignored. A combination of both types of reasoning processes in science unifies the theoretical and the practical, which is the basis for the scientific method and research.

Limitations of the Scientific Method in Nursing

Polit and Hungler (1997, p. 11) asserted that the scientific method is the "most sophisticated method of acquiring knowledge that humans have developed." Many authorities believe that using any other method is to be avoided. There are at least four reasons, however, why the scientific method has limitations when applied to nursing.

The first and most obvious drawback is that health care settings are not comparable to laboratories. There are realities and priorities operating in health care settings that must take precedence over laboratory protocols. The safety and security of human patients are of the utmost importance and cannot be jeopardized.

Second, human beings are far more than collections of parts that can be dissected and subjected to examination or experimentation. A strength of nursing is its ability to view patients holistically, whereas the basis of the scientific method is to divide a problem into manageable problem statements, each of which can be tested. Because humans are complex organisms with interrelated parts and systems, the classic scientific method loses much of its usefulness.

A third limitation of the scientific method as the only approach to solving patient problems is its objectivity; it fails to consider the meaning of patients' own experiences, that is, their subjective view of reality. Nurses are keenly aware that patients' perceptions of their experiences, or subjective data, are just as important as objective data.

Finally, there are definite ethical implications involved in experimenting with humans that make reliance on the scientific method impractical. The rights of human subjects in research are paramount, as discussed elsewhere in this chapter.

Nursing Research Based on the Scientific Method

For many undergraduates their only exposure to research is in introductory psychology or sociology courses, in which they are subjects in a professor's research project. All they see of research are the boring forms they fill out or the nonsense syllables they memorize. This kind of orientation leads them to wonder what research has to do with their ability to care for patients.

Before students of nursing write off research altogether, they should consider the value of a different kind of research—patient care research. Through patient care research, nursing "seeks to understand and ease the symptoms of acute and chronic illness, to prevent or delay the onset of disease or disability or slow its progression, to find effective approaches to achieving and sustaining good health, and to improve the clinical settings in which care is provided" (Friends of the National Institute of Nursing Research, 1995).

For example, nurses are often the key to life or death for low-birth-weight infants. What do nurses need to know to tip the balance in favor of life for those babies? A group of researchers at the University of Pennsylvania, led by nurse Barbara Medoff-Cooper (Gibson et al., 1998; Medoff-Cooper and Ray, 1995), has considered this question. They are studying neonatal sucking behaviors. According to these researchers, "Effective sucking behaviors or feeding is not only a prerequisite for survival, but also implies that an infant has achieved the neurologic, behavioral, and physiologic maturity required for safe, effective oral feeding" (Medoff-Cooper and Ray, 1995, p. 195). Their finding that for premature or sick infants breast-feeding is easier and requires less energy expenditure than bottle-feeding is important in infant care.

Then there is the question of pacifiers—are they useful or harmful? Known in the research literature as "nonnutritive sucking," pacifier usage for five minutes before feeding has been demonstrated to increase the time infants are awake. This knowledge provided the basis for nurses to experiment with giving pacifiers to infants who were being tube fed. The use of the pacifier was found to help the tube-fed infants move more rapidly to normal oral feedings (Medoft-Cooper and Ray, 1995). Another group studied neonates given sucrose-dipped pacifiers to determine whether the pain from procedures (such as heel sticks to obtain blood samples) would be somewhat ameliorated (Stevens et al., 1999).

Another nurse researcher, Dr. Patricia Becker of the University of Wisconsin, has also studied low-birth-weight infants and the stress they experience during routine feeding, bathing, and intrusive procedures in neonatal intensive care units (NICUs). Her findings are expected to change NICU caregiving routines, thereby reducing complications and improving weight gain (Becker et al., 1993). The sooner the infants gain weight, the sooner they can be discharged to their homes and families. From these examples, it is easily seen that studying newborn behavior yields a great deal of useful information that can improve nursing care and ultimately improve the health of infants. This is only one area in which evidence-based nursing practice benefits patients (see News Note).

Another example of nursing research that makes a difference is the study of falls in geriatric patients. Some older persons lose strength in their lower extremities or lose their balance from time to time, leading to hip fractures and other injuries suffered during falls. Fractures can be set and hips surgically replaced, but it would be better if older people did not fall.

Elizabeth McNeely, a nurse who specializes in working with older persons, collaborated with researchers from other disciplines to study falls in elderly individuals. A group of older persons were taught tai chi, a form of martial arts, to see whether they would fall less often than those who did not practice tai chi (Kutner et al., 1997; Wolf et al., 1996). The moves performed in tai chi exercises promote balance and strengthen muscles. When elderly

"Beyond Tender Loving Care, Nurses Are a Force in Research"

The Florence Nightingales of the nation are busily adding a Louis Pasteur research component to their profession. And nursing's distinctly human, low-tech studies are bringing better and less costly medical care to millions of patients as well as helping relatives who care for them at home.

Since Congress established the National Center for Nursing Research over President Reagan's veto, federally financed studies by nurses have made important strides toward closing gaps in patient care that often lead to physical and emotional complications, prolonged hospital stays or failure to adapt to disease or its treatment.

. . . Nurse researchers at the University of Rochester found that when nurses or family members provided moral support for heart patients during their transfer out of the coronary care unit, fewer cardiovascular complications occurred and the patients stayed in the hospital an average of four days fewer than similar patients who weathered the transfer without added support.

A study by nurses at Ohio State University showed that several weeks of aerobic exercise before surgery and chemotherapy for breast cancer speeded the patient's ability to return to normal activities.

. . . A recent analysis of 84 studies conducted by nurse researchers among a total of 4146 patients prompted Dr. Barbara S. Heater, associate professor of nursing at the University of Missouri in St. Louis, to conclude that "research-based nursing interventions can produce 28 percent better outcomes for 72 percent of patients" and save money by shortening hospital stays . . . .

. . . [N]urse researchers are carving out new territories in health promotion and disease prevention that have been all but ignored by physicians. Studies by nurses look, for example, at factors that help patients follow doctor's orders, to change their living habits after a heart attack, reasons many elderly patients fail to take influenza seriously, ways to help families cope with high cholesterol levels in children, and circumstances that keep women from following an exercise routine.

people have better balance and greater strength, they are not as likely to fall, and they may avoid breaking bones. This study is expected to have an impact on the health of the elderly in the future.

Another example is provided by nurses who work with children. These nurse researchers use imagery to decrease the nausea and vomiting of children receiving cancer treatment. Imagery involves creating positive mental images that counteract unpleasant experiences and is sometimes used in stress reduction exercises. The nurse researchers design individual imagery programs for the children with whom they work. They make a tape with the child's favorite music in the background and talk the patient into relaxing while listening to the music. For children who have a favorite recording artist, the nurses play that artist's recordings and talk the children through a sequence of pleasant mental images. Children who have cancer respond in a positive way to music and images to which they can relate and thereby tolerate their treatments better (Hochenberry, 1989).

The rest of this chapter describes some basic concepts of **nursing research.** The purpose is to introduce nursing research, demonstrate its merit, and provide a basic vocabulary. The ultimate goal is for nurses to participate in the research process and apply research findings to clinical practice. This is what is known as **evidence-based practice.**

What Is Nursing Research?

Nursing research is the systematic investigation of **phenomena** (events or circumstances) related to improving nursing care. When nurses have a question they believe they must answer to provide better care for patients, and they have the time, money, skill, and energy to study that question, they should do nursing research. Although the chosen research topic may be in a new area of investigation, there is much to be gained from choosing research problems that are connected to work already done. This builds nursing knowledge in an orderly way.

Research problems should be pursued if they meet all three of the following tests:

1. There is a conceptual framework; that is, the researchers' ideas about the problem fit logically and dovetail with what is already known about the topic.
2. The proposed research project is based on related research findings published in professional journals or is networked with similar ongoing research in other settings, thereby building nursing knowledge.
3. The proposed research is carefully designed so that the results will be applicable in similar situations.

In addition to building nursing knowledge, studies that build on previous work are more likely to receive financial support. Research is expensive and often requires funding beyond what one nurse, hospital, or university can supply. Nurses who want to do research usually find it necessary to obtain outside funding or compete with other aspiring researchers for limited internal (from within the agency) funding. Therefore, to receive funding, nurses must do research that interests others and that a funding agency is willing to support.

The agencies that fund nursing research look for ideas that build on and advance nursing knowledge. Thus, although nursing research may be broadly defined as anything that interests nurses and helps them provide better care, controversy exists over what can legitimately be included. When choosing a research question, the wise nurse researcher considers the practical issues of background and financial support.

Research is different from **problem solving.** Problem solving is specific to a given situation and is designed for immediate action, whereas research is **generalizable** (transferable) to other situations and deals with long-term solutions rather than immediate ones. For example, Mrs. Abney is an elderly patient who frequently was found wandering in the halls of the nursing home, unable to find her way back to her room. This was quite distressing to her and time-consuming for the nursing staff who helped her find her way "home." A nurse noticed that Mrs. Abney had no difficulty recognizing her daughter, so she taped a photograph of the daughter to Mrs. Abney's door. Now Mrs. Abney can find her room easily. She is less agitated, and the nursing staff time can be spent on other priorities.

This is an example of problem solving. It is effective in one set of circumstances and has immediate application. But the solution that worked for Mrs. Abney may not work for all confused patients. Indeed, it may not continue to work for Mrs. Abney if her cognitive abilities decline further. Table 12–1 compares problem solving and research.

Research Process

The nursing research process is the same as any other research process; it simply addresses a nursing-related problem. Research starts with a problem or stimulus. The stimulus for a research project may be the feeling that something needs to be addressed, that something is not right. It may be that there are insufficient data for resolving a problem, or the literature is unclear, or the data presented in the literature are conflicting. When there is a need for more information and no adequate information exists, research is in order.

There are two major categories of research: quantitative and qualitative. **Quantitative research** is generally considered objective and uses data-gathering techniques that can be repeated by others and verified. Data collected are quantifiable; that is, they can be counted, measured with standardized instruments, or observed with a high degree of agreement among observers.

Qualitative research is more subjective. Finding may be presented from more than one perspective (multiple realities) and the report may be a rich

---

TABLE 12-1
Comparison of Problem Solving and Research

Characteristic	Research	Problem Solving
Type of problems addressed	Widely experienced	Situation specific
Conceptual basis	Theoretical framework	Often none; trial and error
Knowledge base needed	Extensive review of literature to determine latest thinking and research	Practical knowledge, common sense, and experience
Scope of application	Generalizable to similar situations	Useful in immediate situation; transferability must be determined

narrative (Streubert and Carpenter, 1999). Questions that cannot be answered by quantitative designs must be addressed by qualitative methods. Answering "why" questions requires the use of qualitative approaches. Why do persons with diabetes choose not to follow the diet prescribed for them? Why do chronically mentally ill individuals choose not to take the medications that would reduce psychotic symptoms? Qualitative research is useful in understanding the perceptions, feelings, and motivations of the research subjects.

Whether quantitative or qualitative, all research must be rigorously planned, carefully implemented, and scrupulously analyzed. Therefore, most research follows a formal process known as the **research process.** Students in baccalaureate nursing programs often take a semester-long course in nursing research in which both qualitative and quantitative methods are described, so this chapter will serve as a brief introduction to the research process.

First, the several steps (listed below) in the quantitative research process are presented, then the importance of research for nursing theory and practice and general considerations in doing research are discussed.

1. Identification of a research problem.
2. Review of literature.
3. Formulation of the research question or hypothesis.
4. Design of the study.
5. Implementation.
6. Drawing conclusions based on findings.
7. Discussion of implications.
8. Dissemination of findings.

Identification of a Research Problem

Problems generally come from three sources: clinical situations, the literature, or theories. Clinical situations are rich sources for research problems. Nurses want to prevent elderly clients from wandering off the unit and getting lost. How can they do it? Asking this question can lead to a research problem. Or perhaps a nurse wonders if a time-honored method of providing care is, in fact, the best way. A research problem may result from her curiosity.

Sometimes researchers become interested in a problem because it has been written about in the literature. They may decide to **replicate** (repeat) the study or may design a similar one to test part of the original study in a new way.

The third source of research problems, theory, relates to testing theoretical models. Chapter 11 discussed several models of nursing theory that have been developed. If a theoretical model is designed to predict patients' responses to nursing actions, whether or not it actually does predict patients' responses can be tested through research. The researcher can create certain conditions and determine whether, in fact, the events happen as the theoretical model predicted. Most ideas for nursing research projects come from one of these three sources.

Review of Literature

Once a problem is identified, the professional literature must be reviewed. A review of the literature is comprehensive and covers all relevant research and supporting documents in print. Doing a thorough review of the literature requires a lot of library time or computer search efforts and detective work. Computer-generated searches of the literature can assist tremendously with this step but cannot totally replace the efforts of a dedicated researcher.

The literature review is essential to locate similar or related studies that have already been completed and upon which a new study can build. The review is helpful in creating a **conceptual framework,** or organization of supporting ideas, upon which to base the study. The review of literature answers the question, "What have other researchers and theorists written about this problem?"

Formulation of the Research Question or Hypothesis

Once researchers have identified a research problem, are intimately acquainted with the relevant literature, and have chosen a conceptual framework that helps to focus the topic, they need to formulate the **research question.** The question may be stated in one of three forms: a statement, a question, or a hypothesis. If researchers are going to describe something, they may make a statement, such as, "The purpose of this study is to identify the five most frequently expressed needs of family members in intensive care unit waiting rooms." They could also ask a question, such as, "What are the characteristics of mothers who have difficulty bonding to their newborn babies?" If comparing the relationship of two variables, a question might be asked such as, "What is the relationship of time spent studying and grade point averages?" If conducting an experiment, researchers must have a **hypothesis** (educated guess) as to what the outcome will be so that hypothesis-testing statistics may later be applied. For example, "First-time mothers who attend childbirth classes will demonstrate earlier bonding with their newborn babies than mothers who do not attend the classes" is a testable hypothesis. Whatever the form used, the research question must be expressed succinctly and clearly. It answers the question, "Exactly what am I trying to determine with this study?"

Design of the Study

Once the research question is identified, the study must be designed. There are two broad categories of research **designs: experimental** and **nonexperimental.** If the researcher influences the subjects in any way, the research is experimental. If not, the research is nonexperimental. There are numerous types of research under each of these two categories, but the main difference between experimental and nonexperimental research is whether the researcher manipulates, or influences, the subjects.

True experimental designs provide evidence of a cause-and-effect relationship between actions. For example, testing the hypothesis "Patients who receive preoperative teaching need less pain medication in the first 72 hours postoperatively than those who do not" would provide evidence of a cause-

and-effect relationship between teaching and pain. Sometimes it is impossible to conduct a true experimental study with human beings because to do so might endanger them in some way. In those instances, modified experimental studies are used.

Nonexperimental designs are frequently referred to as *descriptive designs* because the researcher describes what the situation is or was at some point in the past. There are many types of nonexperimental designs: surveys, descriptive comparisons, evaluation studies, exploratory studies, and historical-documentary research.

Whether the researcher chooses an experimental or nonexperimental design influences the data-collection process. The data-collection process includes selection of data collection instruments, design of the data collection protocol, the data analysis plan, subject selection, and informed consent and institutional review plans. It answers the question, "How will we conduct the study?"

Data Collection Instruments. When designing a study, researchers must consider how the data will be collected. Data collection instruments, sometimes called data collection tools, range from simple survey forms to complex radiographic scanning devices. The instrument used must be **reliable,** or accurate. A reliable instrument is one that yields the same values dependably each time the instrument is used to measure the same thing. The tool must also be valid, which, when applied to a research instrument, means that it must measure what it is supposed to be measuring.

If body temperature is being measured, a thermometer is an obvious data collection tool. When measuring an abstract factor, such as anxiety or depression, the best data collection tool is not as clear. The selection of a data collection instrument answers the question, "What tool(s) will we use to collect the data?" To minimize measurement errors, beginning researchers should choose published instruments with established reliability and validity, rather than designing their own.

Data Collection Protocol. Another aspect of designing the study is deciding on the data collection **protocol** (procedure). The quality of the data depends on strict adherence to the plan. If, for example, the plan calls for administering a questionnaire to renal dialysis clients after dialysis, the data collectors must be sure to give the questionnaires to all subjects only after their treatments. The data collection protocol answers the question, "How will we go about gathering our data?"

Data Analysis Plan. It may seem premature to decide how the data will be analyzed before it is even collected, but careful planning for the analysis is important. The research design is developed with data analysis in mind. The analysis must be part of the planning process because the data and the protocols for collecting them depend on how the data will be analyzed. Unless the nurse researcher is an expert in statistics or there is one on the research team, consultation with a statistician well versed in human subject research is recommended in designing the data analysis plan, which answers the question, "What will we do with the data once we gather it?"

Subject Selection. Once the researcher knows what is to be done, the specifics of who is to be included are decided. The individual people or laboratory animals being studied are known as research **subjects.** If the researchers plan to study pain control in postoperative patients, for example, they have to decide the specific type of surgery and the age, sex, ethnicity, and geographic location of the patients as well as a variety of other factors in planning the subject selection (Fig. 12–1). Subject selection answers the questions, "Who qualifies to be a participant in this study?"

In the past, women have not been well represented as research subjects. Today there is recognition that women must be included as study subjects if the research findings are to be applicable to women. This is considered such a high priority that the National Institutes of Health, a major funding source for health-related research, has established a policy regarding inclusion of women as study subjects. The policy is available online at http://www4.od.nih.gov/orwh/inclusion.html. See Box 12–2 for further information about including women in research.

Figure 12–1
Research subjects are selected based on factors such as age, gender, condition, and location. They must then be informed about certain aspects of the proposed research in order to make a decision about participating. That decision, which is written and signed, is known as "informed consent" (Courtesy of Memorial Hospital, Chattanooga, Tennessee).

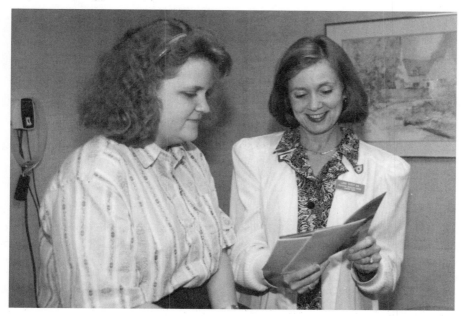

BOX 12-2
Including Women in Research

Nurses have a responsibility to apply appropriate ethical standards as they incorporate research findings into practice. Additionally, qualified nurses conducting research must do so in an ethical manner. While these two statements may seem obvious, the practice is not as obvious or as easy as one might think.

For example, women have traditionally been excluded as subjects from research for seemingly appropriate reasons: a) the drugs being tested in some experiments could be harmful to fetuses if women in the study were or became pregnant during the study; and b) the recognition that women might react differently to some experiments due to hormonal changes was a deterrent in some studies.

There have been more serious problems with the misuse of women as subjects in research. An example was the use of gynecological patients in a pilot study to test antibody reaction to transplanted cancer cells without obtaining written permission from the subjects (although signed permission was obtained from male prison volunteers who were the healthy subjects). Another example was a study to determine the side effects of hormone contraceptives. Most of the women subjects were poor and from an ethnic/minority population who were seeking effective contraceptive measures after having had several pregnancies. More pregnancies resulted in the placebo group. It was determined that the women were not adequately informed about the risk of pregnancy before participating in the study.

Such examples provided the stimulus for the National Institutes of Health to publish guidelines for including women and minorities in research. The guidelines mandate:

- The inclusion of women and members of minorities in all human research.
- The inclusion of women and minorities in clinical trials to the degree that differences in intervention effect can be accomplished in the statistical analysis.
- The exclusion of cost as an acceptable reason to exclude groups.
- The initiation of programs and support for outreach efforts to recruit these groups into clinical studies.

The nurse's increased awareness of these potential dilemmas and subsequent action to prevent biased and discriminatory treatment can result in decreased vulnerability and oppression for women.

From Pinch, W. J. (1994). Women and research. *ANA Center for Ethics and Human Rights Communique*, 3(3), 4–5. Used by permission.

Rarely, all subjects in a particular group are studied. The term **population** refers to all subjects who meet the selection criteria. Usually, researchers have to use a **sample** (subgroup) of the entire population, however, and valid results can be obtained if the sample is properly selected.

Variations in Design: Qualitative Methods of Inquiry. The planning and design of the second type of research process, qualitative research, is more fluid and dynamic than the process of quantitative research. Polit and Hungler (1997) emphasized the need for considerable advanced planning, although the researcher must be flexible. The researcher typically does not seek to control research conditions but tries to observe natural environments. Some of the strategies used to collect information are focus groups, interviews, and field notes (Streubert and Carpenter, 1999).

Phenomenological research is a frequently used qualitative approach. The focus of this method is what people experience in regard to a particular phenomenon and how they interpret those experiences. The main source of data is extensive interviews with the subjects. The researcher poses planned and follow-up questions depending on the subjects' responses, modifying the investigation according to the responses of the subjects. A major difference between quantitative and qualitative methods is that with qualitative methods the subject is generally more aware of the aims of the research. While researchers do not attempt to influence subjects, they are coparticipants in the experience (Polit and Hungler, 1997).

Informed Consent and Institutional Review. Next, researchers who use human subjects must plan to protect the rights of those subjects by asking them to sign an **informed consent** form that describes the details of the study and what participation means. Any risks involved in participating must be explained. No one should be pressured in any way to participate, and the **confidentiality** (privacy) of participants must be assured.

A related step when using human subjects is submitting the proposal to the institution, such as a hospital or clinic, where the research will take place. It must be approved by the **institutional review board.** Usually composed of individuals from different disciplines, these boards exist to ensure that research is well designed and ethical and does not violate the policies and procedures of the institution or the rights of the subjects. Only after the institutional review board approves the proposal can the study begin.

Implementation

Up until this point, only planning has taken place. Careful planning is, however, the key to a successful study. In the implementation phase, the actual study is conducted. The two main tasks during this phase are data collection and data analysis.

Data Collection. **Data** (research-generated information) should be collected only by those who are thoroughly familiar with the study. All research assistants should understand the purpose of the data and the importance of accuracy and careful record keeping. No matter who is collecting the data the integrity of the project is ultimately the responsibility of the primary researcher.

Data Analysis. If all goes well, the data are analyzed exactly as proposed. In analyzing the data, most researchers use the same statistical consultants who assisted in planning the study. The researcher is well advised to work closely with the statistician in interpreting as well as analyzing the data. The nurse researcher is in charge, however, and he or she has the final word on what interpretations are made.

Analyzing the findings of qualitative research presents formidable challenges for several reasons. First the data are voluminous, often consisting of lengthy dialogues between researchers and subjects. Next, dialogues must be transcribed verbatim, yielding hefty stacks of pages. Then comes the task of organizing the transcripts, identifying themes, and organizing the themes into meaningful patterns. Fortunately, there now exist computer programs to assist in this process.

Drawing Conclusions Based on Findings

In writing the research report, the findings directly related to the research question are presented first. Findings are presented factually—without value judgments. The facts must speak for themselves. Simple presentation of the facts is the only requirement. After findings related to the research question are reported, unexpected findings can be reported. Conclusions are then drawn. Conclusions answer the question, "What do these findings mean?" Here researchers can be more subjective and inject some of their own thinking but should stay within the boundaries of the study.

Discussion of Implications

Researchers are always alert to the implications of their studies. Implications are suggestions of things that should be done in the future. Every good study raises more questions that it answers. In nursing studies, there may be indications for modifications in nursing education or nursing practice. Nearly every study has implications for further research, and if the findings turn out as expected, almost all studies should be carefully replicated. Replication can answer these and other questions: "What needs to be known to develop more confidence in the findings? Will the research instrument produce similar results in a similar population in a different geographic location? Will the procedure be effective with patients having a slightly different diagnosis, condition, or type of surgery? Will age make a difference? Will cultural beliefs make a difference? What else do we need to know to improve the care of patients?"

Dissemination of Findings

A research study is not useful unless the results are communicated to others who may use them. Most funding agencies want to know in advance how the researcher plans to **disseminate** the findings. The two major vehicles for dissemination of knowledge are articles published in professional journals and presentations at conferences. Examples of nursing research journals include *Clinical Nursing Research, Journal of Nursing Scholarship, Nursing Research, Research in Nursing and Health Care,* and the *Western Journal of Nursing Research.* Because there are relatively few research journals in nursing, the competition for publishing might seem fierce, but editors say they have great difficulty getting well-written manuscripts on topics of interest to readers. A review process, called **peer review,** is the method most journals use to determine whether or not to publish a research report. During peer review, a manuscript is circulated to a review panel consisting of one or more experts in the area of study. They evaluate its appropriateness and accuracy and recommend that it be published, resubmitted with changes, or rejected. Most research that is carefully conceived, conducted, and presented can get published, although the researcher must be persistent and resilient in taking criticism and reworking manuscripts.

A somewhat easier, yet still discriminating, route to dissemination is presentation at one or more of the numerous nursing research conferences. Many research conferences also use the peer review process. In general, however, the proportion of abstracts (summaries of research) chosen for presentation at conferences is higher than the proportion of manuscripts chosen for publication.

Whether research is published or presented, it is important to disseminate research results to other nurses who may choose to use them either to improve patient care practices or to replicate the study (Fig. 12–2).

Figure 12–2

Dissemination of findings is an essential aspect of the research process. Here nurse researcher Maureen Killeen presents her findings at a psychiatric nursing conference (Courtesy of Maureen Killeen).

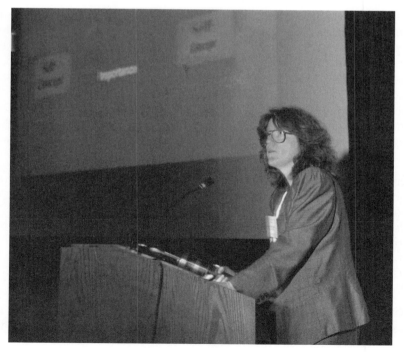

Interviews with Nurse Researchers

The field of nursing research is growing, with many nurses actively involved in it. In this section, two nurse researchers talk about their work (Interviews 12–1, 12–2).

These interviews demonstrate how two nurse researchers feel about the work they do. Nationwide there are hundreds of nurses who, like Killeen and McNeely, are excited about nursing research and the contributions it makes to improving nursing through evidence-based practice.

Relationship of Nursing Research to Nursing Theory and Practice

Relationships among nursing research, practice, and theory are circular. As mentioned earlier, research ideas are generated from three sources: (1) clinical practice, (2) literature, and (3) theory.

Questions about how best to deal with patient problems regularly arise in clinical situations. As shown in the example of Mrs. Abney, the elderly lady who could not find her room, problems often can be "solved" for the present. When the same questions recur, long-term answers may be needed. Research develops solutions that can be used with confidence in different situations.

Published articles about nursing research often generate interest in further studies. If there is published research on a particular nursing care problem, other researchers may be stimulated to investigate the subject further and refine the solutions. This is how nursing knowledge builds.

Nursing theorists also generate research ideas. They piece together postulates or premises that "explain" what has been discovered. The explanation is "tested" to determine whether it is robust or strong enough to be useful. If so, there may be more implications for applications in clinical practice.

Nursing research journals are full of clinical studies that have made a difference in patient care. A few examples of changes in nursing practice stimulated by research include the following:

1. Improved care of patients with skin breakdown from pressure ulcers.
2. Decreasing light and noise in critical care units to prevent sleep deprivation.
3. Using caps on newborns to decrease heat loss and stabilize body temperature.
4. Positioning patients following chest surgery to facilitate respiration.
5. Scheduling pain medication more frequently following surgery.
6. Preoperative teaching to facilitate postoperative recovery.

Nursing research findings not only improve patient care but also affect the health care system itself. For example, research studies have demon-

Research on Self-Esteem in Children

This interview is with Maureen Killeen, an associate professor of nursing at the Medical College of Georgia.

Interviewer: Maureen, your research is with children and self-esteem; exactly what do you do?

Researcher: I go into people's homes and ask children about themselves, and I ask the parents about the children. I ask the children, "What kinds of things are you good at?" And I ask them how important certain words are to them.

Interviewer: What are some examples of the important words?

Researcher: Pretty, smart, honest, messy, lazy, active, careful, happy—things like that. In another study, I am interested in the relationship between obesity and self-esteem. I go into a fifth-grade classroom and give everyone a self-concept scale and measure height and weight. I ask if they are heavier or thinner than others their age.

Interviewer: How do you happen to be doing this kind of work?

Researcher: I read about research on self-esteem in a "Social Psychology and the Self" course I took in graduate school. I read a lot of studies, and every study indicated that if you think of yourself in a certain way, this leads to certain behaviors. But there was nothing about how people come to think of themselves in certain ways. What are the characteristics or traits that get people thinking that way? I wanted to know the answer to that question.

Interviewer: What impact do you hope your research will have on the care of children?

Researcher: If we can figure out how other people affect children's ideas about themselves, how talk about children and talk to children affects them, then we can teach parents how to talk more effectively with their children. We can increase the relevance of treatment and therapy. We will know how to change how people feel about themselves. That is the treatment implication of this research.

Interviewer: What has been most helpful to you in the process of becoming a nurse researcher?

Researcher: Mentoring by more experienced researchers. I have benefited from the kindness of senior researchers who shared ideas. Experience is the best teacher, and I have been fortunate to have had good mentoring. Also, getting a funded grant to pay the bills while I do research has helped a lot!

Interviewer: With regard to your professional life, what is the most enjoyable for you?

Researcher: Some aspects of research are enjoyable, but teaching is close behind. If I can use my research in teaching—that's a *lot* of fun!

Interviewer: What do you least enjoy in your work as a researcher?

Researcher: Writing. Writing is hard because there are constant revisions.

Sometimes it seems it will never be finished.

Interviewer: What are some of your recent research activities?

Researcher: Recently I have been collecting preliminary data for a study of perinatal depression. As a result of my work on self-esteem, I became interested in examining maternal perceptions of their children.

I am conducting the study at a nurse-midwifery clinic. We collect data during pregnancy and at six to ten weeks postpartum. Through questionnaires, interviews, histories, and videotaping, we are trying to answer the question of whether depression in mothers and their ability to recognize infant facial expressions influences their interactions with their babies. There is some evidence that depressed women have difficulty identifying facial emotional expressions and in parenting.

If difficulty in recognizing facial expressions is linked to depressed mothers' parenting difficulties, then we may be able to develop interventions targeted at helping mothers recognize infants' nonverbal cues and respond appropriately to them.

Interviewer: What would you like to say to nursing students about research?

Researcher: Research can be a lot of fun. Find a mentor who believes it's fun and who asks interesting research questions. Nursing research is a very exciting field!

Research on Decreasing Falls in the Elderly

The second nurse researcher interviewed was Elizabeth McNeely, who did the tai chi research with older people mentioned earlier. McNeely was an assistant professor in Emory University's Nell Hodgson Woodruff School of Nursing and is currently a gerontological nurse practitioner in private practice. Her research collaborators were in the Emory School of Medicine and the Atlanta Veterans Administration Medical Center.

Interviewer: How did you happen to become a nurse researcher?

Researcher: Accidentally. It was the last thing I envisioned. I happened to have a specialization in a field [gerontology] where research was growing. I became recognized as an expert in that field. One day my supervisor told me to go to a meeting where my expertise was needed. The meeting turned out to be a planning meeting for the multidisciplinary research I do now.

Interviewer: How do you believe your research has contributed to better patient care?

Researcher: There are so many things health care professionals do because they "know" they work. But this knowledge doesn't get communicated beyond the walls of the institution. With hard data that comes from research, the information can be published so others can know how to do it. This improves patient care.

Interviewer: What are some examples?

Researcher: This tai chi grant. They have been doing tai chi in China for hundreds of years. But thousands of testimonials to the benefits won't lead to its being recommended by medical professionals in this country. We have to study the effects systematically before it will be supported by the medical profession.

Interviewer: How do you like your work as a nurse researcher?

Researcher: It's intriguing. Everyone needs to realize the importance of getting hard data to support practice.

Interviewer: What do you like best about your work?

Researcher: The air of excitement and discovery that comes when we see that some of our ideas are working. Also, my association with other researchers and the opportunities for thinking.

Interviewer: What do you like the least?

Researcher: There is a lot of tedium. It's hard to realize how long it takes to get from idea to publication. You have to be "long-term" oriented.

Interviewer: What would you like to say to nursing students?

Researcher: I would tell them that nurses have a unique contribution to make to the multidisciplinary research team. The problems are complex and require complex approaches, including the nursing perspective. As a clinician in a multidisciplinary practice, I have seen the concept of interdisciplinary clinical practice become more and more acceptable, especially in the present managed care environment. As a result, the number of interdisciplinary research studies conducted and published has increased. The combination of the knowledge and skills from several disciplines has enhanced health care toward a more holistic approach. The health care consumer has benefitted from this trend.

strated the cost-effectiveness of nurses as health care providers. This is discussed further in Chapter 16.

Another contribution of nursing research to practice is in the area of power. A person who possesses knowledge that is useful to others has power. Nurses gain much knowledge through clinical practice. Yet practical knowledge, as important as it is, lacks the power of research-validated knowledge. Research can be used to demonstrate, for example, that one nursing action is more effective than another. When knowledge from practice is validated through research, that knowledge is more powerful. Thus, it could be said that research empowers practice.

BOX 12-3
Relating Nursing Research to Practice and Theory

Behavior theory suggests that behavior can be modified with reinforcement (reward or punishment). Incontinence is behavior characterized by involuntary urination before the patient can get to the bathroom or get positioned on a bedpan or with a urinal. Some researchers wondered, "Can incontinence be modified with positive reinforcements such as a special treat or additional time in the television room?" Specifically, they believed that patients could be "taught" to control urination if effective reinforcers were applied. Several subsequent studies suggest that patients can learn to control incontinence in specific situations. In this case, a theory—behavior theory—was useful in planning research, the results of which enable nurses to improve the clinical nursing care of incontinent patients.

A final point about the influence of research on practice has to do with professionalism. In Chapter 6, the characteristics of professions were given. One of the criteria commonly mentioned is a scientific body of knowledge that is expanded through research. Nursing research enhances the status of nursing as a profession by expanding nursings' scientific knowledge base. A brief example that may clarify the interplay between nursing research, practice, and theory is found in Box 12-3.

Collaboration in Nursing Research

The history of nursing research spans almost 40 years. Beginning in the 1960s with awareness of the need for a nursing body of knowledge based on research, nursing research today has matured to the level of collaboration with other disciplines to generate knowledge that would be limited if done only by members of one discipline. The Open Letter to Nursing Students from nurse researcher Larry Scahill (Box 12–4) illustrates the effectiveness and excitement of collaborative research relationships.

Another example of collaborative research relationships is found in the research partnerships of Judith Noble Halle (Goldsmith, 1995). Halle, a doctoral student at the University of California at Los Angeles School of Nursing, worked with women who were experiencing difficult pregnancies. Halle's concern was for the health of the infant, and she did physiological research to develop methods for preventing brain damage due to a lack of oxygen at birth. Her research was based on a major finding of a physician with whom she collaborated. Other major collaborators included another nurse, Christine Kasper, who administered a nursing cell physiology laboratory, and the director of a pediatric neurosurgery research laboratory.

According to Kasper, "Many of the unique questions that nurses ask when they begin to address new areas of research are supported by existing fields of

BOX 12-4
Open Letter to Nursing Students Regarding Research in Child Psychiatry

Child psychiatry is in the midst of tremendous change. Recent findings from several related fields, including neuroanatomy, developmental neuroscience, pharmacology, genetics, molecular biology, and epidemiology have propelled this change. Because no one discipline can embrace all of these fields, research in child psychiatry is increasingly multidisciplinary. Although nursing education does not prepare students for careers in basic biological research, nurses can and do collaborate in clinical research. What is clinical research in child psychiatry and what part do nurses play in clinical research?

Clinical research refers to research endeavors that are closely connected to the care of patients. In child psychiatry, this might include a medication trial in children with autism, an evaluation of a cognitive-behavioral intervention program in attention-deficit hyperactivity disorder, a neuroimaging study of brain function in Tourette's syndrome, or a family genetic study in obsessive-compulsive disorder. Each of these research studies requires comprehensive assessment of subjects, careful management of the data collected, and analysis of results.

As with other fields of research, clinical research usually involves a question about the relationship between two things. The research question may emerge from theory or from clinical practice. For example, the question of whether the vulnerability for obsessive-compulsive disorder is inherited emerged because clinicians noticed that it recurred in families at a higher than expected rate compared to the general population. To investigate the relationship between childhood obsessive-compulsive disorder and family history, researchers interview family members to ascertain the frequency of obsessive-compulsive disorder in the family and the pattern of inheritance. By contrast, the neuroimaging study of Tourette syndrome evolved from a theory that dysregulation of specific brain circuits underlies this disorder.

Another area of increasing importance in child psychiatry is psychopharmacology. The proliferation of pharmacologic agents for the treatment of psychiatric disorders of childhood offers hope for children afflicted with mental illness. Despite the promise of this growing list of medications, however, the scientific support for their use is limited. Indeed, only a few of the drugs commonly used in child psychiatry have demonstrated efficacy in rigorous studies. The method for showing that a medication is effective for a given problem is the randomized controlled trial. For some, studies of this sort are questionable because a child may receive a placebo rather than the active treatment. On the other hand, in the absence of clear evidence that a given medication is effective in children, there may be ethical concerns about exposing children to an untested psychotropic medication. Thus, the value of placebo-controlled trials is that they provide information about the efficacy and safety of a medication from which the risks and benefits can be evaluated.

Research involves the systematic investigation of the relationship between two or more phenomena. Research in child psychiatry is expanding and embraces a wide range of disciplines from basic scientists to clinicians. Especially relevant for nurses is clinical research, such as placebo-controlled medication trials. These studies require careful assessment, close monitoring during the trial, and accurate assessment of outcome. The future of child psychiatry will increasingly rely on neuroscience, psychopharmacology, and clinical measurement. Nurses interested in these fields can consider a career in clinical research in child psychiatry.

Larry Scahill, M.S.N., M.P.H.
Yale University

science, such as cell physiology, or the behavioral sciences. Rather than reinventing the wheel, collaborating with scientists outside of nursing contributes to nursing science, and nursing contributes to others" (Goldsmith, 1995, p. 7). As the experiences of these nurses illustrate, interdisciplinary collaboration can be a rewarding aspect of nursing research.

Support for Nursing Research

Nursing research is expensive, and support takes many forms. It can include encouragement, consultation, computer and library resources, money, and release time from researchers' regular work responsibilities. Each of these forms of support is important, but none alone is adequate. Early in the development of nursing research, encouragement was often the only support available, and not all nurse researchers had that. Gradually over the years, funding sources have developed, but financial support is still difficult to obtain, particularly for new researchers.

The National Institute of Nursing Research was created in 1992 from what had been the National Center for Nursing Research (NCNR), part of the National Institutes of Health. The purpose of the NINR is to provide structure for selecting scientific opportunities and initiatives and to promote depth in developing the knowledge base for nursing practice. In the years of NCNR/NINR's existence, its budget has quadrupled, but it still is able to fund only a small portion of the proposals it receives. To establish priorities for funding, the National Nursing Research Agenda (NNRA) was launched in 1987. The research priorities in the first phase of the NNRA were selected in 1988 and included the following:

- Low birth weight: mothers and infants.
- Human immunodeficiency virus (HIV) infection: prevention and care.
- Long-term care for older adults.
- Symptom management: pain.
- Nursing informatics: enhancing patient care.
- Health promotion for older children and adolescents.

The NNRA, phase 2, began in 1995 with the following priorities for the five-year period:

- Community-based nursing models (1995).
- Effectiveness of nursing interventions in HIV infection/acquired immunodeficiency syndrome (1996).
- Cognitive impairment (1997).
- Living with chronic illness (1998).
- Biobehavioral factors related to immunocompetence (1999).

These new priority areas were refined by a multidisciplinary priority expert panel (Friends of the National Institute of Nursing Research, 1995).

A May 10, 1999, draft of the NINR document Strategic Planning for the 21st Century included the following objectives:

- End of life/palliative care research.
- Chronic illness experience.
- Quality of life issues and quality of care issues.
- Health promotion and disease prevention research.
- Symptom management research.
- Telehealth interventions and monitoring.
- Implications of genetic advances.
- Cultural and ethnic disparities in health and illness.

Input was sought from a wide audience to help shape the NINR research agenda for the new millennium.

Several other federal agencies accept proposals that meet their funding guidelines when submitted by qualified nurse researchers. These include the National Institute on Aging, the National Cancer Institute, the National Institute of Mental Health, the National Institute of Alcohol Abuse and Addiction, the National Institute on Drug Addiction, and the Centers for Disease Control and Prevention. Competition with researchers from other disciplines is keen, however, and generally only experienced nurse researchers are successful in obtaining funding from these sources.

Nursing associations also fund nursing research. The American Nurses Foundation, Sigma Theta Tau, and many clinical specialty organizations provide research awards, even for novice researchers. State and local nursing associations sometimes have seed money for pilot projects. Universities, schools of nursing, and large hospitals also may provide small amounts of research funds. Generally, however, finding adequate funding for large-scale studies continues to be a problem faced by researchers.

Roles of Nurses in Research

The *Code for Nurses* states: "The nurse participates in activities that contribute to the ongoing development of the profession's body of knowledge" (American Nurses Association, 1985). Ideally, every nurse should be involved in research, but practically, all nurses should, as a minimum, use research results to improve their practices. Evidence-based nursing practice requires staying informed about current literature, especially studies done in one's own specific area of clinical practice.

As seen in Table 12–2, in addition to using research to improve practice, all professional nurses can contribute to one or more aspects of the research process. Baccalaureate nurses can read, interpret, and evaluate research for applicability to nursing practice. Through clinical practice, they can identify nursing problems that need to be investigated. They can participate in the implementation of scientific studies by helping principal researchers collect data in clinical settings or elsewhere. These beginning researchers must know enough about the purpose of the research to follow the research protocols explicitly or know when it is necessary to deviate from the protocol for a patient's well-being. Baccalaureate nurses also can help disseminate research-based knowledge by sharing useful research findings with colleagues.

The master's-prepared nurse may be ready to replicate studies that have been previously conducted. Researchers cannot be sure that their findings are true until studies are repeated with similar results. Nurse researchers have learned that it is not necessary (or even desirable) always to generate a totally new and disconnected idea to do research. As mentioned earlier, to be most useful, research must be based on a conceptual framework and related to previous research.

Depending on education, clinical and research experiences, and interests, some nurses at the master's level are better prepared to conduct research than others. In addition to education and experience, a crucial factor is the support system the nurse has available. To do research, nurses need time, money, consultation, and subjects. With rich resources in a research environment, master's-prepared nurses can and do make vital research contributions.

Usually, to be a nationally recognized researcher and obtain federal funding for a research program, nurses need doctoral and even postdoctoral prepa-

---

TABLE 12–2
Levels of Educational Preparation and Levels of Participation in Nursing Research

Level of Preparation	Level of Research Participation
Student nurse	Consumer
BSN nurse	Problem identifier
	Data collector
MSN nurse	Replicator
	Concept tester
Doctoral nurse	Theory generator
Postdoctoral nurse	Funded program director

BSN, bachelor of science in nursing; MSN, master of science in nursing.

ration. Researchers across the United States in all professions compete for a limited pool of research dollars available each year. Only those nurses with strong academic and experiential backgrounds and the best proposals succeed in obtaining federal funding.

Nurses who aspire to careers as competitive nurse researchers should plan a specific program of research. This means limiting one's research to a defined set of phenomena. For example, May Wykle (Wykle, 1995; Wykle, 1986; Dunkle and Wykle, 1988; Fitzpatrick, Wykle, and Morris, 1990), who is at Case Western Reserve, has a research program producing stimulating studies about persons who care for their elderly dependent relatives. Sandra Dunbar of Emory University is focusing her research program on ways to help patients who are experiencing heart failure to participate in the management of their care (Dunbar, Jacobson, and Deaton, 1998). These researchers realize that only by becoming specialists in a particular area of research can they receive the kind of funding they need to support their research and the national recognition it takes to get the results of their studies published so that they can have the desired impact—better nursing care for patients through evidence-based practice.

Summary of Key Points

- The scientific method is the name given to a systematic, orderly process of solving problems. It has been used for centuries and is applicable in many different situations.
- Knowledge can be categorized as either pure knowledge, that is, knowledge that is not immediately useful, or applied knowledge, that is, knowledge that can be used in a practical way.
- Much of the scientific knowledge we take for granted today was discovered through use of the scientific method.
- The scientific method has been particularly useful in the fields of medicine and health care, and human existence has been profoundly affected by discoveries made through its use.
- The scientific method uses two types of logic: inductive and deductive reasoning.
- Both inductive and deductive reasoning are necessary to combine the theoretical and the practical aspects of the scientific method.
- For safety and ethical reasons, there are limitations on the use of the scientific method with human beings.
- Nursing research is defined as the systematic investigation of phenomena related to improving nursing care.
- The major steps in the research process are identification of a research problem, review of the literature, formulation of the research question, design of the study, implementation, drawing conclusions based on findings, discussion of implications, and dissemination of findings.
- Nurse researchers have made significant contributions to improvements in nursing care practices.

- Nursing research is related to and informed by nursing theory and nursing practice and in turn influences them.
- There is a research role for nurses of all educational backgrounds.
- Evidence-based nursing practice is the goal of nursing research.

Critical Thinking Questions

1. Why is nursing called an applied science? Explain why you agree or disagree with this description.
2. Name and describe the two types of reasoning used in the scientific method. Explain why neither alone is adequate to advance knowledge.
3. List and discuss each step of the scientific process.
4. Explain why a purely experimental model is an inadequate one for nursing.
5. Go to the college library and see which nursing research journals are in the collection. Thumb through some recent issues and notice the types of studies reported. Compare them to studies done 20 years ago. What similarities and differences do you note?
6. Read a research article that interests you. See if you can identify each of the steps in the research process. If not, what is missing? Discuss with your teacher and class what the significance of the missing steps might be.
7. Find out what research is being done in your school or hospital. If possible, talk with those involved, including data collectors, data analysts, research directors, subjects, families of subjects, and nurses who work on units where research is being conducted. What do they know about the research? What are their concerns? What do they hope will be learned from the research?
8. Obtain job descriptions for nurses at varying experience levels at different agencies. Are research functions included in the job descriptions? If not, what research functions do you think might be appropriate to include?
9. Of the following studies, identify which are nursing research and which are not, giving your rationale for each:
   a. The investigation of optimum staffing patterns in a long-term care facility.
   b. A study of effective methods of clinical supervision of nursing students.
   c. A comparison of two behavioral techniques for managing incontinence in spinal cord–injured patients.

Web Resources

Medline, http://www.nlm.nih.gov/medlineplus/medline.html

National Institute of Health's Policy on Inclusion of Women in Research, http://www4.od.nih.gov/orwh/inclusion.html

National Institute of Nursing Research (NINR), http://www.nih.gov/ninr

Decade of Behavior Initiatives, http://www.nih.gov/ninr/decade_behavior.htm

Mission, http://www.nih.gov/ninr/NINRMission.htm

Strategic Plan, http://www.nih.gov/ninr/strategicplan.htm

References

American Nurses Association (1985). Code for nurses with interpretive statements. Kansas City, MO: American Nurses Association.

Becker, P. T., Grunwald, P. C., Moorman, J., and Stuhr, S. (1993). Effects of developmental care on behavioral organization in very-low-birth-weight infants. *Nursing Research,* 42(4), 214–220.

Dunbar, S. B., Jacobson, L. E., and Deaton, C. (1998). Heart failure: Strategies to enhance patient self-management. *AACN Clinical Issues 1998,* 9(2), 244–256.

Dunkle, R. E., and Wykle, M. L. (1998). *Decision making in long-term care: Factors in planning.* New York: Springer.

Fitzpatrick, J. J., Wykle, M. L., and Morris, D. L. (1990). Collaboration in care and research. *Archives of Psychiatric Nursing,* 4(1), 53–61.

Flexner, S. B., Stein, J., and Su, P. Y. (Eds.) (1980). *The Random House dictionary.* New York: Random House.

Friends of the National Institute of Nursing Research. (1995). *Nursing research: Advancing science for health.* Washington, D. C.: Friends of the National Institute of Nursing Research.

Gibson, E., Medoff-Cooper, B., Nuama, I. F., Gerdes, J., Kirkby, S., and Greenspan, J. (1998). Accelerated discharge of low birth weight infants from neonatal intensive care: A randomized, controlled trial. The Early Discharge Study Group. *Journal of Perinatology,* 18(6), 17–23.

Goldsmith, J. (1995). Newborn research depends on partnerships. *Sigma Theta Tau International Reflections,* 21(3), 6–8.

Hockenberry, M. H. (1989). Guided imagery as a coping measure for children with cancer. *Journal of the Association of Pediatric Oncology Nurses.* 6(2), 29.

Kuhn, T. S. (1970). The structure of scientific revolutions. In O. Nurath (Ed.). *International encyclopedia of unified science* (2nd ed., vol. 2). Chicago: University of Chicago Press.

Kutner, N. G., Barhart, H., Wolf, S. I., McNeely, E., and Xu, T. (1997). Self-report benefits of Tai Chi practice by older adults. *Journal of Gerontological Behavioral Psychological Science and Social Science,* 52(5), 242–246.

Medoff-Cooper, B., and Ray, W. (1995). Neonatal sucking behaviors. *Image: Journal of Nursing Scholarship,* 27(3), 195–200.

Pinch, S. J. (1994). Women in research. *ANA Center for Ethics and Human Rights Communique,* 3(3), 4–5.

Polit, D. F., and Hungler, B. P. (1997). *Essentials of nursing research: Methods, appraisals, and utilization* (4th ed.). Philadelphia: J. B. Lippincott.

Streubert, H. J., and Carpenter, D. R. (1999). *Qualitative research in nursing: Advancing the humanistic imperative* (2nd ed.). Philadelphia: J. B. Lippincott.

Stevens, B., Johnson, C., Franch, L., Petryshen P., Jack, A., and Foster, G. (1999). The efficacy of developmentally sensitive interventions and sucrose for relieving procedural pain in very low birth weight neonates. *Nursing Research,* 48(1), 35–41.

Ware, C. F., Panikkar, K. M., and Romein, J. M. (1966). *The twentieth century: History of mankind, cultural and scientific development* (vol. 6). New York: Harper & Row.

Wolf, S. L., Barnhart, H. X., Kutner, N. G., McNeely, E., Coogler, C., and Xu, T. (1996). Reducing frailty and falls in older persons: An investigation of Tai Chi and computerized balance training. *Journal of the American Geriatric Society*, 44(5), 489–497.

Wykle, M. L. (1995). Geriatric mental health interventions in the home. *Journal of Gerontological Nursing,* 21(3), 47–48.

Wykle, M. L. (1986). Mental health nursing: Research in nursing homes. In M. S. Harper and B. Lebowitz (Eds.). *Mental illness in nursing homes: A research agenda* (pp. 221–234). Rockville, Md.: U.S. Department of Health and Human Services.

The Health Care Delivery System

Karen J. Wisdom[*]

13

Key Terms

Capitation
Chief Executive Officer
Chief Nurse Executive
Chief of Staff
Continuous Quality Improvement
(CQI)
Cross-Functional Team
Decentralization
Dietitian
For-Profit Agency
Gatekeeper
Governmental (Public) Agency
Health Maintenance Organization
(HMO)
Health Promotion
Home Health Agency
Illness Prevention
Institutional Structure
Interdisciplinary Team
Long-Term Care
Managed Care
Managed Care Organization
Multi-Skilled Worker
Not-for-Profit Agency
Organizational Structure
Paramedical

Patient-Focused Care
Physician Hospital Organization
(PHO)
Point-of-Service Organization (POS)
Preferred Provider Organization
(PPO)
Primary Care
Reengineering

Rehabilitation Services
Secondary Care
Social Services
Subacute Care
Tertiary Care
Therapists
Voluntary (Private) Agency

Learning Outcomes

After studying this chapter, students will be able to:

- Describe the four basic types of services provided by the health care delivery system.
- Identify the three main classifications of health care agencies.
- Explain the traditional internal structures of health care agencies.
- Identify the key members of the interdisciplinary health care team and explain what each contributes.
- Describe how managed care has changed the health care delivery system.
- Explain the impact of changes in consumers' expectations on the health care delivery system.
- Describe how health care organizations have changed through re-engineering.
- Relate two major mechanisms used to maintain quality in health care agencies.

The health care delivery system in the United States has traditionally provided care for illness. Its complexity, with multiple types of financing and many different places where patients can receive services, has resulted in a fragmented system that is difficult to understand and navigate. Although this country has the best technology and the most sophisticated procedures in the world, many people do not have access to even the most basic care. Dur-

[*] The author wishes to acknowledge the contributions of Jennifer Jenkins in the preparation of this chapter.

ing the last decade, the system, for financial and health reasons, has undergone major reform.

This chapter describes the present health care delivery system and makes some predictions about its future. Most planners believe that one of the essential parts of an improved health care system will be an emphasis on prevention, early detection of disease, and wellness. Active participation of patients in their own health choices will be encouraged as health care services increasingly emphasize the importance of holism and treatment of the whole person, not just the diseased part.

The delivery system of the future will be more efficient than the current one. Life-threatening illnesses and injuries will continue to be treated in centers where technology and intensive care services are available. Primary care, or basic health services, however, will be provided in a variety of settings such as workplaces, schools, homes, and community-based facilities like neighborhood clinics. Health care workers will be educated to provide holistic, efficient, and cost-effective care.

A system that answers the following questions will ensure that these objectives are met:

1. What services does the patient need and want?
2. Who can best provide these services (patient, health care worker, family, others)?
3. Where is the most effective and efficient place to provide these services?
4. How will these services affect the quality of care, the cost, and both patient and health care worker satisfaction?

The U. S. government has not yet devised a definitive national health policy. An important first step, however, has been taken. As discussed in Chapter 10, a consortium of nearly 300 national health organizations, the U. S. Public Health Service, and state health departments met in 1990 to establish goals and objectives for improving the health of U. S. citizens by the year 2000. The resulting report, *Healthy People 2000: National Health Promotion and Disease Prevention Objectives,* set out three broad goals:

1. Increase the span of healthy life for Americans.
2. Reduce health disparities among Americans.
3. Achieve access to preventive services for all Americans (U. S. Department of Health and Human Services, 1990).

Many specific objectives and priorities were accomplished toward these goals, but health practices and technology changed dramatically during the 1990s. Policymakers agreed that these changes necessitated updating the *Healthy People 2000* objectives to reflect the impact of managed care on the system and of the changing demographics of the United States, which created an older and more culturally diverse population. The new plan, *Healthy People 2010: Healthy People in Healthy Communities,* emphasized community involvement and focused on the responsibility of consumers, individuals, and families. (U. S. Department of Health and Human Services, 1999). With this brief look at the future, let us now take a look at today's health care delivery system and build a framework for understanding tomorrow's system.

Major Categories of Health Care Services

Regardless of the setting in which services are provided—clinics, hospitals, homes, primary care provider's offices—there are basically only four major categories of health services: health promotion, illness prevention, diagnosis and treatment, and rehabilitation and long-term care. Each is briefly explained below.

Health Promotion

Health promotion services assist patients to remain healthy, prevent diseases and injuries, detect diseases early, and promote healthier lifestyles. These services require patients' active participation and cannot be performed solely by a health care provider. Health promotion services are based on the assumption that patients who participate in lifestyle changes are likely to avoid heart attacks, lung cancers, certain infections, and other lifestyle-related diseases.

An example of health promotion services is prenatal classes. By learning good nutritional habits, an expectant mother can take care of both herself and her baby during pregnancy and after delivery. This increases the chances of a normal pregnancy and the birth of a healthy baby. Other examples include aerobic exercise and smoking cessation classes aimed at increasing the health of an individual's cardiovascular and respiratory systems.

Health promotion also includes the detection of warning signs indicating the presence of a disease in early stages. Early detection often allows the treatment to be minimal and less costly and results in a good outcome.

Illness Prevention

With the identification of risk factors such as a family history of heart disease, **illness prevention** services assist patients in reducing the impact of those risk factors on their health and well-being. These services also require the patient's active participation.

Prevention services differ from health promotion services in that they address health problems after risk factors are identified, whereas health promotion services seek to prevent development of risk factors. For example, a health promotion program might teach the detrimental effects of alcohol and drugs on a person's health to prevent the person from using alcohol and drugs. Illness prevention services are used when the patient has been using alcohol or drugs and is at risk for developing health problems as a result. The boundary between health promotion, early detection, and illness prevention is often blurred. Box 13-1 gives examples of activities in these three areas.

BOX 13-1
Illness Prevention, Early Detection and Health Promotion Activities

Illness Prevention

- Community health programs.
- Promotion of healthy lifestyles to counteract risk factors.
- Occupational safety programs (use of eye guards for work that endangers the eyes).
- Environmental safety programs (proper disposal of hazardous waste).
- Legislation that prevents injury or disease (seat-restraint laws).

Early Detection

- Mammograms.
- Cholesterol screening.
- Periodic histories and physical examinations.
- Blood glucose screening.

Health Promotion/Maintenance

- Health education programs (prenatal classes).
- Exercise programs.
- Health fairs.
- Wellness programs (worksite/school).
- Proper nutrition.

Diagnosis and Treatment

Traditionally, in the U. S. health care system there has been heavy emphasis on diagnosis and treatment. Modern technology has enabled the medical profession to refine methods of diagnosing illnesses and disorders and to treat them more effectively than in the past. Newer scientific advances permit many tests and treatments to be performed noninvasively, that is, without cutting into the body. Examples include the use of ultrasonography to examine unborn fetuses to determine if they are developing normally and lithotripsy, which disintegrates kidney stones so they can be expelled in the urine. The future promises more "high-tech" noninvasive technologies.

Laparoscopic instruments have transformed surgery techniques, allowing incisions of one inch or less. This technology has reduced pain postoperatively, reduced hospital stays from days to hours, and enabled individuals to return to normal function much more rapidly.

Unfortunately, high-tech services can lead patients to feel dehumanized. This occurs when the caregivers focus on machines rather than on patients. Nurses must remember that patients benefit most when they understand their diagnoses and treatments and when they can be active participants in the development and implementation of their own treatment plans. You may recall that partnering with patients is a recurring theme in the nursing philosophies, models, and theories discussed in Chapter 11.

Rehabilitation and Long-Term Care

Rehabilitation services help restore the patient to the fullest possible level of function and independence following injury or illness. Rehabilitation programs deal with conditions that leave patients with less than full functioning, such as strokes, broken bones, or severe burns. Both patients and their families must be active participants in this care if it is to be successful. Rehabilitation services should begin as soon as the patient's condition has stabilized after an injury or stroke. These services may be provided in institutional settings such as hospitals, in special rehabilitation facilities, in long-term care facilities such as nursing homes, or in the home and the community. The objectives are to assist patients to achieve their full potential and to return them to a level of functioning that permits them to be contributing members of society.

Long-term care is provided in residential facilities such as assisted-living homes, skilled and intermediate nursing homes, and personal care homes. Each facility is tailored to provide services that the patient or family cannot provide but at a level that maintains the individual's independence as long as possible. With the aging of the population, and with more patients surviving severe trauma and disease with impairments in physical or mental functioning or both, these long-term care facilities are expected to experience rapid growth.

Classifications of Health Care Agencies

There are many agencies involved in the total health care delivery system. Organizations that deliver care can be classified in three major ways; as governmental or voluntary agencies; as not-for-profit or for-profit agencies; or by the level of health care services they provide.

Governmental (Public) Agencies

There are many **governmental (public) agencies** that contribute to the health and well-being of U. S. citizens. All are primarily supported by taxes, administered by elected or appointed officials, and tailored to the needs of the communities served.

Federal Agencies
Federal agencies focus on the health of all U. S. citizens. They promote and conduct health and illness research, provide funding to train health care workers, and assist communities in planning health care services. They also de-

velop health programs and services and provide financial and personnel support to staff them. They establish standards of practice and safety for health care workers and conduct national health education programs on subjects such as the benefits of nonsmoking, prevention of acquired immunodeficiency syndrome (AIDS), or the need for prenatal care. Examples of federal agencies are the U. S. Public Health Service (PHS), the National Institutes of Health (NIH), the U. S. Department of Health and Human Services (DHHS), the Occupational Safety and Health Administration (OSHA), and the Centers for Disease Control and Prevention (CDCP).

As a result of the changing health care delivery system, complementary and alternative medicine are now recognized by the federal government. In 1998 under provisions of the Omnibus Appropriations Bill, the NIH established the National Center for Complementary and Alternative Medicine. The center serves as a public information clearinghouse and a research center (National Institutes of Health, 1999).

State Agencies

State health agencies oversee programs that affect the health of citizens across the state. Examples of state governmental health agencies include state departments of health and environment, departments that regulate and license health professionals such as state boards of nursing, and those that administer Medicaid insurance programs for the poor. These agencies are not typically involved in providing direct patient care but support local agencies that do provide direct care.

With increasing influence from managed care organizations, the federal government has transferred responsibility for managing governmental health care funds to some states, at the request of the states. This move was justified by the rationale that states would be able to exercise more flexibility in designing and administering health care programs tailored to the needs of citizens. The danger existed that traditional "safety nets" of federal mandates for services for the poor, elderly, or disadvantaged would be lost. The long-term outcome would be patients who put off seeking care until they were so sick that their diseases are even more expensive to treat, thus defeating the purpose of state control. In fact, these fears were realized during the early days of state control of Medicaid funds.

Local Agencies

Local agencies serve one community, one county, or a few nearby counties. They provide services to both paying and nonpaying citizens. Public health departments are examples of local governmental agencies found in almost every county in the United States. All citizens, whether or not they can pay, are eligible for health care through local public health departments. These services usually include immunizations, prenatal care and counseling, well-baby and well-child clinics, sexually transmitted disease clinics, tuberculosis clinics, and others. Public health nurses sometimes make home visits as well.

Voluntary (Private) Agencies

Citizens often voluntarily support agencies working to promote or restore health. When private volunteers support an agency providing health care, it is called a **voluntary (private) agency.** Support is generally through private donations, although many of these agencies apply for governmental grants to support some of their activities.

Voluntary agencies often begin when a group of individuals band together to address a health problem. Volunteers may initially perform all their services. Later, they may obtain enough donations to hire personnel, staff an office, and expand services. They may be able to secure ongoing funding through grants or organizations such as the United Way. Examples of voluntary health agencies are the Visiting Nurses Association, the American Heart Association, Hospice, the American Cancer Society, and the Mental Health Association (Fig. 13–1).

Not-For-Profit or For-Profit Agencies

The second major way to classify health service delivery agencies is by what is done with the income earned by the agency. A **not-for-profit agency** is one that uses profits to pay personnel, improve services, advertise services, provide educational programs, or otherwise contribute to the mission of the

Figure 13–1
Private, not-for-profit agencies, such as the American Heart Association, provide a variety of health-related services to the citizens of their communities (Photo by Kelly Whalen).

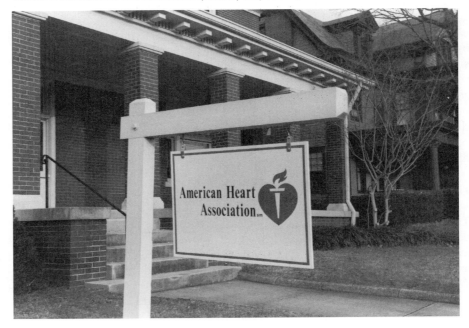

agency. A common misconception is that not-for-profit agencies do not ever make a profit. Actually, they may make profits, but the profits must be used for the improvement of the agency. Most voluntary agencies, such as the ones listed previously, are not-for-profit, as are many private hospitals.

Proprietary agencies, or **for-profit agencies,** may distribute profits to partners or shareholders. The growth in for-profit health care agencies has mushroomed over the past two decades. Health care is big business and has the potential to be very profitable.

For-profit agencies include numerous home health care companies that send nurses and other health personnel to care for patients at home. There are also several large national chains of for-profit health care providers that have demonstrated that it is possible to provide quality patient care and make a profit while doing so. Examples include national nursing home networks, specialty outpatient centers for ambulatory surgery, heart hospitals, and re-habilitation centers. An issue hotly debated is that for-profit health care orga-nizations do not typically treat nonpaying patients. These people must go to publicly funded facilities that are rapidly becoming overburdened with pa-tients who are unable to pay their bills.

Level of Health Care Services Provided

The third major way health care services are classified is by the level of health care services provided. The levels have traditionally been primary care, sec-ondary care, and tertiary care. A new level, subacute care, has recently emerged. These four levels are all discussed.

Primary Care Services

Care rendered at the point at which a patient first enters the health care system is considered **primary care.** This may be in a student health clinic, health cen-ters in the community, an emergency department, physicians' offices, nurse prac-titioners' clinics, or health clinic at work sites. Aydelotte (1983, p. 812) defined the major goals of the primary health care system as providing the following:

1. Entry into the system.
2. Emergency care.
3. Health maintenance.
4. Long-term and chronic care.
5. Treatment of temporary malfunctioning that does not require hospital-ization.

In addition to treating common health problems, primary care centers are, for many citizens, where much of prevention and health promotion takes place. These centers are plagued by many problems, such as lack of adequate financing, staffing, space, and community support. However, this pattern is changing, in large part because of the increasing influence of managed care. Access to primary care in the least costly setting is now mandated by man-aged care organizations.

Secondary Care Services

Secondary care involves assisting in the prevention of complications from disease, treating temporary dysfunction requiring medical intervention such as hospitalization, evaluating long-term care or chronic patients who may need treatment changes, and providing counseling and therapy that are not available in primary care settings (Aydelotte, 1983).

Although hospitals have traditionally been associated with this level of care, agencies that increasingly provide secondary health services are **home health agencies,** ambulatory care agencies, skilled nursing agencies, and surgical centers. These agencies offer skilled personnel, easy access, convenient parking, compact equipment and monitoring systems, medications and anesthesia services, and a financial reimbursement program that rewards shorter lengths of stay and home or community care.

It is expected that the trend toward providing community-based secondary care will continue. However, reimbursement has decreased as the terms of the Balanced Budget Act of 1997 were implemented, eliminating many home health services and skilled nursing care previously covered. The full effect of that act on this segment of the health care industry has yet to be evaluated.

Tertiary Care Services

Tertiary care services are those provided to acutely ill patients, to those requiring long-term care, and to those needing rehabilitation services. Tertiary care also includes provision of care to the terminally ill. It usually involves many health professionals working together on interdisciplinary teams to design treatment plans.

Examples of tertiary agencies are specialized hospitals such as trauma centers and specialized pediatric centers; long-term care facilities offering skilled nursing, intermediate care, and supportive care; rehabilitation centers; and hospices, where care is provided to the terminally ill and their families in the hospital, in the home, or in special centers.

Subacute Care Services

A growing segment of health care, **subacute care** services emerged in the 1990s. According to the Joint Commission on Accreditation of Health Care Organizations (JCAHO), subacute care is defined as:

> goal-oriented, comprehensive, inpatient care designed for an individual who has had an acute illness, injury, or exacerbation of a disease process. It is rendered immediately after, or instead of, acute hospitalization to treat one or more specific, active, complex medical conditions or to administer one or more technically complex treatments in the context of a person's underlying long-term conditions and overall situation. Generally, the condition of an individual receiving subacute care is such that the care does not depend heavily on high technology monitoring or complex diagnostic procedures.
>
> Subacute care requires the coordinated services of an interdisciplinary team, including physicians, nurses, and other relevant professional disciplines who are knowledgeable and trained to assess and manage these specific conditions and perform the necessary procedures. It is given as part of a specifically defined program, regardless of the site.

Subacute care is generally more intensive than traditional nursing facility care and less intensive than acute inpatient care. It requires frequent (daily to weekly) patient assessment and review of the clinical course and treatment plan for a limited time period (several days to several months), until a condition is stabilized or a predetermined treatment course is completed (Joint Commission on Accreditation of Health Care Organizations, 1995, p. 3).

Subacute care lies between hospital care and long-term care. By the mid-1990s, this was one of the fastest-growing segments of the health care delivery system and provided employment opportunities for nurses and other health care team members who lost jobs when hospitals downsized. The goal was to provide lower-cost health care and create a seamless transition for patients moving through the health care system. By the end of the decade, growth in the subacute care sector had slowed, owing to two major factors: increasing government regulation had driven the costs up; and lower third-party reimbursement for services rendered in subacute settings made them less profitable.

Traditional Internal Structures of Health Care Agencies

The health care delivery system consists of agencies such as hospitals, clinics, associations, long-term care facilities, and home health services that provide any of the four major types of health services.

Institutional Structure

Institutional structure refers to how an agency is organized to accomplish its mission. The institutional structure of most agencies includes a governing body, a board of trustees, which may also be called a board of directors.

Board of Trustees

In the past, board members were often chosen from two groups: community philanthropists, who were expected to donate generously to the facility, and physicians who practiced in the institution. Boards were large, met infrequently, and had mainly ceremonial functions.

But as the health care environment became more complex, board members were chosen to represent various business and political interests of the community. They were expected to bring knowledge and expertise from the business world as well as to have an appreciation and understanding of health care agencies and how they operate.

Boards now tend to be smaller and carry significant responsibility for the mission of the organization, the quality of services provided, and the financial status of the organization. Boards are not involved in the day-to-day running of the agency, but they are legally responsible for establishing policies governing operations and for ensuring that the policies are executed. They delegate responsibility for running the agency to the chief executive officer (CEO). Box 13–2 outlines a typical hospital board's primary responsibilities.

Chief Executive Officer

The **chief executive officer** is the individual responsible for the overall operation on a daily basis. He or she usually has a master's degree in business or hospital administration. The CEO's responsibilities include making sure that the institution runs efficiently, is cost-effective, and carries out the policies established by the board. The CEO also has an important external role addressing health care issues in the community. The CEO usually sits on the board of trustees and reports to the board. A chief operating officer (COO) often assists the CEO in larger organizations.

Nurses with advanced degrees and experience in administration, business, and health care policy increasingly occupy both of these positions. Boards, who are responsible for hiring CEOs, have found that the broad holistic education and clinical experience of nurses prepares them unusually well for these positions.

Medical Staff

A medical staff consists of physicians, who may be either employees or independent practitioners. In either case they must be granted privileges by the board of trustees to see patients at that particular institution. They cannot simply decide to admit patients to an institution. A credentials committee, composed of members of the medical staff, performs the credentialing process. They are charged with the responsibility of assuring the board of trustees that every physician admitted to the medical staff of that facility is a qualified and competent practitioner and that, over time, each one keeps his or her skills and knowledge updated.

The medical staff, through its credentials committee, is often charged with the responsibility for credentialing nonphysician providers who admit or

---

BOX 13–2

Board of Directors' Responsibilities

- Mission development and long-range planning.
- Ensuring high quality care.
- Oversight of medical staff credentialing.
- Financial oversight.
- Selection and evaluation of the hospital chief executive officer.
- Board self-evaluation and education.

From American Hospital Association (1999). Welcome to the board: An orientation for the new health care trustee. Chicago: AHA Press.

consult with patients. These include advanced practice nurses, psychologists, optometrists, podiatrists, and others.

In large organizations, medical staffs are usually organized by service (e. g., department of surgery, department of medicine, and department of obstetrics). The entire medical staff usually elects a **chief of staff.** The chief of staff and the chiefs of the various services work together with the chief executive officer and other administrative representatives through the medical executive committee to make important decisions about medical policy for the institution. The rules and regulations that govern these activities are call by-laws. The board of trustees, to whom the physicians are responsible, must approve the actions of the medical staff.

Service on committees and leadership positions of the medical staff are time-consuming activities; therefore, some institutions pay members of the medical staff a fee for special services in recognition that time away from seeing patients reduces their income.

Nursing Staff

The senior administrative nurse in an organization is known as the **chief nurse executive** or officer, vice president for nursing, or director of nursing. Once excluded from broad institutional decision making, nurse executives today are often members of the board of trustees. Many organizations now consider the nurse executive and the chief of the medical staff of equal importance.

The educational preparation of nurse executives usually includes a master's degree in nursing administration or business administration or a joint master's of science in nursing and master's of business administration (MSN/MBA). Nurse executives are responsible for overseeing all the nursing care provided in the institution and serve as clinical leaders as well as administrators. Since there is a need to coordinate patient care and outcomes among all disciplines, the role of the nurse executive has been expanding during recent years to include administrative responsibilities with departments other than nursing, such as pharmacy, respiratory therapy, and social services.

The nursing staff consists of all the registered nurses, licensed practical nurses/licensed vocational nurses, nursing assistants, and clerical assistants employed by the department of nursing. They are usually organized according to the units on which they work.

Each patient care unit has its own budget and staff for which the manager is responsible. The manager, who is usually a nurse, is also a communication link between the staff and the next level of management.

In large or networked organizations, there may be an additional level of management between the nurse executive and the manager of a unit. These are middle managers, known as clinical directors or supervisors. In most cases, they are also nurses, but they may come from other clinical disciplines or from a business background. They have responsibility for multiple units or for specific projects or programs. These directors ensure that nursing and all other services they manage are integrated with other hospital services. They serve as the communication link between the unit managers and the executive staff.

Other nurses combine direct patient care responsibilities with research, education, and management responsibilities, such as nurse educators, nurse researchers, clinical nurse specialists, and infection control nurses. Nurses in these roles support direct care nurses and serve as expert resources to them in their area of specialization.

Others

Physicians, nurses, and all the other individuals who work with patients are called the health care team, or **interdisciplinary team.** They are supported in their work by a number of other departments, such as nutrition services, environmental services, and laundry. Other key health providers are discussed next in this chapter.

Health care organizations are complex facilities. The way they are organized may vary, but each has an organizational chart that shows its unique structure and explains lines of authority. When considering employment in a health care organization, you can learn a great deal by examining its organizational chart to see how nursing is governed and relates to senior management and the board of directors.

The Health Care Team

Within the almost dizzying array of health care settings discussed in this chapter are the people who provide care to patients — the health care team. At one time, physicians and nurses were the only members of the health care team, but as health care became complex and technology expanded, a number of other health disciplines developed. Today, there are many different health care team members who come from a variety of backgrounds. The decision about which of these various personnel should to be involved in the care of a patient depends on the desired patient outcomes.

In the past physicians were the only coordinators of patient care. In contemporary practice, the coordination of services is likely to be led by a case manager. Case managers, who may be nurses, recognize the contribution of each discipline in achieving the desired outcomes and bring a team together to plan, deliver, and evaluate such care in the most cost-effective manner. Case managers are utilized in many health care settings other than in managed care organizations, as previously described. The case management model is discussed more fully in Chapter 14.

Key Members of the Health Care Team

In addition to nurses, there are dozens of health care workers who serve from time to time on interdisciplinary health care teams. Several of the key members who are most likely to be involved in the care of patients are listed below.

Physicians

Physicians have completed college and three or four years of medical school and are licensed by a state board of medical examiners. Although a hospital residency is not required to practice medicine in all states, most physicians have completed one, and many do postgraduate work in a specialty area and then take examinations to become board certified in the specialty area.

Physicians are responsible for the medical diagnosis and therapies designed to restore health. Although physicians have traditionally been involved mainly in restorative care, many are beginning to recognize the value of illness and injury prevention and health promotion. Most insurance companies have not reimbursed these activities, and until recently there has been little financial incentive to do so. But now managed care plans have dramatically increased reimbursement for preventive care. Some physicians are also integrating nontraditional or alternative treatment choices such as chiropractic medicine, acupuncture, herbal treatments, and massage therapy into their practices.

Dietitians

Many patients require management of their nutritional intake as part of the healing process. Others need to know how to prepare and eat a healthy diet (Fig. 13–2). **Dietitians** have baccalaureate degrees and may have completed internships. They understand how the diet (oral or intravenous) can affect a patient's recovery and promote and maintain health. They focus on the therapeutic value of foods and on teaching people about therapeutic diets and healthful nutrition.

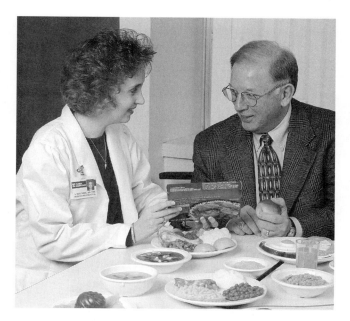

Figure 13–2
Dietitians assist patients to facilitate their own healing and health maintenance through therapeutic diets and healthful nutritional practices (Photo courtesy of Hamilton Medical Center, Dalton, Georgia).

Pharmacists

Pharmacists prepare and dispense medications, instruct patients and other health workers about medications, monitor the use of controlled substances such as narcotics, and work to reduce medication errors. The number and complexity of drugs available today necessitates special education and training in their preparation and dispensing and in monitoring the effects on patients. Clinical pharmacists spend time on hospital units working closely with physicians and nursing case managers to coordinate complex chemotherapy drug administration. They assist in monitoring the drug interactions resulting from a patient taking many different medications because some medications can be rendered ineffective when given with another drug (Fig. 13–3).

Pharmacists may pursue either a bachelor's degree in pharmacy, which takes five years, or a doctor of pharmacy, which takes six years. Depending on state licensing requirements, they may also be required to complete an internship. Pharmacy technicians assist them.

Figure 13–3
Pharmacists are responsible for preparing and dispensing drugs and monitoring their effects on patients, in addition to numerous other duties (Photo courtesy of Hamilton Medical Center, Dalton, Georgia).

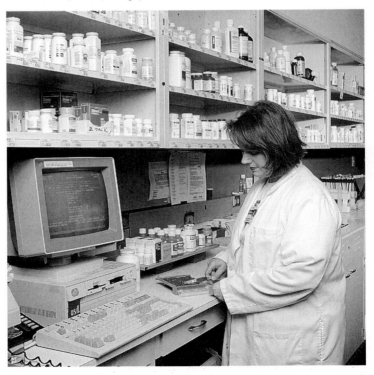

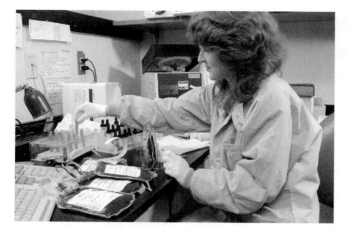

Figure 13-4
This laboratory technologist works in a critically important setting—a blood bank. Here she prepares several units of blood for administration (Photo courtesy of Hamilton Medical Center, Dalton, Georgia).

Paramedical Personnel

A number of personnel are educated to assist physicians in the diagnosis of patient problems. This connection with medicine identifies them as **paramedical** staff.

Laboratory technologists handle patient specimens such as blood, sputum, feces, urine, and body tissues to be examined for cancer or other abnormalities (Fig.13–4). Laboratory technologists carefully subject these body substances to various tests to determine whether or not the patient needs treatment. Technologists have at least a bachelor's degree and are often assisted by laboratory technicians, who have two-year degrees. They must pass a licensing examination to practice.

Radiology technologists perform x-ray procedures. Although patients still need routine x-ray studies, technology in this field has become sophisticated. Subspecialties such as computed tomography (CT), magnetic resonance imaging (MRI), and positron-emission-tomography (PET) have developed (Fig. 13–5). These techniques are all ways of "seeing" what is going on inside the body without surgery. All require specially educated technicians who operate multimillion-dollar equipment. Although some radiology technicians are still trained "on the job," most are educated in formal programs lasting from one to four years. Radiology technologists have a bachelor's degree. They must be registered with the state in which they practice.

Respiratory Technologists

Acutely ill or injured patients often require assistance in breathing. Respiratory technologists operate equipment such as ventilators, oxygen therapy devices, and intermittent positive-pressure breathing machines. They also perform some diagnostic procedures such as pulmonary function tests and, in some facilities, blood gas analysis. With the increase in respiratory care in the home and community, these health care team members are working closely

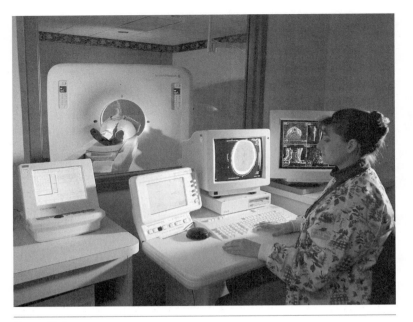

Figure 13–5
Advances in radiology include a new generation of magnetic resonance imaging (MRI), seen here. Radiological technologists are prepared to operate multimillion-dollar equipment such as this in addition to assisting patients during procedures (Photo courtesy of Hamilton Medical Center, Dalton, Georgia).

with home health agencies and community health centers. They must complete either a two-year (technician) or four-year (technologist) educational program; in some states they must complete an internship.

Social Workers

The **social services** worker is specifically educated and trained to assist patients and their families as they face the impact of illness and injury. They help patients and their families deal with financial problems caused by interruption of work or inadequate insurance benefits, and direct them to the appropriate community support systems or facilities for home health care or long-term care.

Social workers hold either a bachelor's or master's degree. They serve as liaisons between hospitalized patients and the resources and services available in the community. In addition, social workers frequently are called on to assist other health care personnel to cope more effectively with the stresses associated with caring for patients in crisis.

Therapists

Several types of **therapists** help patients with special challenges. Physical therapists, or physiotherapists, assist patients to regain maximum possible physical activity and strength. They focus on assessing preillness or preinjury function, current damage, and potential for recovery. They then develop a long-term plan for gradual return to function through exercise, rest, heat, and hydrotherapy. Physical therapists, who have a minimum of a bachelor's degree, also supervise physical therapy assistants, who hold associate degrees.

Occupational therapists work with physical therapists to develop plans to assist patients in resuming the activities of daily living after illness or injury. They may help patients learn to cook, carry out their personal hygiene, or drive a specially equipped car. In addition, they assist patients to learn skills to return to their previous jobs or retrain patients for new employment options. Occupational therapists have bachelor's degrees. Other types of therapists include recreational therapists, art and music therapists, speech therapists, and massage therapists.

Administrative Support Personnel

In all organizations, administrative support personnel are needed for clerical jobs like answering phones, directing visitors, scheduling patient tests, payroll, billing, filing insurance claims, filing forms, paying bills, and other support functions. These activities require considerable time. Hiring administrative staff frees the clinical staff to concentrate on direct patient care.

Keeping complete and accurate medical records is an extremely important administrative function that ensures proper insurance billing and legal protection of the hospital and its staff. Registered records administrators are vital members of the administrative staff. These professionals staff the medical records department, (Fig. 13–6). Many organizations today now refer to the medical records departments as "health information services."

The administrative staff ensures that the operations of the facility run smoothly and that clinicians have the resources necessary to meet patient needs. They also educate the clinical staff on financial constraints and work with the staff to find ways to provide quality care at the lowest possible cost.

Forces Changing the Health Care Delivery System

The last decade of the twentieth century has been described as the most turbulent time of transition and reform in the United States health care system has ever experienced. Total expenditures on health care in the United States exceeded $1 trillion for the first time in 1996. During the last decade, health care spending grew twice as fast as the gross national product (GNP). In 1999, health care services consumed 13.5 percent of the GNP, which is almost double what other nations spend on health care (Bell, 1999). As escalating costs of delivery of services hit record levels, a major change in reimbursement for services took place. During that same period, the explosion of information technology contributed to a revolution in consumer knowledge and changing expectations for information and treatment options.

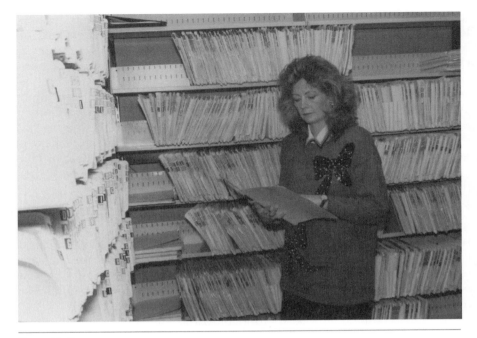

Figure 13–6
This registered records administrator is a highly trained professional whose work is vital to the health care agency by which she is employed (Photo by Kelly Whalen).

Managed Care

The term **managed care** is used to describe a wide variety of organizations and activities that attempt to control health care costs. Issues of access and quality are key factors in determining the success of various managed care strategies. Interestingly, managed care has health promotion, not illness treatment, as one of its primary goals. As the 1990s progressed, several factors led to the development of a variety of managed care models (Fig. 13–7). These included the rising cost of providing health care benefits, growing taxpayer unrest about the expense of tax-funded health care programs, unequal access to services, and concerns about quality.

Types of Managed Care Organizations

Managed care organizations (MCOs) can be categorized into four basic models: health maintenance organizations (HMOs), preferred provider organizations (PPOs), point-of-service plans (POSs), and physician hospital organizations (PHOs).

Health Maintenance Organizations

In contrast to the traditional fee-for-service system, the **health maintenance organization (HMO)** is a system in which a defined group of people receives

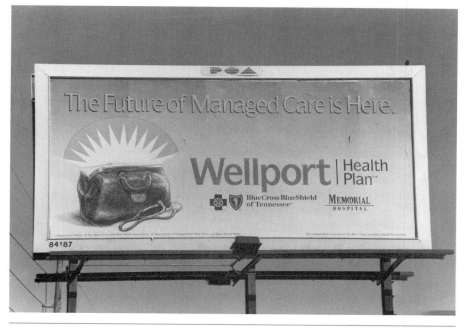

Figure 13–7
Managed care has created a highly competitive health care market, as this billboard illustrates (Photo by Kelly Whalen).

health care services for a predetermined fixed fee. This method of financing is called **capitation,** and it is paid on a per-member per-month basis. The same amount is paid to the provider each month regardless of whether services were provided or how much the services cost. The fee is usually negotiated for a period of one to three years. The patient's access to services is coordinated and managed by a primary care provider. The primary care provider, sometimes called a **gatekeeper,** is responsible for all referrals for tests and to specialists. Keeping patients healthy means that the primary care provider gets to keep more of the fee. Some people worry that this will discourage gatekeepers from ordering diagnostic tests and referring patients to specialists, even when indicated.

Preferred Provider Organizations

The **preferred provider organization (PPO)** contracts with independent providers such as physicians and hospitals for a negotiated discount for the services provided its members.

Point-of-Service Organizations

The **point-of-service (POS) organization** is a form of a MCO with more options. Members may choose to receive services within the defined network, or they may go outside the network and pay a higher deductible or copayment.

Physician Hospital Organizations

As managed care organizations penetrated the market and threatened the financial viability of hospitals and many physicians' practices, the providers of health services created another type of organization, **physician hospital organizations (PHOs).** The PHO is a separate corporation formed by a hospital and a group of its medical staff for the purpose of joint contracting with managed care organizations. This structure allows hospitals and physicians to work together to negotiate fees for services directly with self-insured employers and managed care organizations.

In spite of this collaboration, both hospitals and physicians continue to face cutbacks in reimbursement. Physicians have begun to fight against the high profits of managed care organizations. In June 1999, the physicians of the American Medical Association voted to develop a national labor union. Their claim was that such action was necessary to help them more effectively treat patients. Committed to remaining faithful to the ethical traditions of professionalism in the practice of medicine, physicians assured their patients there would be no strikes (Smoak, 1999).

Hospitals have similar concerns. They have seen reimbursement shrink both from managed care and as a result of the Balanced Budget Act of 1997. The Balanced Budget Act outlined progressive cuts in services and reimbursement rates over a five-year period. In preparation for the declining revenues, mergers and acquisitions between hospitals have taken place at a staggering rate during the last decade. These strategies have consolidated services and cut costs.

Registered nurses are utilized extensively throughout the managed care system. Many HMOs utilize advanced practice nurses in the primary care role in ambulatory and community settings. Another key role for the registered nurse is that of case manager. The case manager coordinates care for a patient throughout the health care system to decrease fragmentation, contain costs, and enhance the quality of life. Nurses also serve in a triage role, deciding the most appropriate course of intervention. Nurses are often employed as utilization reviewers to determine the most appropriate and cost-efficient level of care. This role often facilitates moving a patient out of the hospital and into a rehabilitation center, a nursing home, or home, with home health services.

The consumers' perspective toward managed care and their experiences with it vary. Some consumers have good access, a full range of services, providers they trust, and lower costs. Others have experienced access problems, denial of treatment, and limited coverage. As consumers have become more educated, they have begun to fight for their rights to health care through political reform and the legal system. The collective power of consumers has created changes in the health care system, mainly in terms of safeguards to prevent such abuses as "drive through deliveries."

Changes in Consumers' Expectations

The computer age has afforded access to global information at an explosive rate. Society has embraced the information technology age and has become increasingly dependent on instant global news, information, and service. By the end of the twentieth century consumers had instant service touching every area of life, such as drive-through banking, fast food, and car maintenance and one-hour eyeglass prescriptions and photography services. The proliferation of Internet web sites has also affected the knowledge and expectation of health care consumers.

In 1998 more than 22 million U. S. adults reported using the Internet to obtain health information. Experts predicted that in 2000 more than 33 million will have researched health issues online. "We're seeing a remarkable transition in health care," says Mitchell Morris, a surgeon and vice president at the University of Texas' M. D. Anderson Cancer Center in Houston. "The Internet is going to irrevocably affect how patients and doctors interact. This is not going to go away." (*USA Today,* July 14, 1999, p. 1A) See the accompanying News Note for more on this topic.

Health related web sites offer a wide range of topics, such as wellness, nutrition, general health information, live surgery and births, women's health, medication reference books, government health agencies, professional associations, referrals and information about hospitals, physicians, managed care, patient rights, and libraries filled with medical textbooks and journals. Live interactive web sites even offer diagnosis, treatment, and medication prescription services without a hands-on assessment and examination. Long-term outcomes of electronic care have not been researched and documented at this time.

Physicians today are not surprised when patients come to their offices with complete research, a potential diagnosis, and treatment options from the Internet. This has led some health care leaders to be concerned about consumers' ability to discern the quality of information from such a vast array of choices. The Federal Trade Commission (FTC) cracked down on companies

---

N E W S   N O T E

"Net Empowering Patients: Millions Scour the Web to Find Medical Information"

In ever-growing numbers, patients clutching Internet printouts and a list of smart questions are marching into doctor's offices nationwide, sometimes knowing more about their disease and ways to treat it than their physicians.

This explosion of medical knowledge—and misinformation—among lay people is causing a dramatic shift in the balance of power between doctor and patient, changing how medicine is practiced more profoundly than anything since the advent of managed care.

"That is going to change the whole paradigm we've been used to in medicine," says former surgeon general C. Everett Koop, whose site is the most popular medical area on the Web. "Patients are getting more and more control because of the knowledge they have . . . which enables them to make decisions with their doctor about diagnosis, procedures, and treatment.

and individuals posting misleading health information on the Internet in 1998 after investigators found 800 web sites making fraudulent claims. In June 1999 the FTC launched Operation Cure.All, a campaign to stop false health information on the Internet. The FTC now monitors health sites on the Internet on an ongoing basis (Flaherty, 1999).

Health Care's Response to Managed Care and Consumer Expectations

The impact of managed care and advanced information technology has forced the health care system to undergo massive transformation to meet the demands of new reimbursement structures and consumer expectations. The reengineering of health care organizations has included not only the redesign of patient care delivery but also of the **organizational structures** necessary to support the changes.

Reengineering

During the 1990s, health care organizations recognized the full impact of managed care and changes in consumer expectations. Hospitals were so complex, bureaucratic, and convoluted that many were failing to deliver high-quality products and services consistently. In health care, for example, it was not unusual for a patient staying five to seven days in a typical hospital to travel by wheelchair or stretcher eight or nine miles during that stay. A simple laboratory test might require 40 to 60 separate activities or steps before results could be reported. Excessive and duplicative paperwork and trivial tasks burdened care providers and left patients dissatisfied and angry. The patient was no longer the center of the system. At times, it seemed patients and families were nuisances that got in the way of bureaucratic activities.

Health care organizations recognized that becoming more efficient was imperative for survival. The challenge to provide high quality care at the right cost with the expected outcome has become the focus of the last decade of the twentieth century. A dramatic new paradigm was needed. The continuous quality improvement movement had laid the groundwork and provided the tools necessary to transform patient care from being designed around various specialized departments to an integrated process-driven system. **Reengineering** is the "fundamental rethinking and radical redesign of business processes to bring about dramatic improvement in performance" (Hammer and Stanton, 1995). **Patient-focused care,** also known as patient-centered care, means placing the patient at the center of activity and designing processes that efficiently and effectively attain desired patient outcomes.

Management experts believe that reducing layers of management is an essential component of any reengineering initiative. One key to the new organization and structure is **decentralization.** Decentralization empowers staff, allowing them to exercise their own good judgment rather than waiting to be told what to do. Decision-making authority is given to those most affected by the decision, rather than being limited to a few executives or managers. This means fewer layers in an organizational chart and is in agreement with the philosophy that all professionals should be encouraged to use their talents fully.

For empowerment to be effective, the board of trustees and top executives must clearly articulate their vision, goals, and expectations so that all employees understand the direction of the organization and their roles in it. Decentralization and empowerment involve the development and use of many skills, including consensus, decision making, positive discipline, worker independence and interdependence, negotiation, collaboration, and critical thinking.

Reengineering and patient-focused care are accomplished by **cross-functional teams,** who are involved with all aspects of achieving a specific patient-focused outcome. Cross-functional teams are composed of people from all areas of the organization who contribute to a particular process and outcome. They redesign, from scratch, how the work will be done and who will do it and in what time frame and location. In some new models staff are cross-trained to be able to complete several different tasks, each of which was formerly performed by a different worker. Workers who are cross-trained to perform different tasks are also known as **multi-skilled workers.** For example, a single worker may be trained to collect admission demographic information, draw blood for tests ordered, and take an electrocardiogram. Patient satisfaction is typically higher than with the older fragmented bureaucratic methods.

When done well, reengineering addresses the purpose of the business; the organizational culture needed for success, processes, and performance; and the people, knowledge, and skills needed to accomplish the redesigned work. When done poorly, reengineering is often a euphemism for downsizing or staff reductions or layoffs. Although it is true that as the work is redesigned fewer people may be needed, staff reduction is not the main goal of reengineering.

Downsizing without proper work redesign simply leaves fewer people to accomplish already inefficient and ineffective work. Unfortunately, many companies, both in and outside health care, take this shortsighted approach to reengineering. The result is poor morale, loss of competent staff, lower-quality outcomes, patient dissatisfaction, and loss of market share. Box 13–3 lists key components for successful reengineering.

Tomorrow's health care workers are facing a different work environment. They will probably have seven to ten different jobs during an average work career rather than the three jobs or fewer held by previous generations. Even when employed in the same position, they should expect that it will undergo major evolution and change. How can you thrive in this constantly changing environment? The following suggestions should help you keep your options open, even as the health care system changes.

BOX 13-3
Keys to Successful Reengineering

- Strong leadership.
- Support from the top (financial, cultural, time, resources).
- Team members who love ambiguity, creativity, risk taking, and holism.
- An *irreverence* for the past.
- Optimism, persistence.
- Ability to answer the questions: What is our business? What culture do we want? How do we need to do our work? What people do we want to work with?

- Take every opportunity to learn new skills.
- Read widely both inside and outside your field.
- Identify emerging trends and new opportunities.
- Find new ways to apply your knowledge and skills.
- Volunteer for community activities that will stretch your skills, help you learn new ones, and meet people who can be helpful to you.
- Keep your resume current, but do not change jobs too often because this implies instability.
- Develop flexibility, including openness to new challenges.

Hospitals Respond with New Organizational Models

At the turn of the century, following a decade or more of restructuring efforts in hospitals, there were several basic organizational models in use, each with numerous variations. Five representative structures are described below. Readers should recognize that the models overlap and few "pure" models are in use.

Functional Model
The traditional functional model clearly defines each major function of the organization and establishes clear lines of managerial authority. Examples of the major functions are inpatient care, outpatient care, surgery, professional services, facility operations, marketing and planning, and human resources.

Service Line Model
The service line model establishes management responsibilities around specific types of services wherever they occur in the hospital or in its associated clinics and offices. Examples of major service lines include cardiology, orthopedics, oncology, obstetrics, ambulatory services, and behavioral health.

Matrix Model
The matrix model is a complex model with multiple authority and support systems. Consider this model as a blend of the functional and service line models. In the matrix model there is one overall manager who directs dual

RESEARCH NOTE

Nursing administrators are interested in evaluating how redesigning patient care delivery and organizational restructuring affect the quality of patient care. Eighteen months after Lehigh Valley Hospital, Allentown, Pa., completed restructuring, a study of how the redesign affected patient and nurse satisfaction, cost of care, and clinical quality was conducted on four medical-surgical units. The redesign efforts had included the following: facility changes to improve the convenience of the location of supplies, nurses' stations, and patient records; enhanced telecommunication and information systems; and redesign of all work processes and many staff roles.

Using the Press-Ganey Patient Satisfaction Survey, seven dimensions of nursing care were measured in the evaluation of patient satisfaction: friendliness, promptness, taking problems seriously, attention to special needs, being informative about tests, technical skill, and consideration of patients as individuals.

The clinical quality outcomes measured were patient falls, medication errors, hospital-acquired infections, and intravenous-related complications. Hospital mortality data, length of stay, and the costs of care were also evaluated.

Results of the study revealed that patient satisfaction scores declined during implementation of changes, but after eighteen months, scores increased significantly on three of the four units. Nurses also experienced improved collaboration with physicians following the restructuring. All of the clinical quality outcomes were either improved or maintained at the time of the 18-month follow-up. Hospital mortality data could not be completely linked to redesign initiatives, but the data indicated that the restructuring had not adversely affected patient outcomes. There were varied results in the degree to which costs and length of stay declined. Overall results on the four pilot units were positive enough that nursing leaders decided to expand the redesign initiative to other parts of the hospital.

The researchers pointed out a lack of comprehensive research analyzing long-term effects of hospital restructuring. They also observed that nursing journals have published numerous articles about organizational redesign and concluded that according to many reports, results of organizational redesign have been disappointing They stress the importance of establishing goals and outcomes for restructuring prior to implementation and the need to evaluate changes systematically over a period of time to obtain scientific evidence about the impact on patient care.

From Bryan, Y. E., Hitchings, K. S., Fuss, M. A., Fox, M. A., Kinneman, M. T., and Young, M. J. (1998). Measuring and evaluating hospital restructuring efforts. *Journal of Nursing Administration*, 28(9), 21–27.

lines of authority. It is a team concept with one manager overseeing the specialized functional areas and another manager providing the expertise to the particular service. In this model some employees report to two managers. For example, the housekeeping supervisor in the surgical department would report to both the head of housekeeping and the director of the surgical services.

Process Model

The process model is a newer approach that organizes management of care around phases in the process of health care delivery. These phases include access, treatment, transition, and evaluation. Responsibilities of managers in the process model cut across all departments.

Regional Model

The regional model is another new approach that addresses more complex health care systems that emerged through the expansion of services and organizations beyond the single hospital. It is organized according to the individual service providers. Examples include hospital functions, home health, nursing homes, managed care organizations, rehabilitation centers, and smaller hospitals that have been acquired as part of a larger system.

Maintaining Quality in Health Care Agencies

Maintaining high quality services should be the goal of every health care agency. As pressure increases to control costs, it becomes even more important to ensure that quality is not sacrificed simply to save dollars. This can be accomplished in a variety of ways, chiefly through accreditation and quality care initiatives.

Accreditation of Health Care Agencies

As you learned in Chapter 2, schools of nursing may choose to participate in a process called accreditation. Health care organizations such as hospitals, home health agencies, and long-term care facilities are also accredited. Their accrediting body is the Joint Commission on the Accreditation of Health Care Organizations. Accreditation by JCAHO is important and requires that a number of standards be met in every department. The goal of accreditation is to improve patient outcomes. Considerable agency resources of time and money are spent making sure accreditation criteria are met. Another strategy

---

Figure 13–8
This group of professionals works together to implement continuous quality improvement processes in an acute care hospital with the goal of improving efficiency and patient care while reducing costs (Photo by Wilson Baker).

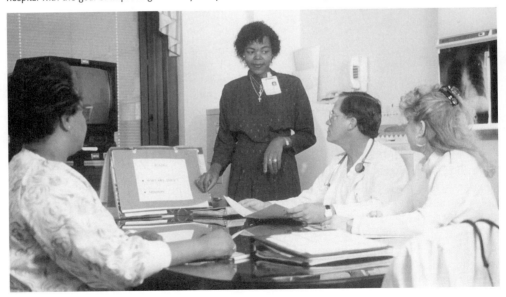

INTERVIEW 13-1

Interview with Pamela G. Stelmack, RN, BSHA, CPHQ, Director Performance Improvement/Utilization Management, Hamilton Medical Center, Dalton, Georgia.

Interviewer: What does a utilization management nurse do?

Stelmack: My primary duties in utilization management are to provide clinical information concerning the patient's admission to third party payers to obtain reimbursement for services. We review all inpatient and observation admissions for both appropriateness and quality of care provided. We review both commercially insured patient records and Medicare, Medicaid, and other payer categories. We are responsible for obtaining the precertification authorization for all emergency, inpatient Medicaid admissions, which is required for both the hospital and physician to get reimbursed.

Interviewer: How has managed care changed your role as a nurse?

Stelmack: I have seen the role of nursing expanding as a result of managed care. We used to focus only on the clinical issues surrounding patient care, not the reimbursement aspects. With today's emphasis on cutting costs in health care while maintaining quality, nurses need to understand the financial impact of providing care for their patients. Patients may not have access to or be able to afford the care they need to maintain optimal health or prevent readmission to the hospital. In our role as patient advocates, nurses try to minimize the financial impact of the condition or disease process.

Interviewer: How can nurses serve as patient advocates in minimizing the financial impact of a patient's illness? Is nursing documentation on the patient's record used in receiving approval for a hospitalization or continued stay?

Stelmack: Yes, definitely. In doing these reviews, we are looking at what is documented in the record to support severity of illness, intensity of service, and discharge criteria. Admission assessments, which include vital signs, symptoms, onset of those symptoms, previous medical history, and discharge, help to support the severity of illness. Intensity of service refers to the treatments/medications ordered for the patients. Nursing documentation should focus on the patient's response to treatment and what additional needs they have. When we review the record, the nursing documentation is a key component in supporting the need for the admission and determining when it is appropriate to consider an alternate level of care. If the documentation does not support the need for services, then either the organization does not get reimbursed or the patient will be responsible for a larger portion of the bill than they might expect. This can have a significant impact on the patient/family's ability to cope with the situation. So you see, nursing documentation is very important.

Interviewer: Managed care organizations have received a lot of negative press. Are they really interested in quality of care? If so, what are some examples of quality indicators they monitor?

Stelmack: Managed care organizations are definitely interested in quality of care. They have a national organization, the National Committee for Quality Assurance (NCQA), that assesses healthcare plans and managed care organizations in a manner similar to JCAHO surveys. They serve as a watch dog for the organizations to help assure quality patient care. Managed care organizations monitor patient outcomes by tracking physician practice patterns and various organizational indicators such as mortality rates, nosocomial [hospital acquired] infections, and c-section rates. Managed care organizations also are judged by their coverage for preventive or early detection health services such as cervical cancer screening, diabetic eye exams, and prenatal care.

through which most organizations choose to work toward improvement in patient outcomes is continuous quality improvement.

Continuous Quality Improvement/Total Quality Management

The concept of **continuous quality improvement (CQI)** was first developed by management expert W. Edwards Deming in the 1940s when he suggested that managers in industry should rely on groups of employees, which he called *quality circles,* as they made decisions about how work was to be done. His work was not widely accepted in this country; but when the Japanese government asked him to help them rebuild their workplaces after the devastation of World War II, Deming went to Japan. His ideas revolutionized Japanese industry, which became superior to American industry in many ways by the 1970s, leading to a belated acceptance of Deming's ideas in this country.

In today's health care systems, one of the most important management concepts borrowed from industry is CQI, also called total quality management (TQM). Rather than trying to identify mistakes after they have occurred, these systems focus on establishing procedures for assuring high-quality patient care. Using quality improvement concepts, groups of employees from different departments decide how care will be provided (Fig. 13–8). They decide what outcomes are desired and design systems and assign roles and activities to create those outcomes. Every effort is made to anticipate potential problems and prevent their occurrence. Management delegates authority to the providers of services to plan and carry out quality improvement programs. Programs in CQI/TQM reinforce the belief that quality is everyone's responsibility.

Nurses are actively involved both in quality improvement and in accreditation processes, but these activities are not the responsibility of nursing alone. They are institution-wide initiatives, and everyone at all levels gets involved. Working together to improve patient care builds cooperation among departments and clinical disciplines and boosts morale (Interview 13-1).

Summary of Key Points

- The health care delivery system in the United States is a complex system that provides health promotion, illness prevention, diagnosis and treatment, and rehabilitation and long-term care.
- Health care agencies may be classified as governmental or voluntary, for-profit or not-for-profit, or according to level of care provided. A single agency may fit into all three categories.
- Health care agencies have traditionally been structured with boards of trustees, chief executive officers, medical and nursing staffs, and members of a variety of other disciplines.
- An interdisciplinary health care team consists of an array of professionals, including physicians, nurses, dietitians, pharmacists, paramedical personnel, respiratory technologists, social workers, various therapists, and administrative support personnel. Each member has an important part to play in ensuring the best patient outcomes.
- Managed care has forced major changes in the health care delivery system.
- Information technology leading to increased consumer expectations has contributed to revolutionary change that will continue into the future and will affect professional nursing in many ways, most of which are yet unknown.

- As a result of managed care and changes in consumer expectations, organizations have gone through reengineering, reducing layers of management, and empowering the workforce to take part in decision making.
- New organizational structures for hospitals include functional, service line, matrix, process, and regional models.
- Accreditation and continuous quality improvement are efforts to ensure public safety and institutional effectiveness and accountability.

Critical Thinking Questions

1. Using the yellow pages of your telephone directory or a directory of social services, identify local health services in the following areas: health promotion, illness prevention, diagnosis and treatment, rehabilitation, and long-term care. Judging from the number of agencies for each service, where does the health care emphasis seem to be? What implications does this have for citizens of your community?

2. Obtain the organizational chart of a health care facility. Determine how it compares to one of the organizational structures described. Examine it to see how nursing fits into the overall structure. Who reports to the nurse executive, and to whom does the nurse executive report? What other administrative staff members are on the same level with the nurse executive?

3. Hold a panel discussion on reimbursement. Invite representatives from government, a managed care organization, a hospital, a major employer, and a nonprofit charity to discuss how managed care has affected their organizations.

4. Interview a nurse and one or more nonnurse health professionals. Ask them to share some of their experiences as members of interdisciplinary health care teams during reengineering or restructuring of their institutions. What impact have these initiatives had on the way they care for patients?

5. Go to the Internet and search for sites that provide information on menopause and hormone replacement therapy. Include sites on prevention, wellness, and alternative medicine. Search for a virtual hospital, referrals to physicians, and patient rights. Analyze the information to determine how many different options for diagnosis and treatment were found. How might patients use this information as they interact with health care professionals?

Web Resources

Complementary and alternative medicine, http://www.nccam.nih.gov

Dr. Koop's Website, http://www.DrKoop.com

Joint Commission on Accreditation of Health Care Organizations, http://www.jcaho.org

NurseWeek Online Journal, http://www.nurseweek.com/new/00-7/36d.html

WebMD, http://www.WebMD.com

References

American Hospital Association (1999). *Welcome to the board: An orientation for the new health care trustee*. Chicago: AHA Press.

Aydelotte, M. K. (1983). The future health care delivery system in the United States. In N. L. Chaska (Ed.), *The nursing profession: A time to speak*. New York: McGraw-Hill.

Bell, C. T. (Ed.) (1999). *Modern healthcare's by the numbers*, July 19(29), 17–24.

Bryan, Y. E., Hitchings, K. S., Fuss, M. A., Fox, M. A., Kinneman, M. T., and Young, M. J. (1998). Measuring and evaluating hospital restructuring efforts. *Journal of Nursing Administration, 28*(9), 21–27.

Davis, R., and Miller, L. (1999): Net empowering patients: Millions scour the Web to find medical information. *USA Today*, July 14, 1A.

Deming, W. E. (1982). *Quality, productivity, and competitive position*. Cambridge, Ma.: Massachusetts Institute of Technology, Center for Advanced Engineering Study.

Deming, W. E. (1986). *Out of the crisis*. Cambridge, Ma.: Massachusetts Institute of Technology, Center for Advanced Engineering Study.

Flaherty, M. (1999). FTC targets Internet health fraud. *Nurse week/Health Week*, July 5, 1999. Available from http://www.nurseweek.com/new/00-7/36d.html.

Hammer, M., and Stanton, S. (1995). *The reengineering revolution*. New York: Harper Business.

Joint Commission on Accreditation of Health Care Organizations (1995). *Survey protocol for subacute programs*. Oakbrook Terrace. Ill.: Joint Commission on Accreditation of Health Care Organizations.

National Institutes of Health (1999). National center for complementary and alternative medicine: General information. Available from http://www.nccam.nih.gov.

Smoak, R. D. (1999). American medical association news release. Available from http://www.ama-assn.org/advocacy/statemnt/990623s.htm.

U. S. Department of Health and Human Services (1990). *Healthy people 2000: National health promotion and disease prevention objectives*. Washington, D. C.: Government Printing Office.

U. S. Department of Health and Human Services (1999). *Healthy people 2010, Fact sheet: Healthy people in healthy communities*. Washington, D. C.: Government Printing Office.

Nursing Roles in the Health Care Delivery System

Karen J. Wisdom *

14

Key Terms

Accountability
Autonomy
Case Management Nursing
Change Agent
Collaboration
Delegate
Differentiated Practice
Entrepreneur
Functional Nursing
Patient Advocate
Primary Nursing
Professional Accountabilities
Shared Governance
Team Nursing

Learning Outcomes

After studying this chapter, students will be able to:

- Differentiate among four nursing care delivery systems.
- Discuss a variety of roles for the nurse in the health care delivery system.
- Discuss the purpose of differentiated levels of practice.
- Describe five professional accountabilities.
- Describe the shared governance council model in nursing organizational structure.
- Identify skills the nurse needs when working with interdisciplinary teams.

Chapter 13 covered aspects of our changing health care delivery system, discussed the organizational structure of health agencies, and explained the impact of managed care and how health care organizations are re-designing their work processes. It also reviewed the classifications of health care agencies and responsibilities of the various members of the health care delivery team. This chapter takes a closer look at nursing both from a historical perspective and at how nursing is integral to the interdisciplinary health care delivery team of today and into the future.

Types of Nursing Care Delivery Systems Used in Hospitals

Before World War I, nurses visited the sick in their homes to care for them. As hospital care improved and nursing education evolved, more sick people were treated in hospitals. Providing care to groups of patients rather than to indi-

* The author wishes to acknowledge the contributions of Jennifer Jenkins to the preparation of this chapter.

viduals required nurses to be efficient and use their time effectively. An organizing structure was needed, and various types of care delivery systems were designed to meet the goals of efficient and effective nursing care. Several types of patient care delivery systems are in use today. Four systems—functional nursing, team nursing, primary nursing, and case management nursing—are reviewed in this chapter.

Functional Nursing

By the 1930s, advances in medical technology had evolved to a point at which hospital treatment surpassed that which could be provided at home. As more patients were admitted to hospitals, more nurses were employed to care for them.

The functional approach to nursing care grew out of a need to provide care to large numbers of patients. It focused on organizing and distributing the tasks, or functions, of care. Trained nurses provided care that required high skill levels, and untrained workers with little skill or education performed many less complex tasks.

In **functional nursing,** personnel worked side by side, each performing the assigned task. The goal of functional nursing was efficient management of time, tasks, and energy. Although this practice saved hospitals money, patient care was fragmented, and patients had to relate to many different people. There was no one person they could call, "My nurse."

Case Study: Functional Nursing

A registered nurse (RN) on the evening shift at a local nursing home has been assigned to administer special skin care treatments to bed-bound patients, change dressings, and give all medications. A licensed practical nurse (LPN) monitors all patient temperatures and blood pressures, weighs patients, records the amount they eat and drink, and monitors the blood sugar of diabetic patients. The nursing assistants have each been assigned a different group of patients for whom they are responsible during the shift. They help these patients with personal hygiene, see that they receive their meals and snacks, and assist them with eating, toileting, and other tasks. Because it is evening, the head nurse is not there. In her place is a charge nurse, who signs all charts, indicating that care was administered; talks with physicians and family members; and orders supplies and medications. As they go about their work, there is infrequent interaction. Often they can be heard telling a patient who asks for something, "I'm not assigned to do that tonight. I'll tell the other nursing assistant that you need something."

Today, functional nursing is still used in some settings. It is particularly useful when there are few personnel available, such as at night, on weekends, and on holidays. It often is combined with another method, however, and is rarely used as the sole care delivery method (Bernhard and Walsh, 1990).

Table 14–1 lists advantages and disadvantages of functional nursing.

| TABLE 14-1 |
| Advantages and Disadvantages of Functional Nursing |

Advantages

Efficient—can complete many tasks in a reasonable time frame.
Workers do only tasks they are educated to do and become very efficient.
Promotes organizational skills—each worker must organize his or her own work.
Promotes worker autonomy.

Disadvantages

Lack of holistic view of patient—emphasis on task, not person.
Lacks continuity—patients often do not know who their nurse is.
Registered nurses have little time to talk with patients or render personal care.

Team Nursing

In response to the frustration some nurses felt when using the functional approach to patient care, Lambertson (1953) designed **team nursing.** She envisioned nursing teams as democratic work groups with different skill levels represented by different team members. They were assigned as a team to a group of patients

Team nursing has been widely used in hospitals and long-term care facilities. The team usually consists of a registered nurse, who serves as team leader, a licensed practical nurse, and one or more certified nursing assistants (Fig. 14-1).

The team leader is ultimately responsible for all the care provided but **delegates** (assigns responsibility for) certain patients to each team member. Each member of the team provides the level of care for which he is best prepared. The least skilled and experienced members care for the patients who require the least complex care, and the most skilled and experienced members care for the sickest patients who require the most complex care.

Team nursing allows the team leader to shift, match, and redistribute patient assignments to team members according to their level of education and expertise. For example, because of the acuity level (extent of illness) of a group of patients, a team leader may "trade" another team leader a nursing assistant for an additional registered nurse. The nursing assistant works on the team with less acutely ill patients, and the team with the sickest patients has an extra registered nurse.

Team nursing enables the team leader to supervise, coordinate, and manage the care given to all the team's patients for the assigned shift. Often the team approach is closer to functional nursing because the team leader delegates without overseeing the care given by team members or patient outcomes. The team leader reports to the head nurse.

Today, team nursing is still used, but the model is usually modified. Many of the patient-focused care models implemented during patient care redesign

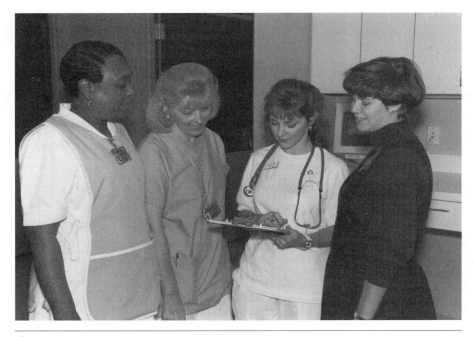

Figure 14–1
Communication and coordination are keys to effective use of team nursing as a model of nursing care delivery. Here team members brief the team leader on their patients (Photo by Kelly Whalen).

use registered nurses as team leaders coordinating care for a group of patients and supervising multiskilled workers who have been trained to perform a variety of comfort measures, such as positioning, and technical procedures, such as taking vital signs or drawing blood.

Case Study: Team Nursing

The team leader for 12 patients on a medical-surgical unit during the night shift has one licensed practical nurse and one certified nursing assistant (CNA) on his team. First, the registered nurse team leader makes visits to all patients' rooms to assess their conditions.

Based on those assessments, he assigns the licensed practical nurse to five patients. Three patients had surgery within the past three or four days and are recovering without complication. The other two have routine conditions.

The nursing assistant is assigned to two patients who are ready for discharge tomorrow, two more who are within two days of discharge, and one newly admitted patient who will have surgery tomorrow.

One patient has had surgery that day and has intravenous fluids as well as a lot of pain. There is a family member spending the night with him. The team leader takes this patient assignment but does not take an overload of patients because he needs the flexibility to assist where needed and to supervise the other team members. During the night, the team leader also develops and updates nursing care plans on all the team's patients.

In team nursing, the registered nurse team leader oversees all care for a particular shift, makes assessments, and documents responses to care. The licensed practical nurse team member provides direct care by performing treatments and procedures and reports patient responses to the team leader. The certified nursing assistant provides routine direct, personal care. If multiskilled, nonlicensed workers are used, the role of the licensed practical nurse or certified nursing assistant is often eliminated.

As with functional nursing, team nursing has both advantages and disadvantages; these are presented in Table 14–2.

Primary Nursing

Developed by Manthey (1980), **primary nursing** was designed to promote the concept of an identified nurse for every patient during the patient's stay on a particular unit. The goal of primary nursing is to deliver consistent, comprehensive care by identifying one nurse who is responsible, has authority, and is accountable for the patient's nursing care outcomes for the period during which the patient is in a unit.

In primary nursing, each newly admitted patient is assigned to a primary nurse. Primary nurses assess their patients, plan their care, and write the plan of care. While on duty they care for their patients and delegate responsibility to associate nurses when they are off duty. Associate nurses may be other registered nurses or licensed practical nurses.

Patients are divided among primary nurses in such a manner that each nurse is responsible for the care of a group of patients 24 hours a day. Unless there is a compelling reason to transfer a patient, the primary nurse cares for the patient in the unit from the time of admission to the time of discharge.

TABLE 14–2
Advantages and Disadvantages of Team Nursing

Advantages

Potential for building team spirit.
Provides comprehensive care.
Each worker's abilities are used to the fullest.
Promotes job satisfaction.
Decreases nonprofessional duties of registered nurses.

Disadvantages

Constant need to communicate among team members is time-consuming.
All must promote teamwork or team nursing is unsuccessful.
Team composition varies from day to day, which can be confusing and disruptive and decreases continuity of care.
May result in blurred role boundaries and resulting confusion and resentment.

These nurses know their patients well and can enjoy a feeling of accomplishment and completion when the patients leave the hospital.

Primary nursing is similar to practice in other professions because there is a continuing relationship between the professional nurse and the patient. It promotes both **autonomy** and **accountability** because one nurse is responsible for all the nursing care for the patient. The primary nurse may be assisted by other care providers (such as other nurses, aides, and technicians) but retains accountability for care outcomes 24 hours a day while the patient is in the unit. Some organizations have implemented the primary care model with registered nurses assuming total care for the patient, thereby eliminating the need for other care providers. The primary nurse communicates effectively with associate nurses caring for the patient on other shifts and with primary nurses in other units when the patient is transferred (e.g., to the operating room and intensive care unit).

Today, primary nursing is still used in a variety of settings. As the restructuring of patient care delivery has occurred, it also has evolved and has been modified. Many of the hospitals using only registered nurses as primary nurses found the cost too great as managed care and lowered reimbursement rates forced organizations to reduce the costs of providing care. Adding non-licensed personnel to assist the registered nurse in a variety of tasks has been widely adopted. Instead of bringing back the nursing assistant role, the newer role of the multiskilled worker was adapted to fit the organizational redesign. The registered nurse may still be the primary nurse but no longer does everything for the patient.

Case Study: Primary Nursing

A primary nurse in a rehabilitation hospital is assigned a new patient. He is a 25-year-old man who sustained a spinal cord injury in a diving accident. He has been in a trauma intensive care unit, and now that his condition has stabilized, he has been transferred. He is paralyzed from the shoulders down.

In addition to providing direct care and writing the care plan, the primary nurse assesses the emotional status of the patient's wife of two months and discovers she has few sources of emotional support and is growing anxious about the future. In addition, the wife feels guilty about her anger and frustration over this dramatic change in their life plans.

The primary nurse acknowledges and discusses these feelings. She explains that patients and family members often have angry feelings under similar circumstances. She refers the couple to a rehabilitation psychologist who works with them in replanning and reprioritizing their life goals.

Primary nursing has several advantages. A major advantage is that owing to the amount of time they spend with patients, primary nurses are in a position to care for the entire person—physically, emotionally, socially, and spiritually. Other advantages and disadvantages of primary nursing are listed in Table 14–3.

Case Management Nursing

The most recent evolution in nursing care delivery systems is **case management nursing.** In many ways, it is a return to the type of nursing practiced before patients were cared for primarily in hospitals. Begun in the late 1980s

TABLE 14–3
Advantages and Disadvantages of Primary Nursing

Advantages

High patient and family satisfaction.
Promotes registered nurse responsibility, authority, and accountability.
Patient knows nurse well, and nurse knows patient well.
Promotes patient-centered decision making.
Increases coordination and continuity of care.
Promotes professionalism.
Promotes job satisfaction and sense of accomplishment for nurses.

Disadvantages

Difficulty hiring all registered nurse staff.
Expensive to pay all registered nurse staff.
Nurses do not know other patients—difficult to "cover" for each other.
May create conflicts between primary and associate nurses.
Stress of round-the-clock responsibility.
Heavy responsibility, especially for new nurses.

as another attempt to improve the cost-effectiveness of patient care, case management ensures that patients receive the services they need from the entire health care team in an efficient manner while holding costs down (Fagin, 1990). In many case management systems, nurses serve in the role of case manager (Interview 14–1).

In 1995 the Case Management Society of America (CMSA) established standards of practice for case management, which have become nationally recognized in defining case management, the functions, settings for services, relationships with patients, and the standards of care and performance. The CMSA has approved the definition of case management as follows:

"a collaborative process which assesses, plans, implements, coordinates, monitors and evaluates options and services to meet an individual's health needs through communication and available resources to promote quality and cost-effective outcomes" (Case Management Society of America, 1995).

Two models of case management nursing have evolved over time. These are characterized by either an "internal" focus, in which the case manager works within a treatment facility, or an "external" approach, in which the case manager oversees patients and the delivery of services over the continuum of an illness or long-term disease. Although different in scope, the principles for both are the same.

Key functions of the case manager role include assessor, planner, facilitator, and advocate. Box 14–1 describes these roles. Key skills for nurses in these roles include critical thinking, communication, advocacy, negotiation, holistic planning and evaluation, and the ability to set both long-term and short-term goals.

INTERVIEW 14-1

Interview with Hiroko Pellom, RN, Director Case Management, and Carlton D. Lancaster, Jr., MD, Medical Consultant, Hamilton Medical Center, Dalton, Georgia.

Interviewer: Why was case management implemented at your hospital?

Pellom: The goal was to improve coordination of the discharge planning and to reduce fragmentation in patient care.

Interviewer: How was the program started?

Pellom: First, the selection of the case managers for this new role was very important. The nurses selected had demonstrated expertise in their clinical knowledge, experience, clinical judgment, and their coordination and communication skills. Secondly, time was invested to enhance relationships with our physicians, since collaboration as a team was critical to success. Thirdly, clinical data collection was a priority, so we provided each case manager with a laptop computer. Then we formed multidisciplinary teams, which included physicians. Over the next one and one-half years we developed and implemented 22 clinical pathways. We also developed patient versions of the pathway to educate patients and their families and to encourage their active participation.

Interviewer: What would you say have been the benefits of clinical pathways in your facility?

Lancaster: Clinical pathways have reduced variation in care, and this was our main goal. In many cases there have been other benefits, including decrease in length of stay and resource utilization, and decrease in time required for the physician to complete orders. Case management is also helping with our disease management programs.

Interviewer: What are your next steps with case management?

Pellom: After we were comfortable with clinical pathways, it was time for us to begin coordinating the care of the high-risk, high-cost patients. We have integrated social workers and the chaplain into the case management department to provide a stronger multidisciplinary team approach. We have also expanded case management into focused areas of disease management, such as asthma, that reaches patients in the community and physician's offices.

Interviewer: How will case management benefit patient care in the future?

Lancaster: As we transition from inpatient clinical pathways to disease management, involving management of care across the continuum, case management will be the clinical core which coordinates this process. We expect to see progressive involvement in quality of care even as we strive to hold down the cost of delivering that care. We feel that combining a patient focused approach with ongoing refinement of our clinical processes will offer improved patient outcomes.

The New England Medical Center and the Center for Case Management in Boston, Massachusetts, developed the internal approach using the nursing case manager to coordinate care for select patients—about 20 percent of the hospital population—whose care is either complex or requires the use of many health care resources (Bower, 1992). These nursing case managers are primary nurses on various units, usually medical-surgical units. They not only care for these patients while on their assigned units but also manage the plans of care from admission to discharge, crossing interdepartmental lines. Although nursing case managers do not physically provide care in all units, they actively collaborate with primary nurses assigned to the patients in those units. This model is similar to the one used by a family practice physician who coordinates medical care for a hospitalized patient but defers to the expertise of a specialist physician if the patient is in the intensive care unit.

In this nursing model, critical paths are used for all patients. A critical path, such as the congestive heart failure CareTrac shown in Appendix B, is an

BOX 14–1
Case Manager Functions

Assessor
- Gathers all relevant data and obtains information by interviewing client/family and performing careful evaluation of the entire situation.
- Evaluates all information related to the current treatment plan objectively and critically to identify barriers, clarify or determine realistic goals and objectives, and seek potential alternatives.

Planner
- Works with client/family to develop a treatment plan that enhances the outcomes and reduces the payer's liability.
- Includes the client/family as the primary decision maker and goal setter.
- Incorporates contingency plans for each step in the process to anticipate treatment and service complications.
- Initiates and implements plan modifications as necessary through monitoring and reevaluation to accommodate changes in treatment or progress.

Facilitator
- Actively promotes communication between all team members, client, family, provider, and all parties involved.
- Collaborates between the client and the health care team to maximize outcomes.
- Coordinates the health delivery process by eliminating unnecessary steps and by promoting timely provision of care.

Advocate
- Incorporates the client's individualized needs and goals throughout the case management process. Supports and educates the client to become empowered and self-reliant in self-advocacy.
- Obtains consensus of all parties to achieve optimal outcomes.
- Promotes early referral to provide optimum care and cost containment.
- Represents the client's best interest through advocacy for necessary funding, treatment alternatives, coordination of health services, and frequent reevaluation of progress and goals.

Reprinted with permission of the Case Management Society of America, 8201 Cantrell Road, Suite 230, Little Rock, Arkansas 72227-2448; www.cmsa.org.

interdisciplinary agreement showing who will provide care in a given time frame to achieve agreed-upon outcomes. The use of critical paths is intended to standardize patient care and allow hospitals to plan staffing levels, lengths of stay, and other factors that heretofore could not be anticipated. Variances in the path are identified. Using continuous quality improvement methodology, health care team members review data periodically to determine if variations are patient induced, staff induced, or system induced. Once identified, they attempt to plan solutions to reduce variances.

The external model of case management nursing began at Carondelet St. Mary's Hospital and Health Center in Tucson, Arizona (Bower, 1992). The nurse case managers spend about 30 percent of their work time in the hospital and 70 percent outside the hospital. Similar to their counterparts in New England, they are partners with their patients. Other similarities include a professional practice model of nursing that uses principles of shared governance, acuity-based billing for nursing care, and salaried, rather than hourly, pay status for the case managers. The nurse case manager in this "multi-setting case management model" is part of a large network (i.e., hospital, clinic, home health agency, long-term care) and may provide services anywhere in the system (Fig. 14–2).

Other case management models may be found in health maintenance organizations (HMOs), managed care organizations (MCOs), third-party payers (e.g., insurance companies), public health departments, physicians' offices, home health agencies, and long-term care facilities. As can be seen from the type of activities in which they engage, case managers do complex and challenging work. Nurses generally need about five years of clinical experience to fill this role effectively. Social workers, psychologists, rehabilitation counselors, or other professionals may also serve as case managers. All case managers, regardless of their discipline, work to reduce the cost of providing services through coordination of providers across the continuum of care.

Case Study: Case Management Nursing

A registered nurse case manager is working with a patient scheduled for a modified mastectomy the following day. He explains the sequence of events to the patient and family and tells them what to expect. He gives the patient and family a tour of the hospital, including the surgical suite and postanesthesia care unit.

As the patient's case manager, he follows the patient after surgery and may or may not provide direct nursing care. He makes sure a "Reach to Recovery" volunteer from the American Cancer Society is called to visit his patient before she leaves the hospital and that she has a follow-up home visit

Figure 14–2
The case management nurse's responsibilities continue following the patient's discharge. This case manager follows up with one of her patients at home (Photo courtesy of Hamilton Medical Center, Dalton, Georgia).

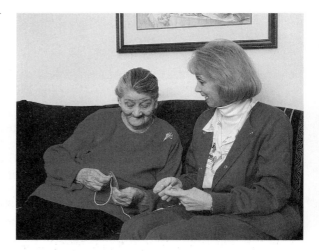

TABLE 14-4
Advantages and Disadvantages of Case Management Nursing

Advantages

Promotes interdisciplinary collaboration.
Increases quality of care.
Cost-effective.
Eases patient's transition from hospital to community services.

Disadvantages

Nurse has increased responsibility.
Requires additional training.
Requires nurses to be off the unit for periods of time.
Time consuming.
Most useful only with high-risk/high-cost/high-volume patients.

---

planned with the volunteer. He talks with the patient's family members, especially her spouse, to help them understand their own feelings and anticipate those of the patient.

Before his patient is discharged, he provides any discharge planning or teaching she may need. He makes sure she has a follow-up appointment scheduled with the surgeon and that she has transportation to the appointment. After she is discharged, he makes a home visit to check on her progress and report back to the physician. If indicated, he refers her to an ongoing support group, such as Y-ME.

Advantages and disadvantages of case management nursing are shown in Table 14–4.

The Patient's Definition of Excellent Nursing Care

It is important for nurses to understand how patients describe quality nursing care. Although patients probably could not name any model of patient care delivery, the levels of practice, the various roles of registered nurses, or nurses' professional accountabilities, they have a clear idea about what they expect from nursing care. While these models and roles provide a framework for practice, it is critical to stay focused on patients' perceptions of what makes a good nurse. The accompanying Research Note describes a study that quantified eight qualities of good nursing as defined by patients.

Differentiating Levels of Practice: An Ongoing Debate

A continuing issue in the delivery of nursing care is differentiating among the levels of nursing practice. Historically, nurses with different levels of education were used interchangeably in hospitals. Nursing graduates qualify for the

---

RESEARCH NOTE

Researcher Laurel Radwin, PhD, RN, an assistant nursing professor at the University of Massachusetts, Lowell, believes that most professionals have a good idea of what constitutes good quality nursing care but that they do not stop to ask patients what they think often enough. Radwin's study quantified eight qualities of good nursing as defined by patients. She interviewed 22 oncology patients, asking them what characteristics make a good nurse. They responded with these eight qualities:

- Attentiveness (promptness).
- Care coordination (communication with other providers).
- Caring.

- Continuity (same nurse as often as possible).
- Individualized care (humanized approach).
- Partnership (shared decision making).
- Professional knowledge (including technical competence).
- Rapport (human connection).

Radwin reported that the effect of quality care was profound. Patients who felt they received excellent care were more optimistic about the future and felt a greater sense of fortitude to fight their illness. The study also found that good nurses inspired a sense of "authenticity," helping the patient feel

comfortable about being honest and open.

The study also demonstrated a change in the type of personal attachment nurses have with their patients. Nurses are no longer trained to maintain a purely clinical relationship with their patients, a change from the days when divulging any personal information was considered unprofessional. Patients appreciate it when nurses have experience that can be related to them.

From Schreiber, C. (1999). A closer look: Patients explain what they think makes excellent nursing. *Nurse Week/Health Week*. June 10. Available from http://www.nurseweek.com/features/99-6/ptswant.html.

---

same license, and in many settings, diploma, associate degree, and baccalaureate nurses all function under the same job description. This sometimes creates a discrepancy between the competencies nurse managers expect of new graduates and their actual competencies.

The goal of **differentiated practice** is to define two levels of practice, implying two levels of education and possibly leading ultimately to two levels of licensure.

Clearly differentiating two levels of practice would promote understanding of nursing practice in terms of technical skills needed to provide care, interpersonal skills needed to facilitate care, and leadership skills needed to manage care. In the mid-1980s, a group of donors, including the Kellogg Foundation, funded the South Dakota Statewide Project for Nursing and Nursing Education, which lasted two years. The project participants differentiated the competencies for the associate degree in nursing (ADN) and the bachelor of science in nursing (BSN) as follows:

> The BSN cares for focal clients who are identified as individuals, families, aggregate, and community groups. The level of responsibility of the BSN is from admission to postdischarge. The unstructured setting is a geographical and/or situational environment that may not have established policies, procedures, and protocols and has the potential for variation requiring independent nursing decisions. The ADN cares for focal clients who are identified as individuals and members of a family. The level of responsibility of the ADN is for a specified work period and is consistent with the identified goals of care. The ADN is prepared to function in a structured health care setting. The struc-

tured setting is a geographical and/or situational environment where the policies, procedures, and protocols for the provision of health care are established and there is recourse to assistance and support from the full scope of nursing expertise (Primm, 1988, p. 2).

Table 14–5 compares selected competencies of nurses with associate degrees in nursing versus those with a bachelor of science in nursing.

Only one state, North Dakota, has adopted a model of differentiated nursing education and practice. There, associate degree nursing graduates are licensed practical nurses and baccalaureate-nursing graduates are registered nurses. Although this model has been in place since the early 1990s, other states have been slow to follow. This is an issue that creates great division within the ranks of nursing itself.

During the 1990s an issue that affected differentiated levels of practice moved to center stage: mutual recognition for licensure. This means that nursing licensure would move from the current single-state model to a system that would be similar to the one used for a driver's license: multistate regulation (MSR). Reasons to change the current system were identified in 1995 through the Pew Task Force on Health Care Work Force Regulation. Since then the National Council of State Boards of Nursing (NCSBN) has evaluated the work of the Pew Task Force and added additional supportive arguments for reform. In 1997 the NCSBN endorsed the mutual recognition model, approved a 10-step implementation model, agreed that no interstate model would be implemented until after January 1, 2000, and that implementation would be contingent on an electronic database and the supporting technology required to support the system. If the mutual recognition model is implemented, it further complicates support for differentiated levels of licensure (Chaffee, 1998).

TABLE 14-5
Comparison of Differentiated ADN and BSN Competencies

Clients

ADN: Individuals and family members
BSN: Individuals, families, aggregate and community groups

Level of Responsibility

ADN: For a specified work period
BSN: From admission to after discharge

Type of Setting

ADN: Structured; other personnel available
BSN: Unstructured; other personnel may not be available

ADN, associate degree in nursing; BSN, bachelor of science in nursing.
From Primm, P. (1987). Differentiated practice for ADN and BSN prepared nurses. *Journal of Professional Nursing,* 3(4), 218–225.

You can read more about the issue of multistate regulation in the *Online Journal of Issues in Nursing* at http://www.nursingworld.org.

Five Professional Accountabilities

Regardless of the setting in which nursing care is delivered or whether differentiated practice becomes a reality, all professional nurses have five **professional accountabilities** for which they are responsible. These accountabilities are practice, quality improvement, research, education, and management and are described in Box 14–2. Each accountability takes on more or less importance depending on the role a nurse assumes in a particular setting. For example, staff nurses' accountabilities are primarily in the areas of clinical practice and quality improvement. They also may have secondary accountabilities in other areas if, for example, they advise managers about management of resources, precept new nurses, or join a research discussion group to learn about research being done by other nurses.

Nurse managers have primary accountability to manage resources so that the clinical staff has what they need to provide care. They also advise the clinical staff in areas of practice and quality improvement. They collaborate with nurse educators on staff orientation and continuing education programs. They may also work with nurse researchers to identify needs for research to define new and better nursing practices.

Novice nurses usually concentrate on the accountabilities central to their jobs. Later, as they gain confidence and competence, they gradually expand their scope to include all five professional accountabilities.

The Nurse's Role on the Health Care Team

Whatever the setting, nurses fulfill a number of roles on the health care team. As the health care delivery system experienced major change during the 1990s, the evolving role of the registered nurse required new competencies and skills in each of the roles described below.

Provider of Care

Nurses provide direct, hands-on care to patients in all health care agencies and settings. As providers, they take an active role in illness prevention and health promotion and maintenance. They offer health screenings, home health services, and an array of health care services in schools, workplaces, churches, clinics, physicians' offices, and other settings. They are instrumental in the high survival rates in trauma centers and newborn intensive care units. Nurses with advanced nursing degrees are increasingly providing care at all levels of the health care system. Managed care has created opportunities for nurses to provide direct care as gatekeepers in primary care settings. Their breadth and depth of knowledge, their ability to care holistically for patients, and their natural partnership with physicians are making them some of the most sought after care providers.

BOX 14–2
Five Professional Accountabilities Inherent in the Role of the Professional Nurse

Practice
- Define standards of care (patient outcomes).
- Define standards of practice (interventions).
- Define standards of performance (job/position descriptions and expectations).
- Management of interdisciplinary collaborative relationships.
- Define career advancement criteria.
- Select and manage the conceptual framework and/or care delivery system.

Quality Improvement
- Develop measurement tools and methods for applying to standards of care, standards of performance, standards of practice, and career advancement.
- Develop and administer the nursing plan for continuous quality improvement referring to the appropriate group or individual for resolution of variances.
- Integrate unit-based quality improvement activities.

Research
- Review the literature for nursing research pertinent to current work environment.
- Identify opportunities for nursing research.
- Develop mechanisms and forums for validating current practice.
- Develop mechanisms for studying ways to improve care through new nursing interventions and/or new ways of applying existing interventions.
- Disseminate information on nursing research to the nursing staff.
- Review requests for nursing research and approve as appropriate, ensuring safety of clients and staff, full disclosure, and minimized risk.

Education (Competency)
- Foster a positive environment for learning and teaching.
- Evaluate need for and develop competency-based educational programs (orientation, inservice, continuing education).
- Measure the outcomes of nursing education programs.
- Manage the relationship between schools of nursing and the care facility.
- Monitor effectiveness of nursing's communication and develop interventions for improvement as needed.
- Recognize that both the individual and the organization have responsibility for ensuring competency.

Management
- Coordinate, allocate, and manage human, fiscal, material, support, information, and system resources needed to deliver care to patients and to foster healthy, productive relationships.

Adapted with permission of Porter O'Grady, T. (1992). *Shared governance implementation manual*. St. Louis: Mosby; Jenkins, J. (1991). Professional governance: The missing link. *Nursing Management*, 22(8), 26–28, 30.

Educator

Nurse educators teach patients and families, the community, other health care team members, students, and businesses. In hospital settings as patient and family educators, nurses provide information about illnesses and teach about medications, treatments, and rehabilitation needs. They also help patients understand how to deal with the life changes necessitated by chronic illnesses (Fig. 14–3) and teach how to adapt care to the home setting when that is required.

In community settings, nurses offer classes in injury and illness prevention and health promotion. Often, these classes are jointly taught with other health care team members. For example, a nutritionist and a nurse may teach a group of expectant parents how to prepare formula and feed their infants. School settings offer opportunities for nurses to fulfill aspects of several roles inherent in professional practice, as illustrated in the accompanying News Note. Nurses also have a responsibility to understand and teach how a healthful or unhealthful environment may affect both the short-term and long-term health of the community.

Another community setting for nurse educators is parish nursing. Discussed in Chapter 5, parish nursing has grown to become a discipline that offers educational opportunities with a holistic emphasis in a setting that is ideal for ongoing education.

Nurses are often the key educators on the health care team. They teach other team members about the patient and family and why different interventions may have varying degrees of success. Nurses help other team members find cost-effective, quality interventions that are desired and needed by

Figure 14–3
In the role of teacher, this nurse educates a newly diagnosed diabetic patient about insulin self-administration (From Lindeman, C. A., and McAuthie, M. (1999): Fundamentals of Nursing Practice (p. 229) Philadelphia, Penn.: W. B. Saunders).

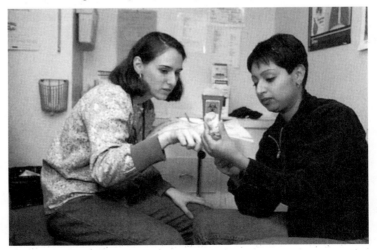

NEWS NOTE

"Nurse Honored, Helps Pregnant Students"

Keeping pregnant teenagers in school is Ann Richey's goal, but it isn't achieved by following a pat formula. Mrs. Richey is a Hamilton County school nurse who serves the system's three Teen Learning Centers and three other schools that have parent support groups.

She was named Nurse of the Year by the Tennessee Association of School Nurses in recognition of her excellence in school nursing practice and leadership in school health. Her specific jobs include talking to classes about issues related to adolescent pregnancy and health issues, doing health assessments and home visits and participating in WIC (Women, Infants and Children program) and immunization clinics for teen mothers and their infants.

Not all Mrs. Richey's work is directed at teenage parents or parents-to-be. She sees other students if the need arises. "Sometimes I see 20 or 30 people in a day and I have to make judgments," she said. And she finds herself juggling a variety of things all at once.

Reprinted with permission of McDonald, E., *Chattanooga Times/Free Press*, June 8, 1999, B1.

the patient rather than wasting resources on ineffective, inefficient, undesired, or unneeded services.

Nurses also serve as teachers of the next generation of nurses. Nursing students need educators who set high standards and ideals and who help students understand the ethical choices that all health care providers must make.

As discussed in Chapter 13, the Internet is transforming the access and dissemination of information. Nurses can play an important role in assisting patients to use the Internet as an enhancement to traditional education. "Nursing is about information and the transmission of that information from professional to healthcare consumer. There's an increasing number of information resources on the Internet that provide far more current information than we're seeing in the literature", said Carol Bickford, RN, MS, a certified informatics nurse with the American Nurses Association. "To become Internet savvy, nurses don't need to be informatics specialists. They just need to learn to surf the Net," she said during a recent interview. Tips from the experts for referring patients to the Internet are found in Box 14–3.

Counselor

People who experience illness or injury often have strong emotional responses. It is clear that the relationships among the emotions, the mind, and the body are critical to promotion of and restoration to health. As counselors, nurses provide basic counseling and support to patients and their families.

Using therapeutic communication techniques, nurses encourage people to discuss their feelings, to explore possible options and solutions to their unique problems, and to choose for themselves the best alternatives for action. They also serve as bereavement counselors to terminally ill patients and

BOX 14-3
Referring Patients to the Internet: Advice from the Experts

- Familiarize yourself with Internet resources in your field.
- Refer patients to sites you know have reputable information.
- Caution patients to consider the source before believing online information.
- Encourage patients to print out what they find and bring it to their next appointment.
- Answer patients' questions about information they've gleaned from the Web.
- Advise patients not to make decisions based solely on what they've read in cyberspace.

From Federwisch, A. (1999). Plugged in: Point your patients to the Web for health information. *NurseWeek/HealthWeek*, 5/27/99. Available from http://www.nurseweek.com/features/99-5/webuse.html.

their families. Nurses may, with advanced education and certification, provide psychotherapy services that extend beyond the basic counseling role.

The nurse's role as counselor often overlaps with the roles of social workers, psychiatrists, spiritual advisers, and mental health specialists. Because nurses spend more time with patients than these other professionals, they have opportunities to respond to the emotional needs of patients as they occur.

Manager

The effective management of nursing resources is essential. With budgets ranging from hundreds of thousands to many million dollars, nurse managers of patient care units in hospitals manage "businesses" larger than many small companies. Nurse managers must have strong leadership, financial, marketing, system design, outcome research, and organizational behavior skills.

Chief nurse executives may manage more than 1,000 employees and multimillion-dollar budgets. They interact with other top executives and community leaders, often sitting on the health care organization's board of directors. Nurse executives must ensure the quality of nursing care within financial, regulatory, and legislative constraints. As noted in Chapter 13, nurses frequently serve as patient care executives, chief operating officers, and chief executive officers.

In their daily work, all nurses are managers. The bedside staff nurse must manage the care of a group of patients and decide priorities, which staff members to assign to patients, and how to accomplish all the activities during an 8- or 12-hour period. Nurses are also involved in case management or managed care. In this role, nurses review patient cases and coordinate services so that quality care can be achieved at the lowest cost.

Researcher

As discussed in Chapter 12, whether or not research is a nurse's primary responsibility, all nurses should be involved in nursing research. Nurse researchers investigate whether current or potential nursing actions achieve their expected outcomes, what options for care may be available, and how best to provide care. Nursing research looks at patient outcomes, the nursing process, and the systems that support nursing services.

Outcome research has become an integral part of the health care delivery system. Managed care organizations and regulatory agencies require outcome data related to quality of care, which requires research by nurses. Participation by all nurses in research is essential to the growth and development of the nursing profession.

Collaborator

With so many health care workers involved in providing patient care, **collaboration** among the professions is important. The collaborator role is an important one for nurses to ensure that everyone agrees on the same patient outcomes. Multidisciplinary teams require collaborative practice, and nurses play key roles as both team members and team leaders. Collaboration requires that nurses understand and appreciate what other health professionals have to offer. They must also be able to interpret to others the nursing needs of patients. More about collaboration with professional colleagues is in Chapter 18.

An often-overlooked collaborative function of nurses is collaboration with patients and families. Involving patients and their families in the plan of care from the beginning is the best way to ensure their cooperation, enthusiasm, and willingness to work toward the best patient outcomes.

Change Agent (Intrapreneur)

When changes are needed in the nursing system, nurses themselves can serve as agents of change. Most professional nursing education programs include change theory as part of their management courses, and graduates are prepared to become change agents in their work settings. The role of change agent is one that requires a combination of tact, energy, creativity, and interpersonal skills. Change is often resisted, particularly if people are comfortable with the "old way" and believe it works. The role of **change agent** within a health care organization has been dubbed *intrapreneurship* (Manion, 1990) in the belief that it requires the same kind of initiative and risk taking that entrepreneurship requires (Box 14–4).

Entrepreneur

Nurse **entrepreneurs** are becoming more common. As you learned in Chapter 5, nurses now have businesses of their own that provide direct patient services in hospitals, community settings, businesses, schools, homes, and many

BOX 14-4

Self-Assessment: How Intrapreneurial Are You?

If you answer "yes" to more of these questions than you answer "no," you have the personality characteristics to become an intrapreneur.

- Do you like to spend time thinking of ways to make things work better?
- Are you willing to take risks that you view as reasonable?
- Do you enjoy ambiguity because it stimulates your creativity?
- Do you think of new ideas while driving to work, taking a shower, or exercising?
- When you have a new idea, can you visualize the steps to take to get it done?
- Do you have more energy than most people you know?
- Do you like the challenge of new tasks and projects?
- Are you willing to work extremely hard at problems or tasks when you believe you can make a difference in how they turn out?
- Are you good at influencing others to accept new ways of doing things?
- Do you have a good sense of humor? Can you laugh at yourself?
- Do you like to consider the possibilities rather than the limitations in a situation?
- Can you mobilize the necessary resources (time, energy, people, and materials) when a job needs to be done?
- Can you work collaboratively with others on your ideas?
- Do you learn from your failures?
- Have you found ways to give yourself positive feedback so you are less reliant on the feedback of others?

Adapted with permission of Manion, J. (1991). Nurse intrapreneurs: The heroes of health care's future. *Nursing Outlook*, 39(1), 18–21.

other settings. Nurse entrepreneurs provide consultation and education services to nurses and other health team members. They provide services to businesses by conducting work site wellness programs and by advising human resource staff on how to provide high-quality health benefits to employees while reducing costs.

Patient Advocate

Rules and regulations designed to help a complex hospital run efficiently can often get in the way of a patient's treatment, and an impersonal health care system frequently infringes on the patient's rights.

Health care institutions often have special positions for **patient advocates.** Nurses who occupy these positions know how to cut through the levels of bureaucracy and red tape and will stand up for the patient's rights, advocating his best interests at all times. They must value patient self-determination, that is, patient independence and decision making. In this role, nurses sometimes help patients bend the rules when it is in the patient's best interests and doing so will harm no one else. Patient advocates are nurses who re-

---

BOX 14–5
Nursing Roles

- Provider of care
- Teacher
- Counselor
- Manager
- Researcher

- Collaborator
- Change agent
- Entrepreneur
- Patient advocate

---

alize that policies are important and govern most situations well but occasionally can, and should, be broken. For example, special care units often have strict visiting hours. Family members may be allowed in to see the patient for only 10 minutes each hour. If a patient's recovery will be faster if the family is present, the nurse, serving as a patient advocate, will allow the family members more generous visitation than the policy provides. Whether or not a nurse is employed as a patient advocate, every nurse should advocate for patients daily. Box 14–5 lists roles nurses fulfill.

Nursing Organization Governance Structure

In most health care agencies, nurses have a nursing staff organization. In some settings it serves mainly as a communication vehicle. In other more enlightened settings, nurses are expected to govern themselves through the organization, much as the medical staff is expected to govern itself through the medical staff organization. The concept of **shared governance** is founded on the philosophy that employees have both a right and a responsibility to govern their own work and time within a financially secure, patient-centered system. Nursing has led the way and been the most successful in implementing the shared governance model. This structure consists of councils that are modeled after the five professional accountabilities discussed earlier and five of the core roles of a professional nurse—manager, educator, researcher, care giver, and evaluator.

There is a management council made up of the chief nurse executive and the chairpersons of four subcouncils (clinical practice council, education council, research council, and quality council). The management council establishes management practices, sets broad goals and objectives, oversees resources, and facilitates communication about nursing's vision. This group also ensures that successes are shared and that learning rather than punishment is the result of risk taking.

The other councils have the responsibility, authority, and accountability within their designated areas—clinical, research, education, and quality of practice—for setting the standards, policies, procedures, and behaviors necessary for nurses to carry on their work. Each council works closely with the others to ensure that decisions are well thought out. At the patient care unit level, a unit committee (or council) is elected by the staff to represent all jobs and shifts on that unit. This group is authorized to translate the organizational council decisions at the unit level.

Shared governance promotes decentralization and participation at all levels in nursing. This form of organizational structure in nursing has been successful in improving patient outcomes and enhancing job satisfaction among nurses.

Team-Building Skills

For years nurses have tried to implement care teams that included all disciplines providing care to a particular patient and that would discuss, agree on, and deliver complex care. Too often, nurses were frustrated in their attempts by a variety of problems: a lack of skill in developing and managing teams, a lack of incentive for other health care team members to participate, and a failure of the system to sanction, support, create, and encourage opportunities for this type of team work.

Figure 14–4
This multidisciplinary team is trained to stop the progression of strokes and rehabilitate stroke patients. The team includes paramedics, nurses, care managers, imaging technologists, laboratory technologists, physical therapists, chaplains, neurologists, emergency physicians, and volunteers. The nurse is required to use all his or her team building skills to work successfully with the group (Courtesy of Memorial Hospital, Chattanooga, Tennessee).

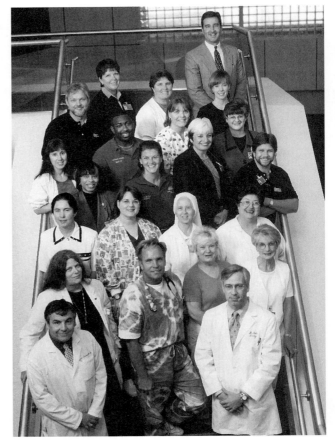

Because of the emphasis on continuous quality improvement, re-engineering, restructuring, and changing reimbursement patterns, nurses now find themselves at the center of interdisciplinary teams. Nurses managing interdisciplinary teams must know how to manage people as equals and not as subordinates because other team members are frequently experts in their fields (radiology technicians, physicians, social workers, physical therapists, or laboratory technicians, for example). Nurses must be prepared to participate both as leaders and as members of these teams and to assume and relinquish the leadership role to meet best the needs of patients and the team.

Managing this diverse group requires tact, diplomacy, a genuine respect for the contribution of each team member, flexibility, and the ability to "think outside the box." The last-mentioned quality is demonstrated when a person's mind is open to solutions that are nontraditional and challenge current thinking and practice. For many nurses who have fought hard for their "turf," sharing it with others is intimidating. For others, it is a freeing experience that permits them to experience truly collaborative relationships on equal footing with other professionals (Fig. 14–4).

Leaders in health care organizations have recognized that special leadership training is necessary for employees to assume both leadership and team member roles on multidisciplinary teams. Training is often provided in several sessions to equip participants with the understanding of what it takes to

---

BOX 14–6

Key Components in Highly Effective Teams

- Team goals are as important as individual goals; members are able to recognize when a personal agenda is interfering with the team's direction.
- The team understands the goals and is committed to achieving them; everyone is willing to shift responsibilities.
- The team climate is comfortable and informal, people feel empowered, individual competitiveness is inappropriate.
- Communication is spontaneous and shared among all members; diversity of opinions and ideas are encouraged.
- Respect, open-mindedness, and collaboration are high; members seek win/win solutions and build on each other's ideas.
- Trust replaces fear, and people feel comfortable taking risks; direct eye contact and spontaneous expression are present.
- Conflicts and differences of opinion are considered opportunities to explore new ideas; the emphasis is on finding common ground.
- The team works on improving itself constantly by examining its procedures, processes, and practices and experimenting with change.
- Leadership is rotated; no one person dominates.
- Decisions are made by consensus and have the acceptance and support of members.

From Harrington-Macklin, D. (1994). *The Team Building Tool Kit*. New York: American Management Association, p. 21.

develop a successful team. Training includes how to structure meetings, rules of conduct, use of the tools available in data gathering and decision making, and conflict resolution. Box 14–6 identifies the characteristics that are necessary for a highly effective team.

Summary of Key Points

- There are a number of systems of nursing care delivery, each of which has advantages and disadvantages.
- Functional nursing is task oriented, often impersonal, but efficient.
- Team nursing makes use of the skills of team members, who are assigned as a team to care for a group of patients.
- Primary nursing promotes the concept of having an identified nurse for every patient.
- Case management nursing involves collaboration between nurse and patient and coordination of services to meet health needs in a cost-effective manner.
- There are many variations and combinations of the major nursing care delivery systems in use today.
- Satisfaction or frustration can result from the match between nurses' expectations and the system of care in use in the employing agency.
- When interviewing for a position, nurses must assess the delivery system carefully to make sure it is congruent with their values about nursing practice.
- Nurses use a variety of roles, such as provider of care, teacher, counselor, manager, researcher, collaborator, change agent, and patient advocate in meeting patients' needs.
- As members of interdisciplinary care teams, nurses are often in leadership roles.
- n An understanding of team building skills is critical to working effectively with interdisciplinary teams.

Critical Thinking Questions

1. Compare and contrast the four types of nursing care delivery systems from the viewpoint of the patient. If you were a consumer of nursing care, which system would you prefer? Why?
2. Look at the same question from the standpoint of the nurse. Which system would you find most satisfying in terms of your practice? Which would you like least?
3. Talk to a practicing nurse and find out which systems he or she has used to deliver care. What were the strong and weak points?
4. Interview nurses in practice in your community to determine how they apply the five professional accountabilities on a daily basis. Which roles emphasize different accountabilities?
5. From your own experiences as a consumer of nursing care, identify all the nursing roles you have encountered. Share these with at least one classmate.

6. If possible, interview nurses from different countries. How does their approach to providing nursing care differ from nursing in the United States? In what ways is it similar?

Web Resource

Case Management Society of America, http://www.cmsa.org

Health-related web sites, http://www.nurseweek.com/features/99-5/webuse.html

Mutual recognition updates, http://www.ncsbn.org/files/mutual/mrnews.asp

Online Journal of Issues in Nursing, http://www.nursingworld.org

References

Bernhard, L. A., and Walsh, M. (1990). *Leadership: The key to the professionalism of nursing.* (2nd ed.) St. Louis: Mosby.

Bower, F. A. (1992). *Case management by nurses.* Washington, D. C.: American Nurses Publishing.

Chaffee, M. (1998). Changes proposed for RN licenses. *Pediatric Nursing,* 24(1/2), 75–77.

Case Management Society of America (1995). *Standards of practice for case management* (pp. 8–12). Little Rock, Ark.: Case Management Society of America.

Fagin, C. M. (1990). Nursing's value proves itself. *American Journal of Nursing,* 90(10), 17–30.

Federwisch, A. (1999). Plugged in: Point your patients to the Web for health information. *NurseWeek/HealthWeek,* 5/27/99. Available from http://www.nurseweek.com/features/99-5/webuse.html.

Friese, C. G., Flevrant, S., Sanders, S., Hilman, B., Ulmen, K. T. (1998). Nursing council coordination within decentralization. *Nursing Management,* 29(3), 40–41.

Harrington-Mackin, D. (1994). *The team building tool kit.* New York: American Management Association.

Lambertson, E. (1953). *Nursing team organization and functioning.* New York: Columbia University.

McDonald, E. (1999). Nurse honored; Helps pregnant students. *Chattanooga Times/Chattanooga Free Press,* June 8, B1.

Manion, J. (1990). *Change from within: Nurse intrapreneurs as health care innovators.* Kansas City, Mo.: American Nurses Association.

Manthey, M. (1980). *The practice of primary nursing.* Boston: Blackwell Scientific Publications.

Porter O'Grady, T. (1992). *Shared governance implementation manual.* St. Louis: Mosby.

Primm, P. L. (1987). Differentiated practice for ADN and BSN prepared nurses. *Journal of Professional Nursing,* 3(4), 218–225.

Primm, P. L. (1988). Differentiated nursing care management/patient care delivery system. *Kansas Nurse,* (April, 1988), 2.

Schreiber, C. (1999). A closer look: Patients explain what they think makes excellent nursing. *Nurse Week/Health Week,* 6/10/99. Available from http://www.nurseweek.com/features/99/ptswant.html.

Critical Thinking, the Nursing Process, and Clinical Judgment

Kay K. Chitty[*]

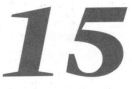

Key Terms

Affective Goal
Analysis
Assessment
Clinical Judgment
Cognitive Goal
Consultation
Critical Path
Defining Characteristics
Dependent Intervention
Evaluation
Implementation
Independent Intervention
Interdependent Intervention
Long-Term Goal
North American Nursing
    Diagnosis Association
    (NANDA)
Nursing Diagnosis
Nursing Intervention Classification
    (NIC)
Nursing Order
Nursing Outcome Classification
    (NOC)

Nursing Process
Objective Data
Outcome Criteria
Patient Interview
Planning
Primary Source
Protocol
Psychomotor Goal

Reflective Thinking
Secondary Source
Short-Term Goal
Signs
Subjective Data
Symptoms
Tertiary Source

Learning Outcomes

After studying this chapter, students will be able to:

- Define critical thinking in nursing.
- Contrast the characteristics of "novice thinking" with those of "expert thinking."
- Explain the purpose and phases of the nursing process.
- Differentiate between nursing orders and medical orders.
- Explain the differences between independent, interdependent, and dependent nursing actions.
- Describe evaluation and its importance in the nursing process.
- Define clinical judgment in nursing practice.
- Develop a personal plan to use in developing sound clinical judgment.

Almost every nurse-patient encounter is an opportunity for the nurse to assist the patient in moving to a higher level of wellness. Whether or not this actually happens depends in large measure on the nurse's ability to think critically about the patient's particular needs and how best to meet them. It also depends on the nurse's ability to use a reliable problem-solving approach that leads to sound clinical decisions about the patient's priority nursing needs. Underlying this admittedly simplistic description is the assumption that patients are not passive recipients of nursing care but active participants in care to the extent of their ability.

[*] The author wishes to acknowledge the contributions of Barbara Norwood to earlier editions of this chapter.

This chapter explores several important approaches to thinking and decision making in nursing: critical thinking, the nursing process, and clinical judgment.

Critical Thinking in Nursing

The ability to think critically can be learned. It involves paying attention to how one thinks and making thinking itself a focus of concern. A nurse who is exercising critical thinking asks, "What assumptions have I made about this patient?" "How do I know my assumptions are accurate?" "Do I need any additional information?" and "How might I look at this situation differently?" Nurses just beginning to pay attention to their thinking processes may ask these questions after nurse-patient interactions *have ended.* This is known as **reflective thinking.** After practice, however, nurses can learn to examine their thinking processes *during* the interaction as they learn to "think on their feet."

Critical thinking in nursing involves more than good problem-solving strategies. It is a complex process that has specific characteristics that make it different from run-of-the-mill problem solving. Critical thinking in nursing involves a purposeful, disciplined process, consciously developed, to improve patient outcomes. It is motivated by the needs of the patient and family, and determined in part by elements of the scientific method. Critical thinking in nursing is undergirded by the standards and ethics of the profession. Nurses who think critically seek to build on patients' strengths while honoring patients' values and beliefs (Alfaro-LeFevre, 1999). They are engaged in a process of constant evaluation, redirection, improvement, and increased efficiency. Box 15–1 summarizes these characteristics.

BOX 15–1

Characteristics of Critical Thinking in Nursing

- Is purposeful, disciplined, and consciously developed.
- Improves patient outcomes.
- Is motivated by patient needs.
- Builds on knowledge, skill, and experience.
- Utilizes informed intuition and the scientific method.
- Is undergirded by standards and ethics.
- Builds on patient strengths.
- Honors patient values and beliefs.
- Is continuously evaluated and improved.
- Increases efficiency.

From Alfaro-LeFevre, R. (1999). *Critical thinking in nursing.* Philadelphia: W. B. Saunders.

In other chapters you read about Dr. Patricia Benner (1984), who studied the differences in expertise of nurses at different stages in their careers, from novice to expert. So it is with critical thinking; novices think differently than experts. Novices tend to act as soon as they recognize a pattern, while experts may spend time gathering more information before acting, recognizing that other patterns may emerge. For example, when confronted with a patient who has not voided postoperatively, the novice might want to intervene by catheterizing. The expert, before intervening, may palpate the patient's suprapubic area for distention, check the chart to see how much intravenous fluid the patient has received, assess the amount of vomiting, if any, and determine how long the patient was kept on a nothing by mouth (NPO) order prior to surgery before considering catheterization. Box 15–2 summarizes the differences in novice and expert thinking.

The Nursing Process in Historical Perspective

The **nursing process** is a method used by nurses in solving patient problems in professional practice. It is an outgrowth of the scientific method and can be used as a framework for approaching almost any problem. Yura and Walsh (1983) defined the nursing process as "a designated series of actions intended to fulfill the purposes of nursing—to maintain the patient's wellness—and, if this state changes, to provide the amount and quality of nursing care the situation demands to direct the patient back to wellness." They continued to state that, "if wellness cannot be achieved, then [the purpose of the nursing process is] to contribute to the patient's quality of life, maximizing his resources as long as life is a reality" (p. 71).

A simple example of using a process approach to problem solving is illustrated by examining a daily decision that you and most other people face every day: how to dress for the day. Before putting on your clothes, there are several factors you need to consider. What is the expected temperature? Will it be clear, raining, or snowing? How much time will be spent outdoors? Are there any activities planned that require special dress? Next, you probably look at the possible clothing choices. Some clothes may be out of season, and others need repairs, are too dressy or casual, or don't fit quite right. After considering the environmental factors, the day's activities, and your mood, you select the day's clothing. After dressing, you may look in a mirror to evaluate how you look. You may then modify your outfit based on your image in the mirror. At this point, you have solved the problem of clothing yourself. You have identified a problem, considered various factors related to the problem, identified possible actions, selected the best alternative, evaluated the success of the alternative selected, and made adjustments to the solution based on the evaluation. This is the same general process nurses use in solving patient problems through the nursing process.

For individuals outside the profession, nursing is commonly defined in terms of what nurses do (i.e., give injections). Even within the profession, the

BOX 15–2
Novice Thinking Compared with Expert Thinking

Novice Nurses	*Expert Nurses*
Knowledge is organized as separate facts. Must rely heavily on resources (texts, notes, preceptors). Lack knowledge gained from actually doing (e.g., listening to breath sounds).	Knowledge is highly organized and structured, making recall of information easier. Have a large storehouse of experiential knowledge (e.g., what abnormal breath sounds sound like, what subtle changes look like).
Focus so much on *actions*, they tend to forget to *assess* before acting.	*Assess* and think things through before *acting*.
Need clear cut rules.	Know when to bend the rules.
Are often hampered by unawareness of resources.	Are aware of resources and how to use them.
Are often hindered by anxiety and lack of self-confidence.	Are usually more self-confident, less anxious, and therefore more focused.
Must be able to rely on step-by-step procedures. Tend to focus more on *procedures* than on the *patient response* to the procedure.	Know when it's safe to skip steps or do two steps together. Are able to focus on both the parts (the procedures) and the whole (the patient response).
Become uncomfortable if patient needs preclude performing procedures exactly as they were learned.	Comfortable with rethinking procedure if patient needs require modification of the procedure.
Have limited knowledge of suspected problems; therefore, they question and collect data more superficially.	Have a better idea of suspected problems, allowing them to question more deeply and collect more relevant and indepth data.
Tend to follow standards and policies by rote.	Analyze standards and policies, looking for ways to improve them.
Learn more readily when matched with a supportive, knowledgeable preceptor or mentor.	Are challenged by novices' questions, clarifying their own thinking when teaching novices.

From Alfaro-LeFevre, R. (1999). *Critical thinking in nursing.* Philadelphia: W. B. Saunders. Reprinted with permission.

intellectual basis of nursing practice was not articulated until the 1960s, when nursing educators and leaders began to identify and name the components of nursing's intellectual processes. This marked the beginning of the nursing process.

During the 1970s and 1980s, debate about the use of the term *diagnosis* began. Up until that time, diagnosing was considered to be within the sphere of practice of physicians only. Nurses were not supposed to diagnose patients. All this began to change in 1973 when the National Group for the Classification of Nursing Diagnosis, now called the **North American Nursing Diagnosis Association (NANDA)** published its first list of nursing diagnoses. The purpose of this group was (and is) to identify terminology and definitions that may be used and tested as nursing diagnoses.

The nursing process as a method of clinical problem solving is taught in nurse curricula across the United States, and many states refer to it in their nursing practice acts. The operations of the nursing process are described in detail in the American Nurses Association's (ANA) *Standards of Clinical Nursing Practice* (1998), which serves as the profession's guide to a national standard of care. It was once so widely accepted that the Joint Commission on the Accreditation of Healthcare Organizations (JCAHO) expected there to be evidence in each patient's record that nurses used the elements of the nursing process as the basis for clinical decision making (Joint Commission on Accreditation of Healthcare Organizations, 1992). The emphasis of the JCAHO has now shifted to the multidisciplinary approach (1997), however, which many facilities find more accurately reflected by critical paths.

In recent years some nursing leaders have questioned the use of the nursing process, describing it as linear, rigid, and mechanistic. While it can be taught, learned, and used in that manner, it can also be used as a creative approach to thinking and decision making in nursing. Since the nursing process is an integral aspect of nursing education and practice nationwide, learning to use it as a dynamic approach to patient care and a tool for critical thinking is a worthwhile endeavor.

If you are a beginning student wondering about the value of the nursing process, read the letter in Box 15–3. It is from a student nearing graduation and describes her thoughts about the nursing process and how they have changed since she first began using it. If you are a registered nurse who has returned to school to pursue a bachelor's degree, read this chapter's Research Note to find out how other nurses feel about the nursing process.

The ANA's 1995 revision of *Nursing's Social Policy Statement* includes the following statements (p. 9):

> Nurses identify the human responses to actual or potential health problems they observe and name their conceptualization of the diagnosis using a variety of classification systems. Diagnoses facilitate communication among health care providers and the recipients of care and provide for initial direction in choice of treatments and subsequent evaluation of the outcomes of care.

The *Statement* goes on to describe nursing assessments, interventions, and evaluation of outcomes—all of which are phases in the nursing process. In spite of debate within and outside the profession about its usefulness, the nursing process remains a cornerstone of nursing practice and should be well understood by every nurse.

BOX 15-3
Letter to Beginning Nursing Students

Dear Nursing Students:

I recall sitting in my first nursing class wondering how long my professor would lecture about the "nursing process." I didn't want to learn about problem-solving techniques. I didn't want to get bogged down in all the time-consuming paperwork. I wanted to save lives. You know what I mean—I was only interested in learning about the diseases, traumas, and surgeries I was sure I would be dealing with on a daily basis. What was all this assess, diagnose, plan, etc., stuff? I was impatient to be finished with this material and thought that once I got through the exam covering the nursing process, I would be home free. I was so naive!

I can also remember the day I realized that the nursing process had become as natural to me as walking and talking. It was during my acute care rotation when I walked into a patient's room to find him experiencing respiratory difficulty. I immediately assessed the patient and began to take steps to alleviate his distress. I admit I felt a little anxious, yet I was able to take the necessary steps to bring the situation under control. If not for my knowledge of the nursing process, I am positive that I would have been unable to organize my thoughts and actions in an efficient manner while under pressure.

So my message to you is this: Relax and don't resist learning the nursing process. I guarantee this tool will help you feel more self-confident and better able to organize your time and thoughts.

Good Luck!

At the time this was written, Elizabeth Baird was a senior nursing student at The University of Tennessee, Chattanooga (Courtesy of Elizabeth Baird).

RESEARCH NOTE

What do nurses who provide direct patient care have to say about the nursing process? This question was posed by Patricia A. Martin and five of her colleagues as they conducted a multifaceted study of the use of the nursing process. A survey instrument entitled the "Dayton Attitude Scale toward Care Planning" was developed and sent to more than 3,000 nurses practicing in nine acute care hospitals in midwestern metropolitan areas.

A total of 1,096 surveys were returned. Statistical analysis of the surveys revealed that a relatively positive attitude existed toward the nursing process and nursing diagnosis. Nurses with a bachelor of science in nursing and nurses who had been practicing longer had higher positive attitudes than other nurses. The most common barrier to using the nursing process was lack of time, with 30 percent stating that they did not like the way care planning was done in their facility. The study suggests that improving the systems for implementing care planning would increase both the use of and positive attitudes toward the nursing process.

Adapted with permission of Martin, P., Dugan, J., Freundl, M., Miller, S., Phillips, R., and Sharritts, L. (1994). Nurses' attitudes toward nursing process as measured by the Dayton Attitude Scale. *The Journal of Continuing Education in Nursing,* 25(1), 35–39.

Phases of the Nursing Process

As in the scientific method, a series of steps is involved in the nursing process. Identifying phases makes the process clear and concrete but can cause nurses to use them rigidly. Keep in mind that this is a process, that progression through the process may not be linear, and that it is a tool to use, not a road map to slavishly follow. For example, if a newly hospitalized patient is experiencing a great deal of pain, the expert nurse would realize that performing an initial assessment under those circumstances would not contribute to the patient's well-being and would instead reposition, massage, or administer medication first.

Phase 1: Assessment

Assessment is the beginning phase in the nursing process. During this phase, information or data about the individual patient, family, or community are gathered. Data may include physiological, psychological, sociocultural, developmental, spiritual, and environmental information. The patient's available financial or material resources also need to be assessed and recorded in a standard format; each institution usually has a slightly different instrument for recording assessment data.

Types of Data

There are two types of data that nurses obtain about patients: subjective and objective. **Subjective data** are obtained from patients as they describe their needs, feelings, strengths, and perceptions of the problem. Subjective data are frequently referred to as **symptoms.** Examples of subjective data are statements such as, "I am in pain" and "I don't have much energy." The source for these data can be only the patient. Subjective data should include physical, psychosocial, and spiritual information. Subjective data can be very private. Nurses must be sensitive to the patient's need for confidence in the nurse's trustworthiness.

The second type of patient data is **objective data.** These are data that the nurse obtains through observation, examination, or consultation with other health care providers. These data are factual, not colored by patients' perceptions, and include patient behaviors observed by the nurse. Objective data are frequently called **signs.** An example of objective data that a nurse might gather includes the observation that the patient, who is lying in bed, is diaphoretic, pale, and tachypneic and holding his hand to his chest.

Objective data and subjective data usually are congruent; that is, they usually are in agreement. In the situation just mentioned, if the patient told the nurse, "I feel like a rock is sitting on my chest," the subjective data would substantiate the nurse's observations (objective data) that the patient is having chest pain. There are times, however, when subjective and objective data are in conflict. An example of incongruent subjective and objective data would be an emaciated teenager stating, "I'm too fat." In this example, the conflict reveals a perceptual error by the patient.

Sources of Patient Data

Patient data can be obtained from many sources (Fig. 15–1). The patient is considered the only **primary source.** Sources of data such as the nurse's own observations or reports of family and friends of the patient are considered **secondary sources. Tertiary sources** of data include medical records and information gathered from other health care providers such as physical therapists, physicians, or dietitians.

Methods of Collecting Patient Data

A number of methods are used when collecting patient data. An important one is the **patient interview.** This usually involves a face-to-face interaction with the patient and requires the nurse to use the skills of interviewing, observation, and listening. The environment in which the interaction occurs or other internal and external factors can influence the amount and the type of data obtained. For example, when interviewing a patient who is having difficulty breathing, the verbal data obtained by the interview may be limited, but observation and listening can reveal much about the patient's condition. Likewise, if an interview takes place in a cold, noisy, or public place, the type of data obtained may be affected.

A second method of obtaining data is through **consultation.** Consultation is discussing patient needs with health care workers and others who are di-

Figure 15–1
Patient data come from primary, secondary, and tertiary sources.

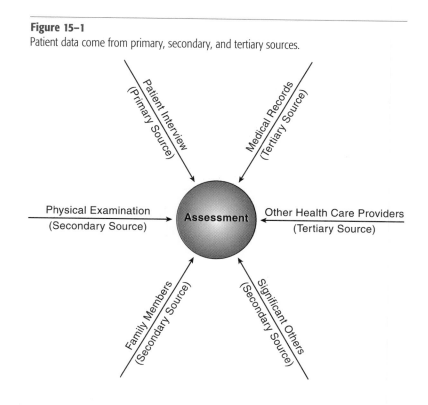

rectly involved in the care of the patient. Nurses also consult with patients' families to obtain background information and their perceptions about the patients' needs. Physical examination is the third method for obtaining data. Nurses utilize physical assessment techniques of inspection, auscultation, percussion, and palpation to obtain these data (Fig. 15–2).

Organizing Patient Data

Once patient data have been collected, they must be sorted or organized. A number of methods have been developed to assist nurses in organizing patient data. They include Abdellah's 21 nursing problems, Henderson's 14 nursing problems, Yura and Walsh's human needs approach, and Gordon's 11 functional health patterns. Contemporary nursing theorists continue to develop other organizing frameworks, including those of Madeleine Leininger, Sister Callista Roy, Dorothy Orem, and others (Marriner-Tomey, 1994). Nurses choose different methods of organizing patient data depending on personal preference and the method used in the agencies where they are employed.

Confidentiality of Patient Data

A word of caution is needed in regard to patient data. Earlier, it was mentioned that patients confide personal information to nurses only if they believe the nurse is trustworthy. Patients need to know and trust that nurses

Figure 15–2
Physical examination is one source of objective assessment data (Photo courtesy of Hamilton Medical Center, Dalton, Georgia).

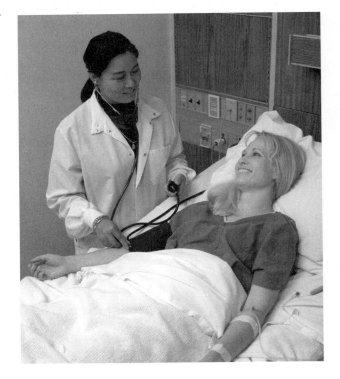

share such information only with the other treatment team members. Nurses must respect patients' privacy rights and should never discuss patient information with anyone who does not have a work-related need to know.

A complicating factor in ensuring patients' privacy in this age of information technology is that vast amounts of patient data may be stored and retrieved relatively easily. Although the issues of confidentiality and access to data have yet to be fully resolved, each nurse should commit himself or herself never to violate a patient's privacy by revealing patient information except to other members of that patient's treatment team.

Phase 2: Analysis

As mentioned, during the data-gathering phase of the nursing process, nurses obtain a great deal of information about their patients. These data must be validated, then compared with norms to sort out data that might indicate a problem or identify a pattern. Next, the data must be clustered or grouped so that problems can be identified and their cause discerned. This process is known as data analysis and results in the identification of one or more nursing diagnoses. Knowledge from the biological sciences, social sciences, and nursing enables nurses to analyze relationships among various pieces of patient data.

Nursing Diagnosis

Nursing diagnosis was defined by Gordon (1976) as "actual or potential health problems which nurses, by virtue of their education and experience, are capable and licensed to treat" (p. 1299). In 1990, the NANDA defined nursing diagnosis as "a clinical judgment about individual, family, or community responses to actual or potential health problems/life processes . . . (which) provide the basis for selection of nursing interventions to achieve outcomes for which the nurse is accountable" (North American Nursing Diagnosis Association, 1990).

NANDA Diagnoses

For two decades the NANDA has worked to develop a comprehensive list of nursing diagnoses. The composition of the NANDA includes nursing educators, theorists, and practitioners from the United States and Canada who first met in 1973 to develop standard terminology, content, and format for nursing diagnoses. The group has continued to meet every two years to revise the original list of approved diagnoses. After each revision, new diagnoses are tested by nurses in practice settings to evaluate their appropriateness and usefulness. This is a continuing process. Membership in the NANDA is open to all nurses interested in advancing nursing diagnosis. Appendix D contains the 1999–2000 list of the NANDA's nursing diagnoses.

All nursing diagnoses must be supported by data, which the NANDA refers to as **defining characteristics.** These defining characteristics are also known as signs and symptoms. Remember that a sign is observable, whereas a symptom is reported by the patient.

Writing Nursing Diagnoses

A format that can be used to write the diagnostic statement is called the PES format and was developed by Gordon (1987) (Box 15–4). In this format, the P stands for the concise description of the problem using the NANDA diagnostic label, for example, ineffective breathing pattern. The E part of the statement stands for etiology and begins with the words *related to*. These related factors are conditions or circumstances that can cause or contribute to the development of the problem. To follow the example, "ineffective breathing pattern related to anxiety" explains that the cause of the ineffective breathing pattern is the patient's high anxiety level. If the cause were decreased energy or fatigue rather than anxiety, the nurse would need to select different nursing actions to solve the problem.

The last part of the diagnostic statement is S, which stands for signs and symptoms or as the NANDA calls them, defining characteristics. Thus, the complete diagnostic statement for the diagnosis could be "ineffective breathing patterns related to anxiety as manifested by dyspnea, nasal flaring, shallow and rapid respirations, and use of accessory muscles of respiration."

Prioritizing Nursing Diagnoses

After diagnoses are identified, the nurse must put them in order of priority. There are two common frameworks used to establish priorities. One of these considers the relative danger to the patient. Using this framework, diagnoses that are life-threatening are the nurse's first priority. Next come those that have the potential to cause harm or injury. Last in priority are those that are related to the overall general health of the patient. Thus, a diagnosis of "ineffective airway clearance" would be dealt with before "sleep pattern disturbance," and "sleep pattern disturbance" would have priority over "knowledge deficit."

Another framework that may be used to prioritize diagnoses is Maslow's (1970) hierarchy of needs (see Fig. 10–3). When this framework is used, there is an inverse relationship between high-priority nursing diagnoses and high-level needs. In other words, highest priority is given to diagnoses related to basic physiological needs. Diagnoses related to higher-level needs such as love and belonging or self-esteem, although important, have lower priority.

Except in life-threatening situations, nurses should take care to involve patients in identifying priority diagnoses. Because varied sociocultural factors have a great impact on the manner in which patients prioritize problems,

---

BOX 15–4

Writing Nursing Diagnoses

P = Problem
E = Etiology
S = Signs and symptoms (defining characteristics)

nurses must be aware of these factors and take them into consideration when planning patient care.

Medical Diagnosis and Nursing Diagnosis

Nursing diagnosis is different from medical diagnosis and was never intended to be a substitute for it. Rather than focusing on what is wrong with the patient in terms of a disease process, a nursing diagnosis identifies the problems the patient is experiencing as a *result* of the disease process.

Another important difference between nursing diagnosis and medical diagnosis is nursing diagnoses cover patient problems that nurses can legally treat. It would do little good for nursing diagnoses to include "appendicitis" because appendicitis is a medical diagnosis requiring surgery, and it is not legal for nurses to perform surgery. An appropriate nursing diagnosis for a patient after an appendectomy might be "ineffective airway clearance related to incisional pain." Because it is legal in all states for nurses to provide comfort measures and to assist patients, to cough and deep breathe, this would be both appropriate and a legal nursing diagnosis.

Phase 3: Planning

Planning is the third phase in the nursing process. **Planning** begins with the identification of patient goals. These are goals that are used by the patient and the nurse to guide the selection of interventions and to evaluate patient progress.

Just as nursing diagnoses are written in collaboration with the patient, goals should also be agreed on by both nurse and patient unless collaboration is impossible, such as when the patient is unconscious. In that event, family members or significant others can collaborate with the nurse. Goals give the patient, family, significant others, and nurse direction and make them active partners.

Writing Patient Goals and Outcomes

The terms *goal* and *objective* are frequently used interchangeably. These terms are statements of what is to be accomplished and are derived from the diagnoses. Because the problem or diagnosis is written as a patient problem, the goal should also be in terms of what the patient will do rather than what the nurse will do. The goal begins with the words "the patient will" or "the patient will be able to." The goal sets a general direction, includes an action verb, and should be both attainable and realistic for the patient.

Outcome criteria are specific and make the goal measurable. Outcome criteria define the terms under which the goal is said to be met, partially met, or unmet.

Each diagnosis has at least one patient goal, and each patient goal may have several outcome criteria. Effective outcome criteria state under what conditions, to what extent, and in what time frame the patient is to act. A sample patient goal with outcome criteria might be "The patient will demonstrate effective bowel elimination as evidenced by having one soft, formed stool every other day without the use of laxatives or enemas within two weeks." It is easy to see that this goal is written in terms of what the patient will do (have a bowel movement at least every other day), is measurable (one soft, formed stool), gives conditions (without the use of laxatives or enemas), and has a specified time frame for accomplishment (two weeks).

Types of Patient Goals. There are three types of patient goals: psychomotor, cognitive, and affective goals. A goal that requires motor skills or actions by the patient is a **psychomotor goal,** for example, "The patient will walk 10 feet in the hallway with a walker three times per day within one day after surgery." **Cognitive goals** deal with a desired change in a patient's knowledge level. An example of a cognitive goal might be "The patient will list three effects of a high cholesterol level on the heart prior to discharge from the hospital." **Affective goals** involve a change in mood, values, attitudes, or belief systems. An example of an affective goal is "The patient will express an increased sense of well-being after participating in an exercise program for one month." A single patient may have a combination of psychomotor, cognitive, and affective goals (Fig. 15–3).

Establishing Time Frames for Patient Goals. One aspect of goal setting not yet discussed is the estimated length of time needed to accomplish the goal. **Short-term goals** may be attainable within hours or days. They are usually specific and are small steps leading to the achievement of broader, long-term goals. For example, "The patient will lose two pounds" is a short-term goal, and the time limit for accomplishment can be brief, perhaps a week or 10 days.

Figure 15–3
Patient goals may be in one or more of three domains: cognitive, psychomotor, or affective.

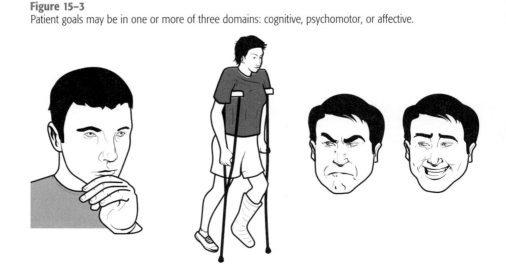

Long-term goals usually represent major changes. A goal such as "The patient will lose 75 pounds" may take months or perhaps even years to accomplish, and the time frame should be set accordingly.

It is extremely important to assist patients to set realistic goals for themselves. Setting their sights too high causes frustration and discouragement in patients, families, and nurses.

Nursing Outcomes Classification (NOC). Although not yet in nationwide use, a system of classification of patient outcomes sensitive to nursing interventions has been developed by a group of researchers at the University of Iowa. They sought to evaluate the effects of nursing care, believing that this was essential if nursing was to become "a full participant in clinical evaluation science along with other health disciplines" (The Center for Nursing Classification, 1999). The work began in 1991 with a team of 43 nurses from all aspects of nursing—service, education, and research. As the work progressed, they were funded by a grant from the National Institute of Nursing Research (NINR). From 1993 through 1997, these researchers identified, labeled, validated, and classified nursing outcomes and tested them in the field. Their work is ongoing. **Nursing outcomes classifications** are the result.

There are 260 standard NOC outcomes, each with a label, definition, and a set of indicators and measures to determine achievement of the outcome. Examples of outcome include ambulation, mobility level, and cognitive orientation.

You can learn more about NOC online at http://www.nursing.uiowa.edu/noc.

Selecting Interventions and Writing Nursing Orders

After short-term and long-term goals are identified through collaboration between nurse and patient, the nurse writes nursing orders. **Nursing orders** are actions designed to assist the patient in achieving a stated goal. Every goal has specific nursing orders, which may be carried out by a registered nurse (RN) or delegated to other members of the nursing staff.

Nursing orders and medical orders differ. Nursing orders refer to interventions that are designed to treat the patient's response to an illness or medical treatment, whereas medical orders are designed to treat the actual illness or disease. An example of a nursing order is "Teach turning, coughing, and deep-breathing exercises prior to surgery." These activities are designed to prevent postoperative respiratory problems due to immobility. They are appropriate nursing orders because prevention of complications due to immobility is a nursing responsibility. Nursing orders may include instructions about consultation with other health care providers, such as the dietitian, physical therapist, or pharmacist.

Types of Nursing Interventions. Nursing interventions are of three basic types: independent, dependent, or interdependent. **Independent interventions** are those for which the nurse's intervention requires no supervision or direction by others. Nurses are expected to possess the knowledge and skills to carry out independent actions safely. An example of an independent nursing intervention is teaching a patient how to examine her breasts for lumps. The nursing practice act of each state usually specifies general types of independent nursing actions.

Dependent interventions do require instructions, written orders, or supervision of another health professional, usually a physician. These actions require knowledge and skills on the part of the nurse but may not be done without explicit directions. An example of a dependent nursing intervention is the administration of medications. Although a physician or advanced practice nurse must order most medications, it is the responsibility of the nurse to know how to administer them safely and to monitor their effectiveness.

The third type, **interdependent interventions,** are actions in which the nurse must collaborate or consult with another health professional before carrying out the action. One example of this type of action is the nurse implementing orders that have been written by a physician in a protocol. **Protocols** define under what conditions and circumstances a nurse is allowed to treat the patient as well as what treatments are permissible. They are used in situations in which nurses need to take immediate action without consulting with a physician, such as in an emergency department, a critical care unit, or a home setting.

Nursing Interventions Classification (NIC). Classification research conducted at the University of Iowa College of Nursing resulted in the development of the **Nursing Intervention Classifications.** These describe the treatments that nurses perform in all specialties and in all settings. There is a list of 433 interventions. Each is defined and includes a set of activities that a nurse performs to carry out the intervention. Interventions are coded and organized for ease of computerization. Examples of interventions include acid-base management, anxiety reduction, shock management, fall prevention, exercise promotion, and emergency cart checking. Note that the last is an indirect care intervention. You can learn more about NIC at http://www.nursing.uiowa.edu/nic.

Writing the Plan of Care

Once interventions are selected, a written plan of care is devised. Some health care agencies use individually developed plans of care for their patients. The nurse creates and develops a plan for each patient. Others use standardized plans of care that are based on common and recurring problems. The nurse then individualizes these standard plans of care. One of the advantages of using standardized plans is that they can decrease the time spent in generating a completely new plan each time a patient is seen. These plans are easily computer generated, with the nurse making selections from menus to individualize the plan to the particular patient. The amount of time needed to update and document these plans is thereby vastly decreased. Computer use also facilitates data collection for research.

Because of the decreasing average length of stay for patients in health care facilities, the increasing focus on achieving timely patient outcomes in the specific time frame permitted by reimbursement systems, and the

JCAHO's emphasis on multidiciplinary care, many agencies have adopted the use of multidisciplinary plans of care known as **critical paths,** care tracks, or care maps. See Appendix B, which contains a critical path for congestive heart failure. Multidisciplinary care plans such as critical paths are written in collaboration with physicians and other health care providers and establish a sequence of short-term daily outcomes that are easily measured. This type of care planning facilitates communication and collaboration among all members of the health care team. It also permits comparisons of outcomes between treatment plans as well as among health care facilities.

The development of appropriate plans of care depends on the nurse's ability to think critically. Nurses must be able to analyze information and arguments, make reasoned decisions, recognize many viewpoints, and question and seek answers continuously. At the same time, nurses must be logical, flexible, and creative and take initiative while considering the holistic nature of each patient.

Phase 4: Implementation of Planned Interventions

When nursing orders are actually carried out, the fourth phase of the nursing process, **implementation,** begins. Most people think of nursing as "doing something" for or to a patient. Notice, however, that in using the nursing process, nurses must do a great deal of thinking, analyzing, and planning before the first actual nursing action takes place.

Nurses who skip the essential first three phases of the nursing process and jump immediately into action are not behaving in a responsible, professional manner. Patients feel a greater sense of trust in a nursing staff if both physicians' and nurses' orders are carried out in an orderly, planned, and competent manner.

It is difficult to make general statements about this phase of the nursing process because interventions vary widely, depending on the nursing diagnosis and patient goals. Typical nursing interventions include such actions as monitoring patients' responses to medications, patient teaching, and performing certain procedures, such as changing dressings on a wound. As the nurse carries out planned interventions, he or she is continually assessing the patient, noting responses to nursing interventions and modifying the care plan or adding nursing diagnoses as needed. Integral to the implementation phase of the nursing process is the documentation of nursing actions.

Very sick patients require intense nursing care. As patients improve, however, they are gradually able to assume responsibility for their own care. It is important for nurses to allow patients to do as much for themselves as their illnesses allow. Patient independence is an important step in recovery.

To implement the plan of care, nurses must possess a triad of skills: thinking, or cognitive skills; doing, or psychomotor skills; and communicating or interpersonal skills. If any one set of skills is lacking, the nurse's ability to implement the nursing process is significantly decreased. Implementation involves performing actions, delegating, teaching, counseling, consulting, reporting, and documenting, all while continuously assessing.

Phase 5: Evaluation

The next phase in the nursing process is **evaluation.** In this phase, the nurse examines the patient's progress in relation to the goals and stated outcome criteria to determine if a problem is resolved, is in the process of being resolved, or is unresolved. In other words, the outcome criteria are the basis for evaluation of the goal. Evaluation may reveal that data, diagnosis, goals, and nursing interventions were all on target and that the problem is resolved.

Evaluation may also indicate a need for a change in the plan of care. Perhaps inadequate patient data were the basis for the plan, and further assessment has uncovered additional needs. The nursing diagnoses may have been incorrect or placed in the wrong order of priority. Patient goals may have been inappropriate or unattainable within the designated time frame. It is possible that nursing actions were incorrectly implemented.

Evaluation is a critical phase in the nursing process and one that is often slighted. It is not enough to continue to do the "right things" if the patient is not improving in the expected manner. If, on evaluation, the problem has not been resolved, the nursing care plan must be revised to reflect the necessary changes, and the process must begin again.

In addition to evaluating the individual plan of care, nurses are responsible for evaluating the quality of care that all patients receive. As discussed in Chapter 13, many terms are currently used for this process including *total quality management* (TQM), *continuous quality improvement* (CQI), and *quality improvement* (QI). Regardless of the terminology, the goal is the same: to improve health care and the way in which it is delivered.

Dynamic Nature of the Nursing Process

Although the phases in the nursing process are discussed separately here, in practice they are not so clearly delineated. Nor do they always proceed from one to another in a linear fashion. As seen in Figure 15–4, the nursing process is dynamic, meaning that nurses are continuously moving from one phase to another and then beginning the process again. Often a nurse performs two or more phases at the same time, for instance, observing a wound for signs of infection (assessment) while changing the dressing on the wound (intervention)

Figure 15–4
The nursing process is a dynamic, non-linear tool for critical thinking.

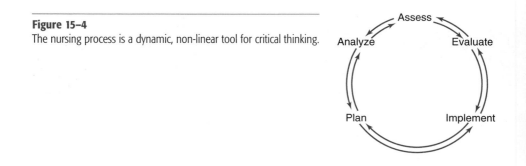

and asking the patient whether pain has been relieved by the pain medication (evaluation).

Now that you have reviewed the phases of the nursing process, let us look back at the opening scenario. The problem that was identified was the necessity to don appropriate clothing. Data, both objective (the temperature outdoors) and subjective (the mood one is in), were gathered. Selection was made and implemented, and an evaluation of the implementation was carried out by looking in the mirror. This comparison reveals that problem solving is something each person does every day. The use of the nursing process simply provides professional nurses with a patient-oriented framework with which to solve clinical problems.

An example of using the nursing process in a clinical situation is found in Box 15–5. This case study demonstrates how using the nursing process becomes so natural that experienced nurses go through the phases fluidly and automatically.

BOX 15-5
Nursing Process Case Study

You have just received a report from the day shift about Mr. Burkes. You were told that he had been admitted with a diagnosis of cancer of the tongue and that he had had a radical neck dissection. He has a tracheostomy and requires frequent suctioning. He is alert and responds by nodding his head or writing short notes.

When you enter his room, you note that he is apprehensive and tachypneic, and is gesturing for you to come into the room. You auscultate his lungs and note coarse crackles and expiratory wheezes. You can see thick secretions bubbling out of his tracheostomy. He has poor cough effort.

Based on these data, you realize that a priority nursing diagnosis is *ineffective airway clearance*. You immediately prepare to perform tracheal suctioning. As you are suctioning, you watch the patient's nonverbal responses and note that he is less apprehensive when the suctioning is completed. You also auscultate the lungs and note that decreased crackles and the expiratory wheezes are no longer present. Mr. Burkes writes "I can get my breath now" on his note pad.

I. Assessment
  A. Subjective data
    1. None due to inability to speak
  B. Objective data
    1. Tracheostomy with copious, thick secretions
    2. Tachypnea
    3. Gesturing for help
    4. Coarse crackles and expiratory wheezes
    5. Poor cough effort

(continued)

BOX 15–5
Nursing Process Case Study (*Continued*)

II. Analysis
   A. Ineffective airway clearance related to copious, thick secretions
III. Plan
   A. Short-term goal: Patient will maintain patent airway as evidenced by absence of expiratory wheezes and crackles.
   B. Long-term goal: Patient will have patent airway as evidenced by his ability to clear the airway without the use of suctioning by the time of discharge.
IV. Implementation
   A. Assess lung sounds every hour for crackles and wheezes
   B. Suction airway as needed
   C. Elevate head of bed to 45 degrees
   D. Teach patient abdominal breathing techniques
   E. Encourage patient to cough out secretions
V. Evaluation
   A. Short-term goal: Achieved as evidenced by decreased crackles and absent wheezes when auscultating the lungs.
   B. Long-term goal: To be evaluated prior to discharge.

BOX 15–6
Clinical Judgment: Nine Key Questions

1. What major outcomes (observable beneficial results) do we expect to see *in this particular person, family,* or *group* when the plan of care is terminated? Example: The person will be discharged infection free, able to care for himself, three days after surgery. Outcomes may be addressed on a standard plan or you may have to develop these outcomes yourself. Be sure that you check to make sure any predetermined outcomes in standard plans are *appropriate* to your patient's specific situation.
2. What problems or issues must be addressed to achieve the major outcomes? Answering this question will help you set priorities. You might be faced with a long list of actual or potential health problems. You need to narrow down your list to those that *must* be addressed.
3. What are the circumstances? *Who's* involved (e.g., child, adult, group)? How urgent are the problems (e.g., life threatening, chronic)? What are the factors influencing their presentation (e.g., when, where, and how did the problems develop)? What are the patient's values, beliefs, and cultural influences?
4. What knowledge is required? Knowledge required includes problem-specific facts (e.g., how health problems usually present, how they're diagnosed, what their common causes and risk factors are, what common complications occur, and how these complications are prevented and

managed); nursing process and related knowledge and skills (ethics, research, health assessment, communication, priority setting); related sciences (anatomy, physiology, pathophysiology, pharmacology, chemistry, physics, psychology, sociology). You must also be clearly aware of the circumstances, as addressed in question three above.

5. How much room is there for error? In the clinical setting, there is usually minimal room for error. However, it depends on the health of the individual and the risks of interventions. Example: In which of the following cases do you think you have more room for error? (1) You're trying to decide whether to give a healthy child a one-time dose of acetaminophen for heat rash without checking with the doctor. (2) You have a child who's been sick for three days with a fever and the mother wants to know if she should continue giving acetaminophen without checking with the doctor. If you thought the *first one* above, you're right. In the *second* case, the symptoms have continued for three days without a diagnosis. If you continue to give acetaminophen without checking with a physician, you might be masking symptoms of a problem requiring medical management.

6. How much time do I have? Time frame for decision making depends on (1) the urgency of the problems (e.g., there's less time in life-threatening situations, such as cardiac arrest) and (2) the planned length of contact (e.g., if your patient will be hospitalized only for two days, you have to be realistic about what can be accomplished, and key decisions need to be made *early*.).

7. What resources can help me? Human resources include clinical nurse educators, nursing faculty, preceptors, more experienced nurses, advance practice nurses, peers, librarians, and other health care professionals (pharmacists, nutritionists, physical therapists, physicians). The patient and family are also valuable resources (usually they know their own problems best). Other resources include texts, articles, other references, and computer databases and decision-making support; national practice guidelines, facility documents (e.g., guidelines, policies, procedures, assessment forms).

8. Whose perspectives must be considered? The most significant perspective to consider is the patient's point of view. Other important perspectives include those of the family and significant others, caregivers, and relevant third parties (e.g., insurers).

9. What's influencing my thinking? Be sure you identify personal biases and any other factors influencing your critical thinking.

From Alfaro-LeFevre, R. (1999). *Critical thinking in nursing: A practical approach* (2nd. ed.). Philadelphia: W. B. Saunders. Reprinted with permission.

Developing Clinical Judgment in Nursing

Becoming an effective nurse involves more than critical thinking and the ability to use the nursing process. It depends heavily on developing what is known as **clinical judgment.** Clinical judgment consists of both informed

BOX 15–7
Self-Assessment: Developing Sound Clinical Judgment

Answer the following questions honestly. When finished, make a list of the items you need to work on in your quest to develop sound clinical judgment. Keep the list with you and review it frequently. Seek opportunities to practice needed activities.

1. Use References
- Do I look up new terms when I encounter them to make them part of my vocabulary?
- Do I familiarize myself with normal findings so I can recognize those outside the norm?
- Do I bother to find out why abnormal findings occur?
- Do I learn the signs and symptoms of various conditions, what causes them, and how they're managed?

2. Use the Nursing Process
- Do I always assess before acting, stay focused on outcomes, and make changes as needed?
- Do I always base my judgments on fact, not emotion or hearsay?

3. Assess Systematically
- Do I have a systematic approach to assessing patients to decrease the likelihood that I will overlook important data?

4. Set Priorities Systematically
- Do I evaluate both the problem and the probable cause before acting?
- Am I willing to obtain assistance from a more knowledgeable source when indicated?

5. Refuse to Act Without Knowledge
- Do I refuse to perform an action when I don't know the indication, why it works, and what risks there are for harm to this particular patient?

6. Use Resources Wisely
- Do I look for opportunities to learn from others—teachers, other experts, even my peers?
- Do I seek help when needed, being mindful of patient privacy issues?

7. Know Standards of Care
- Do I read facility policies, professional standards, school policies, and state board of nursing rules and regulations to determine my scope of practice?
- Do I know the clinical agency's policies and procedures affecting my particular patients?
- Do I attempt to understand the rationales behind policies and procedures?
- Do I follow policies and procedures carefully, recognizing that they are designed to help me use good judgment?

8. Know Technology and Equipment
- Do I routinely learn how to use patient technology such as IV pumps, patient monitors, computers?
- Do I learn how to check equipment for proper functioning and safety?

9. Give Patient-Centered Care
- Do I remember always the needs and feelings of the patient, family, and significant others?
- Do I value knowing my patients' health beliefs and values within their own cultural contexts?
- Do I "go the extra mile" for patients?
- Do I demonstrate the belief that every patient deserves my very best efforts?

Adapted with permission from Alfaro-LeFevre, R. (1999). *Critical thinking in nursing: A practical approach* (2nd. ed.) (pp. 88–92). Philadelphia: W. B. Saunders.

opinions and decisions based on theoretical knowledge and experience. Nurses develop clinical judgment gradually as they gain a broader, deeper knowledge base and clinical experience. There is no substitute for direct patient contact in developing clinical judgment.

Critical thinking and clinical reasoning used in the nursing process are both important aspects of clinical judgment. A nurse who has developed sound clinical judgment knows what to look for (elevation of temperature in a surgical patient), draws valid conclusions about what the signs mean (possible postoperative infection), and knows what to do about it (listen to breath sounds, assess for dehydration, check incision for redness and drainage, seek another opinion, notify the physician, and so forth). Developing sound clinical judgment requires recalling facts, recognizing patterns in patient behaviors, putting facts and observations together to form a meaningful whole, and acting upon the resulting information in an appropriate way.

An important aspect of clinical judgment is knowing the limitations of your expertise. Most nurses have an instinctive awareness of when they are approaching their limits and should seek consultation with another professional. Your state's nurse practice act, health agency policies, school policies, and the professions' standards of practice all provide guidance in making the decision about nursing actions within your scope of practice. Nursing students, whether new to nursing or registered nurses in baccalaureate programs, must consider policies and standards in determining their scope of practice in any given nursing situation.

Rosalinda Alfaro-LeFevre (1999) developed a list of nine key questions to consider when seeking to improve clinical judgment. These are found in Box 15–6.

Nurses are responsible for developing sound clinical judgment and are accountable for their decisions. You may want to devise a personal plan for improving your own clinical decision making. Thoughtfully completing the self-assessment in Box 15–7 will help you begin.

Summary of Key Points

- Critical thinking in nursing is a purposeful, disciplined, active process designed to improve patient care.
- Thinking by novice nurses is different from that of expert nurses in identifiable ways.
- The nursing process is a systematic problem-solving strategy that is based on the scientific method. It is used by nurses when delivering patient care.
- The phases of the nursing process are assessment, analysis, planning, implementation, and evaluation.
- Properly used, the nursing process is cyclic and dynamic rather than rigid and linear.
- Nurses may initially find that using the nursing process feels awkward or slow. After practice, however, most find it becomes a natural yet organized way to approach patient care.
- When all nurses use the nursing process, patient care is consistent, comprehensive, and coordinated.
- Through the use of the nursing process, nurses are able to work toward resolving patient problems in a systematic manner, thus advancing both the scientific basis of nursing and professionalism.
- Critical thinking, creative use of the nursing process, current knowledge about health, illness, and scope of practice, and abundant clinical experience combine to create sound clinical judgment.

Critical Thinking Questions

1. Explain the characteristics of critical thinking in nursing.
2. List at least four ways in which novice thinking and expert thinking differ.
3. Describe the phases in the nursing process and the activities of each phase.
4. List a short-term personal goal and a long-term personal goal using all the essential elements of effective goals. Evaluate your progress toward these goals.
5. Compare the nursing process with the scientific method (Chapter 12) and state how they are similar and how they differ.
6. Explain the difference between independent, dependent, and interdependent nursing interventions and give an example of each.
7. Describe the PES format for writing a nursing diagnosis.
8. Explain the difference between medical and nursing diagnoses.
9. Describe what is meant by the statement "the nursing process is a cyclic process."
10. Describe how nurses develop sound clinical judgment.

Web Resources

Foundation for Critical Thinking, http://www.sonoma.edu/cthink

North American Nursing Diagnosis Association (NANDA), http://www.nanda.org

Nursing Interventions Classification (NIC), http://www.nursing.uiowa.edu/nic

Nursing Outcomes Classification (NOC), http://www.nursing.uiowa.edu/noc

References

Alfaro-LeFevre, R. (1999). *Critical thinking in nursing: A practical approach* (2nd ed.). Philadelphia: W. B. Saunders.

American Nurses Association (1980). *Nursing: A social policy statement.* Kansas City, Mo.: American Nurses Association.

American Nurses Association (1995). *Nursing's social policy statement.* Washington, D. C.: American Nurses Association.

American Nurses Association (1998). *Standards of clinical nursing practice.* Washington, D. C.: American Nurses Association.

Benner, P. (1984). *From novice to expert.* Menlo Park, Calif.: Addison-Wesley.

Center for Nursing Classification (1999). Nursing outcomes classification. Online at http://www.nursing.uiowa.edu/noc.

Gordon, M. (1987). *Nursing diagnosis: Process and application* (2nd ed.). New York: McGraw-Hill.

Gordon, M. (1976). Nursing diagnosis and the diagnostic process. *American Journal of Nursing, 76*(5), 1298–1300.

Joint Commission on Accreditation of Healthcare Organizations (1997). *Comprehensive accreditation manual for hospitals: The official handbook.* Oakbrook Terrace, Ill.: Joint Commission on Accreditation of Healthcare Organizations.

Joint Commission on Accreditation of Healthcare Organizations (1992). *Accreditation manual for hospitals.* Oakbrook Terrace, Ill.: Joint Commission on Accreditation of Healthcare Organizations.

Marriner-Tomey, A. (1994). *Nursing theorists and their work.* St. Louis, Mo.: Mosby.

Martin, P., Dugan, J., Freundl, M., Miller, S., Phillips, R., and Sharritts, L. (1994). Nurses' attitudes toward nursing process as measured by the Dayton Attitude Scale. *The Journal of Continuing Education in Nursing, 25*(1), 35–39.

Maslow, A. (1970). *Motivation and personality.* New York: Harper & Row.

North American Nursing Diagnosis Association (1990). *Nursing diagnoses: Definitions and classifications, 1999–2000.* St. Louis: North American Nursing Diagnosis Association.

Yura, H., and Walsh, M. B. (1983). *The nursing process: Assessing, planning, implementing, evaluation.* (4th ed.) Norwalk, Conn.: Appleton-Century-Crofts.

Financing Health Care

Frances A. Maurer

16

Key Terms

Acuity
Capitation
Certificate of Need (CON)
Copayment
Cost Containment
Deductible
Diagnosis-related Groups (DRGs)
Gatekeeper
Health Care Financing
  Administration (HCFA)
Health Care Network
Health Maintenance Organization
  (HMO)
Hill-Burton Act
Managed Care Organization
  (MCO)
Medicaid
Medicare
Out-of-pocket Payment
Patient Classification System (PCS)
Personal Payment
Point-of-Service (POS)
Preferred Provider Organization
  (PPO)
Premium

Private Insurance
Professional Review Organization
  (PRO)
Prospective Payment System
  (PPS)
Quality Management

Retrospective Reimbursement
Self-insurance
Skill Mix
Third-party Payment
Universal Care
Worker's Compensation

Learning Outcomes

After studying this chapter, students will be able to:

- Explain the economic principle of supply and demand and its relevance to health care costs.
- Cite examples of causes of health care cost escalation.
- Describe the major methods of payment for health care.
- Explain cost-containment efforts since 1975 and their impact on nursing practice.
- Describe the impact of managed care on cost containment and health care consumers.
- Describe the relationship between cost containment and quality management initiatives.
- Identify current and proposed strategies aimed at changing segments of the health care delivery system.
- Identify general guidelines for evaluating national health insurance proposals.

The 1990s ended with renewed vigor in the public debate over financing health care in the United States. Health care costs continued to climb, as did the number of uninsured citizens. Legislative reforms and managed care efforts had mixed success at cutting health care costs and increasing access to health care. The dilemma faced by the nation was, and remains, how to provide high-quality health care services to all citizens while keeping costs down.

In 1997, the nation's health care expenditures reached $1.1 trillion and consumed 13.5 percent of the gross domestic product (GDP). This percentage has doubled since 1960, making health care the largest single budget item (Braden et al., 1998). Estimates for the year 2007 indicate that health care costs are expected to reach $2.1 trillion (Smith et al., 1998). If this trend is allowed to continue until the year 2010, one-third of all national resources will be spent on health care. Yet the health of American citizens is not as good as it should be. As a result, almost everyone agrees that there is a crisis in health care and that reform is needed.

Evidence of public concern about rising health care costs are not new. For example, the cover story entitled "MediScare" in the September 18, 1995, issue of *Newsweek* magazine featured the statement: "Young Versus Old: Who Will Carry the Burden?" (Fineman, 1995). Accompanying that statement was a cover photograph of a young man struggling to hold an older woman in a wheelchair over his head. Today the public's concern is about the ability of our health care system to maintain the Medicare program, provide for the growing number of uninsured, and ensure the quality of managed care. It seems that at a time when health care breakthroughs are at an all-time high, public support for the system that created those breakthroughs is eroding.

Most Americans believe that health care is a right, not a privilege. In 1993 President Bill Clinton attempted national health care reform because of rising health care costs and restricted health care coverage for many Americans. His plan, designed by a task force headed by Hillary Rodham Clinton, was heavily attacked by various special interest groups and failed to pass Congress. Since then, debate and confusion about the exact nature of reform and its impact on the population has tempered enthusiasm and public support for governmental action to change the health care structure.

Despite governmental inaction, major changes in health care access and delivery were forced by business interests. Corporations and other large employers were in the vanguard of efforts to reduce health care costs, primarily because health care benefits represent a significant cost to employers. For example, in 1996 health benefits cost employers an average of $3,821 per employee (Knight-Ridder, 1996). General Motors alone spent $4.8 billion, or $1,200 per vehicle built in the United States, to provide health coverage for employees, their dependents, and retirees (Lowes, 1997).

The cost-reduction strategies implemented by businesses placed limits on employees' treatment options and altered the payment structure of health care for many employed Americans. Even without planned, organized, comprehensive change in the structure of the health care system, significant change nevertheless continued. Finding a solution to the health care finance dilemma while maintaining quality and improving access to services remains a challenge that will not easily be achieved.

Nurses and nursing practice are profoundly affected by financial issues. Therefore, students of professional nursing need to understand the overall economic context in which nursing care is provided. The financial component of health care affects nurses both professionally, in their nursing practice, and personally, in the type of insurance and health services they and their families, are able to afford. This chapter explores several major concepts necessary to understanding health care finance: basic economic theory, a brief historical review of the causes of health care cost escalation, current methods of payment, cost-containment efforts, the economics of nursing care, and the impact of cost containment on nursing care. Criteria to evaluate health reform proposals are summarized.

Basic Economic Theory

Nursing school curricula do not typically require undergraduates to take courses in economics, yet there is an urgent need for nurses to understand the economic context in which they practice. Economics influences the type and quality of health services provided as well as employment opportunities for nurses.

Supply and Demand

A basic economic theory is the *law of supply and demand*. According to this theory, a normal economic system consists of two parts: suppliers, who provide goods and services, and consumers, who demand and use goods and services. In a monetary environment, that is, one in which money is used as a unit of exchange, consumers exchange money for desired goods and services.

In an efficient marketplace, the market price of goods and services serves to create an equilibrium in which supply roughly equals demand, and demand roughly equals supply. When demand exceeds supply, prices rise. When supply exceeds demand, prices fall. The relationship between price and equilibrium can be seen at the clothing store. During an unusually mild winter for example, the demand for heavy coats is likely to be low. Because demand is low, manufacturers cut back on production, and retailers stop ordering coats and place their current stock of coats on sale. If the sale price is low enough, however, people will continue to buy coats. Through fluctuations in supply and demand, created by price, equilibrium is approached. This example illustrates the principle of price sensitivity, that is, a change in demand for goods or services is a function of the change in the price of those goods or services (Feldstein, 1998). Figure 16–1 illustrates the relationships among price, supply, and demand.

Difficulty with Basic Economic Theory in Health Care

There are problems associated with applying basic economic theory in the health care market. This chapter highlights a few of those problems.

Health Care as a Right or Privilege?

In a free-market economy, consumption of any good or service is determined by an individual's ability to pay. In a pure free market, a portion of the population would be denied health care if they were unable to pay. People who

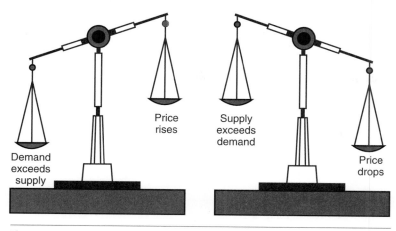

Figure 16–1
Price sensitivity in a normal economic environment.

support this position consider health care a privilege. Others believe that everyone should have access to basic health care and consider health care a right.

Despite the United States's leanings toward a free-market economy in general, health care is largely considered a right, not a privilege. Rather than allowing economically disadvantaged citizens to do without health services, the federal government has taken steps to ensure certain groups access to health care services through publicly funded programs such as **Medicare** and **Medicaid.** Although this is generally considered an ethical policy, it is nevertheless a policy decision that interferes with the functioning of free-market principles.

Price Sensitivity in Health Care

In the days before health insurance existed, when people paid their own medical bills, physicians and hospitals set their fees with some sensitivity to what patients could pay. When costs were high, patients complained. Health insurance created an indirect payment structure, **third-party payment,** that removed price sensitivity from the concern of most health care consumers because they pay only a small portion of the real costs; a third party (the employer, insurance company, or government) pays the rest. If someone other than the consumer pays, demand can increase because the consumer is *insensitive* to cost. This is an important point to keep in mind when reviewing the history of health care finance. History has demonstrated that when there is little or no out-of-pocket expense to the consumer, economic equilibrium is upset because consumers use more health care services (Feldstein, 1998).

Additional Influences on the Health Market

Economists have identified a number of other factors that affect the health care market in ways that violate the assumptions surrounding an effective free-market system. For example, consumers cannot always control demand for health care services. With other products, a consumer can delay an ordinary purchase until there is a sale or forego the purchase altogether. Health care is different because often health care needs are immediate. The consumer might suffer serious injury or even death by a delay in seeking services. Box 16–1 summarizes some of the other factors that reduce the efficient functioning of free-market economics in the health care market.

Current Methods of Payment for Health Care

There are four major methods of payment for health services in use today: personal payment, Medicare, Medicaid, and private insurance. Worker's compensation is an additional mechanism for financing some health care services. Figure 16–2 represents the proportion each of the four major methods contributes to the purchase of health care.

Personal Payment

Personal payment for services is the least common method. Few people can afford **out-of-pocket payment** for more than the most basic health services. At today's prices, an illness or injury severe enough to require hospitalization can quickly exhaust a family's financial reserves, forcing them into bankruptcy. Generally, only those people without access to some form of private group insurance or public insurance rely on personal payment.

Medicare

Medicare, or Title XVIII of the Social Security Act, is a nationwide federal health insurance program established in 1965. Medicare is available to people aged 65 and over, regardless of the recipient's income. It also covers certain disabled individuals and people requiring dialysis or kidney transplants. Medicare has two separate but coordinated programs. The first, known as Part A, is a hospitalization insurance program. Part B is a supplementary medical insurance program that covers visits to physicians' offices and other outpatient services. Originally intended to be a no-cost or low-cost program for the elderly, the cost of participating in Medicare has risen steadily. By 1999, Part A required participants to pay a $768 deductible for hospitalization, and Part B required an annual $100 deductible and a monthly premium of $45.50 (The *Medicare Handbook,* 1999). Although originally designed to be all-inclusive, many elderly people now find they cannot afford to participate in Medicare. Ironically, some elderly are so poor that they qualify for Medicaid assistance in paying their Medicare premiums.

BOX 16–1
Barriers to a Free Market Economy in Health Care

Poor Consumer Information
Individual consumers are not accustomed to "shopping" for the best available prices for medical services, supplies, and equipment. Even when the consumer is motivated to compare costs, getting that information from the suppliers of health care is difficult and time-consuming. Most consumers require services quickly and cannot afford long delays to seek information, even if they have the expertise to search out the needed information.

Ineffective Pricing System
When the price of services is based on "reasonable and customary costs of similar services" in an area, health care providers have an incentive to continue to increase their prices rather than compete by lowering prices. Eventually the new, higher price becomes the "reasonable and customary" price. Reform efforts have had some success at reducing the impact of this phenomenon by establishing prospective funding and capping reimbursement for the cost of selected services.

Health Care Providers' Imperfect Agents—Interests
Conflict with Consumers'
Health care providers have economic interests that can be in opposition to consumer interests. Physicians, for example, act both as suppliers of health care and demanders of patient services. When physicians are partners or stockholders in services, such as laboratories or radiographic facilities, they are more likely to order such tests, according to studies by the Department of Health and Human Services. Conversely, HMO or PPO physicians who receive incentives for not referring patients to specialists are less likely to do so.

Cost Efficiency Is Not Always a Motivator for Suppliers
Although businesses are expected to operate with cost efficiency, others, particularly some nonprofit organizations, may be influenced by other factors. By law, nonprofits cannot have a profit or surplus of funds at the end of the fiscal year, but there is no law that dictates how they spend their money. Most nonprofits operate efficiently and at the lowest cost to consumers; others have been found to use their funds to provide amenities and perks for staff and board members, such as plush exercise facilities, all-expense-paid trips, or purchase of private boxes at sports stadiums.

Reprinted with permission of Maurer, F. A. (2000). Financing of health care: Context for community health nursing. In Smith, C., and Maurer, F. A. (Eds.). *Community health nursing: Theory and practice* (2nd ed). Philadelphia: W. B. Saunders.

Medicaid

Medicaid, or Title XIX of the Social Security Act, is a group of jointly funded federal-state programs for low-income, elderly, blind, and disabled individuals. It, too, was established in 1965. There are broad federal guidelines, but states have some flexibility in how they administer the program. People must

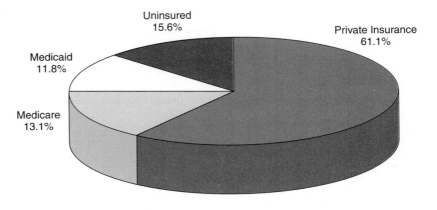

NOTE: Adds to more than 100% because some individuals have double health coverage.

Figure 16–2
Sources of financing for medical coverage: U. S. population 1997 (Data from *Statistical abstract of the United States*. [1998]. Washington, D. C.: Government Printing Office).

meet eligibility requirements determined by each state. Eligibility depends on income and varies from state to state. Rates of payment also vary, with some states providing far higher payments than others. The amount the federal government contributes to Medicaid varies from a minimum of 50 percent of total costs to a maximum of 75 percent. The differences in eligibility and payment rates lead to wide variations in the level of care provided to the poor in different states. In contrast to those on Medicare, people who receive Medicaid are not required to pay any fees to participate. Table 16–1 highlights the similarities and differences in the Medicare and Medicaid programs.

Private Insurance

Private insurance, also called voluntary insurance, is a system wherein insurance premiums are either paid by insured individuals or their employers or shared between individuals and employers. Periodic payments (**premiums**) are paid into the insurance plan, and certain health care benefits are covered as long as the premiums are paid. Early in the development of private insurance, many treatments were covered only if they were performed in an inpatient (hospital) setting. This was one of the features that tended to drive up the cost of services. Today most insurers stipulate that costs of hospitalization are reimbursable only if treatment cannot be performed on an outpatient basis.

Worker's Compensation

Worker's compensation constitutes a small proportion of insurance coverage. The program varies from state to state but generally covers only workers who are injured on the job. It usually covers both treatment for injuries and

TABLE 16-1
Facts About Medicare and Medicaid

Medicare	Medicaid
Funding	
Federal government	Federal and state governments
Administration	
Federal government	State governments
Eligibility	
People over 65 and certain others	Selected poor and disabled (includes some elderly)
Level of benefits	
Same nationwide	Varies from state to state
Payment by recipients?	
Required	Not required
Coverage	
Hospitalization; outpatient care; no prescriptions, custodial nursing care, or optical care	Comprehensive, including prescriptions and optical care

From Health Care Finance Administration (1998).*Medicare and Medicaid statistical supplement.* Washington, D. C.: Government Printing Office.

weekly payments during the time the worker is absent from work for injury-related causes. In the case of accidental death, the worker's family receives compensation. Companies are required by law to contribute to a compensation fund from which money is withdrawn when accidental injuries or deaths occur at work.

History of Health Care Finance

Before 1940, more than 90 percent of Americans either paid directly from their own pockets for health care or depended on charity care. Few had private health insurance. Public insurance programs, such as Medicare and Medicaid, did not exist. Following World War II, most industrialized countries began publicly financed health care systems that provided care for all citizens. The United States, however, did not adopt a public, universal access system, choosing instead to continue the private, fee-for-service system.

Growth of Private Insurance

In 1943, the Internal Revenue Service (IRS) ruled that health benefits paid by employers were not taxable as income. Employers began to offer health benefits as a reward to employees. States granted tax-exempt status to private insurance companies, such as Blue Cross and Blue Shield, and private insurers grew dramatically. By 1960, two-thirds of nonelderly Americans had private health insurance, mostly paid for by employers.

Hill-Burton Act

In 1946, the U. S. Congress passed the Hospital Survey and Construction Act (the **Hill-Burton Act**). This law called for and funded surveys of states' needs for hospitals, paid for planning hospitals and public health centers, and provided partial funding for constructing and equipping them. The Hill-Burton Act spurred community hospital construction. With accessible, new, well-equipped hospitals in many towns and employer-paid health insurance a standard job benefit, the stage was set for increased consumer demand leading to dramatic increases in the utilization of hospitals and health care services.

Rise of Public Insurance Programs

The problem of paying for health care for the unemployed and the elderly was not solved by private insurance, and many continued to receive inadequate care. In 1965, Congress approved two public insurance programs to cover these groups: Medicare, which is for the elderly and certain disabled people, and Medicaid, which is for the poor. They were designed to ensure that citizens who were uninsured by employers and unable to afford their own private health insurance would be protected. At that point in time, a unique public-private partnership system of insurance that would care for all seemed to be in place. Unfortunately, that partnership has not lived up to anyone's expectations, and universal health care coverage for all Americans is still an elusive goal.

Retrospective Reimbursement

Originally, both public and private insurance plans were based on **retrospective** (after-the-fact) **reimbursement.** This meant that when Patient Doe went to the hospital with pneumonia, a request for reimbursement for whatever services were rendered (chest radiographs, blood work, physical examinations, antibiotic therapy) was sent to the insurer. Depending on the terms of her insurance policy and the level of Patient Doe's **deductible** (the portion she has to pay yearly before insurance coverage begins), the hospital was reimbursed for much, or even most, of the charges. **Copayments** (the percent of charges the patient pays) were low, often as low as 10 percent. Using retrospective reimbursement, the cost of services to insured consumers of health care was extremely low or zero. Because neither the orderers of health care (physicians) nor the consumers (patients) were concerned about cost, the demand for health care services became virtually insatiable, driving costs up dramatically (Feldstein, 1998).

Early Cost-Containment Initiatives

In the late 1960s, new federal legislation required states to develop comprehensive health planning. At least one agency per state was established and empowered to review the health care needs of communities in order to reduce costs and duplication of service. A **certificate of need** (CON) had to be approved by the health planning agency before new building or expansion of existing facilities was permitted. Only projects that could demonstrate a real need were issued CONs. The result was a dramatic slowing in the construction and expansion of hospitals and public health facilities nationwide (Lampe, 1987).

By 1975, additional serious cost-containment efforts were underway, stimulated by the concerns of politicians, consumer groups, and employers about costs. Some states initiated rate setting, placing limits on reimbursement to health care providers for services. One important strategy was a move toward replacing retrospective payment for services to **prospective payment systems** (PPS). In prospective payment systems, providers, such as physicians and hospitals, receive payment on a per case basis, regardless of the cost to the provider to deliver the services. Prospective payment systems were developed because of escalating costs in the Medicare and Medicaid programs. It became apparent that basic changes in payment mechanisms were needed. Box 16–2 contains information about the dramatic increases in costs to taxpayers of Medicare and Medicaid since they were implemented in 1967.

BOX 16–2

Medicare and Medicaid Costs, 1967 and 1997

Medicare

1967[*]   1997

$5 billion $213.6 billion

- Those helped equal 95 percent of the elderly regardless of family resources and persons receiving social security because of disability.

Medicaid

1967[*]   1997

$2.3 billion $166 billion ($94 billion federal; $72 billion state)

- Those helped in 1980 equal 65 percent of the poor.
- Those helped in 1997 equal 43.3 percent of the poor.
- Medicaid is the fastest-growing spending program in the United States.

[*] First full year of operation for medicare and medicaid (data from Organization for Economic Cooperation and Development (1989). *Health care expenditures and other data: An international compendium*. Washington, D. C.

Health Care Finance Administration (1998). *Medicare and Medicaid statistical supplement*. Washington, D. C.: Government Printing Office; Bennefield, R. L. (1998). Health insurance coverage: 1997. *Current Population Reports* (pp. 60–202). Washington D. C.: U. S. Bureau of the Census.

The passage of the Tax Equity and Fiscal Responsibility Act (TEFRA) in 1982 dramatically restructured the payment method for Medicare to a prospective payment system based on **diagnosis-related groups (DRGs),** which are described later in this chapter. Prospective payment was designed to create more competition and resulted in an emphasis on efficiency, cost-effectiveness, and financial accountability. It also stimulated competition among health care providers by awarding incentives to those who operated in a cost-effective manner. Because prospective payment has the potential to encourage providers to undertreat patients to reduce costs, quality management initiatives were implemented to protect consumers.

Continued Escalation of Health Care Costs

Despite those early comprehensive cost planning efforts, health care costs continued to rise in the 1980s and 1990s. In addition to the imperfect operation of a market economy in health care, other factors have affected costs. Some of the most important ones are inflation, improved technologies, increasing demand for health care services, and the impact of fraud and abuse.

Inflation generally affects all business sectors but has tended to escalate faster in health care than in other segments of the economy. Even during economic climates of low to moderate inflation, health care costs continue to consume a greater portion of the GDP, limiting what can be spent on other segments of the economy.

Another reason for the rise in costs is related to the development of and demand for technology. In fact, many believe it is the primary cause of increasing health care costs (Fuchs, 1996). Modern medical care depends on advanced technologies that were not even dreamed of a few decades ago. New drugs, new equipment such as magnetic resonance imaging, and new procedures such as angioplasty and hip replacement are commonplace. The demand for Viagra (a male potency drug) is expected to add $1 billion to health care costs in the next few years (Fuchs, 1999). New technologies are extremely costly: A single x-ray machine can cost up to $250,000, and more advanced types of diagnostic imaging machines can cost up to $2 million each (Roddy, 1996, personal communication).

Demographics also play a role in escalating health care costs. The United States has experienced increases in both the aging and the uninsured nonelderly populations. Medicare and Medicaid have improved access for the poor and elderly, two groups that previously had limited access because of inability to pay. Because older persons are more likely to have chronic illnesses, their demand for health care services exceeds that of younger segments of the population. The elderly population is expected to continue to rise, thus increasing the demand for health care services. Although in 1996 only one in eight Americans was over 65 years of age, by 2030, this figure will increase to one in five, or 20 percent of the population (U. S. Bureau of the Census, 1996).

Fraud and abuse of payment systems account for part of the problem as well. An estimated $75 billion of the United States's annual health expenditures may be due to fraud, including as much as 20 percent of all worker's compensation claims and 10 percent ($17 billion) in Medicare losses (Duston, 1996).

Health care providers such as physicians, clinics, and hospitals are on the honor system, but some intentionally cheat the system with "little fear of getting caught" (Duston, 1996, p. 2B). The Department of Health and Human Services developed Operation Restore Trust to combat fraud in the Medicare program. In 1997, those efforts returned $1 billion in fraudulent payments to Medicare (Shalala and Reinhardt, 1999). In 1999, for example, Beverly Enterprises, the largest U. S. nursing home chain announced it had settled a Medicare fraud suit brought by the Justice Department and set aside $225 million for the fine (*Baltimore Sun,* 1999).

The result of upwardly spiraling costs, fueled by technology, demand for services, and fraud, is that health care costs accounted for an increasing portion of U. S. resources. Most economists believe that this trend cannot continue without damaging the nation's economy.

Cost-Containment Measures Revisited

The continuous escalation in health care costs during the 1980s and 1990s caused both public and private insurers to rethink past containment strategies and to institute a variety of newer measures designed to reduce costs. There are several cost-containment entities and legislative efforts of which students should be aware.

Public and Private Sector Cost-Containment Efforts

Both public and private health care entities have a vested interest in containing costs. Sometimes alone, sometimes in tandem with one another, and frequently with one sector leading and the other following, new initiatives have been developed. Several are reviewed briefly.

Health Care Financing Administration

The Health Care Financing Administration (HCFA) is a federal cost-containment agency created to administer the Medicare and Medicaid programs. Its purpose is to establish standards and monitor care in both programs. It has the authority to enforce these standards for hospitals, nursing homes and other long-term care facilities, laboratories, clinics, and other health facilities that care for Medicare and Medicaid patients. It is responsible for establishing regulation and oversight of any changes legislated by Congress to either program.

The HCFA contracts private insurance agencies, such as Blue Cross and Blue Shield, to service the Medicare program. When patients or their families have questions about coverage or payments, nurses advise them to contact the insurer who administers the program in their area, not the HCFA. While retaining oversight of the Medicaid program, the HCFA has ceded administration of that program to the states. Publications of the HCFA are a good source of information on health care costs, government share of funding, descriptions of the populations served by both programs, and evaluations of program effectiveness for nurses and nursing students interested in these topics.

Professional Review Organizations

Professional review organizations (PROs) are designed to monitor the quality of care received by health care consumers and to ensure that care meets professional standards. The peer review process is a combined public and private effort. These organizations are usually private, but their functions in certain situations are a requirement of federal regulation. Peer review started as a voluntary review process that brought prestige to hospitals passing review.

Professional review organizations became mandatory as a result of Medicare regulations, which stipulated that all hospitals receiving Medicare payments had to submit to peer review. Medicare demanded that hospital admissions and length of stay be examined to ensure that a patient's health and treatment needs were best met in a hospital environment; as a result PROs expanded. If a patient is hospitalized unnecessarily or for a period of time longer than the PRO determines to be appropriate or if procedures are performed that the PRO determines are unnecessary, the hospital is denied Medicare reimbursement for the extra days and the unnecessary procedures. This causes hospitals to be careful about who they admit, how long they allow patients to stay, and what procedures are performed while patients are hospitalized.

Professional review organizations first concentrated on care delivered in hospitals because that was Medicare's emphasis for peer review. Private sector insurance companies expanded the peer review process into other areas, such as outpatient and community-based services. In addition, managed care organizations developed a peer review process. The National Committee for Quality Assurance (NCOA) developed a set of quality measurements (HEDIS) based on clinical outcomes and patient satisfaction (Thompson et al., 1998). What started as a voluntary annual review process became a required protocol for Medicare, Medicaid, and private insurance reimbursement contracts (Buppert, 1999; Grimaldi, 1999).

Diagnosis-Related Groups

Diagnosis-related groups (DRGs) were developed as part of the reform of Medicare payments into a prospective payment system. They place diagnoses with similar resource consumption and length-of-stay patterns into a single category. Diseases are grouped into 495 DRGs, or categories, for reimbursement purposes. For each DRG, the Medicare system has predetermined a fair price for hospital services based on averages. This represents the amount the hospital is paid by Medicare to treat patients in that particular DRG. If the hospital's costs exceed the preestablished reimbursement rate, it loses money. If the hospital is able to treat the patient successfully for less than the established reimbursement rate, it can keep the excess.

Private insurers have benefited from this cost-containment initiative because they tend to establish private reimbursement rates at the same level the federal government uses for reimbursing hospitals for Medicare DRGs.

Block Grants

Combined with the enactment of DRGs and prospective payment, federal reform efforts in the 1980s included block grants to states. Block grants changed the funding mechanism the federal government employed to supply monies for combined federal-state programs. Instead of sharing the expense of a program, such as matching a state's expenditures on Medicaid, the block grant program gave the state a set amount of money. The state government then decided how to spend the federal and state dollars on behalf of Medicaid patients.

Since inception, block grants have reduced the proportion of health program costs paid by the federal government, while the states' shares have increased. At the same time, states have been mandated by federal requirements to provide specific health services to Medicaid patients, such as poor children and the elderly. Block grants have dramatically increased the number of dollars state budgets have been required to expend on health care, thereby forcing either tax increases or reductions in other state-funded programs. Reform proposals in the mid-1990s brought further reductions in federal block grants and frequent proposals to lower federal standards for mandated care, such as in nursing homes. Concerned health professionals believed that such changes would place the poor, especially children and the elderly, at greater risk of reduced access to care and to a lower quality of care (Berman, 1995).

Rapid Expansion of Managed Care

Private insurers and employers have increasingly relied on the managed care concept to lower their health care costs. By 1997, more than 100 million Americans were enrolled in some form of managed care program (Waid, 1998). Managed care programs limit consumers' choices of treatment options or provider of care (or both) but are not intended to reduce quality of care. As reviewed in Chapter 14, they include **health maintainance organizations** (HMOs), **preferred provider organizations** (PPOs), **point-of-service** (POS) **providers,** and **health care networks.** Box 16–3 provides a listing of various types of managed care organizations.

Federal attempts at health care reform, although unsuccessful, spurred the reliance on managed care in employer-provided health plans and the formation of large health networks. Business interests, determined to survive in the changing health care market, merged and consolidated assets into larger systems. For example, Helix Health System and MedAtlantic Healthcare Group merged to form BWHealth, which is now one of the largest health care systems in the United States (Guidera, 1996). Most managed care organizations are for-profit arrangements, whereas some are nonprofit. For example, the Henry Ford Health System, a large nonprofit in Michigan, serves 800,000

BOX 16-3
Types of Managed Care Organizations

Health Maintenance Organizations

Networks or groups of providers who agree to provide certain basic health care services for a single predetermined yearly fee, called a **capitation** fee, constitute a health maintenance organization (HMO). The voluntarily enrolled participants in HMOs pay the same amount regardless of the amount and kind of services they actually receive. Health maintenance organizations have an incentive to promote health and prevent illness in the enrolled participants. They benefit financially when their patients stay well because they receive the same fee whether patients use services or not.

Preferred Provider Organizations

Groups of physicians or institutions who contract with insurance companies to provide services at discounted prices characterize preferred provider organizations (PPO). Policy holders are provided a list of *preferred providers* from which to choose. If they choose to use providers not on the list, they usually must pay a larger share of the costs of care. Insurers save money through PPOs because services are provided at discounted rates.

Point-of-Service Organizations

A hybrid of the PPO concept, these have a provider network of physicians. The consumer selects a primary care physician who acts as a **gatekeeper** and makes decisions about clients' needs for specific health services and referrals. Consumers may seek care from other sources within or outside the provider network but may incur additional costs, unless they have the express permission of the primary care physician. Some plans do not pay for services not approved by the primary physician. Some may even pay physicians bonuses for reducing the number of services used by their patients. Insurers save money through providers by discounted services, reducing services, and eliminating unnecessary specialist referrals.

Health Care Networks

A corporation with a consolidated set of facilities and services intended to provide comprehensive health care to its consumers is a health care network. This is a private health care system. Referrals for almost all services are made within the network. Managed care and other cost-containment efforts are a significant part of any health network operation. A well-developed network includes the following components (Nornhold, p. (1995). What networks mean to you. *Nursing 95*, 25(1), 49–50):

- A major hospital.
- Several small hospitals.
- A long-term care facility.
- A rehabilitation center.
- A home health care agency.
- A subacute center.

people. It offers a comprehensive package of services including preventive services, primary care, specialty care, and acute and long-term care (Whitelaw and Warden, 1999).

Although the private sector initiated managed care for consumers, the public sector soon followed. The Medicare program has allowed seniors to use managed care organizations for some time, and in 1998 unveiled several new health care options for seniors with a managed care emphasis. Federal legislation allowed states to pilot the use of managed care in the Medicaid program, and legislation in 1997 expanded that use to most of the clients in Medicaid programs. These two initiatives will be discussed in detail in the next section.

Recent Legislation in Health Care Reform

Although the Clintons' plan for wholesale health care reform was rejected in 1993, several pieces of federal legislation designed to improve consumer access to health care services and reduce the federal share of health care costs were subsequently enacted. Three important measures are reviewed briefly.

Kassebaum-Kennedy Act 1996

Also known as the Health Insurance Accountability and Portability Act, this bill placed new restrictions on insurance companies. Its provisions included the following:

- Portability of health insurance for people who change jobs.
- Limits on exclusions for preexisting conditions.
- Improved access to health insurance coverage for small employers and their employees.

This legislation had limited impact on consumers. Portability only applied to workers who moved from one job to another. If the new employer had an insurance plan, the new worker was covered immediately, eliminating waiting periods. If the employer did not offer insurance, the employee was forced to purchase an individual plan and the bill did nothing to control the costs of these plans. Individual plans can cost from $2,600 to $5,100 annually, with family plans ranging from $6,200 to $11,800, making it difficult for most consumers to purchase this type of coverage (Government Accounting Office, 1997, 1998). The bill did not require employers to offer health insurance, and few small employers added coverage as a result of this legislation.

Balanced Budget Act of 1997

A major piece of legislation, the Balanced Budget Act (BBA) was enacted in hopes of saving $115 billion dollars over five years (Wilensky and Newhouse, 1999). It concentrated on Medicare reforms, although it did address several other issues. The main features were as follows:

- Provided a Medicare+Choice (Part C) program with new optional features, including a Medicare PPO, private contracts with physicians (outside Medicare regulations), medical savings accounts, and provider-sponsored organizations (PSO) a new hybrid form of managed care.
- Expanded the prospective payment system to include hospital outpatient, home care, and skilled nursing facilities.
- Adjusted capitation rates to reduce geographic variations.
- Shifted home visits from Medicare Part A to Medicare Part B.
- Funded new preventive measures.
- Established the Children's Health Insurance Program to increase access to health care for uninsured children.

Many of the reforms dictated by BBA were not operational until 1998 and 1999. They caused considerable turmoil in home care, skilled nursing facilities, and outpatient care as well as with Medicare patients needing home care, who had to bear greater out-of-pocket expenses (Government Accounting Office, 1999a). The full impact of these initiatives on consumers and providers of health care has not yet been determined. There is some concern the BBA will merely shift the cost of services from the federal government to individual consumers, health care businesses, and state governments rather than actually saving dollars. The shifting of costs is illustrated in the accompanying case study (Box 16–4).

Children's Health Insurance Program

Part of the Balanced Budget Act of 1997, this program provided federal funds to states in an effort to increase health care services to at-risk children not previously covered by public or private health insurance. As of 1998, there were at least 11 million children who were uninsured and at risk (Weinick, Weigers, and Cohen, 1998).

The State Children's Health Insurance Program (SCHIP) provided $24 billion in federal grants over five years. States could enroll at-risk children in Medicaid or establish a new health program. It is too early to evaluate the SCHIP, but preliminary information suggests enrollment efforts have been slow to identify and provide coverage to targeted children (Halfon et al., 1999). A major concern is the funding mechanism and time limit set by the legislation. Questions such as "What will happen after five years when federal funding ends?" and "Will the states be left with the decision to cover all costs or discontinue CHIPs, or will the federal government renew commitment to the program?" remain unanswered.

Current Issues of Concern

Despite public sector efforts to improve health care access, there remains a substantial group of people at risk. These individuals either have no health insurance or are in danger of losing employer-provided health coverage.

BOX 16–4
Case Study: The Changing Face of Health Care Finance—One Person's Story

Situation
Mrs. Martin is an 80 year old widow who lives alone. She has just returned home from a skilled nursing home. She was transferred there after her hospitalization and treatment for a fractured hip. She is hypertensive and diabetic and takes oral medications for these conditions, including a beta blocker. As the home health nurse, you visit Mrs. Martin to determine how she is adjusting.

Assessment
- Mrs. Martin is able to ambulate and perform all activities of daily living without difficulty.
- She is very upset, having just received notice that her Medicare health maintenance organization (HMO) will no longer cover her.
- She does not know what to do because she is on a fixed income, consisting of social security benefits of $600 per month ($8,388 per year,) which is the average widow's social security benefit.
- Although she changed to the current HMO because it included a prescription drug benefit and reduced her insurance paperwork, she is willing to change again to another HMO.
- Her prescription drugs will cost $125 per month ($1,500 per year) if she must pay out of pocket for them.
- Her daughter lives in the area, but she is not financially able to assist with her mother's expenses.

Continued Assessment
After you leave Mrs. Martin's home, you investigate further and discover that no other HMO is willing to enroll her, and therefore, she will have to return to the basic Medicare program.

- She will need Medigap insurance to cover her Medicare deductibles and copayments.
- Her out-of-pocket expenses for basic health care costs, even if she has no other medical emergencies or hospitalizations, will be as follows: Medicare part A is free but requires a deductible per hospitalization or skilled nursing facility stay. Medicare part B equals $646 in yearly premiums as well as copayments for service. Note: Premiums are expected to increase to $1,172 by 2006; prescription drugs are $1,500 annually; and Medigap policy costs $1,461 annually. The total is $3,607, or 43 percent of her total annual income.
- Mrs. Martin will not be able to pay this much for health care because she has to pay for food, clothing, and shelter. Even without the Medigap insurance, the cost would be 26 percent of her total annual income, and she would have no coverage for her copayments and deductibles if she has another sustained health care need.

(continued)

BOX 16-4

Case Study: The Changing Face of Health Care Finance—One Person's Story (*Continued*)

Plan of Care

Your employer has restricted you from helping Mrs. Martin with her financial issues because they are not considered nursing services, and the agency cannot bill Medicare for them. So you problem solve with her during your regular follow-up visits for the hip fracture and medication assessments and establish the following plan:

- Arrange to meet with Mrs. Martin's daughter and enlist her help in completing the activities below. Validate that she is unable to assist financially.
- Mrs. Martin must apply to Medicaid for assistance to low income Medicare patients. If she is eligible, she will not need to purchase Medigap insurance. This will require much paperwork and waiting for approvals.
- Mrs. Martin should investigate the possibility that a pharmaceutical company might assist her in obtaining her medications at low or no cost. This will require many phone calls and more paperwork.
- Mrs. Martin should contact her local Office on Aging. They may be able to provide additional financial assistance, some social work support to negotiate the Medicaid system, and transportation to various offices as needed.

*American Association of Retired Persons's Plan C rates

Significant Pool of Uninsured and Underinsured

The number of uninsured Americans continues to grow. In 1997, an estimated 43.4 million Americans, more than 16 percent of the population, had no health insurance (Bennefield, 1998a). When the temporarily uninsured are added to the count, the number of persons without health insurance is even greater. Between 1993 and 1996, 71.5 million Americans, or one of every 3.3 citizens, was uninsured for some or all of that period (Bennefield, 1998b). The poor, near poor, foreign-born, and young adults (between 18 and 24) are in greatest danger of having no health insurance.

Because most nonelderly Americans are insured by job-related policies, they are at risk if they change or lose their jobs or if their employer chooses not to offer health insurance benefits. It is myth that people do not have health insurance because they do not work. Some uninsured people do not work, but most have part-time or full-time jobs. Davis and Schoen (1994) report that 84 percent of the uninsured are employed or are family members of employed individuals. Fifty percent of all poor workers are uninsured (Bennefield, 1998a). Poor workers are less likely to be insured than poor non workers, perhaps because many poor nonworkers may be eligible for government-sponsored health care such as Medicaid.

In addition to the uninsured, there are many Americans who are under-insured because their insurance plan either requires large out-of-pocket expenses or limits coverage for catastrophic illnesses. In 1995 the size of this at-risk group was estimated at around 29 million people (Short and Banthin, 1995).

Reduction or Elimination of Employer-provided Health Insurance

One reason for the growth of the uninsured population is changes in employer-provided health insurance. Because of increased costs, some employers have left the system and insured their own employees (called **self-insurance**), scaled back or eliminated health benefits, limited the employees' choice of in-surance plans, or passed more of the costs of insurance on to employees.

Employers led the charge to managed care, and now many employers limit their health insurance plan to managed care options. At the same time employers have increased the employee share of premium costs, making health insurance unaffordable to many workers (Government Accounting Office, 1997). Health insurance programs sponsored by employers continued to decline throughout the 1990s.

In 1979, 15.1 percent of workers did not have health insurance; by 1995, 23.3 percent did not (Kronich and Gilmer, 1999). Smaller firms, nonunion-ized work places, and service industries were more likely not to provide in-surance. In 1995, 50 percent of workers in firms with under 10 employees had employer-based health coverage, while 82 percent of workers in firms with 1,000 employers had health insurance (Government Accounting Office, 1997).

Employers are also dropping coverage for their retirees. Between 1993 and 1996, approximately 1 in every 10 retirees were dropped from their em-ployer-provided plan (Government Accounting Office, 1998). In 1996, for ex-ample, Pabst Brewing Company canceled health benefits for 750 retirees. This is particularly burdensome for young retirees who are not yet eligible for Medicare and must pay for individual health coverage, often only available at very high costs, or go without.

Impact of Managed Care on Health Services

During the 1990s, the rapid growth of HMOs and related managed care orga-nizations raised concerns that quality of care might suffer. Care decisions, for-merly based on the needs of the patient, were increasingly influenced by busi-ness interests. Physicians, hospitals, and other providers were being forced to provide services for less. These conditions created shock waves in the health care industry, resulting in limits on choice and services, a drive to expand managed care to vulnerable populations, and physician gags and financial in-centives to limit services.

Limits on Choice and Services

In the past decade many employers have limited employees' choice of health plans. Some managed care plans increased the cost (copayments or deductibles) to consumers who used out-of-plan providers and services. Some plans refused to pay any part of out-of-plan services.

Managed care plans set stricter limits than other health insurance plans on the types of services covered. Expensive new therapies, such as bone marrow transplants for breast cancer, and costly treatments for rare conditions were often denied, as were referrals, especially outside the plan (Larson, 1996; Mechanic, 1997). Routines services, such as hospitalization after childbirth, were also cut. News Note 16–1 describes congressional reaction to such cuts. As managed care became widespread, concern also developed about managed care practices toward patients with psychiatric illnesses, as denials and limits on coverage for chronic problems became routine (Purdy, 1995; Sharpfstein, 1996.)

Drive to Expand Managed Care to Vulnerable Populations

Federal and state initiatives to reduce costs have been designed to enroll large segments of the Medicare and Medicaid populations in managed care health plans. Critics voiced concern that these two vulnerable populations, who traditionally had poorer health status than employed adults, would not be well served by managed care. Pilot programs with Medicare HMOs reported that seniors were less satisfied and disenrolled more frequently than consumers covered by employer-provided managed plans.

States experimenting with using managed care to control Medicaid expenses reported that some plans practiced fraud and misrepresentation in efforts to enroll Medicaid patients by overstating available benefits and services. In addition to abuses, there was some evidence that Medicaid patients had difficulty negotiating the **gatekeeping** process to access services. They often needed to call several times to succeed in getting an appointment or were given appointments at geographically inaccessible sites (Khanna, 1995).

By the late 1990s many states required Medicaid patients to be enrolled in managed care; for Medicare clients, however, managed care was still an option. Many seniors liked the managed care option because prescription drugs were included and they had little or no paperwork associated with filing health insurance claims. By 1998 there were 7 million Medicare clients in managed care programs and around 11 million in Medicaid managed care (Braden et al., 1998; Government Accounting Office, 1999b). At the end of the decade, however, many managed care organizations were rethinking their participation in Medicare and Medicaid. Some, for example, Aetna/U. S. HealthCare, Humana, and Kaiser-Permanente, disenrolled Medicare clients in certain geographic areas. An estimated 400,000 Medicare patients were involuntarily dropped from managed care in 1999 (Inglehart, 1999). In the mean-

NEWS NOTE 16-1

Getting Tough on Drive-through Delivery

Government intervention is necessary to stop insurers from forcing mothers and newborns from the hospital too soon after delivery, Kathryn Moore, director of government relations for the American College of Obstetricians and Gynecologists, said Dec. 13 [1995].

Moore spoke at a panel discussion on the issue at a National Conference of State Legislatures meeting in Washington.

About half of the states have introduced or passed maternity-stay legislation since Maryland adopted the first such law earlier this year, Moore said.

The trend is a reaction to so-called "drive-through" deliveries—a growing insurer practice of limiting maternity-stay coverage to 24 hours or less after delivery. The obstetrician/gynecologist group and the American Academy of Pediatrics recommend 48–hour stays following a normal vaginal delivery and 96 hours for a cesarean section.

"We have a situation of insurers limiting consumers' coverage, of insurers pressuring doctors, ignoring medical guidelines and not producing any conclusive data that their practice is safe," Moore said.

Getting Tough

In some cases, insurers are overruling physicians' decisions to keep women in the hospital longer than their coverage allows, she said. Some insurers also threaten to cut physicians from the insurance panel unless they release women and infants early, she added.

State maternity-stay laws are a reaction to market forces' inability to change insurer practices, Moore said.

"Given all of these factors, government intervention is necessary," she said.

E. Neil Trautman, manager for health care policy for the U. S. Chamber of Commerce, disagreed.

"If we encourage the marketplace to respond to consumer demands, we can do better," he said.

The chamber opposes insurance-benefit mandates, Trautman said. Each mandate makes insurance less affordable and could price health coverage out of some Americans' reach, he added.

Supporters of maternity-stay legislation maintain that its price would be low.

According to Colleen Meiman, legislative assistant to Sen. Bill Bradley (D-NJ), maternity-stay legislation would only add $1.13 a year to insurance premiums. Bradley, along with Sen. Nancy Kassebaum (R–KS), sponsors federal maternity-stay legislation currently before Congress.

Bradley is looking for a measure to attach the legislation to a vote. Kassebaum said she prefers to hold hearings on the measure first and then bring it before the Senate next year.

Like the Bradley/Kassebaum bill, most maternity-stay legislation requires that insurers follow national guidelines. Many measures, including the federal proposal, permit early discharges if the physician and woman approve, and if follow-up care is provided.

Maryland has had trouble enforcing its new law, which took effect Oct. 1, 1995.

Insurers are forcing doctors to discharge women early with follow-up care, rather than giving physicians and women a choice, said Maryland Delegate Marilyn Goldwater (D-Bethesda). State lawmakers are trying to close that loophole, she said.—G.A.

time, managed care organizations with Medicaid clients complained of financial losses, slowed or eliminated their efforts to enroll Medicaid patients, and lobbied state and federal governments to increase capitation fees (McCue, 1999). Some of the financial difficulties for managed care organizations may be because both Medicaid and Medicare clients need more medical services because of the health risks associated with poverty, near poverty, or advancing age.

Physician Financial Incentives to Limit Services

In 1996, a serious development came to light about managed care efforts to regulate physicians who advised their patients about treatment options. Physicians were sometimes discouraged or forbidden by their managed care contracts to mention treatment options that were expensive or not covered by a patient's managed care plan (Larson, 1996). Because of intense publicity, physician gag rules have been largely discontinued either through voluntary means or by state regulation. Other incentives to limit service persist.

Some plans offered physicians bonuses for limiting services and referrals for their patients. U. S. HealthCare, for example, offered physicians bonuses if they were able to reduce hospital stays, limit emergency department use, limit use of costly prescription drugs, and reduce referrals to specialists (Gray, 1996; Hillman et al., 1999). Such bonuses placed physicians in conflict between the best interests of patients and their own economic best interests. Physicians who called attention to bonus plans or exceeded average costs for services could be terminated by the plans (Gray, 1996; Larson, 1996). These practices evoked concern by organized medicine, organized nursing, consumer groups, and the U. S. Congress.

Economics of Nursing Care

Traditionally, nurses were unconcerned with the cost of care, believing all patients were entitled to high-quality nursing care regardless of ability to pay. Until fairly recently, few efforts were made to determine the actual cost of nursing care. The average hospital bill included the cost of nursing services in the general category of "room rate," just as housekeeping services are included in the room rate. In the past, the hospital census (number of patients) was used to determine the number of nurses needed. This worked fairly well when payment was retrospective. With the advent of prospective payment, however, it was imperative for hospitals to determine their staffing needs more efficiently.

It has long been recognized that different patients require different amounts of nursing time, depending in large part on how sick they are. **Patient classification systems (PCS)** were developed to identify patients' needs for nursing care in quantitative terms in order to help hospitals determine the need for nursing resources. Patient classification systems have been developed that depend on patient **acuity,** or degree of illness, and the resulting amount and complexity of nursing care required.

Initiatives called *costing nursing services* have been used to determine precisely the cost of nursing care. Not knowing the exact costs of nursing services limits nurses' ability to determine what high-quality nursing care costs and to calculate the number of hours of nursing care it takes to provide service for each DRG. Determining the best **skill mix,** that is, the ratio of registered nurses to licensed practical nurses and nursing assistants in each hospital unit, is also impaired when the cost of nursing care is unknown.

In the past, it was assumed that the cost of nurses was a major part of hospital expenses. During tough economic times, the first cost reduction efforts were therefore aimed at nursing. Studies in the mid-1980s found that nursing accounted for only 20 to 28 percent of the costs of hospitalization for two-thirds of the DRGs examined (McKibben, 1985). Costing nursing services and developing standardized reimbursements based on costs were expected to enhance the ability of nurse managers to control nursing resources and negotiate for a fair share of hospital financial resources.

There is some concern, however, that costing nursing services may not be beneficial to nursing. Costing strategies may make nursing more vulnerable to labor substitution efforts as hospital administrators experience increasing pressure to reduce costs. Isolating nursing costs might also lead to efforts to devalue nursing services by reducing wages or impeding salary increases (salary compression) (Buerhaus, 1995a). In fact, there is some evidence to suggest that managed care and other cost-containment efforts have had a direct negative impact on nurse staffing and salaries (Buerhaus and Staiger, 1999).

Impact of Cost Containment on Nursing Care

When the drive to provide high-quality nursing care meets the constraints of cost containment head-on, something has to give. What nurses hope, as both providers and consumers of health care, is that quality will not suffer because of the emphasis on "the bottom line." To many, this is a forlorn hope. Yet the financial realities that affect the institutions in which 60 percent of nurses practice—hospitals—cannot be ignored. To stay in business, hospitals must make at least enough money to pay personnel, maintain buildings and equipment, and pay suppliers of goods and services. One cost-reduction strategy has been to reorganize and restructure the delivery of hospital nursing services, reduce nursing personnel, and substitute unlicensed assistive personnel for registered nurses (Curtin, 1994; Buerhaus and Staiger, 1999). This strategy was explored in Chapter 13.

There is some evidence that hospitals, after years of reducing nursing personnel, are now in need of additional nurses, especially clinical specialists. In a 1998 survey, 80 percent of hospitals reported they have or anticipate a shortage of nurses in the near future (The Hay Group, 1998).

The leadership of the American Nurses Association (ANA) has been outspoken in their assertion that overzealous cost-containment efforts have led to lower quality hospital care. In 1996, the ANA president called on professional nurses to inform family members, friends, and acquaintances about the "eroding quality in acute care" (Betts, 1996, p. 4). The ANA's "Every Patient Deserves A Nurse" campaign is a concrete step taken by the professional organization to educate the public about these concerns. Accompanying News Note 16–2 elaborates on the effects of overemphasizing cost reductions in hospitals and other health care facilities.

As hospital employment opportunities for nurses leveled off, the dispersal of health care services into community settings had improved opportuni-

NEWS NOTE 16-2

Who's Taking Care of Mama?

The delivery of health care in America has changed a great deal. Unless you are very young, you probably remember doctors making house calls. We knew our doctors quite well and the nurses who worked with them. Those days are long gone, and with them, it's sad to say, is much of the trust that we reposed in our health care delivery system. Now, we must all ask who's taking care of mama when she goes to the hospital?

Nursing's Proud History

As a child, I dreamed of being a professional nurse. Caring for others who were not able to care for themselves was a calling for me as it has been for generations of nurses. There is simply no reward like that received for serving another human being who is depending upon you for their recovery or even their life.

Through the years, I have witnessed changes in our nursing profession that are both exciting for the professional nurse and essential for our patients. Nursing has made strides educationally and professionally that have brought it to the forefront of the national health care debate. Every-day, there is more evidence that the professional nurse is the key to successful and cost-effective health care delivery.

Research shows that when there are more nurses in a health facility, there will be lower mortality rates, shorter lengths of stay, lower costs and fewer complications. In addition to boosting health outcomes, professional nurse staffing levels are tied closely to a hospital's ability to provide care in the least costly, most highly effective means possible.

Opportunities Stifled

Despite this, changes in the health care community are stifling the opportunities that the professional nurse brings to health care delivery. Many external and internal forces, ranging from political and economic to social, are driving the health care industry to make sweeping but not yet fully evaluated changes in how, where and by whom health services are delivered.

These forces have been escalating rapidly over the past few years and include a heightened scrutiny by consumers and insurers about rising costs, pressure to move services to less expensive environments and embarrassing public health statistics. In addition, continually tightening federal reimbursement guidelines for Medicare and Medicaid have spawned a myriad of managed care networks that have resulted in even more changes.

I am disappointed to say that these forces have culminated in an institutional mentality in hospitals that is driven much more by the bottom line than by health outcomes. Health care facilities, in what they perceive as a scramble to survive, are borrowing cost-containment strategies utilized by other industries. These strategies include "downsizing" or "right-sizing" the work force to cut labor costs, and then crosstraining or "multi-skilling" remaining workers to maximize their productivity. Facilities are merging, closing and forming networks to better utilize existing services and resources—all in an effort to self-regulate and limit external controls and, perhaps, public accountability.

Dangers of Change

Professional nurses are greatly concerned about the implications of these changes in health care. Highest on the list of concerns is the impact on patient safety and quality of care and the current lack of data collection and sophisticated quality measurements to quantify these concerns. Nurses are concerned about the "deskilling" of nursing, the fragmentation of comprehensive care into a series of tasks and the assignments of these tasks to unlicensed individuals. When a hospital staff is diluted to a staff mix of as few as 50 percent registered nurses, the facility is risking increased mortality. When the hospital assigns more and more administrative functions to professional nurses, patient care also will suffer.

Hospitals have now reached the point that, in too many cases, the personnel tending its patients' needs are neither qualified nor trained adequately to perform the duties assigned to them. They are instead unlicenced employees who, while dressed appropriately, are not professional nurses at all. In some hospitals, professional nurses are told not to wear any identification indicating they are registered nurses (RNs) so that patients will not know the difference between the professional staff and the unlicensed, untrained staff. That is simply shocking!

Yet, these are exactly the kinds of changes that we are witnessing today, and it could not come at a more critical time in our history—a time when there is an increasing growth of an aging patient population that dictates an increased, rather than decreased, nursing service.

Consumer Education

As professional nurses, we feel obligated to tell our friends, families and the public that hospital care must be sought and procured with apprehension and diligence. No patient should be admitted to hospital care without an informed and active advocate, whether a relative or friend. Health care in America has changed dramatically and the public must change with it, or change it. Until then, America's professional nurse must educate consumers by issuing the warning that it is critical to ask: "Who's taking care of mama?"

Reprinted with permission of Morris, E. A. (1996). Who's taking care of Mama? *The American Nurse*, 28(1), 4.

ties for community-based nursing services, such as home care. However in the past five years the home care market has also demonstrated a reduced demand for nursing services. Managed care appears responsible for a significant portion of the reduced demand. In areas where managed care organizations are more concentrated, employment rates and wage scales for nurses are lower than in areas with fewer of these care models (Buerhaus and Staiger, 1999). Medicare's expansion of prospective payment systems into community-based settings such as home care and skilled nursing facilities is likely to increase pressure to reduce costs and may also adversely affect the prospects for nursing employment.

Quality of care is expected to become a more important competitive feature among managed care and health network providers. Nurses are more favorably regarded as care providers when compared with other health professionals. Eighty percent of Americans believe nurses do a good job, whereas only 65 percent believe doctors and hospitals do. Only 34 percent believe that managed care organizations are doing right by the consumer (Blendon et al., 1998). To the extent that the nursing profession can link quality of care with nursing care, the demand for nursing services will continue to flourish (Buerhaus, 1995b).

Cost Containment and Quality Management

Most people agree that there is potential for disaster if cost reduction is the only outcome that matters in the health care system. The challenge is to balance the cost-effectiveness and quality of patient care. Concern for maintaining high-quality services in the face of cost constraints has led to the development of a new health care initiative called **quality management.** As discussed in Chapter 13, this field is growing and changing rapidly and creating change within hospitals. The accompanying interview (Interview 16–1) with two nurses involved in quality management gives insights into the complexities and satisfactions of participation in quality management initiatives (Robertson, 1996; Alexander, 1996).

Health Care Reform and National Health Insurance

In 1999, the United States and South Africa were the only two industrialized nations not providing universal access to health care to all citizens. Despite the fact that 1997 health care expenditures in this country averaged $3,925 per person, infant mortality ranked eighteenth of 24 among developed countries, lower than many countries with far fewer national resources (Anderson, 1997). Two-thirds of inner-city children under four years of age did not have the full series of immunizations that could protect them from preventable childhood diseases (Burner and Waldo, 1995). There was no established minimum set of health services available to the entire population, and access to health care was not universal.

Concerns about health care in the United States are not new. In the 1992 presidential campaign, candidates in both political parties, as well as nonpartisan groups, advocated some type of health care reform. These groups included nursing organizations, the American Association of Retired Persons, labor unions, the American College of Physicians, the National Leadership Coalition for Health Care Reform, and members of the U. S. Congress. Most of these groups put forward specific plans for reform, including "Nursing's Agenda for Health Care Reform," discussed in Chapter 4. Despite widespread public support for reform, the effort failed. Lack of legislation on health care reform was aided by powerful interest groups such as the pharmaceutical, health insurance, and health equipment industries; the American Medical Association; and the American Hospital Association.

Today concerns about access to health care, the quality of care, and limits on consumer choice in managed care have fueled a new debate about health care in this country. There is the question about what to do with the millions of people who have no insurance and limited access to health care. In addition, there is a growing concern about consumer choice restrictions in MCOs. A 1999 Time/CNN poll reported that 85 percent of Americans think patients should be able to select their own doctor, and 61 percent think patients should be allowed to sue their MCO for medical malpractice (Miller, 1999, p. 61). A

Quality Management and Cost Containment

JoAnn Alexander, MSN, RN, is chief operations officer, and Charlene Robertson, MSN, RN, is chief nursing officer, at a private not-for-profit hospital in a mid-sized city in the southeastern United States.

Interviewer: Tell me a little about the hospital—its size, services, and the number of nurses employed there.

Robertson: This is a 365-bed hospital. We have all services, including obstetrics, pediatrics, and behavioral health. There are 596 members on the nursing staff, which includes 464 RNs [registered nurses], 38 LPNs [licensed practical nurses], and 94 nursing assistants.

Interviewer: What specific cost-containment programs have been started here in the past few years that have influenced nursing care?

Robertson: Specific cost-containment programs began in 1992 with intensive education of physicians, nurses, and support staff on continuous quality improvement strategies, managed care strategies, and cost containment. The implementation of continuous quality improvement enhanced several multidisciplinary clinical groups to achieve good outcomes. For example:

- The pneumonia group reduced length of stay by four days and cost per discharge.
- A multidisciplinary CareTrac [clinical pathway] tool was implemented housewide with physician support.
- A short-stay, one-stop unit for PTCA [percutaneous transluminal coronary angioplasty] patients was implemented. Patient care was also redesigned with a combination of an RN and cardiac tech who make up a "care pair." This approach has reduced cost by $1,400 per case, with high patient and physician satisfaction.

Interviewer: What has been done to relieve nurses of nonnursing tasks?

Robertson: Improvement in documentation comes immediately to mind, with charting by exception, bedside charting, computerized Kardexes and MAR, and the implementation of CareTracs, which has reduced redundant documentation. Other strategies include the formation of care pairs in the cardiac short-stay unit, cross-training in the operative suite, and implementation of the Pyxis system.

Interviewer: What is the goal of quality management?

Alexander: The focus of continuous quality improvement is to view our hospital system from our patient, physician, and family perspective. Multidisciplinary cross-functional teams identify barriers to service and systematically implement change using the PDCA [plan, do, check, and act] approach.

Interviewer: Who participates in quality management?

Alexander: All members of the health care team, including physicians, nurses, and support and clinical services associates participate in quality management. The cross-functional team allows all persons to have an active role. Customer service is everyone's responsibility.

Interviewer: How are nurses involved in quality management?

Robertson: About five years ago, we reorganized nursing and decentralized certain functions. The director of each unit has the responsibility of quality management and continuous quality improvement activities for that unit. When our hospitalwide and unit-specific quality monitoring programs reveal a problem, an action plan is developed either on the unit or by the nursing council. For example, the response on a hospitalwide patient satisfaction survey showed that patients felt that the call lights were not being responded to in a timely manner for pain medication or other needs. The nursing staff was apprised of this concern and, as a means of addressing this concern, a nurse pager system was implemented. Patient care needs are communicated immediately. The pager dials in directly to the nurse who provides that care. This response is monitored internally by placing a phone call to the patient after discharge, and the unit secretary completes periodic monitoring of actual time frames of nurse response to patient call lights. By increasing the sensitivity of the patient's need for immediate call-light response and by implementing the new pager system, the patient satisfaction in this area has greatly increased.

The hospital is organized around a service line structure. The chief nursing officer is accountable for nursing wher-

(*continued*)

Quality Management and Cost Containment (*Continued*)

ever nursing is practiced. Nursing leads some of the cross-functional teams and was involved with the development of the CareTracs. Most of the care managers are nurses who manage patients daily through the system and are starting to establish a method to manage across the continuum.

Interviewer: How does quality management affect the way nursing care is provided?

Alexander: The CareTracs eliminate the need for nurses to be mind readers of other disciplines involved in the care of the patient. It allows better dialogue with the disciplines and the patient. It makes the truly collaborative model easier to live with on a daily basis. It also gives nurses more objective outcome data to measure the effectiveness of their care.

Interviewer: What would you say about cost containment and quality management to students of professional nursing around the United States?

Alexander: It is important for nurses to adopt a philosophy of rather than finding fault, find a remedy. The public will not accept a continued escalation in cost, and nurses are in a good position to broaden their skills outside of the hospital and be primary care providers. I believe that the cross-functional team is the model that will provide productivity with time. Be a risk taker and have the initiative to try something different and remember that cost and quality can be measured.

Courtesy of Charlene Robertson and JoAnn Alexander.

Patient's Bill of Rights has stalled in Congress every year since 1997. Many of its most vocal opponents are the same groups who opposed President Clinton's plan for health reform.

In the present political climate, it seems unlikely that a systematic and comprehensive reform of the entire health care system is possible. Instead, we can expect to see incremental efforts to address specific issues of concern. Box 16–5 identifies some of the proposals under consideration in the year 2000 and beyond. Most experts agree that reform efforts are doomed unless they are projected to reduce, or at least not increase, the cost of health care.

Guidelines for Evaluating Reform Proposals

Despite wide-ranging differences of opinion about the specifics of health care reform proposals, there are areas of general agreement. Some form of health care reform will ultimately be enacted. Some general guidelines to look for in evaluating reform proposals are the following:

1. Is there a uniform minimum set of benefits for all citizens, otherwise known as universal care?
2. Are coverage and benefits continuous and not dependent on where people live or work?
3. Are there mechanisms for controlling costs, especially administrative expenses?

BOX 16-5

Potential Health Care Reform Initiatives: Some Predictions Based on Anticipated Changes to Health Insurance Laws and Regulations

Employer-provided Health Insurance

- Employers will be required to provide health insurance for all employees, including part-time workers.
- Employees might be given an allowance and expected to purchase their own insurance. (Hawaii is the only state currently requiring health insurance coverage for all employees.)

Universal Health Insurance

- Every American will be covered by health insurance.
- Government will expand health insurance funding for all vulnerable populations, including those currently not covered.
- Employees will be covered by employer-provided plans.

Catastrophic Limits

- Catastrophic coverage will be part of every health insurance plan, and lifetime limits on costs of care will be increased or limits eliminated altogether.

Medicare

- Medicare payments for services will continue to decline.
- Copayments or deductibles will rise.
- Increased pressure to enroll all Medicare recipients in managed care plans is likely.
- Well-off seniors may pay more in premiums than those who are less affluent.

Medicaid

- Expansion of states requiring managed care enrollment for Medicaid recipients will occur.
- Changes in the standard set of health services paid for by the program will occur, with most likely reductions in services.
- Reduction in federal oversight will occur, freeing states to change eligibility standards for service.
- Some states might continue existing eligibility criteria; others might expand or reduce criteria.
- Minimal copayments for services may be added.

Block Grants

- Expect to see more federal funds distributed in block grants, less federal oversight of funded programs, and greater state autonomy in selection of services and populations served by federal funds.

(continued)

BOX 16-5

Potential Health Care Reform Initiatives: Some Predictions Based on Anticipated Changes to Health Insurance Laws and Regulations (*Continued*)

Managed Care and Health Networks
- The proportion of the population covered by managed care will continue to expand.
- Health care providers will continue to merge into large health networks.

Managed Care and Vulnerable Populations
- All the cost savings of switching vulnerable populations to managed care have been realized.
- Managed care organizations (MCOs) are finding it difficult to care for Medicare and Medicaid populations for the established capitation fees and are disenrolling or declining new enrollments. This will continue and may accelerate.
- Studies indicate that MCOs have the healthiest of the Medicaid and Medicare populations, (i.e., seniors with few chronic conditions, young mothers, infants, and children) (Braden et al., 1998; Government Accounting Office, 1999).
- If the government persists in continuing MCO enrollment of all, including the less healthy Medicare and Medicaid populations, capitation fees will increase, cost savings will disappear, health care costs for MCOs will increase, and the government will reduce the menu of benefits required of health care providers in order to keep costs down.

Managed Care and Legislation
- If federal legislation regulating MCO practices does not pass, states will pass more laws.
- Consumers will find regulations differ depending on the state in which they live. (In 1999, 39 states had laws providing comprehensive consumer health protection, 22 banned financial incentives to physicians, 47 banned gag clauses in physician contracts, and 37 required direct access for consumers to obstetries/gynecological services [Association of Operating Room Nurses, 1999].)

Patients' Bill of Rights
- Various versions of patients' rights legislation have been considered by Congress every year since 1997. In whatever version ultimately passes, some provisions are expected to be:
- The right to sue your MCO.
- The right to go to the doctor of your choice.
- The right to see appropriate specialists outside the MCO.
- The right to use the emergency room for services any prudent layperson will consider necessary.
- The right for expedited review of denials of health care services.

- The right to be provided with a list of all treatment options for your condition.
- The right to privacy (sharing of health information limited to use for clinical decision making, not to be shared with other insurers).
- Protection for health care professional whistle blowers from retaliation by employers.

Rationing

- Current rationing of care is by ability to pay; insurance coverage ensures care for most.
- Because for-profit structures dominate the health market, there may be additional curtailments on such items as expensive therapies, disputes between providers and payers about what constitutes "experimental procedures," and shortening of allowable hospital recovery times.
- Legislation may be necessary to compel care.
- Unless a minimum standard of care is established at the federal level, each state may need to take action separately to address each inequity. For example, some states have already passed legislation that ensures a new mother's right to extend postdelivery hospital stays to 48 hours. Insurers had been willing to pay for 24 hours or less.

Two-tiered System of Health Care

- Health care services will be based on ability to pay.
- There will be a basic level of benefits established for those with public health insurance (similar to the Oregon Medicaid Plan).
- All other individuals will be free to purchase additional benefits based on ability to pay.
- Private employers might provide only the basic plan, or a range of plans, and employees will be free to chose more costly options and pay the premium difference out of pocket.

Association of Operating Room Nurses (1999). Patient rights still hot topic in Congress and the states. *AORN Journal*, 69(5), 1031–1036; Braden, B. R., Cowan, C. A., Lazenby, H. C., et al. (1998). National health expenditures, 1997. *Health Care Financing Review*, 20(1), 83–126; Government Accounting Office (1999c). Medicare managed care: Better risk adjustment expected to reduce excess payments overall while making them fairer to individual plans (GAO/T-HEHS-99-72, February 25). Washington, D. C.: Government Printing Office.

4. Are provisions made for care to be provided by the most cost-effective personnel, taking quality issues and patient outcomes into consideration?
5. Are the issues of adequate facilities and personnel to ensure access for all addressed?
6. Is there an emphasis on quality care?
7. Are there incentives for healthy lifestyles and preventive care?

A point of particular interest to nurses is the issue of cost-effectiveness of personnel. If care is to be provided by the most cost-effective personnel, it should mean an expansion of the role of nurses as primary care providers (Fig. 16–3). Studies have shown that nurses are cost-effective caregivers and are well ac-

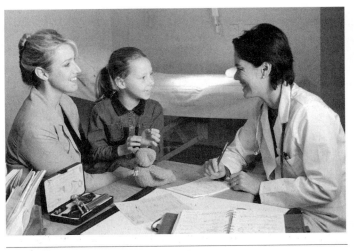

Figure 16–3

Cost-containment initiatives have strengthened the demand for nurse practitioners. Another result has been federal legislation requiring reimbursement of nurse practitioners who care for certain populations. Only sweeping reimbursement reform, however, will allow nurse practitioners, like this family nurse practitioner, to demonstrate their brand of high-quality, cost-effective, primary care and thereby contribute to the nation's efforts to contain health care costs (Photo courtesy of Hamilton Medical Center, Dalton, Georgia).

cepted by the public (Lenz and Edwards, 1992; Harrinton and Estes, 1994; and Scott and Rantz, 1997). Organized medicine, however, actively opposes moves to give clinical autonomy to almost all nonphysician providers (Feldstein, 1998). This is a conflict that must be resolved for true reform to occur, and nurses themselves must be active in its resolution.

Summary of Key Points

- How health care is financed in the United States has changed dramatically from a system dominated by personal payment to one dominated by third-party payment.
- This change created basic economic disequilibrium in health care because people who do not pay directly for health care are not sensitive to the price of care.
- Medicare and Medicaid programs, begun in 1965, created a serious financial drain on federal and state budgets. In response, cost-containment efforts were begun by the federal government in the 1970s.
- Initial cost-containment efforts were unsuccessful, so in 1982 more sweeping reforms were initiated. Retrospective payment was replaced by prospective payment.
- In the early 1990s, systemwide health reform efforts were supported by public opinion but failed to pass the U. S. Congress. Even without govern-

mental action, many Americans have seen substantial changes in their health care plans, stimulated by business interests and employers.

- There has been a dramatic escalation in managed care plans and consolidation of health providers into larger health networks.
- By the late 1990s, governmental action imposed some restrictions on health insurance practices, made an effort to improve health care for a limited number of at-risk children, and encouraged or mandated the enrollment of Medicaid and Medicare clients in managed care.
- The entire health care system, including nurses and nursing services, has been profoundly affected by these changes.
- Further changes are on the horizon. It remains to be seen whether these changes will improve access and maintain quality of health care for all Americans.

Critical Thinking Questions

1. In your view, is access to health care a basic right? Who should pay for it? Be prepared to defend your opinions.
2. List the basic health care services that should be provided to all citizens. Compare your list with the lists of classmates and discuss the reasons for your priorities.
3. Should there be a limit on the percentage of national resources expended on health care? If so, how should the limit be established?
4. What process should be used to determine how health care resources are allocated? List criteria you would suggest to determine whether or not a person should receive a kidney transplant, a hip replacement, or a bone marrow transplant.
5. Should people with healthy lifestyles pay the same for care or insurance as those whose habits result in a greater likelihood of illness? How could such a differentiation be determined?
6. Should there be rationing of extremely expensive procedures, such as heart transplants, even if the patient is able to pay? Give a rationale for your answer.

Web Resources

Children's Health Matters, http://www.childrenshealthmatters.org

Health care costs, http://www.ahepr.gov/data/lcup

Health Care Financing Administration (HCFA), http://www.hcfa.gov

State Children's Health Insurance Programs, http://hcfa.gov/init/children.htm

References

Anderson, G. F. (1997). In search of value: An international comparison of costs, access, and outcomes. *Health Affairs,* 16(6), 163–171.

Ashton, G. (1995). Getting tough on drive-through delivery. *AHA News,* 31(50), 3.

Association of Operating Room Nurses (1999). Patient rights still hot topic in Congress and the states. *AORN Journal,* 69(5), 1031–1036.

The Baltimore Sun (1999). Nursing home giant set to settle fraud case. July 28, D1, D3.

Bennefield, R. L. (1998a). Health insurance coverage: 1997. *Current Population Reports* (pp. 60–202). Washington, D. C. : U. S. Bureau of the Census.

Bennefield, R. L. (1998b). Dynamics of economic wellbeing: Health insurance, 1993–1996. *Current Population Reports* (pp. 70–64). Washington, D. C. : U. S. Bureau of the Census.

Berman, S. (1995). State block grants for Medicaid may increase number of poor children at risk. *JAMA,* 274(18), 1472–1473.

Betts, V. T. (1996). 1996—Speak out for quality care. *The American Nurse,* 28(1), 4.

Blendon, R. J., Brodie, M., Benson, J. M., Altman, D. E., Levitt, L., Hoff, T., and Hugick, L. (1998). Understanding the managed care backlash. *Health Affairs,* 17–17(4), 80–94.

Braden, B. R., Cowan, C. A., Lazenby, H. C., Martin, A. B., McDonnell, P. A., Sensenig, A. L., Stiller, J. M., Whittle, L. S., Donham, C. S., Long, A. M., and Stewart, M. W. (1998). National health expenditures, 1997. *Health Care Financing Review,* 20(1), 83–126.

Buerhaus, P. I. (1995a). Economics and reform: Forces affecting nurse staffing. *Nursing Policy Forum,* 1(2), 8–14.

Buerhaus, P. I. (1995b). Economic pressures building in the hospital employed RN labor market. *Nursing Economics,* 13(3), 137–141.

Buerhaus, P. I., and Staiger, D. O. (1999). Trouble in the nurse labor market? Recent trends and future outlook. *Health Affairs,* 18(1), 214–222.

Buppert, C. (1999). HEDIS for the primary care provider: Getting an "A" on the managed care report card. *The Nurse Practitioner,* 24(1), 84–99.

Burner, S. T., and Waldo, D. R. (1995). National health expenditure projections, 1994–2005. *Health Care Finance Review,* 16(4), 221–242.

Curtin, L. (1994). Restructuring: What works—and what does not! *Nursing Management,* 25(10), 7–8.

Davis, K., and Schoen, C. (1994). Universal coverage building on Medicare and employer financing. *Health Affairs,* 13(1), 7–20.

Duston, D. (1996). Secret witness tells senators of Medicare fraud by hospitals. *Naples Daily News,* February 15, 2B.

Feldstein, P. J. (1998). *Health care economics* (5th ed.). West Albany, NY: Delmar.

Fineman, H. (1995). Mediscare. *Newsweek,* 126 (12), 38–40.

Fuchs, V. R. (1996). Economics, values, and health care reform. *American Economic Review,* March, 1–24.

Fuchs, V. R. (1999). Health care for elderly: How much? Who will pay for it? *Health Affairs,* 18(1), 11–21.

Government Accounting Office (1997). Private health insurance: Continued erosion of coverage linked to cost pressure (GAO-HEHS-97-122, July 27). Washington, D. C.: Government Printing Office.

Government Accounting Office (1998). Retiree health insurance: Erosion in retirement health benefits offered by large employers (GAO-HEHS-98-110, March 10). Washington, D. C.: Government Printing Office.

Government Accounting Office (1999a). Balanced Budget Act: Any proposed fee-for-service payment modifications need thorough evaluation (GAO-HEHS-99-139, June 10). Washington, D. C.: Government Printing Office.

Government Accounting Office (1999b). Medicare managed care plans: Many factors contribute to recent withdrawals; plan interest continues (GAO-HEHS-99-91, April). Washington, D. C.: Government Printing Office.

Government Accounting Office (1999c). Medicare managed care: Better risk adjustment expected to reduce excess payments overall while making them fairer to individual plans. Washington D. C.: Government Printing Office.

Gray, P. (1996). Gagging the doctors. *Time,* 147(2), 50.

Grimaldi, P. L. (1999). Medicare increases managed care's accountability, part 2. *Nursing Management,* 30(2), 10–11.

Guidera, M. (1996). Care system to base in Columbia. *The Baltimore Sun,* January 26, 1C, 3C.

Halfon, N., Inkelas, M., DuPlessis, H., and Newacheck, P. W. (1999). Challenges in securing access to care for children. *Health Affairs,* 18(2), 48–52.

Harrinton, C., and Estes, C. L. (1994). *Health policy and nursing: Crisis and reform in the U. S. delivery system.* Boston, Ma.: Jones and Bartlett.

Health Care Finance Administration (1998). *Medicare and Medicaid statistical supplement.* Washington, D. C.: Government Printing Office.

Health Care Financing Administration (1999). *The Medicare Handbook.* Washington, D. C.: Government Printing Office.

Hillman, A. L., Pauly, M. V., Escarce, J. J., Ripley, K., Gaynor, M., Clouse, J., and Ross, R. (1999). Financial incentives and drug spending in managed care. *Health Affairs,* 18(2), 189–200.

Inglehart, J. K. (1999). Bringing forth Medicare+Choice: HCFA's Robert A. Berenson. *Health Affairs,* 18(1), 144–149.

Khanna, V. (1995). Medicare HMOs: A bad deal for aged. *The Baltimore Sun,* December 3, 6J.

Knight-Ridder/Tribune. (1996). Health benefits and employer costs. January 30, 1996, P1300029.

Kronich, R., and Gilmer, T. (1999). Exploring the decline in health insurance coverage, 1979–1995. *Health Affairs,* 18(2), 30–47.

Lampe, S. (1987). *Costing hospital nursing services: A review of the literature.* Washington, D. C.: U. S. Department of Health and Human Services.

Larson, E. (1996). The soul of an HMO. *Time,* 147(4), 44–52.

Lenz, C. L., and Edwards, J. (1992). Nurse-managed primary care: Tapping the rural community power base. *Journal of Nursing Administration,* 22(9), 57–61.

Lowes, R. L. (1997). GM wants to tune up your practice: The carmaker hopes to apply to medicine the lessons it so painfully learned from its Japanese competitors. *Medical Economics,* 74(18), 193–195.

Maurer, F. A. (2000). Financing of health care: Context for community health nursing. In Smith, C., and Maurer, F. A. (Eds.), *Community health nursing: Theory and practice* (2nd ed.). Philadelphia: W. B. Saunders.

McCue, M. J., Hurley, R. E., Draper, D. A., and Jurgensen, J. (1999). Reversal of fortune: Commercial HMOs with the Medicaid market. *Health Affairs,* 18(1), 223–230.

McKibben, R. C. (1985). *DRGs and nursing care.* Kansas City, Mo.: American Nurses Association Center for Research.

Mechanic, D. (1999). Managed care as a target of distrust. *JAMA,* 277 (22), 1810–1812.

Miller, M. (1999). Political malpractice. *Time,* 164 (4), 60–61.

Morris, E. A. (1996). Who's taking care of Mama? *The American Nurse,* 28 (1), 4.

Nornhold, P. (1995). What networks mean to you. *Nursing 95,* 25 (1), 49–50.

Organization for Economic Cooperation and Development (1989). Health care expenditures and other data. An international compendium. *Health Care Financing Review* (annual supplement, pp. 111–195).

Purdy, R. (1995). Achieving stakeholder participation. *Managing care in the public in-*

terest: *Eleventh annual Rosalynn Carter Symposium on mental health policy* (pp. 30–34). Atlanta Ga.: The Carter Center.

Scott, J., and Rantz, M. (1997). Managing chronically ill older people in the midst of health care revolution. *Nursing Administration Quarterly,* 21 (2), 55–64.

Shalala, D. E., and Reinhardt, U. E. (1999). Viewing the U. S. health care system from within: Candid talk from HHS. *Health Affairs,* 18 (3), 47–55.

Sharpfstein, S. S. (1996). Psychiatry suffers under managed care. *The Baltimore Sun,* February 4, 6J.

Short, P. F., and Banthin, J. S. (1995). New estimates of the underinsured younger than 65 years. *JAMA,* 274, 1302–1306.

Smith, S., Freeland, M., Heffler, S., McKusick, D., and the Health Expenditures Projection Team. (1998). The next 10 years of health spending: What does the future hold? *Health Affairs,* 17 (5), 129–140.

Statistical abstract of the United States (1998). Washington, D. C.: Government Printing Office.

The Hay Group. (1998). *Nursing shortage study.* Walnut Creek, Calif: The Hay Group.

Thompson, J. W., Bost, J., Ahmed, F., Ingalls, C. E., and Sennett, C. (1998). The NCQA's quality compass: Evaluating managed care in the U. S. *Health Affairs,* 17 (1), 152–158.

U. S. Bureau of the Census (1996). 65+ in the United States. *Current population report, special studies* (pp. 23–190). Washington D. C.: Government Printing Office.

Waid, M. O. (1998). Overview of the Medicaid and Medicare programs. *Health Care Financing Review* (statistical supplement, pp. 11–19).

Weinick, R. M., Weigers, M. E., and Cohen, J. W. (1998). Children's health insurance, access to care, and health status: New findings. *Health Affairs,* 17 (2), 127–136.

Whitelaw, N. A., and Warden, G. L. (1999). The Henry Ford Health System. *Health Affairs,* 18 (1), 132–143.

Wilensky, G. R., and Newhouse, J. P. (1999). Medicare: What's right? What's wrong? What's next? *Health Affairs,* 18 (1), 92–106.

Illness and Culture: Impact on Patients and Families

Kay K. Chitty[*]

17

Key Terms

Acute Illness
Anxiety
Chronic Illness
Coping
Cultural
   Assessment
Culturally Competent
   Care
Culture
Dependency
Disease
Ethnocentric
Exacerbation
Hardiness
Illness

Learned Resourcefulness
Personal Space
Remission

Stereotyping
Stress
Stressor

Learning Outcomes

After studying this chapter, students will be able to:

- Differentiate between acute and chronic illness.
- Describe the stages of illness.
- Describe behavioral responses to illness.
- Identify internal and external influences on illness behaviors.
- Discuss the influence of culture on illness behaviors.
- Describe the characteristics of the culturally competent nurse.
- Describe the physical, emotional, and cognitive effects of stress.
- Discuss how family functioning is altered during illness.

Although prevention and health maintenance activities are primary functions of nurses, many nurse-patient interactions center on the management of illness. A unique characteristic of nursing is the emphasis on viewing patients holistically. Nurses recognize that human beings are complex organisms with physical, mental, emotional, spiritual, social, and cultural components, all of which affect how a person responds when ill. The effective nurse takes each of these dimensions into consideration when planning nursing care. This chapter explores the stages of illness, illness behaviors, cultural factors that influence how people behave during illness, and the impact of illness and culture on patients and families.

Illness

Illness is a highly personal experience. It is differentiated from **disease** in that disease is an alteration at the tissue or organ level causing reduced capacities

[*] The author wishes to thank Carolyn Maynard for her contributions to earlier editions of this chapter.

or reduction of the normal life span. **Illness** is usually considered a subjective state. One may feel ill in the absence of a disease. Conversely, one may be unaware of a disease, such as high blood pressure, and not feel ill.

Ellis and Nowlis (1994) discuss the theory of "illness with evidence." This theory proposes that there must be demonstrable evidence of an organic nature for an illness to exist. According to this theory, health care professionals may define a state of illness, such as hypertension, even in the absence of subjective symptoms in the ill person.

People's perceptions of change or loss play a major role in whether or not they see themselves as ill. People with mild arthritic changes who have no decrease in their activities and who need to use only over-the-counter analgesics such as aspirin may not consider themselves ill. To a radiologist looking at a radiography, however, arthritic changes indicating a disease process may be evident.

Whether the presence of illness is determined by the individual or by a health care provider, illness is experienced differently by individuals and their families. Culture plays a powerful role in health beliefs and behaviors; it also determines how individuals and families react to illness. The nurse's responses to patients must be defined in terms of these unique reactions.

Acute Illness

Illnesses can be classified as either acute or chronic. **Acute illness** is characterized by severe symptoms that are relatively short lived. Symptoms tend to appear suddenly, progress steadily, and subside quickly. Depending on the illness, the patient may or may not require medical attention. The common cold is an example of an acute illness that does not usually require a health care provider's attention. Others, such as acute appendicitis, may be fatal without rapid medical intervention. Unless complications arise, people suffering from acute illness usually return rather quickly to their previous level of wellness.

Chronic Illness

Chronic illnesses cannot normally be cured. They develop gradually, require ongoing medical attention, and may continue for the duration of the person's life. Hypertension, diabetes, and Parkinson's disease are examples of **chronic illnesses.**

It is increasingly important for nurses to understand chronic illnesses and their impact because they are one of the fastest-growing health problems in the United States. It is estimated that one-third to one-half of the U. S. population has one or more chronic illnesses. Factors such as changing lifestyles and the aging of the population are expected to contribute to a continued increase in the number of chronically ill Americans for the foreseeable future.

Chronic illnesses are caused by permanent changes that leave residual disability. They vary in severity and outcomes, but there is generally not an end point at which normal health is regained. Some chronic illnesses are progressively debilitating and result in premature death, whereas others are associated with a normal life span even though functioning is impaired. Chronic illnesses typically go through periods of **remission,** when symptoms subside, and **exacerbation,** when symptoms reappear or worsen.

Chronic illnesses often lead to altered individual functioning and disruption of family life. Long-term medical management of chronic illness can create financial hardship as well. Box 17–1 describes how one patient experiences a chronic illness, lupus erythematosis, and describes its impact on her feelings and family responsibilities.

Stages of Illness

Although the behaviors are different for each person, people who are ill tend to progress through certain recognizable stages. Ellis and Nowlis (1994) have identified five stages: disbelief and denial, irritability and anger, attempting to gain control, depression and despair, and acceptance and participation. Nurses encounter patients in each stage, so it is important to have some understanding of the types of behaviors that are associated with each. Remember that a person's culture affects how he or she responds to illness and that Ellis and Nowlis' studies were done with people of individualistic, Western cultures.

BOX 17–1

Comments of a Patient with a Chronic Disease: Lupus Erythematosis

If there is one thing I want to say to nurses who work with patients with chronic disease it is, "Be patient and understand our problems and feelings." When I go to the doctor's office or to the hospital, I usually leave feeling guilty because I have been impatient with everyone I saw. Guilt and anger are the two feelings I seem to have had since I was diagnosed with this disease. I alternate between being angry that I got lupus and feeling that I should be grateful for the fact that I have something I can at least live with when others are not so fortunate.

I guess the thing that bothers me most is that the nurses keep telling me what changes I need to make to take better care of myself. They never seem to understand that I am doing the best I can do. I can't possibly get the amount of rest they seem to think I need, and I can't avoid as much stress as they seem to think I should avoid. Both my husband and I work hard at our jobs, and I hate asking him and my sons to take over my responsibilities at home when I am sick, so I wind up compromising. I ask them to help some and I do more than I should. When I get the lecture from the nurses on how I should take better care of myself, I usually just nod and say that I will even when I know that I probably won't be able to.

Anonymous

Stage I: Disbelief and Denial

According to Ellis and Nowlis (1994), the first stage results from difficulty in believing that the signs and symptoms being experienced are caused by illness. Often, there is a belief that the symptoms will go away. Fear of illness often leads to the hope that the symptoms will subside without treatment.

Denial is a defense mechanism that people sometimes use to avoid the anxiety associated with illness. People who pride themselves on their vigor and health may downplay the significance of symptoms. If this occurs, they may avoid treatment or attempt inappropriate self-treatment. Extended denial can have serious results because some illnesses, left untreated, may become too advanced for effective treatment.

Stage II: Irritability and Anger

As the ability to function is altered by illness, irritability results. Anger is directed toward the body because it is not performing as it should. With the current emphasis on wellness and prevention, anger may be directed inward, and guilt feelings may occur for failing to prevent the illness. Anger may also be directed toward others—spouse, family members, or co-workers.

Stage III: Attempting to Gain Control

In this stage, people may try over-the-counter medications, folk practices, or home remedies. They are aware that they are ill and usually experience some concern or even fear about the outcome. These fears usually stimulate treatment-seeking behavior as a way of gaining control over the illness, but they may lead to further denial and avoidance. Family members may become involved, encouraging the person to seek treatment.

Stage IV: Depression

Depression is perhaps the most common mood that occurs with illness. The ability to work is altered, daily activities must be modified, and the sense of well-being and freedom from pain are lost. Illness results in many types of loss, and depression is a normal response. The severity of the depression varies according to the severity and length of the illness as well as the individual's personality characteristics and coping abilities. Individuals with chronic illnesses often undergo cycles of depression as remissions and exacerbations occur.

Stage V: Acceptance and Participation

By the time this stage occurs, the patient has acknowledged the reality of illness and is ready to participate in decisions about treatment. Active involvement and the hope attached to pursuing treatment usually lead to increased feelings of mastery and serve to decrease depression.

Not all individuals go through every stage, and they do not necessarily go through them at the same rate or in the same order. Individuals may become "stuck" in a stage before reaching the ideal stage of acceptance and participation. Those with acute illnesses may progress through stages in a different way than those with chronic illnesses. As mentioned, culture plays a major role in how people respond to illness. Nevertheless, these stages represent a useful model for nurses to keep in mind.

Illness Behavior and the Sick Role

Although illness is highly subjective and is experienced differently by each individual, a number of factors influence how a particular person will respond. One important factor is the cultural expectation about how people should behave when ill.

Each culture generally requires that certain criteria be met before people can qualify as "sick." Talcott Parsons (1951), a sociologist, identified five attributes and expectations of the sick role that guided the view of illness in Anglo-American society for decades. According to Parsons, the sick person:

1. Is exempt from social responsibilities.
2. Cannot be expected to care for him- or herself.
3. Should want to get well.
4. Should seek medical advice.
5. Should cooperate with the medical experts.

For decades, Parson's sick role expectations were taught and guided the way health care providers viewed patients' reactions to pain and illness. In our multicultural society, however, this view is no longer adequate.

By 2010, whites will be the smallest ethnic minority in the world. Nurses must strive to provide **culturally competent** care to patients of many diverse cultures. With over 66 different categories of race listed in the 2000 U. S. Census, this can seem like an overwhelming task. In fact, it is probably impossible for nurses to master the subtleties of every culture they encounter. Nurses *can* learn about their patients' culturally determined health care and illness beliefs, values, and practices, however, by consistently performing cultural assessments. These instruments will be discussed later in this chapter.

Although the current Anglo-American expectation is that people should accept responsibility for their own care rather than completely submit to health care providers, there continues to be some presumption that ill people should want to get well and should behave in a way that leads to wellness.

This expectation that ill persons should want to get well and return to their normal duties as quickly as possible means that patients should cooperate in the treatment process and, to a great extent, become submissive and compliant, placing themselves in the hands of the caretakers. Persons who refuse to take medications as ordered or who refuse to perform prescribed activities, such as adhering to an exercise program or therapeutic diet, are viewed in a negative light. Their friends and family members may become irritated at their lack of participation in getting well again. Their caregivers call them "noncompliant." Often what is missing is an understanding of the patient's perception of the illness. Shifting from a focus of caring *for* patients to partnering *with* them is helpful in overcoming negative attitudes.

In caring for patients with acute and chronic illnesses, it is important for nurses to refrain from making judgments about patients' lifestyle choices. Emphasis should be on encouraging and reinforcing healthy behaviors. Education and support are important role functions for the nurse, especially in the management of chronic disorders.

Working with patients with chronic illnesses can be particularly challenging for nurses. The inability of modern medicine to cure disease sometimes leads caregivers to feel hopeless and powerless. They may also feel overwhelmed and inadequate at times. Self-aware nurses recognize these feelings and do not allow them to interfere with the nurse-patient relationship.

Influences on Illness Behavior

Although some behaviors are expected of sick people, there is also a wide variation in responses. Each person who is newly diagnosed with diabetes behaves somewhat differently from other people with the same condition. Both internal and external variables affect how an individual acts when ill. An ill individual's personality has a great deal of influence on the response to illness. Past experiences with illness and cultural background also influence illness behaviors.

Internal Influences

Personality structure is an internal variable that determines, to a large extent, how one manages illness. Personality characteristics the nurse should consider when assessing the ill person are dependence/independence, coping ability, hardiness and learned resourcefulness, and spirituality.

Dependence and Independence. Patients' needs for dependence are unrelated to the severity of their illnesses. Some patients adopt a passive attitude and rely completely on others to take care of them. Others deny they are ill or have problems with being dependent and try to continue living as they did before becoming sick.

We have all encountered sick people who have expressed views like, "I don't ask any questions—I know that my doctor and nurses know what is best for me, and I do what they tell me." Perhaps you also know someone who reacted to illness by saying, "They don't know what they are talking about. I don't need to be in bed, and I don't need to take that medicine." These two sentiments are at the opposite ends of the **dependency** continuum.

People who perceive themselves as helpless may be more willing to submit to health care personnel and do what they are told. Those who are used to being in charge and see themselves as independent may resent the enforced dependency of hospitalization and illness. These two different attitudes are illustrated in the following clinical case studies.

Case Study: *Dependency*

Mrs. Johnson has been in the hospital for several days following abdominal surgery. Even after she progressed to the point at which she could feed herself, turn over in bed, and go to the bathroom unaided, she continued to call for assistance when she needed to turn or to get out of bed. She now calls the nurse every few minutes, making some small request that she is quite capable of performing for herself. She is communicating to the nurse that she needs a great deal of assistance and is demonstrating overly dependent behavior.

Case Study: *Independence*

Mr. Thomas has just returned to his room after surgery. The nurse found him trying to get out of bed by himself. He does not call to ask for medication. He says that he is used to doing things for himself and feels uncomfortable asking the nurses for help. Mr. Thomas is demonstrating behavior that is too independent for his current physical status.

Both overly dependent and overly independent behavior can be frustrating to nurses, who sometimes become angry with patients who request help with activities they are capable of doing themselves. The patient who is too dependent requires assistance to assume gradually more responsibility. The patient who needs to be "in charge" may have problems turning control over to caregivers and is often too independent. This patient needs assistance in recognizing limitations and using available resources to get needs met.

Because nurses most often focus on independence, they may react negatively to patients who are exhibiting dependent behavior. It is important for the nurse to be aware of personal feelings about dependent behaviors and to keep in mind that dependent behaviors may be the patient's way of signaling an increased need for security or support. Sometimes independence may not be the desired outcome. For patients with chronic illnesses who must rely on others for assistance in meeting their needs, independence may actually be dysfunctional (Whiting, 1994).

Coping Ability

An individual copes with disease or illness in a variety of ways. **Coping** is the method a person uses to assess and manage demands. With an acute illness, coping is generally short term and leads to a return to the preillness state. With chronic disorders, coping behaviors must be used continuously.

Sick people use coping methods to deal with the negative consequences of the disorder, such as pain or physical limitations. Each individual has a unique coping repertoire that is called into play to achieve a sense of control. With chronic health problems, there is a continuous need for adjustments to maintain well-being and prevent the feelings of despair that can result from high stress conditions (Bowsher and Keep, 1995).

Hardiness and Learned Resourcefulness

Hardiness and **learned resourcefulness** are two concepts that have received attention as personal characteristics related to coping. Hardiness is viewed as a function of resistance to stressful life events (Bowsher and Keep, 1995). The tendency to believe that one can influence the course of events, viewing change as a challenge, and feeling commitment to values or goals are seen as the interrelated dimensions of hardiness.

The person with high levels of hardiness is believed to be better able to manage the changes associated with illness and to have less physical illness resulting from stress. Hardy people are likely to perceive themselves as having some control over a situation, even when ill. This feeling can affect a person's sense of well-being and adaptation to chronic health problems.

Zauszniewski (1995) has described the concept of learned resourcefulness as a characteristic useful in promoting adaptive, healthy lifestyles. Throughout life, individuals acquire a number of skills that enable them to cope effectively with stressful situations. The resulting attitude of self-control can be particularly helpful in reducing the feelings of depression and helplessness that often accompany the numerous stressors of chronic illness.

The nurse can enhance both hardiness and resourcefulness by teaching new coping skills. Stress inoculation and skills in self-regulation, problem solving, conflict resolution, and emotion control are examples of the types of educational interventions the nurse may implement.

Spirituality

The role of spiritual beliefs in health and illness has only recently been formally investigated. A growing number of scholars and health professionals think that spiritual beliefs have psychological, medical, and financial benefits that can be and have been proved scientifically.

One of the leading proponents of the spirituality and healing movement in American medicine is Dr. Herbert Benson, a Harvard Medical School cardiologist. He originated the relaxation-response therapy to reduce stress in patients with hypertension, chronic pain, and other stress-related illnesses. According to Benson, many people use prayer as part of the relaxation response. His Mind/Body Medical Institute of Pathway Health Network in Boston has studied the effects of the relaxation response and claims the following benefits (Larson, 1996):

- A 36 percent reduction in physician visits by chronic pain patients.
- Significantly fewer postoperative complications in open heart surgery patients.
- Lowered blood pressure and decreased use of medications in 80 percent of hypertensive patients.
- A 50 percent reduction in health maintenance organization (HMO) visits by relaxation response users.

Another indication of the priority of meeting patients' spiritual needs in health care settings is the increase in chaplain presence in some inpatient and outpatient settings. More than 90 percent of the patients surveyed believed that having a chaplain available was helpful, and 60 percent were more likely to return to a hospital with a pastoral presence in an otherwise frightening and confusing environment (Larson, 1996).

Nurses are participating in the use of spirituality in healing. St. Francis Hospital's Congregational Nurse Program in Evanston, Illinois, for example, is reaching 15,000 local families in an interfaith health project. Following training as congregational nurses, nurses spend approximately 20 hours weekly at churches and other places of worship providing classes, counseling, and referrals. They dovetail their efforts with the spiritual beliefs and customs of each congregation. As you learned in Chapter 5, the congregational/parish nurse concept is being implemented in numerous communities around the United States. By respecting and treating the whole person, these practitioners are affirming that a key dimension of health and healing is spiritual.

External Influences

External factors that bear on illness behaviors include past experiences and cultural group membership. Both directly influence how an individual perceives and responds to illness. The values that guide feelings about illness and steer a person toward particular methods of treatment are acquired primarily in the family of origin and in the culture.

Past Experiences. Adults who were pampered during childhood illnesses may accept being ill fairly easily. Relying on others for care may not bother them, and they may settle into the sick role easily. Adults who received childhood messages such as "It is weak to be ill" or "One must keep going even when not feeling well" may have difficulty accepting illness and the restrictions that accompany it. Still other adults who were hospitalized as small children or threatened with injections for misbehaving may see hospitals and nurses as threatening. Clearly, these adults behave differently when ill.

Nurses should determine the patient's past experiences with illness and the health care system during a careful admission assessment. They can then use these findings to individualize care.

Culture. **Culture** is a pattern of learned behavior and values that are reinforced through social interactions, shared by members of a particular group, and transmitted from one generation to the next. Culture exerts considerable influence over most of an individual's life experiences, including illness. Meanings attached to illness and perceptions of treatment are affected to a large degree by a person's culture. Culture determines when one seeks help and the type of practitioner consulted. It also prescribes customs of responding to the sick. Culture defines whether illness is seen as a punishment for misdeeds or as the result of inadequate personal health practices. It influences whether one goes to an acupuncturist, an herbalist, a folk healer, or a traditional physician.

Beginning in the early 1970s, schools of nursing began including cultural concepts in their curricula. Increasing numbers of universities and colleges offered graduate programs in transcultural nursing. The Transcultural Nursing Society was legally incorporated in 1981, and in 1988 it began certifying nurses in transcultural nursing. Through oral and written examinations and evaluation of educational background and working experiences, a qualified nurse can become a certified transcultural nurse (CTN) (Andrews, 1992).

The Transcultural Nursing Society began publishing the *Journal of Transcultural Nursing* in 1989. By 1993, a resolution was adopted by the American Nurses Association's House of Delegates to identify and determine strategies to promote diverse and multicultural nursing in the workforce (Kirkpatrick and Deloughery, 1995). Changes in the nursing workforce are needed in order to deal more effectively with commonalities and differences in patients. Clearly, transcultural nursing is an important field of study, practice, and research and an essential one in today's increasingly diverse society.

Knowledge of a patient's culture directs the nurse in understanding behaviors and planning appropriate approaches to patient problems. Because culture may guide the patient's response to health care providers as well as intervention, it is necessary for the nurse to be knowledgeable about cultural influences. Understanding a patient's cultural background can facilitate communication and support establishing an effective nurse-patient relationship. Conversely, lack of understanding can create barriers that impede nursing care.

The shared values and beliefs in a culture enable its members to predict each other's actions. They also affect how members react to each other's behavior. When nurses work with patients from cultures about which little is known, they lack these familiar guidelines for predicting behavior. This can cause anxiety and feelings of distrust in both patient and nurse.

In an effort to predict behavior, the nurse may resort to **stereotyping** patients from different cultures. It is important that nurses refrain from overgeneralizing and stereotyping members of cultures or ethnic groups that are different from their own. Individual assessment is always the best basis for care, whatever the patient's culture or ethnic group.

The nurse should keep in mind that patterns of communication are strongly influenced by culture. The Asian patient who smiles and nods may be communicating politeness and respect rather then agreeing or indicating understanding. Anglo-Americans tend to value a direct approach to problems, but in other cultures, subtlety and indirectness may be valued. Although Western culture values direct eye contact, some cultures view this as impolite, particularly direct eye contact between men and women.

The amount of **personal space** needed is another factor that varies depending on cultural experience. Some cultures use touch as a major form of communication; in others, touching between persons who are not considered family is disrespectful. Culture also has a primary influence on the type of stress its members experience at various points in their lives. Every society places stress on its members at one or more stages of development. For instance, Anglo-American adolescents are typically under great stress as they struggle with independence. Amish adolescents tend to experience less stress because their behavior during this period of development is more rigidly prescribed by their culture.

Values held by the nurse may come into conflict with patients' cultural values. In the Navajo culture, for example, great value is placed on keeping pain and discomfort to oneself. Letting others know how you feel is seen as weak. The nurse who expects patients to ask for medication when in pain may assume that the Navajo patient is comfortable when the opposite is actually the case. A nurse who values suffering in silence may underrate the discomfort of a patient who comes from a culture that proclaims pain loudly and uses dramatic physical gestures to communicate discomfort.

The role expectations of nurses also vary from culture to culture. A common Anglo-American view of nurses is that they treat people as equals, are passive, and take direction from physicians. These patients feel free to ask questions of their nurses. Asians, however, may expect nurses to be authoritative, to provide directives, and to be expert practitioners who take charge. Out of respect for authority, they may not speak until spoken to and may verbally agree with anything nurses propose. The following patient case study illustrates a cultural difference between patient and nurse in expressing pain.

Case study: *Cultural Expression of Pain*

Mrs. L., a 42-year-old Asian woman, became ill and required surgery while visiting her daughter in the United States. Following surgery, she was placed on a patient-controlled analgesia pump (PCA). The nurse explained how she should self-administer medication when she felt pain. Mrs. L. smiled and nodded her head when asked if she understood the instructions. Much later the nurse noticed that this patient appeared to be in great pain. After talking with Mrs. L's daughter, the nurse realized that Mrs. L. had not understood how to use the equipment but felt that she should not ask for additional instructions or complain of pain.

Nurses respond to sick people based not only on their formal education but also on their own socialization and culture. All too often people are unaware of their own biases and tend to be **ethnocentric.** Ethnocentrism is the inclination to view one's own cultural group as superior to others and to view differences negatively. The nurse who identifies how personal beliefs and expectations can influence care is better able to recognize and deal with any prejudices that may impede patient care. Cultural assessment, therefore, begins with self-assessment.

To begin a cultural self-assessment, examine your own values. What behavior do you expect from people who are ill? Toward what groups do you have prejudices or biases? The nurse who is frustrated by the difficulty of caring for a patient from a different culture may benefit from taking a few minutes to imagine what it would be like to be hospitalized in a foreign country. Candidly answering the questions in Box 17–2 will help you begin the important process of self-assessment.

Cultural Assessment.   An important step in meeting the challenge of providing nursing care to diverse patients is the **cultural assessment.** Cultural assessments are used to identify beliefs, values, and health practices that may help

BOX 17–2
Sociocultural Self-Assessment

Directions: Use your answers to these questions to understand your own social and cultural beliefs and expectations better.

1. To what groups do I belong? What is my cultural heritage? My socioeconomic status? My age group? My religious affiliation?
2. How do I describe myself? What parts of the description come from the groups I belong to?
3. What kinds of contact have I had with persons from different groups? Do I assume that others have the same values and beliefs that I have?
4. What about my group affiliations do I feel proud of? Am I ethnocentric in my attitudes and behavior? What about my group affiliations would I change if I could? Why?
5. Have I ever experienced the feeling of being rejected by another group? Did this experience heighten my sensitivity to other cultures or cause me to denigrate others different from myself?
6. When I was growing up, what messages did I get from parents and friends about people from groups different from mine? Do these attitudes cause me any difficulty today?
7. What are the major stereotypes I hold about people from different groups? Do these biases help or hinder me in developing cultural sensitivity?
8. To work effectively with people from different cultural groups, what do I need to change about myself?

or hinder nursing interventions. Dr. Madeleine Leininger, nurse anthropologist, nurse theorist, and founder of transcultural nursing, advocated that nurses routinely perform cultural assessments to determine patients' culturally specific needs. To demystify the process, it may be helpful to think of cultural assessment as "merely asking people their preferences, what they think, who we should talk to in making a decision" (Villaire, 1994, p. 138). There are numerous cultural assessment instruments available. Some of these instruments require indepth interviews and comprehensive data gathering, which may require more time than is available in today's health care settings.

You can continue the process of becoming a culturally competent nurse by using the "Cultural Assessment Checklist" in Box 17–3. It was designed for use by home health nurses but is easily adapted for use in other settings. Its concise yet comprehensive nature takes into account the limited amount of time nurses may have to get to know new patients yet recognizes the necessity of developing a culturally congruent plan of care if desired outcomes are to be achieved.

Culturally competent nurses take cultural differences into consideration, usually interpret patient behavior accurately, and recognize problems that

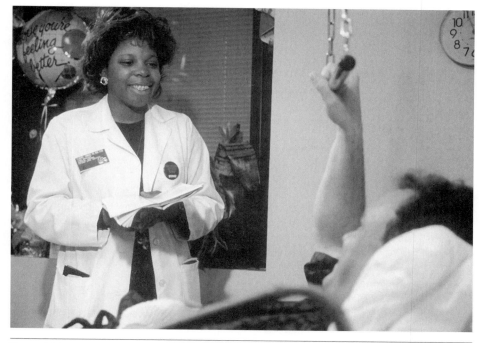

Figure 17–1
The culturally competent nurse recognizes that performing a cultural assessment is an increasingly important measure that improves the effectiveness of the plan of care (Photo by Wilson Baker).

need to be managed. They realize that cultural norms must be included in the plan of care to prevent conflicts between nursing goals and patient/family goals. They recognize that planning culturally congruent care is the most time effective way to achieve the desired goals (Fig. 17-1). In addition, being knowledgeable about other cultures promotes feelings of respect and enhances understanding of attitudes, behaviors, and the impact of illness. The accompanying interview with Dr. Madeleine Leininger provides insights into her vast experience and strongly held beliefs about cultural competence in nursing (Interview 17-1).

Impact of Illness on Patients and Families

Regardless of culture, illness results in a number of changes for both patients and families. Common experiences include behavioral and emotional changes, changes in roles, and disturbed family dynamics. Illness creates stress and other emotional responses.

Severe illnesses that profoundly affect physical appearance and functioning are more likely to result in high levels of anxiety and extensive

BOX 17-3
Cultural Assessment Checklist

Patient-identified cultural/ethnic group _____

Religion _____

Etiquette and Social Customs
- Typical greeting. Form of address: Handshake appropriate? Shoes worn in home?
- Social customs before "business." Social exchanges? Refreshment?
- Direct or indirect communication patterns?

Nonverbal Patterns of Communication
- Eye contact. Is eye contact considered polite or rude?
- Tone of voice. What does a soft voice or a loud voice mean in this culture?
- Personal space. Is personal space wider or narrower than in the American culture?
- Facial expressions, gestures. What do smiles, nods, and hand gestures mean?
- Touch. When, where, and by whom can a patient be touched?

Client's Explanation of Problem
- Diagnosis. What do you call this illness? How would you describe this problem?
- Cause. What caused the problem? What might other people think is wrong with you?
- Course. How does the illness work? What does it do to you? What do you fear most about this problem?
- Treatment. How have you treated the illness? What treatment should you receive? Who in your family or community can help?
- Prognosis. How long will the problem last? Is it serious?
- Expectations. What are you hoping the nurses will do for you when we come?

Nutrition Assessment
- Pattern of meals. What is eaten? When are meals eaten?
- Sick [comfort] foods.
- Food intolerance and taboos.

Pain Assessment
- Cultural responses to pain.
- Patient's perception of pain response.

Medication Assessment
- Patient's perception of "Western" medications.
- Possible pharmacogenetic variations.

Psychosocial Assessment
- Decision maker.
- Sick role.
- Language barriers, translators.
- Cultural/ethnic community resources.

Reprinted with permission of Narayan, M. C. (1997). Cultural assessment in home healthcare. *Home Healthcare Nurse*, 15(10), 663–672.

Dr. Madeleine Leininger, Founder of Transcultural Nursing

Interviewer: Dr. Leininger, please tell us what you mean by the term, "culturally competent."

Dr. Leininger: Culturally competent care has been defined as the culturally based knowledge with a care focus that is used in creative, meaningful, and appropriate ways to provide beneficial and satisfying care to individuals, families, groups, or communities or to help people face death or disabilities. I coined this term in 1962 as the goal of my theory of culture care diversity and universality. The term has caught hold today and is being used by many health care providers. It is now used as a requirement for JCAHO [Joint Commission on Accreditation of Healthcare Organizations] accreditation and with other organizations as essential to work effectively with cultures and their health care needs.

Interviewer: Please describe how a culturally competent nurse's patient care differs from that of one who is not culturally competent.

Dr. Leininger: A culturally competent nurse demonstrates the following attributes and skills: (1) Uses transcultural nursing concepts, principles, and available research findings to assess and guide care practices: (2) understands and values the cultural beliefs and practices of designated cultures so that nursing care is tailor-made or fits individuals' needs in meaningful ways; (3) knows how to prevent major kinds of cultural conflicts, clashes, or hurtful care practices; (4) demonstrates reasonable confidence to work effectively and knowingly with clients of different cultures and can also evaluate transcultural nursing care outcomes.

The nurse who is unable to demonstrate these culturally competent attributes often shows signs of being frustrated and impatient with people of different cultures. Moreover, the nurse who does not practice cultural competencies often shows signs of excessive ethnocentrism, biases, and related problems that impede client recovery and well-being.

Interviewer: How do patients respond differently when nurses take their cultural patterns into consideration when planning and implementing care?

Dr. Leininger: It is most encouraging to observe and listen to clients who have received culturally based nursing care. These clients often exhibit the following behaviors: (1) They show signs of being satisfied and very pleased with nurse's actions and decisions (2) They make coments such as, "This is the best care I or my family members have received from health care providers." Frequently they say, "How did you know about my values, my culture and how to use these ideas in my care? You anticipated my needs well." (3) They appreciate the different ways the nurse incorporates their cultural needs. They express their gratitude to the nurse. (4) Clients appreciate respect for their culture shown by the nurse in care decisions and practices. (5) The clients do not experience racial biases and negative comments about their cultures or familiar lifeways.

Interviewer: With so many cultural groups in this country, knowing all one needs to know about other cultures seems overwhelming. How do you advise nurses to begin the process of becoming culturally competent?

Dr. Leininger: The nurse should first enroll in a substantive transcultural nursing course to learn the basic and important concepts, principles and practices of transcultural nursing. This knowledge base is essential so the nurse becomes aware of common cultural needs and ways to work with a few cultures that are different. A few cultures are studied indepth, focusing on common and unique cultural features. The most frequently occurring cultures in the nurse's home or local region are studied first and then one learns about other cultures over time, becoming sensitive and knowledgeable about these cultures. The nurse can greatly increase her or his knowledge of several cultures or subcultures by reading the literature, or by studying specific cultures when caring for people under transcultural mentors. Gradually, the nurse learns several cultures in a general way and a few indepth. As the nurse becomes increasingly knowledgeable about several cultures, comparative knowledge and competencies become evident.

There is no expectation that professional nurses can know all human cultures, as this would be impossible. An open learning attitude and mind with a sincere desire to learn as much as possible about a few cultures will help the nurse in becoming culturally knowledgeable, competent, and sensitive.

(Continued)

Dr. Madeleine Leininger, Founder of Transcultural Nursing (*Continued*)

Interviewer: What signs can students look for to determine if their nursing programs are preparing them to provide culturally competent care?

Dr. Leininger: Nursing students will find they are able to provide culturally competent care when (or if) the following signs are evident:

- They consistently know, understand, and respect specific cultures and appreciate commonalities and differences among cultures.
- They feel a sense of confidence, creativity, and competence in their nursing care practices and see how their care fits specific cultures and accommodate cultural

differences in meaningful and creative ways.

- They go beyond common sense to actual use of culture-specific knowledge in patient care as shown in the Sunrise Model (*see* figure 11–2).
- They creatively use the clients' beliefs, values, and patterns along with appropriate professional knowledge and skills that meet clients' needs.
- They prevent racial discrimination practices in nursing and in other places; they avoid cultural imposition, ethnocentrism, cultural conflicts, cultural pain, and related negative practices.
- They value and know how to use Leininger's Culture Care Theory and

basic transcultural care concepts, principles, and research findings in their nursing practices to provide culturally congruent care for people's health and well-being.

- They appreciate a global perspective of nursing and value transcultural nursing to meet a growing and intense multicultural world.
- They markedly grow in their professional knowledge and sensitivities, developing a global worldview of transcultural nursing. They reach out to help cultural strangers in different living contexts.

Courtesy Dr. Madeleine Leininger

behavioral changes than are short-term, non–life-threatening illnesses. The impact of a chronic illness is significant and continues for the lifetime of the patient. When planning care, the nurse must take into consideration how the family both influences and is influenced by the illness of a family member.

Impact of Illness on Patients

Illness creates a variety of emotional responses. The most common responses are guilt, anger, anxiety, and stress.

Guilt

Individuals may experience guilt about becoming ill, particularly if the illness is related to lifestyle choices, such as smoking. Guilt may also be associated with the inability to perform usual activities because of illness. A mother who is unable to perform child care tasks or a father who has to take a lower-paying job because of illness may experience considerable guilt. Some cultures view certain illnesses as shameful and people suffering from them as guilty of cultural transgressions. Nurses who identify and encourage patients to discuss guilt feelings may help prevent the depression that can be a consequence of illness-induced alterations in lifestyle.

Anger

Anger is another common emotional response to illness, particularly in the Anglo-American culture. When patients must make sacrifices to manage their illnesses, such as giving up favorite foods or activities, they may experience anger about the changes. At times, they may feel that their bodies have betrayed them, which results in self-directed anger. Anger may also be directed toward caregivers for their inability to produce a cure, reduce pain, or prevent negative consequences of the illness. Nurses must be prepared to accept such angry feelings, to refrain from rejecting or avoiding patients who express their fears through anger, and to encourage the adaptive expression of angry feelings.

Anxiety

Anxiety is a common and universal experience. It is also a common emotional response to illness and hospitalization. Anxiety is an ill-defined, diffuse feeling of apprehension and uncertainty (Ellis and Nowlis, 1994). Anxiety occurs as a result of some threat to an individual's selfhood, self-esteem, or identity.

A number of threats are associated with illness. Illness may alter the way people view themselves. Some illnesses result in a change in physical appearance. Often, ability to function, is affected, altering relationships, work performance, and abilities to meet others' expectations. In addition, there may be concern about pain and discomfort associated with illness or treatment. Because of real and potential threats and changes arising from illness, nurses must develop skills that enable them to help patients recognize and manage anxiety.

Although the responses are similar, there is general agreement that anxiety and fear are different. Fear results from specific, known causes, whereas with anxiety the cause of the feelings is unknown (Ellis and Nowlis, 1994). For example, if you are home alone at night and you hear an unusual noise outside, your heartbeat and respirations increase, your stomach tightens, and you perspire. The emotion in this situation is fear. If you begin to have the same feelings but have heard no noises and cannot identify a source of fear, you are experiencing anxiety. Both emotions may be present at the same time. The patient who is in the hospital for an operation may experience anxiety about the unknown consequences of the surgery and fear of the procedure itself.

Symptoms of Anxiety. Nurses should be familiar with the numerous symptoms of anxiety. They are classified as physiological, emotional, and cognitive. Physiological symptoms include increased heart rate, respirations, and blood pressure; insomnia; nausea and vomiting; fatigue; sweaty palms; and tremors. Emotional responses include restlessness, irritability, feelings of helplessness, crying, and depression. Cognitive symptoms include inability to concentrate, forgetfulness, inattention to surroundings, and preoccupation.

Responses to Anxiety. Responses to anxiety occur on a continuum. Peplau (1963) described four levels: mild, moderate, severe, and panic. A mild level is characterized by increased alertness and ability to focus attention and concentrate. There is an expanded capacity for learning at this stage.

A person with a moderate level of anxiety is able to concentrate on only one thing at a time. Frequently, there is increased body movement and more rapid speech and a subjective awareness of discomfort.

At the severe level, thoughts become scattered. The severely anxious person may not be able to communicate verbally, and there is considerable discomfort accompanied by purposeless movements such as handwringing and pacing.

At the panic level, the person becomes completely disorganized and loses the ability to differentiate between reality and unreality. There are constant random and purposeless movements. The individual experiencing panic levels of anxiety is unable to function without assistance. Panic levels of anxiety cannot be continued indefinitely because the body will become exhausted, and death may occur if the anxiety is not reduced. Box 17–4 lists the characteristics of each level of anxiety.

Because anxiety is such a common response to illness and hospitalization, nurses often encounter patients who are experiencing mild or moderate anxiety and, occasionally, patients who are severely anxious. When interacting with an anxious patient, the nurse should carefully assess the level of anxiety before attempting to develop the plan of care.

According to Peplau (1963), anxiety is communicated interpersonally. In other words, it is "contagious." For this reason, it is crucial that the nurse be aware of and manage personal anxiety so that it is not inadvertently transferred to patients. Self-awareness is also essential to prevent absorbing patients' anxiety.

BOX 17–4
Levels of Anxiety

Mild Anxiety
Increased alertness, increased ability to focus, improved concentration, expanded capacity for learning.

Moderate Anxiety
Concentration limited to one thing, increased body movement, rapid speech, subjective awareness of discomfort.

Severe Anxiety
Scattered thoughts, difficulty with verbal communication, considerable discomfort, purposeless movements.

Panic
Complete disorganization, difficulty differentiating reality from unreality, constant random movements, unable to function without assistance.

Stress

Stress is another internal variable that affects patients. Stress is both a response to illness and an important factor in the development of illness. Because illness and hospitalization involve so many alterations in lifestyle, they tend to cause a great deal of stress.

Stress is an unavoidable and essential part of life. To survive and grow, individuals must cope adaptively with constantly changing demands. The stress related to examinations, for example, motivates most students to grow by studying and learning. Although stress is unavoidable, and even sometimes desirable, some control can be exerted over the number and types of **stressors** encountered, and responses to the stressors can often be managed.

Hospitalized patients are removed from their usual support systems. They lose much of their control because nurses and other care providers make decisions for them. Being ill often means that they are no longer able to perform activities as they did before the illness occurred. Stress is a common response to all these changes.

Differentiating between Stress and Anxiety. Stress and anxiety have some characteristics in common. The physiological responses are similar. Anxiety is a response to some real or perceived threat to the individual, whereas stress is an interaction between the individual and the environment. Stress includes all the responses the body makes while striving to maintain equilibrium and deal with demands.

Case Study: *Stress and Anxiety*

Mary S. is a 32-year-old single mother and a lawyer who was recently hired as the first woman in an established law firm. One morning as she prepares to take her 2-year-old daughter to the child care center, she receives a call saying that the woman who has provided child care was in an accident and will be closing the center indefinitely. Ms. S. experiences both stress and anxiety in this situation. She has a number of demands placed on her from her workplace and from her family that lead to stress. The additional demands caused by the sudden change in her plans results in even higher levels of stress. In addition, even though none of the male lawyers has responsibility for child care, Ms. S. has placed the expectation on herself that she will perform her job exactly like the men in the firm. Being late or missing work because of making new arrangements for child care conflicts with her self-expectations and poses a threat to her self-esteem. This threat leads to feelings of anxiety.

Internal, External, and Interpersonal Stressors. Selye (1956) defined stress as the nonspecific response of the body to any demand made upon it. He named this response the *general adaptation syndrome* and identified three stages through which the body progresses while responding to stress.

Stressors trigger the body's stress response. Stressors are agents, or stimuli, that an individual perceives as posing a threat to homeostasis (Ellis and Nowlis, 1994). Stressors may come from external, interpersonal, or internal sources. External stressors include such things as noise, heat, cold, malfunctioning equipment (such as a car that will not run), or organizational rules and expectations. Interpersonal sources of stress include the demands made by others and conflicts with others. Placing unrealistic expectations on oneself is an example of an internal stressor. In the example of Mary S., an internal stressor is her expectation that her child care responsibilities will not affect the hours she works. It is an unrealistic expectation for any single parent of a small child to expect that the child's needs will never interfere with work.

Responses to Stress. Outward responses to stress are determined by the individual's perception of the stressor. Cognitive appraisal, or the way one thinks about a specific situation, determines the degree to which the situation is considered stressful. For example, adolescents may perceive loud music at a rock concert considerably less stressful than their parents do.

Another factor related to the assessment of threat is whether the individual feels capable of handling the threat, that is, whether the person exhibits hardiness. The person who feels capable can be expected to feel less stress than the person who does not generally feel competent.

Stress affects the physical, emotional, and cognitive areas of functioning just as anxiety does. Physically, there is a feeling of fatigue; muscles are tight and tense. There is an increase in heart rate and respiration. The person who is under prolonged stress may be unable to sleep or eat, or there may be excessive sleeping or eating in an attempt to avoid or cope with the stress.

Emotionally, stressed people feel drained and unable to care for themselves or others. This can result in social isolation and distancing from others. There is difficulty with enjoying life. There may be feelings of hopelessness and of being out of control. Irritability and impatience often occur.

Cognitively, stress causes decreased mental capacity, and problem-solving skills are reduced. Therefore, there is a tendency to have difficulty making decisions.

Stress and Illness. It has been known for some time that stress plays a major role in the development of illness. More recent research has provided better understanding of the links between prolonged stress and body functioning.

The person who is under stress for long periods of time is at risk for a number of physical problems. The exhaustion that results from excessive, unmanaged stress leads to physiological breakdowns and predisposition to a number of problems. Disorders such as peptic ulcers, hypertension, and rheumatoid arthritis are called *stress-related* diseases because they frequently occur in individuals who have been severely stressed.

Stress has been found to be related to a reduction in the immune response, which can delay healing and result in greater susceptibility to infectious disorders such as colds and flu. Long-term studies of persons with medical illnesses revealed that the more stress people experienced in a given year, the more likely they were to develop physical illness.

Coping with Stress. Nurses have a role in helping patients modify their stressors. They should assess patients' abilities to recognize symptoms of stress and their usual methods of coping.

Coping with stress can be direct or indirect. In using direct action, nurses assist patients to identify those situations that can be changed and take responsibility for changing them. The focus is on using problem-solving skills and planning to eliminate or avoid as many stressors as possible. It is important to realize that completely eliminating stress from one's life is neither possible nor desirable.

In helping patients use indirect coping, nurses' actions are aimed at reducing the affective (feelings) and physiological (bodily) disturbances resulting from stress. Patients are taught techniques such as deep breathing, muscle relaxation, and imagery, which help them cope more effectively with stress (Boxes 17–5 and 17–6).

To help patients to manage stress, it is important that nurses be skilled in assessing and managing their own personal stress. Nurses who are feeling stressed themselves have difficulty assisting patients to deal with similar problems. The questions in Box 17–7 can help you identify your own sources of stress and develop self-awareness so you can be effective in helping patients deal with their stress.

Coping with Stress through Learning. Patient education is a major part of nursing practice, and nurses have a professional responsibility to ensure that their patients' learning needs are met. When patients are competent in the knowledge and skills they need to manage their illnesses, they tend to feel more masterful and less stressed.

Nurses can assist patients in acquiring new methods of coping with stressors through learning, but first they must identify factors that can create barriers to learning. One factor is anxiety.

BOX 17–5
Breathing Exercises

1. Sit comfortably with feet on the floor and eyes closed.
2. Inhale slowly and deeply through the nose and fill the lungs completely. As you breathe in, imagine the oxygen flowing to all your cells. Hold your breath while slowly counting to four.
3. Slowly release all the air while thinking the word "calm." As you breathe out, imagine the air taking all the tension out with it.
4. Repeat the cycle four times. Try to banish all thoughts except those related to your breathing, but don't fight them if other thoughts creep in.
5. When you have completed the exercise, open your eyes slowly and sit for a moment before resuming your regular activities.

BOX 17-6
Relaxation Exercises

Get into a comfortable position in a place where you will not be interrupted. First focus on slow, deep breathing. Close your eyes and begin to think about the muscle sensations in your body. Identify where you are feeling tense. Slowly inhale as you stretch like a cat, then exhale and allow the tension to flow out.

Neck and Shoulders
Slowly bend your head forward and backward, then side to side three times. Bring your shoulders up as if you were trying to touch them to your ears. Slowly relax and feel the difference in tension.

Arms and Hands
Make a tight fist in one hand and tighten the muscles throughout your arm. Slowly release the muscles from the shoulder to the hand. Repeat with the other arm and hand.

Head
Make a wide smile and hold for a count of five. Slowly relax your face muscles and let your jaw go loose. Tightly close your eyes and feel the tension. Slowly give up the tension and allow your eyes to remain gently closed.

Stomach
Make your stomach muscles tight by pushing them out as far as possible. Make your stomach hard and feel the tension. Slowly relax your muscles and notice the difference.

Legs and Feet
Holding your leg still, curl your toes down to point to the floor. Do first one leg and then the other. As you tighten your muscles, feel the tension. Then slowly relax.
　　Sit quietly for a few moments and feel the relaxation in your body before you resume your activities.

Mild anxiety improves learning by increasing the ability to focus on the task. As anxiety increases, however, the ability to listen, pay attention, and concentrate decreases. Information is not retained, and the patient is unable to make the cognitive connections that are required for learning to take place.

Physiological factors may also impede learning. Visual or hearing deficits must be overcome. Unmet physiological needs, such as fatigue, shortness of breath, hunger, or thirst decrease the patient's attention to learning. Pain dramatically impairs the ability to learn. Nurses who ensure that patients' physiological needs are met enhance their readiness to learn.

Culture also influences learning. This is especially true when patient and nurse have different languages and patterns of learning. When the nurse works toward an educational goal that is not seen as desirable by a patient of a different culture, their cultural values may be in conflict. Understanding the

BOX 17-7
Personal Stress Inventory

	Very Often	Sometimes	Rarely or Never
1. I feel tense, anxious, and have some nervous indigestion.			
2. People at home, school, or work make me feel tense.			
3. I eat, drink, smoke in response to tension.			
4. I have tension or pain in my neck or shoulders.			
5. I have headaches or insomnia.			
6. I have trouble turning off my thoughts long enough to feel relaxed.			
7. I find it difficult to concentrate on what I am doing because I worry about other things.			
8. I take tranquilizers or other medications to relax or sleep.			
9. I feel a lot of pressure at work or school.			
10. I do not feel that my work is appreciated.			
11. My family does not appreciate what I do for them.			
12. I feel I do not have enough time for myself.			

(*continued*)

BOX 17-7
Personal Stress Inventory (*Continued*)

	Very Often	*Sometimes*	*Rarely or Never*
13. I have difficulty saying "no."			
14. I wish I had more friends with whom to share experiences.			
15. I do not have enough time for physical exercise.			

Scoring: Give yourself 2 points for every check in the *Very Often* column, 1 point for every check in the *Sometimes* column, and 0 points for every check in the *Rarely* or *Never* column. Total the number of points. A score of 20 to 30 represents a high level of stress. If you scored in this range, you should take steps to reduce your stress level. A score from 10 to 19 means that you are experiencing midlevel stress. You should monitor your stress and begin relaxation exercises. A score of 9 or under means that you are experiencing relatively low stress at the present time.

meaning of illness in the patient's culture is necessary. Communicating in language and with handouts (written in the patient's native language and at an appropriate reading level) that the patient can understand is important. Using an interpreter also shows sensitivity to cultural differences.

Lack of motivation and readiness are often significant barriers to education. The patient may not be motivated to learn what the nurse plans to teach. Often, nurses believe that simply pointing out what patients need to know is sufficient to motivate them. It is usually more effective to assist patients to make their own decisions about the knowledge they need. This approach may require greater effort initially, but it is ultimately more efficient to assess patient motivation and readiness first before engaging in patient teaching.

The nurse who is preparing to teach should also assess and manage the environment. A setting that is private, comfortable, and free of distractions is beneficial to the learning process. Boxes 17–8 and 17–9 review several simple principles of adult learning and teaching-learning concepts that are useful in working with patients.

Impact of Illness on Families

Families are best understood as systems, which means that change in one member changes the functioning of the total family. It is important to remember that the entire family system is affected by a member's illness. Whether the ill family member is hospitalized or cared for in the home, illness drastically increases stress in a family and disrupts healthy family function.

BOX 17-8
Principles of Adult Learning

- Prior experiences are resources for learning.

  Example: If the patient enjoys gardening, try to link health maintenance suggestions to preventive maintenance of indoor/outdoor plants.
- Readiness to learn is usually related to a social role or developmental task.

  Example: New parents are usually eager to learn how to care for their first newborn infants.
- Motivation to learn is greater when the material is seen as immediately useful.

  Example: The same new parents are more motivated to learn care of the small infant than they are to learn about disciplining toddlers.

The most important factor in how a family tolerates stress is the individual and group coping abilities. Families already experiencing difficulties may find that their problems are intensified to the point of disruption when acute or chronic illness occurs.

A sick family member has to give up responsibility to other family members. The family must continue to fulfill its usual functions while dealing with the alterations imposed by the illness or absence of a member. Family members who are able to shift and assume different roles, who can share their feelings, and who seek assistance can be expected to adjust to changes better than those who are inflexible.

Both acute and chronic illness cause changes in family functioning. Chronic illness can be particularly stressful because it is never completely cured. Families experience emotional highs and lows as the patient has remissions and exacerbations. Resentment may be experienced. Family members who must take over the sick person's responsibilities may be angry and then feel guilty about their anger. If they cannot deal with feelings of anger, they may displace them onto nurses by becoming critical and demanding.

BOX 17-9
Basic Teaching and Learning Concepts

- A person learns best when there is active involvement.
- Feedback should include positive as well as negative comments.
- The presentation should proceed from simple to complex concepts.
- Practice, or frequent repetition, reinforces skill acquisition.
- Learning is enhanced when multiple senses are used: Seeing, hearing, telling, and doing make the best combination.

Similarly, patients may feel guilty about creating hardships for loved ones. They may become convinced that they are no longer essential because others are capably taking over their roles.

Family members sometimes withdraw from each other because they fear that their negative feelings may not be understood and accepted. This mutual withdrawal leads to feelings of isolation for both patients and family members.

Families are often confused or uncertain about how to treat the sick member. They may have problems accepting and responding appropriately to the patients' dependency needs. As discussed earlier, patients may react to illness with either overly dependent or overly independent behaviors. Nurses need to monitor whether family members foster dependence, thereby keeping the patient from becoming more independent. Nurses should also be aware that some families are uncomfortable with the ill person being in a dependent role and do not allow the necessary dependency for recovery. For example, if a man who is very much in control in a family has a heart attack and is in the coronary care unit, family members may have difficulty seeing the usually strong father in a helpless position. They may continue to bring family problems to him. Other families may find it difficult to shift responsibilities back to the formerly ill member as he or she becomes able to resume role functions, thereby fostering dependence. The accompanying Research Note shows how illness affects family roles.

The nurse needs to recognize the anxiety in the family and take steps to reduce it. Talking with family members, explaining what is happening and what to expect, and teaching them how to participate in their loved one's care can help the family considerably.

The nurse should assess family functioning and the ability of the family to provide support for the patient within the family's cultural context. Observe for feelings of anger, resentment, and guilt and assist the family in identifying

RESEARCH NOTE

Research on how illness affects family roles increases the knowledge base needed to develop effective nursing interventions to meet family needs. Johnson and colleagues undertook a study designed to identify the changes in family roles and responsibilities resulting from the hospitalization of a family member in a critical care unit. They also studied how these changes were affected by the passage of time.

The study involved 52 family members who visited patients in critical care units in a large midwestern medical center. The subjects completed the Iowa ICU Family Scale each day during the first week and weekly thereafter as long as the patient remained in the unit. Family members were asked to describe changes in family roles and responsibilities. Approximately 59 percent reported that they experienced changes in family roles or responsibilities as a result of the hospitalization. Qualitative analysis of their responses identified seven themes: (1) pulling together, (2) fragmentation, (3) increased dependence, (4) increased independence, (5) increased re- sponsibilities, (6) change in routine, and (7) change in feelings. The researchers recommended that further research be conducted to examine how family roles vary within family systems.

Adapted with permission of Johnson, S., Craft, M., Titler, M., Halm, M., Kleiber, C., Montgomery, K., Nicholson, A., and Burkwalter, K. (1995). Perceived changes in adult family members' roles and responsibilities during critical illness. IMAGE: *Journal of Nursing Scholarship*, 27(3), 238–243. Copyright 1995 by Sigma Theta Tau International.

adaptive methods of expressing these feelings. The nurse needs to determine the level of knowledge of the family members and assist them to identify concerns and make realistic plans. Providing information and including the family in the planning can result in increased support for the patient and in effective care.

Nurses must be prepared to accept the anger and distrust that often is directed toward care providers who are unable to cure disease or relieve the negative consequences of illness. Understanding that anger expressed by patients and families is not personally directed can enable nurses to assess patients objectively and respond to feelings expressed in a nondefensive manner.

Despite the numerous stresses and adjustments necessitated by illness of a family member, many families find that there are also positive experiences. Finding new activities to share and working together to meet challenges can lead to feelings of closeness that were not present before. Previously unrecognized individual strengths may be identified as new roles and responsibilities are assumed. New meanings for the entire family may emerge as values are reassessed and priorities are shifted.

Summary of Key Points

- Illness is a highly personal experience.
- Reactions to illness are culturally determined.
- Sick people may progress through stages of disbelief and denial, irritability and anger, attempting to gain control, depression, and acceptance and participation.
- Anglo-American expectations of sick people are that they want to get well, will seek appropriate care, and will cooperate in treatment. In return, they are exempted from some of their usual responsibilities during their illnesses.
- Although every culture has expectations about how sick people should behave, previous experience and personality characteristics also affect individuals' responses to illness.
- Culturally competent nurses perform cultural assessments to determine how best to work with patients and families.
- Because of the stress and anxiety involved with illness, it is important for the individual to have methods of coping.
- Coping ability is enhanced in people who exhibit personality characteristics of hardiness and learned resourcefulness.
- Spiritual beliefs may also play a role in stress reduction.
- Providing holistic care means that nurses must consider their patients' families.
- The family is a system in which a change in one member affects all the other members.
- Illness causes alterations in usual family functioning that can result in feelings of anger and guilt.
- The nurse needs to assess both how the family is influencing the patient and how they are being influenced by the member who is ill.

- An understanding of the cultural factors that affect behaviors associated with illness can provide a better framework for the delivery of nursing care that is both effective and satisfying to patients, families, and nurses.
- As nurses view responses to illness in a cultural context, they are better able to understand and accept the unique ways in which individuals and families react to illness thereby providing more effective nursing care.

Critical Thinking Questions

1. Think of your most recent illness. Can you identify any benefits you gained from being ill? If this seems like a strange question, think about it some more.
2. If you or someone close to you has been hospitalized, how did the nurses encourage or discourage dependent behaviors? Independent behaviors?
3. Would it be easy or hard to allow yourself to be bathed and have other intimate needs met by nurses of the same gender? Of the opposite gender? Of your cultural group? Of a different cultural group?
4. If possible identify your own cultural group's response to illness. What are your family's characteristic responses to illness of a member?
5. Interview someone from another cultural background to learn how he or she perceives illness. Prepare several specific questions to ask about the meaning, causes, treatment, and feelings engendered by both acute and chronic illnesses. How does his or her culture tend to view nurses?
6. Speculate about the potential changes in the family of a husband and father of four small children who has experienced a severe illness and will be unable to work for an extended period. What stresses is this family likely to encounter? How would these stresses be different if the wife and the mother were the sick family member?

Web Resources

American Diabetes Association, http://www.diabetes.org

National Association of Hispanic Nurses, http://www.nahn.org

National Black Nurses' Association, http://www.nbna.org

National Center for Cultural Competence, http://www.dml.georgetown.edu/depts/pediatrics/gucdc/cultural.html

Transcultural Nursing Society, http://www.tcns.org

References

Andrews, M. M. (1992). Cultural perspectives on nursing in the 21st century. *Journal of Professional Nursing,* 8(1), 7–15.

Bowsher, J., and Keep, D. (1995). Toward an understanding of three control constructs: Personal control, self-efficacy, and hardiness. *Issues in Mental Health Nursing,* 16(1), 33–50.

Ellis, J., and Nowlis, E. (1994). *Nursing: A human needs approach* (5th ed.). Philadelphia: J. B. Lippincott.

Johnson, S., Craft, M., Titler, M., Halm, M., Kleiber, C., Montgomery, K., Nicholson, A., and Burkwalter, K. (1995). Perceived changes in adult family members' roles and responsibilities during critical illness. *IMAGE: Journal of Nursing Scholarship,* 27(3), 238–243.

Kirkpatrick, S. M., and Deloughery, G. L. (1995). Cultural influences on nursing. In G. L. Deloughery (Ed.), *Issues and trends in nursing* (pp. 173–197). St. Louis: Mosby.

Larson, L. (1996). Heaven and hospitals: The role of spirituality in healing. *AHA News,* 32(1), 7.

Leininger, M. (1999). Personal communication.

Narayan, M. C. (1997). Cultural assessment in home health care. *Home Healthcare Nurse,* 15(10), 663–672.

Parsons, T. (1951). *The social system.* New York: Free Press.

Peplau, H. (1963). A working definition of anxiety. In S. F. Burd and M. A. Marshall (Eds.), *Some clinical approaches to psychiatric nursing.* New York: Macmillan.

Selye, H. (1956). *The stress of life.* New York: McGraw-Hill.

Villaire, M. (1994). Toni Tripp-Reimer: Crossing over the boundaries. *Critical Care Nurse,* 14(3), 134–141.

Whiting, S. A. (1994). A Delphi study to determine defining characteristics of interdependence and dysfunctional independence as potential nursing diagnoses. *Issues in Mental Health Nursing,* 15(1), 37–47.

Zauszniewski, J. A. (1995). Learned resourcefulness: A conceptual analysis. *Issues in Mental Health Nursing,* 16(1), 13–31.

Communication and Collaboration in Nursing

Kay K. Chitty

18

Key Terms

Acceptance
Action Language
Active Listening
Appropriateness
Clarification
Communication
Congruent
Context
Efficiency
Empathy
Evaluation
False Reassurance
Feedback
Flexibility
Incongruent
Irrational Belief
Message
Nonjudgmental Acceptance
Nonverbal Communication
Nurse-Patient Relationship
Open-Ended Question
Open Posture
Orientation Phase

Perception
Receiver
Reflection
Self-Awareness
Sender
Somatic Language
Stereotypes

Termination Phase
Transmission
Ventilation
Verbal Communication
Working Phase

Learning Outcomes

After studying this chapter, students will be able to:

- Describe therapeutic use of self.
- Identify and describe the phases of the nurse-patient relationship.
- Explore the role self-awareness plays in the ability to use nonjudgmental acceptance as a helping technique.
- Discuss factors creating successful or unsuccessful communication.
- Differentiate between therapeutic and social relationships.
- Evaluate helpful and unhelpful communication.
- Identify key prerequisites of collaboration.
- Explain the impact of cultural diversity on professional relationships.

Interpersonal skills are important to professional nurses. Regardless of the settings in which they work and the roles they assume within those settings, most nurses interact with many people every day. The way in which they relate to patients, families, colleagues, and other professionals and nonprofessionals determines the level of comfort and trust others feel and, ultimately, the success of their interactions. This chapter includes information that can enhance the development of self-awareness, nonjudgmental acceptance of others, communication skills, and collaboration skills, all of which are essential components of effective interpersonal relationships in nursing.

Therapeutic Use of Self

Hildegard Peplau first focused on the importance of the nurse-patient relationship in her 1952 book *Interpersonal Relations in Nursing*. She called using one's personality and communication skills to help patients improve their health status "therapeutic use of self."

The ability to use oneself therapeutically can be developed. Nurses develop this ability by acquiring certain knowledge, attitudes, and skills that assist them in relating effectively to patients, patients' families, co-workers, and other health care professionals.

The Nurse-Patient Relationship

The nursing process can begin only after the nurse and patient establish their initial therapeutic relationship. Awareness of the three identifiable phases of the nurse-patient relationship helps nurses to be realistic in their expectations of this important relationship. Each of three phases—orientation, working, and termination—is sequential and builds on previous phases.

The Orientation Phase

The **orientation,** or introductory, **phase** is the period often described as "getting to know you" in social settings. Relationships between nurses and their patients have much in common with other types of relationships. The chief similarity is that there must be trust between the two parties for the relationship to develop. Nurses cannot expect patients to trust them automatically and to reveal their thoughts and feelings.

During the orientation phase, nurse and patient assess one another. Early impressions made by the nurse are important. Some people have difficulty accepting help of any kind, including nursing care. Putting the patient at ease with a pleasant, unhurried approach is important during the early part of any nurse-patient relationship.

During the orientation phase, the patient has a right to expect to learn the nurse's name, credentials, and extent of responsibility. The use of simple orienting statements is one way to begin: "Good morning, Mr. Davis. I am Jennifer Carter, and I am your nurse until noon today. I am responsible for your total care while I am here."

Developing Trust. The orientation phase includes the beginning development of trust. Notice the use of the term *beginning development*. Full development of trust is slow and may take months of regular contact. A fact of contemporary nursing practice is that patient interactions may be brief, sometimes lasting only minutes. But even in the most abbreviated contacts, nurses must orient patients and help them feel comfortable and as trusting as possible.

Certain behaviors help patients develop trust in the nurse. A straightforward, nondefensive manner is important. Answering all questions as fully as possible and admitting to the limits of your knowledge also facilitate trust. Promise to find out the answers to all questions and report the information to the patient as soon as possible. Meet with patients at the designated times or make arrangements to let them know of a change in plans. Use active listening behaviors and accept the patient's thoughts and feelings without judgment.

Congruence between verbal and nonverbal communication is a key factor in the development of trust. Communicating in a congruent manner requires that nurses be aware of their own thoughts and feelings and be able to share those with others in a nonthreatening manner. The self-assessment of communication patterns in Box 18–1 is the type of activity that can help improve self-awareness.

Developing an initial understanding of the patient's problem or needs also starts in the orientation phase. Because patients themselves often do not clearly understand their problems or may be reluctant to discuss them, nurses must use their communication skills to elicit the information needed in order to make a nursing diagnosis. Communication skills are discussed later in this chapter.

Tasks of the Orientation Phase. By the end of a successful orientation phase, regardless of its length, several things will have happened. First, the patient will have developed enough trust in the nurse to continue to participate in the relationship. Second, the patient and nurse will see each other as individuals, unique from all others and worthy of one another's respect. Third, the patient's perception of major problems and needs will have been identified. And

---

BOX 18–1
Communication Patterns Self-Assessment

Directions: Answer the following true/false questions as honestly as possible, then review your answers and draw at least two conclusions about your habitual communication patterns. Check your conclusions for accuracy with a friend who knows your style of communicating well.

1. I usually listen about as much as I talk.
2. I rarely interrupt others.
3. I pay close attention to what others say.
4. I usually make eye contact with the person I am talking with.
5. I can usually tell if someone is angry or upset.
6. I would hesitate to interrupt someone to ask for clarification.
7. People often tell me personal things about themselves.
8. I find it is best to change the subject if someone gets too emotional.
9. If I can't "make things better" for a friend with a problem, I feel uncomfortable.
10. I am comfortable talking with people much older or much younger than myself.

fourth, the approximate length of the relationship will have been estimated, and the nurse and patient will have agreed to work together on some aspect of the identified problems. This agreement, whether formalized in writing or informally agreed upon, is sometimes called a "contract." An example of a contract that might emerge from the orientation phase of the relationship with a newly diagnosed diabetic patient is an agreement to work together on his ability to calculate and inject his daily insulin requirement.

The Working Phase

The second phase of the nurse-patient relationship is called the **working phase** because it is during this time that the nurse and patient tackle tasks outlined in the previous phase. Because the participants now know each other to some extent, there may be a sense of interpersonal comfort in the relationship that did not exist earlier.

Nurses should recognize that in the working phase patients may exhibit alternating periods of intense effort and periods of resistance to change. Using the example of the diabetic patient, the nurse can anticipate that he will experience some degree of difficulty in accepting the life changes the illness causes. He may show progress in learning to give himself insulin one week but not be able to demonstrate injection technique the next week. Nurses who become frustrated when patients' progress toward self-care is not smooth and sustained must realize that regression is an ego defense mechanism that occurs as a reaction to stress and that regression often precedes periods of positive behavioral change.

It is difficult to make and sustain change. Patience, self-awareness, and maturity are required during the working phase. Continued building of trust, use of active listening, and other helpful communication responses facilitate the patient's expression of needs and feelings during the working phase.

The Termination Phase

The **termination phase** includes those activities that enable the patient and the nurse to end the relationship in a therapeutic manner. The process of terminating the nurse-patient relationship begins in the orientation phase when participants estimate the length of time it will take to accomplish the desired outcomes. This is part of the informal contract.

As in any relationship, positive and negative feelings often accompany termination. The patient and nurse feel good about the gains the patient has made in accomplishing goals. They may feel sadness about ending a relationship that has been open and trusting. People tend to respond to the end of relationships in much the same way they have responded to other losses in life. Feelings of anger and fear may surface, in addition to sadness.

Feelings evoked by termination should be discussed and accepted. Sumarizing the gains the patient has made is an important activity during this phase. The importance of the relationship to both patient and nurse can be shared in a caring manner.

The giving and receiving of gifts at termination has different meanings for different people. The meaning of such behavior should be explored in a sensitive manner, and the agency's policies on gifts should be consulted.

Because termination is often painful, participants are sometimes tempted to continue the relationship on a social basis, and requests for addresses and phone numbers are not uncommon. The nurse must realize that professional relationships are different from social relationships. It is not helpful to stay in touch with patients following termination of a professional nurse-patient relationship. Several other differences between social and professional relationships are outlined in Box 18–2.

During the course of a professional career, every nurse will experience countless nurse-patient relationships, each with its own meaning and duration. If nurses can view each new relationship both as an opportunity to assist another human being to grow and change in a positive, healthful way and as a challenge to grow and change themselves, the rewards of nursing will be rich indeed.

Developing Self-Awareness

Awareness of oneself, called **self-awareness,** is basic to effective interpersonal relationships, especially the nurse-patient relationship. Robert Burns, the eighteenth-century Scottish poet, described the rarity of true self-awareness in his poem "To a Louse": "Oh wad some Power the giftie gie us/To see oursels as ithers see us!" (Barke, 1955).

BOX 18–2
Differences in Social and Professional Relationships

Social	*Professional*
Evolve spontaneously.	Evolve through recognized phases; use planned and purposeful interactions.
Not time limited.	Limited in time with termination date often predetermined.
Not necessarily goal directed; broad purpose is pleasure, companionship, sharing.	Goal directed; systematic exploration of identified problem areas.
Centered on meeting both parties' needs.	Centered on meeting patient needs; does not address nurse's needs.
Problem solving rarely/occasionally a focus.	Problem solving a primary focus.
May or may not include nonjudgmental acceptance.	Includes nonjudgmental acceptance.
Outcome is pleasure for both parties.	Outcome is improved health for patient.

As Burns knew, few people have the innate capacity to recognize their own emotional needs, biases, and blind spots as well as their impact on others. With practice, however, most can become more effective in doing so, thus improving self-awareness.

An important guideline in professional nursing is this: nurses should get their own emotional needs met outside of the **nurse-patient relationship.** When nurses' strong unmet needs for **acceptance,** approval, friendship, or even love enter into their relationships with patients, professionalism is lost, and relationships become social in nature. Becoming aware of one's needs and making conscious efforts to meet those needs in private life make professional, therapeutic relationships with patients possible. As discussed earlier and summarized in Box 18–2, there are important differences in social and professional relationships.

Nurses care for a diverse array of patients whose values, beliefs, and lifestyles may challenge the nurses' own. Patients sometimes are attractive or repellant to nurses. Sometimes nurses find themselves meeting their own needs to be liked or needed through relationships with patients. Nurses who have emotional reactions to patients, positive or negative, sometimes feel disturbed or guilty about these feelings. Part of self-awareness is recognizing one's feelings and understanding that although feelings cannot be controlled, behaviors can. Effective nurses control their behaviors to prevent their own prejudices, beliefs, and needs from intruding into nurse-patient relationships.

Avoiding Stereotypes

Stereotypes and prejudices are attitudes developed through interactions with family, friends, and others in each individual's social and cultural system. It is not uncommon for even well-educated professionals to have stereotypical expectations of groups of people different from themselves. These stereotypes are established through childhood experiences and affect relationships with people in the stereotyped group. Because stereotypes and prejudices tend to persist despite contrary experiences, they are **irrational,** or illogical, **beliefs.**

The subtle intrusion of stereotyped expectations into the nurse-patient relationship can cause disturbed patterns of relating. For example, the expectation that all elderly people are irritable and demanding may cause the nurse to avoid all elderly patients or to treat their complaints as unimportant.

Professional nurses deliver high-quality care to all patients regardless of ethnicity, age, gender, religion, lifestyle, or diagnosis. *The Code for Nurses* (see Appendix A) calls upon nurses to do this. Nurses are not without stereotypes and prejudices, however, and must strive to be aware of their own irrational feelings toward patients. Every professional nurse's goal is to accept patients as individuals of dignity and worth who deserve the best nursing care possible.

Becoming Nonjudgmental

Acceptance is not always easy because prejudices are strong and are often outside our awareness. This makes judging others as "good" or "bad" occur automatically. It is important to remember that acceptance conveys neither approval nor disapproval of patients, their personal beliefs, habits, expressions of feelings, or chosen lifestyles. **Nonjudgmental acceptance** means that nurses acknowledge all patients' rights to be different and to express their "differentness."

Therapeutic use of self begins with the ability to convey acceptance to patients and requires self-awareness and nonjudgmental attitudes on the part of nurses. Ongoing examination of attitudes toward others is both a lifelong process and an essential part of self-awareness and interpersonal growth.

Communication Theory

Communication is the exchange of thoughts, ideas, or information and is at the heart of all relationships. Communication is a dynamic process that is the primary instrument through which change occurs in nursing situations. Nurses use their communication skills in all phases of the nursing process. These skills are vital to effective nursing care and to effective interaction with others in health care.

Jurgen Ruesch (1972, p. 16), a pioneer communications theorist, defined communication as "all the modes of behavior that one individual employs, conscious or unconscious, to affect another: not only the spoken and written word, but also gestures, body movements, somatic signals, and symbolism in the arts."

Communication begins the moment two people become aware of each other's presence. It is impossible not to communicate when in the presence of another person, even if no words are spoken. Even when alone, people routinely engage in "self-talk," which is an internal form of communication.

Levels of Communication

Communication exists on at least two levels: verbal and nonverbal. **Verbal communication** consists of all speech and represents only a small part of communication. The majority of communication is **nonverbal communication**, which consists of grooming, clothing, gestures, posture, facial expressions, tone and volume of voice, and actions, among other things (Fig. 18–1). Because individuals tend to exercise less conscious control over nonverbal communication than verbal communication, the nonverbal component is considered a more reliable expression of feeling.

Consider, for example, a young woman who is angry with her boyfriend. She may "clam up," pout, or otherwise show her displeasure nonverbally but when asked, "What's wrong?" may reply, "Nothing. Nothing at all!" The wise suitor would pay more attention to her nonverbal communication than to the spoken word. If he pays attention only to her words, she may become even more annoyed at his lack of perceptiveness. His job in evaluating her intent is made more difficult by the incongruence between her verbal and nonverbal messages.

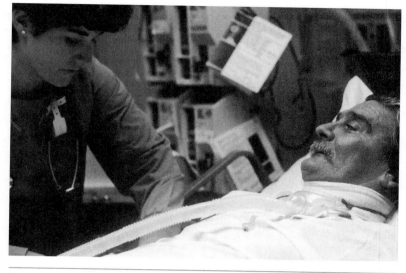

Figure 18–1
Nonverbal communication consists of grooming, clothing, gestures, posture, facial expressions, tone and volume of voice, and actions. Nonverbal communication is particularly important to patients whose ability to speak is impaired (Courtesy of Medical University of South Carolina).

When **congruent** communication occurs, the verbal and nonverbal aspects match and reinforce each other. For example, the words "I'm glad to see you!" spoken in a pleasant tone and accompanied by a smile and a proffered hand represent congruence between verbal and nonverbal behavior. The same words spoken listlessly, in a monotone, and without eye contact convey **incongruent** communication. Incongruent communication creates confusion in receivers, who are unsure to which level of communication they should respond.

Elements of the Communication Process

Ruesch identified five major elements that must be present for communication to take place: a sender, a message, a receiver, feedback, and context. The **sender** is the person sending the message, the **message** is what is actually said plus accompanying nonverbal communication, and the **receiver** is the person receiving the message. A response to a message is termed **feedback.** The setting in which an interaction occurs—the mood, relationship between sender and receiver, and other factors—is known as the **context.** All of these elements are necessary for communication to occur.

Consider the classroom situation. During a lecture, the professor is the sender, the lecture is the message, and students are the receivers. The professor (sender) receives feedback from the students (receivers) through their facial expressions, alertness, posture, and attentiveness. The atmosphere in the classroom is the context. If the atmosphere is a relaxed one of give-and-take between students and professor, the feedback is quite different from feedback in a more formal context. Figure 18–2 shows the relationships among the five elements of communication.

Operations in the Communication Process

In addition to the five elements of communication, Ruesch also identified three major operations in communication: perception, evaluation, and transmission.

Perception

Perception is the selection, organization, and interpretation of incoming signals into meaningful messages. In the classroom situation just described, students select, organize, and interpret various pieces of the professor's message or lecture. Each student perceives the information differently, based on factors such as personal experience, previous knowledge, alertness, sensitivity to subtleties of meaning, and sociocultural background.

Evaluation

Evaluation is the analysis of information received. Is the content of the professor's lecture useful? Is it important or relevant to the students' needs? Is it likely to be on the next test? Each student evaluates the message in a different manner.

Figure 18–2
Elements of the communication process.

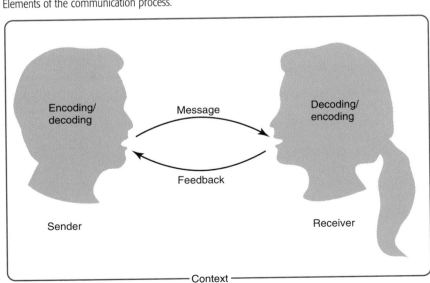

Transmission

Transmission refers to the expression of information, verbally or nonverbally. While the professor is transmitting his verbal message to the students, his nonverbal behavior of excitement about his subject matter also transmits a message to the class.

Factors Influencing Perception, Evaluation, and Transmission

Perception, evaluation, and transmission are influenced by many factors. The gender and culture of the sender and receiver; the interest and mood of both parties; the value, clarity, and length of the message; the presence or absence of feedback; and the atmosphere of the context all are powerful influences. Also involved are individuals' needs, values, self-concepts, sensory and intellectual abilities or deficits, and sociocultural conditioning. Given the variety of factors involved, it is clear that communication is a complex human activity worthy of nurses' attention.

How Communication Develops

People learn to use language (and therefore to communicate verbally) through a certain developmental sequence, which begins in infancy. Infants use **somatic language** to signal their needs to caretakers. Somatic language consists of crying; reddening of the skin; fast, shallow breathing; facial expressions; and jerking of the limbs. The sequence progresses to **action language** in older infants. Action language consists of reaching out, pointing, crawling toward a desired object, or closing the lips and turning the head when an undesired food is offered. Last to develop is verbal language, beginning with repetitive noises and sounds and progressing to words, phrases, and complete sentences.

If a child's development is normal, any one or combination of these forms of communication can be used. Somatic language usually decreases with maturity, but because it is not under conscious control, some somatic language may persist past childhood. A familiar example is facial blushing when embarrassed or angry. The development of communication is determined by inborn and environmental factors. The amount of verbal stimulation an infant receives can enhance or retard the development of language skills. The extent of a caretaker's vocabulary and verbal ability is therefore influential. Some families engage in lengthy discussions on a variety of issues, thereby providing intense verbal stimulation, whereas others are less verbal.

Nonverbal communication development is similarly influenced by environment. Some families communicate through nonverbal gestures such as touch or facial expressions, which children learn to "read" at young ages. Other families ascribe to the adage "Children should be seen and not heard," thus discouraging verbal expression and increasing dependence on nonverbal cues for communicating. The ability to communicate effectively is dependent on a number of factors. Primary among these are the quantity and quality of verbal and nonverbal stimulation received during early developmental periods.

Criteria for Successful Communication

Everyone has had the experience of being the sender or receiver of unsuccessful communication. An example is arriving for an appointment with a friend at the wrong time or wrong place because of a communication mix-up. Unsuccessful communication creates little harm when done under social circumstances. In nursing situations, however, accurate, complete communication is vitally important. Nurses can achieve successful communication on most occasions if they plan their communication to meet four major criteria: feedback, appropriateness, efficiency, and flexibility. Each of these criteria is examined.

Feedback

When a receiver relays to a sender the effect of the sender's message, feedback has occurred. Feedback was identified as one of Ruesch's five elements necessary for communication (see Fig. 18–2). It is also a criterion for successful communication. In making the social appointment mentioned previously, if the receiver of the message had said, "Let's make sure I understand you. We'll meet at 12:30 on Tuesday at Cafe Al Fresco," that feedback could have led to successful communication.

In a nurse-patient interaction, a nurse can give feedback to a patient by saying, "If I understand you correctly, you have pain in your lower abdomen every time you stand up." The patient can then either agree or correct what the nurse has said: "No, the pain is there only when I arise in the morning." Effective nurses do not assume that they fully understand what their patients are telling them until they feed the statement back to the patient and receive confirmation.

Appropriateness

When a reply fits the circumstances and matches the message, and the amount is neither too great nor too little, **appropriateness** has been achieved. In day-to-day conversation among acquaintances passing on the street, most people recognize the question, "How are you?" as a social nicety, not a genuine question. The individual who launches into a detailed description of how his morning has gone has communicated inappropriately. The reply does not fit the circumstances, and the quantity is too great. An appropriate response is, "Fine, and how are you?"

If a patient asks, "When is my lunch coming?" the nurse, knowing that the patient has already eaten lunch, will be alert to other inappropriate messages by this patient that may signal a variety of problems. In this instance, the inappropriate message does not match the context.

Efficiency

Using simple, clear words that are timed at a pace suitable to participants meets the criterion of **efficiency.** Explaining to an adult that she will have "an angioplasty" tomorrow morning probably will not result in successful communication. Telling her she will have "a procedure in which a small balloon is threaded into an artery and inflated to open up the vessel so more blood can flow through" will more likely ensure her understanding. This message would not be an efficient one for a small child, however. Messages must be adapted to each patient's age, verbal level, and level of understanding.

Some examples of patients who require special assistance in evaluating and responding to messages are young children, the mentally ill, some people with neurological deficits, and those recovering from anesthesia. For efficient communication to occur, nurses must recognize patients' needs and adjust messages accordingly.

Flexibility

The fourth criterion for successful communication is **flexibility.** The flexible communicator bases messages on the immediate situation rather than preconceived expectations. When a student nurse who plans to teach a patient about diabetic diets enters the patient's room and finds her crying, the nurse must be flexible enough to change gears and deal with the feelings the patient is expressing. Pressing on with the lesson plan in the face of the patient's distress shows a lack of compassion as well as inflexibility in communicating.

Nurses can learn to use these four measures of successful communication to enhance their effectiveness with patients. The continuing absence or malfunction of any of these four criteria can create disturbed communication and hamper the implementation of the nursing process.

Becoming a Better Communicator

People are not born as good communicators. Communication skills can be developed if you are willing to put forth a moderate amount of time and energy. Becoming a better listener, learning a few basic helpful responding styles, and avoiding common causes of communication breakdown can put you on the path to becoming a better communicator.

Listening

A requirement of successful verbal communication in any setting is listening. **Active listening** is a method of communicating interest and attention. Using such signals as good eye contact, nodding, and "mumbles" (mmhmm) and encouraging the speaker ("Go on." or "Tell me more about this.") help to communicate interest. Facing the speaker squarely and using an **open posture** (arms uncrossed) also communicate interest.

Having someone listen to concerns, even if no problem solving takes place, is considered therapeutic. **Ventilation** is the term used to describe the verbal "letting off steam" that occurs when talking about concerns or frustrations. The experience of feeling "listened to" is becoming so rare in contemporary American society that a columnist in the *Christian Science Monitor* was prompted to write about it (News Note).

NEWS NOTE

Where Did All the Listeners Go?

When everybody learned how to tune out their machines—blabbing-off radio and television ads, hanging up on computer phone calls, and so on—they also learned how to tune out other people.

During the talkiest era ever, nobody listens. Or so it is assumed. In his new novel, *A Tenured Professor*, Harvard economist John Kenneth Galbraith puts it nicely:

"By long custom, social discourse in Cambridge is intended to impart and only rarely to obtain information. People talk; it is not expected that anyone will listen. A respectful show of attention is all that is required until the listener takes over in his or her turn."

But wait. Just as it seems that the glazed-over eye and the numbed ear typify the Age of the Non-Listener, there is heartening news.

In Milwaukee, the Roman Catholic Archdiocese is sponsoring six "listening sessions" to give Catholic women a chance to express their feelings about abortion.

The first session, held last month in a college gymnasium in Fond du Lac, Wis., drew 100 women. While participants gathered in small groups to discuss the volatile issue, Archbishop Rembert Weakland, who organized the event, moved from table to table, listening and reportedly saying little.

Archbishop Weakland, considered one of the more liberal Catholic leaders, has been criticized within his church for his gesture. But as he explained to a reporter, "The polarization about this issue has become so great that I had to admit we needed dialogue about it within the Catholic community."

It is one thing for equals to listen to equals, or for subordinates to listen to those in authority. But it is a high tribute when individuals in power listen to those below them.

Once upon a time, being a "good listener" was considered a social grace. At least 51 percent of the world were "good listeners." They were also called women. A young woman learned by example that her gender role was to listen to what others—especially men—were saying. Her mouth was primarily for smiling at what she heard, with an occasional rhythmic "uh-huh."

Today that "uh-huh" is increasingly likely to come from a stranger. Lending an ear has become a paid profession. As if to signify a national hunger for "listening sessions," an entire industry has sprung up.

Eight-year-olds phone latchkey hotlines for after-school comfort and conversation while Mom—the original "good listener"—is off at work. Bereaved dog and cat owners call on pet grief counselors for animal-loving shoulders to cry on. Even technology offers an ear, this one electronic, as answering machines and voice mailboxes do more and more of the listening.

Then of course there is the biggest listening post of all, the talk show. What does it say about the desperate yearning for an audience, any audience, that guests are willing to bare their souls and share their most intimate secrets not with close friends but with Oprah, Phil, Geraldo—and millions of TV viewers?

Is this what it takes to get a word in edgewise in the late 20th century?

Outside the TV studio, other cameras reveal that finding a "good listener"—or any listener at all—can be a tricky business in classrooms as well, especially for women.

Catherine Krupnick, a researcher at the Harvard Graduate School of Education, videotaped thousands of hours of college classes. She discovered that even when male students made up just one-tenth of a class, the men would do one-quarter of the talking. Other studies over the past two decades confirm Ms. Krupnick's findings, showing that professors are more likely to call on men.

The philosopher Mortimer Adler has called listening "the untaught skill." Those like Archbishop Weakland may be thought of as pioneers in retraining. But the changeover from mouth to ear won't come easily. The thing about listening is that it takes more time and, in fact, more thought than merely talking.

When a reporter, after one of the "listening sessions" in Wisconsin, asked the Archbishop what he thought, he gave the right answer: "I'm still listening."

—Marilyn Gardner

Nurses may have difficulty listening for a variety of reasons. They may be intent on accomplishing a task and be frustrated by the time it takes to be a good listener. They may be planning their own next response and not hear what the patient is saying. Similar to other people, nurses have their own personal and professional problems that sometimes preoccupy them and interfere with effective listening. Nurses must remember that no verbal message can be received if the receiver (the nurse) is not listening.

Three common listening faults include interrupting, finishing sentences for others, and lack of interest. It is important for nurses to remember that what the patient is saying is just as important as what the nurse wishes to say.

Being listened to meets the patient's emotional need to be respected and valued by the nurse. Listening can help avert problems by letting people ventilate about the pressures they feel. Hospitalized patients particularly may feel that their lives are out of control and may need to discuss those feelings with someone who will listen without becoming defensive (Fig. 18–3).

Nurses at all levels find listening a useful skill. Nurse managers often use listening as a tool for dealing with staff members' problems and concerns and find that no other intervention is required. Listening is a talent that can be developed; properly used, it can be an important part of a nurse's communication repertoire.

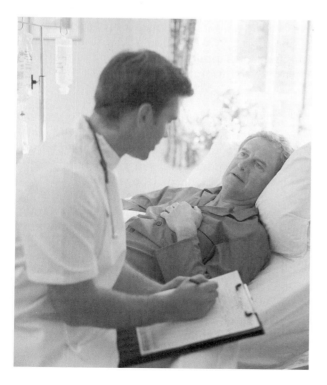

Figure 18–3
Being an active listener is an important part of communication (Courtesy Hamilton Medical Center, Dalton, Georgia).

Using Helpful Responding Techniques

There are many helpful responding techniques nurses can use to demonstrate respect and encourage patients to communicate openly. Helpful responses that have already been discussed in this chapter include being nonjudgmental, observing body language, and active listening. Other useful responses include empathy, open-ended questions, giving information, reflection, and silence.

Empathy

Empathy consists of awareness of, sensitivity to, and identification with the feelings of another person. Nurses can empathize with patients even if they have not experienced an event in their own lives exactly like the one the patient is experiencing. If nurses have had a similar or parallel experience, empathy is possible. For example, the feeling of loss is familiar to most nurses, even though they may not personally have lost a close family member.

Empathy is different from sympathy in that the sympathic nurse enters into the feeling with the patient, whereas the empathic nurse appreciates the patient's feelings but is not swept along with the feelings. "You seem upset about the upcoming procedure" is an example of a nursing statement that demonstrates empathy.

Open-ended Questions

An **open-ended question** is one that causes the patient to answer fully, giving more than a yes or no answer. Open-ended questions are very useful in data gathering and in the opening stages of any nurse-patient interaction. For example, asking a patient, "Are you in pain?" may elicit only a confirming "Yes." Saying to him, "Tell me about your pain" is more likely to elicit information about the site, type, intensity, and duration of the pain and therefore makes the nurse-patient interaction more useful.

Giving Information

An essential part of nursing is providing information to patients and their significant others. Giving information includes sharing knowledge that the recipients are not expected to know. Nurses provide information when they tell patients what to expect during diagnostic procedures, inform them of their rights as patients, and teach them about their conditions, diets, or medications.

An important distinction every nurse needs to make is the difference between providing information and giving opinions. While providing information is a helpful aspect of the nursing role, giving opinions is considered unhelpful. Instead, nurses should encourage patients to consider their own values and opinions as primary in importance. The nurse's opinion is irrelevant.

Reflection

The nurse using **reflection** is serving as a mirror for the patient. Reflection is a method of encouraging patients to think through problems for themselves by directing patient questions back to the patient. Reflection implies respect because the nurse believes the patient has adequate resources to solve the problem without outside assistance. In response to the patient's question, "Do you think I should go through with this surgery?" the nurse can reflect the question: "*Your* thinking on this question is most important. Do *you* think you should have the surgery?"

Silence

Although silent periods in social conversations often feel uncomfortable, using silence in nurse-patient relationships can be a helpful response. Using silence means allowing periods of reflection during an interaction without feeling pressure to "fill the gap" with conversation or activity. For example, when a patient has just been given upsetting news, sitting quietly without making any demands for conversation may be the most therapeutic response a nurse can make at that time. "Being with" patients is often just as valuable as "doing for" them. Professional nurses learn to use both and find time in their busy schedules to be with patients.

There are many more helpful responding styles nurses can use in their interactions with patients. The five discussed here can be a foundation upon which to build.

Culturally Competent Communication

Since communication is the means by which people connect, nurses must take cultural differences into consideration when planning and implementing care. No hard and fast rules can be given because communication practices are unique for each individual and vary widely for people from the same cultural backgrounds. Various elements to assess include dialect, style, volume, use of touch, emotional tone, gestures, stance, space needs, and eye contact (Davidhizar, Dowd, and Giger, 1998).

Culturally competent nurses recognize that even when individuals speak the same language, sender and receiver may perceive different meanings due to unique life experiences. Patients may be unwilling to share certain information with nurses because of cultural taboos. Nurses may inadvertently offend patients or family members by violating cultural norms concerning touch, space, and eye contact.

Box 18–4, found later in this chapter, provides guidelines for communicating effectively with co-workers of different cultural backgrounds. It is easily adapted for use with patients and provides strategies for promoting cross-cultural communication.

Avoiding Common Causes of Communication Breakdown

Just as there are many factors influencing successful communication, unsuccessful communication can occur for many reasons. A sender may send an incomplete or confusing message. A message may not be received, or it may be misunderstood or distorted by the receiver. Incongruent messages may cause confusion in the receiver. In nursing situations, there are several common causes of communication breakdown. They include failing to see each individual as unique, failing to recognize levels of meaning, using value statements, using false reassurance, and failing to clarify unclear messages.

Failing to See the Uniqueness of the Individual

Failing to see the uniqueness of each individual is a frequent cause of communication breakdown. This failure is caused by preconceived ideas, prejudices, and stereotypes. This problem is illustrated by the following interchange between a patient and a nurse:

P: "My back is really hurting today. I can hardly turn over in bed."
N: "I guess we have to expect these little problems when we get older."

This nurse has pigeonholed the patient in a mental group, "old people," and therefore does not react to the patient as an individual. The nurse could have promoted continued communication by responding to the patient as an individual:

N: "Tell me exactly how your back hurts, Mrs. Jameson."

Failing to Recognize Levels of Meaning

When nurses recognize no level of meaning other than the obvious ones, communication breakdown can occur. Patients often give verbal cues to meanings that lie under the surface content of their verbalizations:

P: "It's getting awfully warm in here."
N: (*Responding only to surface meaning*) "I'll adjust the air conditioning for you."

This response does not help the patient express himself fully. A different type of response focuses on the symbolic level of meaning.

N: "Perhaps the questions I am asking are making you uncomfortable."

Although it takes a lot of experience to know when and how to respond to symbolic communication, nurses should be aware of its existence.

Using Value Statements and Clichés

Using value statements and clichés is another communication problem. The use of clichés, which are trite, stereotyped expressions, is common in social conversation. Consider the prevalence of the cliché "Have a good day." This statement has come to have little real meaning. This common error can cut off communication by showing the patient that the nurse does not understand the patient's true feelings.

P: "My mother is coming to see me today."
N: "How nice. Do you want to put on a fresh gown?"

This nurse has failed to verify that the patient actually wishes to see her mother. In fact, the patient and her mother may have a difficult relationship, and the patient may dread the impending visit. By assuming otherwise, the nurse has contributed to communication breakdown. This patient probably will not attempt to discuss her relationship with her mother any further with this nurse. A more helpful response would be:

N: "How do you feel about her visit?"

This allows the patient to ventilate her feelings about her mother's visit, whether positive or negative. The nurse has conveyed a genuine interest in the patient's true feelings.

Giving False Reassurance
Using **false reassurance** is another communication pitfall. It may help the nurse feel better but does not facilitate communication and help the patient.

P: "I'm so afraid the biopsy will be cancer."
N: "Don't worry. You have the best doctor in town. Besides, cancer treatment is really good these days."

For a fearful patient, this type of glib reassurance does not help. This nurse has no way of knowing that the patient's concerns are not legitimate. She may indeed *have* cancer. A more sensitive response would be:

N: "Why don't we talk about your concerns?"

This kind of response keeps the lines of communication open between patient and nurse.

Failing to Clarify
Failing to clarify the patient's unclear statements is a fifth common communication pitfall.

P: "I've got to get out of the hospital. They have found out I'm here and may come after me."
N: "No one will harm you here."

This nurse has responded as if the patient's meaning was clear. A clarifying response might be:

N: "Who are 'they', Mrs. Johnson?"

Confused patients or those with psychiatric illnesses often communicate in ways that are difficult to understand. It is reassuring to patients to know that nurses are trying to understand them, even if they are not always successful. Communication is facilitated by **clarification** responses.

Practicing Helpful Responses

Nurses can practice using helpful responses and avoiding common communication pitfalls with family members, friends, and co-workers as well as in patient contacts. Being a good communicator takes practice and usually feels unnatural at first. Any new behavior takes time to integrate into habitual patterns. By continuing to practice, nurses soon find themselves feeling more natural. They find that these newly acquired skills are beneficial both professionally and personally. Box 18–3 compares different responses in a nurse-patient interaction.

Communication with Professional Colleagues

This chapter has focused on nurse-patient communication as the core of the nursing process and foundation of the therapeutic use of self. In addition to patients and their families, however, nurses must also communicate effectively with a variety of professional and unlicensed personnel such as physicians, other nurses, and nursing assistants. Health care delivery suffers when the members of the health care team experience communication breakdown.

As a general rule, nurses can use with colleagues the same communication skills that have been discussed as part of nurse-patient communication. The attitude of respect for others, regardless of position, is essential. Active listening, acceptance, and nonjudgmentalism are key elements, as are the conscious use of feedback, appropriateness, efficiency, and flexibility.

Communication in Today's Multicultural Workplace

Sensitivity to cultural differences in communication is essential in today's culturally diverse workplace. The composition of the health care workforce is being rapidly transformed by the population demographics of the nation. Diversity in age, race, gender, ethnicity, country of origin, sexual orientation, and disability is present, creating opportunities for nurses to develop skill in transcultural communication.

As discussed in earlier chapters, culture is the lens through which all other aspects of life are viewed. Culture determines an individual's health beliefs and practices. It also affects profoundly the meaning individuals attribute to work. Different cultures view caring for the sick, for example, in such widely varying ways as a divine calling, a religious vocation, or an occupation for the lower classes.

The meaning of work in a given culture also affects how people of that culture communicate. Andrews (1998) pointed out that verbal or nonverbal communication issues are often at the root of conflict in the multicultural health care setting. According to Andrews, the decision to speak directly with someone, send a memorandum, make a phone call, or not to communicate at all should be made only after taking the receiving staff member's cultural preferences into consideration. Strategies for promoting effective cross-cultural communication in the workplace are found in Box 18–4.

Wise nurses do not leave their communication skills at the patient's bedside but use them throughout their personal and professional lives. Using clear, simple messages and clarifying the intent of others constitute a positive goal in all personal and professional communication. As with patients, trust must exist before communication with co-workers can be effective.

BOX 18-3

Case Study: Helpful and Unhelpful Responding Techniques

Directions: Critique both interactions, identifying the helpful and unhelpful responses used by the nurse. Describe how you imagine the patient might feel at the close of each interaction. Identify what the nurse has accomplished in each instance.

Mr. Goodman has been admitted to the hospital for coronary bypass surgery. During the admission process, the following interactions might take place.

Interaction One

N: Mr. Goodman, I am Mrs. Scott. Can I get some information about you now?

P: Okay.

N: You're here for bypass surgery?

P: Yes, that's what they tell me.

N: (Taking blood pressure) Do you have any allergies to foods or medications?

P: Not that I know of. I've never been in a hospital before.

N: Well, your blood pressure looks good (Silence while patient has thermometer in mouth). This is a really nice room—just remodeled. I know you'll be comfortable here. Will your wife be coming to see you tonight? (Removes thermometer)

P: My wife is sick. She hasn't been able to leave home for two years. I don't know what will happen to her while I am here.

N: Gosh, I'm so sorry to hear that. I guess having you back home healthy is what she wants though, isn't it? And you've got a great surgeon. Well, I've got to run now. Check on you later.

Interaction Two

N: Good afternoon, Mr. Goodman. I'm Mrs. Scott, and I'll be your nurse this evening. If this is a good time, I'd like to ask you some questions and complete your admission process.

P: Okay.

N: First, I'll get your temperature and blood pressure, and then we'll talk (Silence while nurse takes vital signs). Everything looks good. Do you have any allergies to foods or medications?

P: Not that I know of. I've never been in a hospital before.

N: Hospitals can be a little overwhelming, especially when you've never been a patient before. Now, would you please tell me in your own words why you are here?

P: Well, the doc tells me I have a clogged artery, and I need a bypass. I guess they'll open up my heart.

N: What exactly do you know about the surgery?

P: Not too much, really. He told me yesterday that I need it right away—and here I am.

N: It sounds like you need some more information about what will happen. Later this evening I will come back, and we'll talk some more. Are you expecting to have visitors tonight?

(continued)

BOX 18-3
Case Study: Helpful and Unhelpful
Responding Techniques (*Continued*)

P: No, my wife can't leave home. I don't know what she will do without me while I'm here. This came up so suddenly.

N: I can see that this is a serious concern for you. We can explore some possibilities when I come back this evening. I'll plan to come around 7:15, if that suits you.

P: Sure, I can use all the help I can get.

Collaboration Skills

Collaboration is a complex process that is related to communication. An often misunderstood concept, collaboration in health care settings is far more than simply cooperation or compromise. Henneman and colleagues analyzed collaboration to understand its complexities better. They asserted that collaboration implies working jointly with other professionals, all of whom are respected for their unique knowledge and abilities, to benefit a patient's wellness or illness needs or to solve an organizational problem. It involves sharing knowledge and authority and is nonhierarchical. For collaboration to occur, a variety of human and organizational factors must be in place (Henneman, Lee, and Cohen, 1995).

Human Factors in Collaboration

Although it may seem obvious, all collaborating parties must be willing to work together if the collaboration is to be successful. They must have attained a level of readiness to collaborate through education, maturity, and prior experience (Henneman, Lee, and Cohen, 1995). They must know what knowledge and expertise they bring to the table and have confidence in the worth of their contributions. They must understand their own limits and their discipline's boundaries while respecting what other professions and professionals can contribute. Above all, they must communicate effectively, trust one another, and be committed to working together (Henneman, Lee, and Cohen, 1995).

Organizational Factors in Collaboration

Just as the people involved must have certain attributes that facilitate collaboration, the organization in which the collaboration takes place also must be supportive. According to Henneman and colleagues, factors supporting collaboration include a flat, as opposed to a multitiered, organizational structure; encouragement and support of individuals to act autonomously; recognition of team accomplishments, as opposed to individual accomplishments; coop-

BOX 18-4
Strategies to Promote Effective Communication in the Multicultural Workplace

- Pronounce names correctly; when in doubt, ask for the correct pronunciation.
- Use proper titles of respect (e.g., doctor, reverend, mister). Be sure to ask for the person's permission to use his or her first name or wait until you are given permission to do so.
- Be aware of gender sensitivities. If uncertain about the marital status of a woman or her preferred title, it is best to refer to her as Ms. (pronounced miz) initially, then at the first opportunity, ask her what she prefers to be called.
- Be aware of subtle linguistic messages that may convey bias or inequality. For example, referring to a white male as mister while addressing an African-American female by her first name.
- Refrain from anglicizing or shortening a person's given name without his or her permission. For example, calling a Russian American "Mike" instead of Mikhael, or shortening the Italian American Maria Rosaria to Maria. The same principle applies to the surname.
- Call people by their proper name. Avoid slang such as "girl," "boy," "honey," "dear," "guy," "fella," "babe," "chief," "mama," "sweetheart," or similar terms. When in doubt, ask whether a particular term is offensive.
- Refrain from using slang, pejorative, or derogatory terms when referring to persons from particular ethnic, racial, or religious groups.
- Identify people by race, color, ethnic origin, religion, or physical handicap/disability only when necessary and appropriate.
- Avoid using words and phrases that may be offensive to others. For example, "culturally deprived" or "culturally disadvantaged" implies inferiority and "nonwhite" implies that white is the normative standard.
- Avoid clichés and platitudes such as, "Some of my best friends are Mexicans" or "I went to school with African-Americans."
- In communications use language that includes all staff.
- Do not expect a staff member to know all the other employees of his or her background or to speak for them. They share ethnicity, not necessarily the same experiences, friendships, or beliefs.
- Refrain from telling stories or jokes demeaning to certain ethnic, racial, age, or religious groups. Also avoid those pertaining to gender-related issues or to persons with physical or mental disabilities.
- Avoid remarks that suggest to staff from diverse backgrounds that they should consider themselves fortunate to be in the organization. Do not compare their employment opportunities and conditions to people in their country of origin.
- Remember that communication problems multiply in telephone communications because important nonverbal cues are lost and accents may be difficult to interpret.

Adapted with permission from Andrews, M. M. (1998). Transcultural perspectives in nursing administration. *JONA*, 28(11), 34.

eration as opposed to competition; and valuing of knowledge and expertise rather than titles or roles. Collaborative organizations have values that support equality and interdependence rather than status and pecking orders. Creativity and shared vision are also valued (Henneman, Lee, and Cohen, 1995).

Outcomes of Collaboration

Collaboration is a positive process that benefits the people involved, as individuals and as a group; the organization in which they work; and health care consumers. Henneman and colleagues identified increased feelings of self-worth, a sense of accomplishment, *esprit de corps,* enhanced collegiality and respect, and increased productivity, retention, and employee satisfaction as positive benefits of collaboration. They suggested that patient outcomes are also improved by collaboration among health care professionals (Henneman, Lee, and Cohen, 1995).

Nurse-Physician Collaboration

Among the most problematic relationships that nurses encounter during practice are those with physicians. Despite rising male enrollments in nursing schools and even more dramatic female enrollments in medical schools, practicing physicians are predominantly male and practicing nurses overwhelmingly female. This leads to differences in styles of communicating and behaving that can cause difficulty in collaborative relationships.

During female-dominated nursing school experiences, most nurses are encouraged to view physicians as teammates and to collaborate with them whenever possible. Male-dominated medical schools, however, tend to instill in their graduates a hierarchical model of teamwork with the physician at the top of the hierarchy. These two divergent cultures, when combined with gender differences in communication and teamwork patterns, further complicate the relationship between the two professions.

Too often, gender differences are interpreted as professional differences, leading to further misunderstanding.

People realize that there are differences in communication styles and behavior among individuals of different cultures. What too few people recognize is that gender is a culture because men and women grow up learning different lessons about what is appropriate adult behaviors. From birth, boy babies and girl babies are dressed differently, given different toys, praised for different types of behavior, and socialized to gender-appropriate behavior in dozens of more subtle ways. Teachers treat boys and girls differently; authors of children's books and television scripts depict men and women differently. Team games and being "coached" are predominantly male experiences (Heim, 1995). Is it any wonder that as adults, men and women have different expectations of professional relationships?

Women tend to treat other people as equal, regardless of their position in the organizational hierarchy. They spend time chatting with others, building and maintaining relationships, and frequently make friends at work. Even when in management roles, they tend to tell people what to do indirectly. They come to meetings expecting to discuss the issues and make decisions depending on the outcome of the discussion. They value the process aspects of decision making as much as the outcome (Heim, 1995).

Men tend to see other workers as above, below, or parallel to them in the organizational structure and to treat them accordingly. They chat less, are friendly but tend not to become friends with co-workers, and are likely to tell subordinates what to do directly. They come to meetings already having discussed the issues, make decisions beforehand, and line up the votes they need to get their decisions approved. They are more goal oriented and pay less attention to process than to outcome (Heim, 1995).

Differences in gender cultures create problems in all aspects of personal and professional life if they are not understood. For insight into how gender culture may affect your working relationships, take the gender culture self-assessment in Box 18–5 and discuss it in a small group composed of both genders.

Collaboration with Assistive Personnel

Relationships between registered nurses and unlicensed assistive personnel, formerly known as nurse's aides or nursing assistants, affect the quality of care given to hospitalized patients. All too often, mutual respect and cooperation are missing in these important relationships, and both groups feel frustrated and unappreciated. In many areas, ethnic and cultural differences complicate the relationship between nurses and unlicensed personnel. Language is often a barrier as are nonverbal and other culturally determined behaviors, such as the value placed on punctuality. Differences in beliefs, values, perceptions, and priorities create conflict, result in poor teamwork, reduce job satisfaction, and ultimately have a negative impact on patient care (Grossman and Taylor, 1995).

Hayes (1994) reported on team building sessions with registered nurses and unlicensed personnel on three general hospital units. The purpose was to identify and align the needs of work-related relationships in both groups with the needs of the nursing unit. This is a key step in team building, which was the model chosen to encourage collaboration between the two groups.

Teams were defined as groups of workers with a fairly stable composition. They worked interdependently and "shared a common purpose" (Hayes, 1994, p. 52). To emphasize that the nurses and unlicensed personnel needed to work cooperatively, each group was asked questions such as, "What do you need from each other to make your day go better?" "What is important for you to have in the way of working relationships on this nursing unit?" "What do you need from the registered nurses?" "What do you need from the nursing assistants?" (Hayes, 1994, p. 52).

Unlicensed personnel reported needing to feel welcome, appreciated, and respected but instead reported feeling unwelcome, unrecognized, and unap-

BOX 18–5
Gender Culture Self-Assessment

Directions: For each of the paired statements, select the one that most accurately expresses your experiences or feelings.

Column One	*Column Two*
I prefer to compete to win.	I prefer to find win-win solutions.
I like work where I know the hierarchy so I know what is expected of me.	I like to work in situations where power is equally shared.
When I lead a meeting, I prefer to sit in front of the group or at the head of the table.	When I lead a meeting, I prefer to sit with the group or in a circle.
In arriving at a decision, I study the options, select one, and move ahead with it.	In arriving at a decision, I usually ask several other people for their opinions.
I define a "team player" as someone who follows orders, supports the leader unquestioningly, and does what is needed no matter how he or she feels.	I define a "team player" as someone who shares ideas, listens even when they disagree, and works collaboratively.
I can disagree or even argue with my friends and not allow it to affect the friendship.	I expect my friends to side with me in disagreements and tend to take it personally if they don't.
In the workplace, competent people don't worry about being nice.	In the workplace it is possible to be both competent and nice.
I spend little time in getting to know my co-workers personally.	It is worthwhile to spend time getting to know my co-workers on a personal level.

Scoring instructions: If most of your checks were in Column One, you have a predominantly male gender style. When you work with women, you can anticipate some difficulties because of differences in behavior and conversational patterns.

If most of your checks were in Column Two, you have a predominantly female gender style. When you work with men, you can anticipate some difficulties because of differences in behavior and conversational patterns.

If your checks were about equally balanced between Column One and Column Two, you have a combination of male and female gender styles. You should be able to work successfully with both men and women.

preciated. They did not realize that registered nurses were expected to plan, supervise, and evaluate the unlicensed personnels' work. The registered nurses expressed the need to feel competent as managers and to have unlicensed personnel comply with requests and give feedback about assigned activities. Some registered nurses reported that they preferred to complete work

BOX 18-6
Colleagues Learn what They Live

If a colleague lives with criticism,
s/he learns to condemn.
If a colleague lives with hostility,
s/he learns to fight.
If a colleague lives with ridicule,
s/he learns to be shy.
If a colleague lives with shame,
s/he learns to feel guilty.
If a colleague lives with tolerance,
s/he learns to be patient.
If a colleague lives with encouragement,
s/he learns confidence.

If a colleague lives with praise,
s/he learns to appreciate.
If a colleague lives with fairness,
s/he learns justice.
If a colleague lives with security,
s/he learns to have faith.
If a colleague lives with approval,
s/he learns to like her/himself.
If a colleague lives with acceptance
   and friendship,
s/he learns to find satisfaction in
   professional nursing.

Adapted with permission of Uustal, D. B. (1985). *Values and ethics in nursing: From theory to practice.* East Greenwich, R.I.: Educational Resources in Nursing and Wholistic Health.

themselves rather than experience embarrassment when unlicensed personnel failed to comply with their requests.

Team-building sessions centered around identifying problematic feelings and misperceptions and correcting them. For example, in response to the unlicensed personnel's belief that their contributions to patient welfare were unappreciated, the registered nurses replied, "We could not run the unit without you" and "What you do makes the difference in how comfortable the patients feel" (Hayes, 1994, p. 53).

During team building with these groups, Hayes reported that misperceptions were aired and discussed, and expectations were clarified. Registered nurses' legitimate authority and responsibility for unlicensed personnel were clarified. The result was an increase in mutual respect and understanding.

To stress the importance of positive working relationships, Diann B. Uustal, clinical ethicist and consultant, adapted the familiar poem, "Children Learn What They Live" (Box 18–6). It reminds us that professional co-workers as much as patients deserve respectful concern.

Summary of Key Points

- The "therapeutic use of self" means using one's personality and communication skills effectively while implementing the nursing process to help patients improve their health status.
- Phases in the nurse-patient relationship include the orientation phase, the working phase, and the termination phase.
- Each phase of the nurse-patient relationship has specific tasks that should be accomplished before progressing to subsequent phases.

- Acceptance of others' values, beliefs, and lifestyles is important in nursing.
- Developing awareness of biases can help nurses to prevent the intrusion of these biases into nurse-patient relationships.
- Communication is the core of all relationships and is the primary instrument through which desired change is effected in others.
- Communication is both verbal and nonverbal and consists of a sender, a receiver, a message, feedback, and context.
- Perception, evaluation, and transmission are the three major operations in communication.
- Communication develops sequentially, beginning with somatic language and progressing to action language and then to verbal language.
- Communication may be successful or unsuccessful. Successful communication meets four major criteria: feedback, appropriateness, efficiency, and flexibility.
- Active listening is a key factor in successful communication.
- Unsuccessful communication is caused by a variety of factors that can be identified and eliminated.
- In addition to communicating well with patients, nurses use communication skills to collaborate effectively with physicians, other nurses, unlicensed personnel, and other members of the health care delivery team.
- Professional nurses must be sensitive to sociocultural factors such as ethnicity and gender that can affect communication and collaboration.

Critical Thinking Questions

1. Explain what is meant by the term "therapeutic use of self."
2. List the phases of the nurse patient relationship and the tasks of each.
3. Explain why nonverbal communication may be more revealing than verbal communication.
4. List as many factors as you can that influence the communication process.
5. Identify a recent interaction you have had in which communication was incongruent. Analyze the effect of the incongruence on the communication. When are people most likely to use incongruent communication?
6. Think of a person with whom you have experienced difficult communication. Identify which of the barriers to successful communication are functioning in that person's communication with you and analyze your responses to that person.
7. Describe a collaborative experience you have had. What factors differentiated it from cooperation or compromise?

References

Andrews, M. M. (1998). Transcultural perspectives in nursing administration. *JONA,* 28(11), 30–38.

Barke, J. (Ed.) (1955). *Burns' poems and songs.* London: Collins.

Davidhizar, R., Dowd, S., and Giger, J. N. (1998). Recognizing abuse in culturally diverse clients. *Health Care Supervisor,* 17(2), 10–20.

Gardner, M. (1990). Where did all the listeners go? *Christian Science Monitor,* April 27, 1990, 14.

Grossman, D., and Taylor, R. (1995). Cultural diversity on the unit. *American Journal of Nursing,* 95(2), 64–66.

Hayes, P. M. (1994). Team building: Bringing RNs and NAs together. *Nursing Management,* 25(5), 52–55.

Heim, P. (1995). Getting beyond "she said, he said." *Nursing Administration Quarterly,* 19(2), 6–18.

Henneman, E. A., Lee, J. L., and Cohen, J. I. (1995). Collaboration: A concept analysis. *Journal of Advanced Nursing,* 21(1), 103–109.

Peplau, H. (1952). *Interpersonal relations in nursing.* New York: G. P. Putnam's Sons.

Ruesch, J. (1972). *Disturbed communication: The clinical assessment of normal and pathological communicative behavior.* New York: W. W. Norton.

Nursing Ethics

Pamela S. Chally
M. Catherine Hough

19

Key Terms

Advance Directives
Autonomy
Beneficence
Bioethics
Code of Ethics
Double Effect
Deontology
Ethical Decision
   Making
Ethics
Justice
Moral
   Development
Morals
Nonmaleficence
Patients' Rights

Personal Value System
Respect for Persons
Utilitarianism

Veracity
Virtue Ethics

Learning Outcomes

After studying this chapter, students will be able to:

- Differentiate between morals and ethics.
- Discuss the importance to nursing of having a code of ethics.
- Identify basic theories and principles central to ethical dilemmas and moral development.
- Describe ethical dilemmas resulting from conflicts between patients, health care professionals, and institutions.
- Describe a model for ethical decision making.
- Discuss the impact of ethical issues on nurses and other health care professionals.

N urses, by the very nature of the work they do, face ethical dilemmas daily. As indicated in the accompanying "Letter to Nursing Students from a Critical Care Nurse," they must decide how to allocate scarce resources, what information to share with patients and their families, how to manage low-functioning colleagues, and how to resolve conflicts between patient wishes and institutional policies (Box 19–1). Preparing to deal with these and other issues requires an understanding of ethical theories and principles and the ability to use an ethical decision-making model that works for the individual nurse in the context of his or her own value system.

To understand ethics and its relationship to health care, the terms *morals, ethics,* and *bioethics* must first be clarified. It is important to recognize that philosophers and scholars have conflicting viewpoints on how to define these terms. **Morals** are established rules in situations in which a decision about right and wrong must be made. Morals provide standards of behavior. These standards guide the behavior of an individual or social group. Morals reflect the *is* or reality of how individuals or groups behave. An example of a moral standard is "Good people do not lie."

BOX 19–1
Letter to Nursing Students From a Critical Care Nurse

Dear Nursing Student,

As you begin your nursing education or return to school to earn your baccalaureate degree, you are probably focused on many learning needs. The resolution of ethical dilemmas and ethical decision-making strategies may be near the end of a long list of things to be learned. Time spent acquiring a solid ethical decision-making foundation, however, will pay dividends to you and your patients throughout your nursing career.

In your nursing career, you will be presented with opportunities to develop your ethical decision-making skills. What are some points to consider when developing these skills? First, take a critical look at yourself. Identify your values and beliefs. Are these values and beliefs firmly entrenched, or are you easily swayed toward change by outside pressure? Are you willing to take a firm advocacy stance on an issue you believe is correct? Are you just as willing to admit if you are wrong and learn from your experiences? Are you comfortable with sensitive or confidential information placed in your possession? Can you comfortably accept both personal praise and criticism from associates? When necessary, can you take a neutral stance and avoid the temptation to give advice?

Like many of these questions, ethical dilemmas cannot always be answered by a simple "yes" or "no." Ethical dilemmas are challenging, with some situations more dramatic than others. You may encounter such situations as supporting a patient or family through a "do-not-resuscitate" decision, the decision to terminate life support systems in a nonviable patient, or organ donation decisions. You may encounter the suicidal patient who confides in no one else. You may encounter chemically impaired or incompetent physicians, nurses, or other health care providers. Most of you will come up against ethical dilemmas almost on a daily basis.

As you gain nursing experience, encountering and resolving ethical dilemmas can prove to be a personally rewarding experience for both you and those who benefit from your abilities. Do not avoid ethical dilemmas. Instead, meet these challenges with confidence and professionalism using principles of moral decision making.

Best wishes as you continue your nursing studies,
Sandra H. Carr, CCRN, BSN

Courtesy of Sandra H. Carr

Morals reflect the *is* of human behavior, whereas **ethics** is a term used to reflect the *should* of human behavior. Ethics identify what *should* be done for individuals to live with one another. Ethics are process oriented and involve critical analysis of actions. If ethicists, people who study ethics, reflected on the moral statement "One should not lie," they would clarify definitions of lying and explore whether or not there are circumstances under which lying might be acceptable.

Despite the fact that differences between ethics and morals are noted by several authors (Davis et al., 1997; Silva, 1990; Thompson and Thompson, 1990), in everyday speech the terms are often used interchangeably.

The application of ethical theories and principles to problems in health care is called **bioethics.** Bioethics as an area of ethical inquiry came into existence around 1970, when health care began to shift its focus from curing disease toward concern for the total patient (Husted and Husted, 1995). A new term, *clinical ethics,* is increasingly being used.

Advances in medicine, science, and technology, while solving some problems, can create ethical dilemmas. For example, people can now be kept "alive" even when there is no higher brain activity. Should they be kept alive under these circumstances just because we now have the technology to do so? This kind of issue mandates that nurses be concerned with what *should* be done for patients under their care. It is important that actions be critically analyzed for their appropriateness because health care professionals possess a good deal of power over those in their care.

Within this context, nurses need to study codes of ethics, ethical theories and principles, moral development, ethical dilemmas, and ethical decision-making models. Such knowledge increases nurses' ability to participate in the resolution of ethical dilemmas. The accompanying interview of respected ethicist Mila Aroskar, RN, EdD, FAAN, highlights some of the reasons why professional nurses need ethical decision-making skills (Interview 19–1).

Nursing Codes of Ethics

As discussed in Chapter 6, an essential characteristic of professions is that they have a **code of ethics.** A code of ethics is an implied contract through which the profession informs society of the principles and rules by which it functions.

Ethical codes help with professional self-regulation. They serve as guidelines to the members of the profession, who then can meet the societal need for trustworthy, qualified, and accountable caregivers. It is important to remember that codes are useful only if they are upheld by the members of the profession.

American Nurses Association Code for Nurses

The *Code for Nurses with Interpretive Statements* (American Nurses Association, 1985) is the nursing profession's expression of its ethical values and duties to the public (Fowler, 1992). The need for a code of ethics was expressed by the Nurses' Associated Alumnae (forerunner of the American Nurses Association [ANA]) as early as 1897 (Veins, 1989). A written code was first adopted in 1950. During the 53-year interval between 1897 and 1950, nursing was emerging as a profession in its own right.

INTERVIEW 19-1

Mila A. Aroskar

Associate Professor
School of Public Health, University of Minnesota
Minneapolis, Minnesota

Interviewer: Who most influenced your thinking about ethics and why?

Aroskar: The foundations were laid by my parents who were wonderful role models for learning personal responsibility, respect for living beings, and concern for the good of the community. Before entering nursing school at Columbia University, I completed a degree in religion at Wooster College in Wooster, Ohio. My professors taught and modeled respect for persons and reflective thinking about significant issues that affected individuals, groups, communities, and nations. Several individuals who have contributed to the field of bioethics over the past three decades have influenced my thinking and work in ethics and nursing. Early influences include the writings of philosophers such as Daniel Callahan, cofounder of The Hastings Center, who writes about priorities and goals of health care, end-of-life decision making, and societal obligations to the elderly; Sissela Bok's writings on lying and truth-telling in the context of individual moral choices and consequences for community; and theologian Paul Ramsey, who wrote about health professionals' obligations to patients and issues in genetics decades before today's Human Genome Project. I am grateful to numerous others working in bioethics who have contributed to my thinking and writing about professional and applied ethics over the past two decades.

Interviewer: Why is ethical decision making so important for nurses?

Aroskar: The societal obligation of the nursing profession is caring for the sick, the healthy, and the worried well. In their professional roles and relationships, nurses offer a holistic perspective of human beings and their health needs in health care and other organizations. Respect for persons, avoiding harm, providing benefits of nursing care for all in need, and promotion of justice in health care are foundational obligations in the practice of nursing as found in the American Nurses Association *Code for Nurses* (American Nurses Associations, 1976, 1985). These ethical principles and values have been and are currently challenged by the power, administrative, and payment structures found in health care institutions and systems. These are not new challenges but put nursing values in even more serious jeopardy with the current emphasis on cost containment in health care. Learning skills in reflective thinking that incorporate consideration of ethical principles and obligations are critical for nurses to be able to respond to the ethical dilemmas and challenges they face at the bedside and in efforts to influence the development of institutional and public policy for health care funding and delivery of services that are accessible to all. Nurses are and can be superb advocates for the health needs of all human beings, including their own physical, psychological, emotional, and spiritual health needs. An ongoing challenge is to main-

tain a level of energy and commitment to doing so as nurse staffing is reduced as a major cost cutting measure in so many settings.

Interviewer: How can nurses prepare to deal with ethical dilemmas?

Aroskar: First, all nursing education programs should include learning opportunities in nursing and health care ethics—to identify ethical issues/problems in practice and learn the skills necessary to respond to these issues in a thoughtful and reasoned way that incorporates attention to the nurses' employment settings, their political and power aspects. There are many excellent workshops and seminars available locally and nationally that enrich nurses' decision making and practice from an ethical perspective. The American Nurses Association and many state nurses associations have an ethics and human rights committee or other resources such as position statements on ethical issues in nursing that help nurses in dealing with ethical concerns in practice. Participation as members of institutional ethics committees, attending their educational programs, and using their consultation resources are other avenues for dealing with ethical practice dilemmas. Nursing journals and bioethics publications contain articles dealing with ethical issues in nursing practice, health care, and organizational ethics. Literature searches via the Web are an additional resource for nurses who do not have easy access to some of the other resources identified here (see Web Resources).

The 1950 *Code* consisted of 17 short, succinct statements depicting the nurse in action (e.g., "The nurse accepts . . . ," "The nurse sustains. . . .") (Veins, 1989). Even in 1950, the broad-spectrum role of the nurse—in illness, prevention and health promotion—was stressed. In addition, this *Code* encouraged nurses to participate in lifelong learning activities. Minor revisions to the first *Code* were agreed upon by delegates to the ANA's conventions throughout the 1950s.

In 1958, the ANA's Committee on Ethical Standards began reviewing the entire *Code,* and in 1960, major revisions were suggested (Veins, 1989). The 1960 *Code* also contained 17 statements, but new statements were added and others deleted. The new statements addressed nurses' responsibilities to participate in the professional organization and the necessity of identifying and upholding professional standards. Another new statement addressed nurses' participation in negotiating terms of employment. This opened the way, in later years, for the ANA to function as a collective-bargaining agent for nurses. An earlier statement, describing nurses' obligations to physicians, was eliminated from the 1960 *Code* (Veins, 1989).

The next major revision of the *Code,* completed in 1976, resulted in 11 statements. The emphasis of the 1976 *Code* was the nurse's relationship to the client. No longer was the word *patient* used. *Client* was adopted in the belief that it was a more inclusive term than *patient.* All gender-related language was eliminated. A paragraph dealing with consequences of breaking the *Code* was also added. Accordingly, the nurse who violated the *Code* could be censured, suspended, or expelled from the ANA. Any violations of civil law would subject the nurse to legal action as well (American Nurses Association, 1976). Clarifying statements were added to each point in the *Code* in the 1976 revision. These interpretations provided definitions of key terms and elaborated on the meaning of each statement.

In 1985, the *Code* was again reviewed. All 11 statements remained the same, but the interpretations were updated. In particular, more emphasis was placed on clients' rights. The 1985 *Code for Nurses* is the latest version of nursing's ethical code. See Appendix A for the *Code for Nurses* (American Nurses Association, 1985). The *Code* is reviewed periodically to ensure that it reflects both nursing's constancy and change (Fowler, 1999). Modification of the *Code* is necessary to meet the ever-changing demands of health care and society.

International Council of Nurses Code for Nurses

The International Council of Nurses (ICN) (1973) also has published a code of ethics for the profession. This document discussed the rights and responsibilities of nurses related to people, practice, society, co-workers, and the profession. The ICN first adopted a code of ethics in 1953. Its last revision in 2000 represents agreement by more than 80 national nursing associations that participate in the international association. Inherent in the *International Council of Nurses Code for Nurses* is nursing's respect for the life, dignity, and integrity of all people in a manner that is unmindful of nationality, race, creed, color, age, sex, political affiliation, or social status (Mitchell and Grippando, 1993).

Ethical Theories

There is no single ethical theory ascribed to by all philosophers or ethicists. Numerous theories have been developed. We discuss three of the primary ethical theories that nurse ethicists have identified as useful.

Utilitarianism

Utilitarianism is one of many consequentialism theories with a fundamental belief that the moral rightness of an action is determined solely by its consequence. **Utilitarianism** theory was first described by David Hume (1711–1776) and was developed further by many notable philosophers, including Jeremy Benthal (1748–1832) and John Stuart Mill (1806–1873). Mill had a significant influence on utilitarian ethics as we know it today.

According to Mill, writing in 1863, a "right action" conforms to the "greatest happiness principle" (Mill, 1985). In other words, it is right to maximize the greatest good for the happiness or pleasure of the greatest number of people. Utilitarian ethics calculates the effect of all alternative actions on the general welfare of present and future generations. Thus, this position is also referred to as "calculus morality" (Davis et al., 1997).

The utilitarian approach to ethics assumes that it is possible to balance good and evil. The goal is that most people experience good rather than evil. Benefits are to be maximized for the greatest number of people possible. In this approach, each individual counts as one.

Professional health care personnel employ utilitarian theory in many situations. The concept of triage, in which the sick or injured are classified by the severity of their condition to determine priority of treatment, is an example of utilitarianism. In triage, those who are so gravely ill or injured that they cannot possibly recover are not treated at all. Although this seems cruel, when there are many more sick and wounded than available facilities to care for them, triage is accepted worldwide as an ethical basis for determining treatment.

Frequently, utilitarianism is the basis for deciding how health care dollars should be spent. For example, money is more likely to be spent on research for diseases that affect large numbers of people than for research on diseases that affect only a few. A difficulty of this approach is that although the appeal is made to the happiness of the majority, the interest of the individual or minority, who also deserves help, may be overlooked.

Deontology

The major proponent of **deontology** was Immanuel Kant (1724–1804). Kant, believed that the rightness or wrongness of an action depended on the inherent moral significance of the action ([1959] 1985). He believed that an act was moral if it originated from good will. Ethical action consisted of doing one's duty. To do one's duty was right; not to do one's duty was wrong. According to Arras and Hunt (1977), the deontologist's belief is that *right* and *wrong* are central concepts in ethical decision making. The moral agent has the duty to do what is right and refrain from what is wrong. Beyond this, nothing is ethically relevant. The outcome or consequences of an action can be desired or deplored, but they are not relevant from an ethical perspective.

Deontology can be further divided into either *act* or *rule* deontology. Act deontologists determine the right thing to do by gathering all the facts and then making a decision. Much time and energy are needed to judge each situation carefully in and of itself. Once a decision is made, there is commitment to universalizing it. In other words, if one makes a moral judgment in one situation, the same judgment will be made in any similar situation.

Rule deontologists emphasize that principles guide our actions. Examples of rules might be "Always keep a promise" or "Never tell a lie." In all situations, the rule is to be followed. Deontologists are not concerned with the consequences of adhering to certain rules or actions. If the principle believed in is "Always keep a promise," the deontologist will keep promises, even if circumstances have changed. For example, if a father has promised that he will take his son to a baseball game and then a close family member becomes critically ill, the baseball game promise will be kept regardless of the changed circumstances.

In nursing, there are many rules and duties that nurses follow. One such rule is "Do no harm" **(beneficence).** Another justifiable rule is "The patient should be allowed to make his or her own decisions" **(autonomy).** Consider the situation of a severely depressed young man who wishes to end his life by committing suicide and asks for the nurse's assistance. Clearly, the rule about doing no harm conflicts with allowing the young man to make his own decisions. You can see that dilemmas cannot always be resolved using theoretical approaches alone.

Virtue Ethics

Virtue ethics was first noted in the works of Plato, Aristotle, and early Christians. According to Aristotle, virtues are tendencies to act, feel, and judge that develop through appropriate training but come from natural tendencies. This suggests that individuals' actions are built from a degree of inborn moral virtue (Burkhardt and Nathaniel, 1998).

Recently, bioethics literature has emphasized the character of the decision maker. Virtues refer to specific character traits, including but not limited to honesty, courage, kindness, respectfulness, and integrity. These virtues become obvious through one's behaviors and are expressions of specific ethical principles. Truthfulness, for example, embodies the principle of veracity. Virtues are beneficial characteristics that have positive effects on the one who possess them and on others as well (Foote, 1993).

Central to the mission of **virtue ethics** is the formation of character. Descriptions of character portray a way of being, rather than the process of decision making. From one's way of being flows a way of acting in both one's personal and professional life (Davis et al., 1997). A certain mental set does not guarantee right behavior, but may predispose to right behavior.

Scott (1995) described how the ethical dimension serves as a foundation for nursing practice, since both nursing and ethics are concerned with the nature of persons relating to one another. It has been recognized that nurses' ways of being and acting are essential to the integrity of nursing practice and patient care. Nurses often practice in challenging circumstances in which they must rely on their own integrity to ensure that care is given conscientiously and consistently. Virtues may be what separates the competent nurse from the exemplary nurse.

Ethical Principles

Respect for persons is the most fundamental human right (Aroskar, 1995). It requires that each person be respected as a unique individual equal to all others. This means valuing every aspect of a person's life, not just the parts that are easy to value because they are congruent with one's own values. Respect for persons is the foundation of all ethical principles.

Justice

The principle of **justice** states that equals should be treated the same and that unequals should be treated differently (Beauchamp and Childless, 1994). In other words, patients with the same diagnosis and health care needs should receive the same care. Those with greater or lesser needs should receive different care.

In health care, the most common concern about justice relates to allocation of resources. How much of our national resources should be appropriated to health care? What health care problems should receive the most financial resources? What patients should have access to health care services? According to the principle of justice, the answer to these questions is based on treating all individuals equally.

Numerous models have been developed for distributing health care resources. These models include the following:

1. To each equally.
2. To each according to merit (They may include past or future contributions to society.).
3. To each according to what can be acquired in the marketplace.
4. To each according to need (Jameton, 1984).

All of these suggestions for distribution have merit and make it difficult to decide who should be treated and for what condition. It would be ideal if all patients could receive all available treatment and resources for their health needs. Unfortunately, this is not possible because of the cost involved.

Justice as a principle often leaves us with more questions than answers. It raises our consciousness about making ethical decisions but certainly does not determine what the answer should be.

Autonomy

The principle of autonomy is based on the assertion that individuals have the right to determine their own actions. Freedom to make one's own decisions is respected under the principle of autonomy. The principle refers to the control individuals have over their own lives. Respect for the individual is the cornerstone of this principle.

Autonomy applies to both decisions and actions. Autonomous decisions have several characteristics. They are based on (1) individuals' values, (2) adequate information, (3) freedom from coercion, and (4) reason and deliberation. Autonomous actions result from autonomous decisions.

The concept of autonomy has featured prominently in ethics and philosophy since the time of the ancient Greeks. Philosophers and lawyers agree that people have a right to make decisions for themselves. Case law established more than 75 years ago that health care professionals should not act against the wishes of an adult human being of sound mind (*Schoendorf v. Society of New York Hospital*, 105 N.E., 92, 1914).

It is almost impossible to disagree with autonomy. Autonomy is a basic principle of the U. S. Constitution. Throughout the history of the United States, people have fought and died for the right of individual autonomy for themselves and others. Disregard for autonomy, however, is glaringly evident in the health care system.

Health care professionals often take actions that profoundly affect patients' lives without adequate consultation with the patients themselves. Incorporating the principle of autonomy in all health care situations is difficult, if not impossible. Patients cannot always make their own choices. Examples of those unable to participate in decisions include infants or small children, mentally incompetent patients, and unconscious patients. Other patients may be unable to participate in decision making because of external constraints, such as financial limitations, lack of necessary information, or the norms of their culture.

Beneficence

Beneficence is commonly defined as "the doing of good." According to Frankena (1988), there are several duties involved with this principle. They include (1) not to inflict harm or evil **(nonmaleficence),** (2) to prevent harm or evil, (3) to remove harm or evil, and (4) to promote or do good.

The first duty, not to inflict harm, takes priority over the three following duties. Even so, all four duties are obligations that must be taken into account. Additional considerations may take precedence when there is conflict about the appropriate course of action. For example, a surgical procedure inflicts harm on the body but potentially has long-term benefits. The procedure may be lifesaving, or it may diminish pain or increase mobility. In this sense, even though it inflicts harm in the short-term, it is justified because of the long-term good that results.

Virtually everyone would agree that causing good and avoiding harm are important to all human beings—and certainly to health care professionals. It is therefore surprising how often conflicts center around this principle. In addition to consideration of both short-term and long-term benefits, the principle of beneficence conflicts with other ethical principles. Consider the elderly patient who has just broken her hip for the second time and refuses to eat. Should she be allowed to decide autonomously not to eat even though it will harm her? The principles of autonomy and beneficence are in conflict in this example.

Nonmaleficence

Nonmaleficence is defined as the duty to do no harm. While this principle is the foundation of the Hippocratic Oath, it is likewise critical to the nursing profession. Inherent in the *Code for Nurses* (American Nurses Association, 1985), the nurse must not knowingly act in a manner that would intentionally harm the patient. While this point appears straightforward, Chulay, Guzzetta, and Dossey (1997) argue that there are some situations in which it is necessary for the nurse to inflict potential harm in an effort to achieve a greater good for the patient. The concept that justifies inflicting harm is referred to as the principle of **double effect.**

The principle of double effect considers the intended foreseen effects of actions by the professional nurse. The doctrine states that as moral agents we many not intentionally produce evil. It is ethically permissible, however, to do what may produce an evil or undesirable result if the intent was to produce an overall good effect (Beauchamp and Childress, 1994).

According to Chulay, Guzzetta, and Dossey (1997), there are four conditions that must be present to justify the use of the double effect principle:

1. The proposed action independent of its consequences must be good or at least morally neutral.
2. The nurse must intend only the good effects; the bad effect can be foreseen but not intended.
3. The unintended or bad effects cannot be a means to the end or good effect.
4. The good effects must proportionately outweigh the bad effects.

A classic example of double effect is found in administering medication for pain to the terminally ill as they near death. The proposed action of administering the medication to relieve pain is intrinsically good. While the nurse intends only the good effect (relief of pain), a bad effect (depression of respiration) may result. The patient and family must be made aware that an undesired and unintended outcome may occur that could further compromise the patient and possibly result in premature death. In this example, the good effects of relief of pain outweigh prolonged pain if the medication were withheld.

Veracity

Veracity is defined as "telling the truth." Truth telling has long been identified as fundamental to the development and continuance of trust among human beings. Telling the truth is expected. It is necessary to basic communication, and societal relationships are built on the individual's right to know the truth.

All communication between individuals has the potential to be misleading. It is easy for information to be misunderstood, misinterpreted, or not comprehended. Usually, these misunderstandings are unintentional. Intentional deception, however, is considered morally wrong.

Despite that well-established fact, much intended deception occurs between health professionals and people seeking health care. Persons seeking health care often are not completely truthful when giving their health histories. For example, they may not reveal the extent of their use of drugs or alcohol.

At the same time, health care professionals are not always truthful in responding to patients' questions. They may choose to answer only part of a question, rather than giving all the known facts. A long tradition of a double standard in truth telling exists in health care (Tschudin, 1993). Health care professionals are not responsible for false information given to them by their patients. They are responsible for information that they give to patients, however.

A number of reasons have been proposed to justify deception by health care professionals. For the most part, the justifications are related to the idea that patients would be better off not knowing certain information or that they are not capable of understanding the information. Based on these justifications, health care professionals often believe they have the right to decide what people should and should not know about their illnesses. If both patient and health care provider are respectful of one another as individuals, it is difficult to accept that deception is ever justified.

Theories of Moral Development

How does a person become moral and thereby able to make decisions about right and wrong? Answering this question moves us into the realm of **moral development.** Moral development describes how a person learns to deal with moral dilemmas from childhood through adulthood. Two major theorists who have worked at understanding this area of human development are Lawrence Kohlberg (1973, 1986) and Carol Gilligan (1982, 1987).

Kohlberg's Levels of Moral Development

Kohlberg (1976, 1986) proposed three levels of moral development: (1) preconventional, (2) conventional, and (3) postconventional.

In the preconventional level, the individual is inattentive to the norms of society when responding to moral problems. Instead, the individual's perspective is self-centered. At the preconventional level, what the individual wants or needs takes precedence over right or wrong. Kohlberg saw this level of moral development in most children under nine years of age as well as in some adolescents and adult criminal offenders.

The conventional level is characterized by making moral decisions that conform to the expectations of one's family, group, or society. When confronted with a moral choice, people functioning at the conventional level follow family or cultural group norms. According to Kohlberg, most adolescents and adults generally function at this level.

The postconventional level involves more independent modes of thinking than previous stages, so that the individual is able to define his or her own moral values. People at the postconventional level may ignore both self-interest and group norms in making moral choices. They create their own morality, which may differ from society's norms. Kohlberg believed that only a minority of adults achieve this level.

Each of Kohlberg's levels is subdivided into two stages. Progression through the stages occurs over varying lengths of time, but each stage is sequential and is characterized by higher capacity for logical reasoning than the preceding stage.

Kohlberg (1976) suggested that certain conditions may stimulate higher levels of moral development. Intellectual development is one necessary characteristic. Individuals at higher levels intellectually are generally more advanced in moral development than those operating at lower levels of intelligence.

An environment that offers people opportunities for group participation, shared decision-making processes, and responsibility for the consequences of their actions also promotes higher levels of moral reasoning. Further moral development is stimulated by the creation of conflict in settings in which the individual recognizes the limitations of present modes of thinking. Students have been stimulated to higher levels of moral reasoning through participating in courses on moral discussion and ethics (Kohlberg, 1973).

Gilligan's Levels of Moral Development

Gilligan (1982) was concerned that Kohlberg did not give adequate acknowledgment to the experiences of women in moral development. She recognized that Kohlberg's theories had largely been generated from research with men and boys. When women were tested using Kohlberg's levels of moral development, they scored lower than men.

Gilligan believed that this was due not to inadequate moral development in women but to the fact that women's identities are largely dependent on relationships with others. Because of the basic difference in the way men and women feel about relationships, Gilligan believed that Kohlberg's theory was inadequate to explain women's moral development.

She suggested that women view moral dilemmas in terms of conflicting responsibilities. The sequence she described included three levels and two transitions, with each level representing a more complex understanding of the relationship of self and others and each transition resulting in a crucial re-evaluation of the conflict between selfishness and responsibility. Gilligan's levels of moral development are (1) orientation to individual survival, (2) a focus on goodness as self-sacrifice, and (3) the morality of nonviolence.

The moral person is one who responds to need and demonstrates a consideration of care and responsibility in relationships. Gilligan described a moral development perspective focused on care. This perspective differed from the orientation toward justice described by Kohlberg (1973, 1976).

More recent work by Gilligan and Attanucci (1988) has attempted to define the relationship between the two moral orientations of justice and care. They determined that both perspectives were present when people faced real-life moral dilemmas, but people generally tended to focus on one set of concerns and paid only minimal attention to the other perspective. As expected, the care focus was more often exhibited by women, and the justice focus was more often exemplified by men.

The justice and care perspectives in themselves are not competing theories but are two separate moral perspectives that organize thinking in different ways (Chally, 1990). The justice perspective strives to treat others fairly, whereas the care perspective is strongly based on relationships with others.

Gilligan, Brown, and Rogers (1988) described a combined care/justice perspective that incorporates both viewpoints as moral deliberations are made. Moral development theory must incorporate all perspectives, some of which may not yet be identified. Analysis of interviews of nurses suggest that nurses at times combine the care/justice perspective when forced to make ethical decisions (Chally, 1995). The accompanying Research Note explores how a preceptor can support ethical decision making by critical care nurses.

Understanding Ethical Dilemmas in Nursing

Ethical dilemmas occur frequently in nursing practice. This is to be expected because nurses focus on life and death issues involving human beings. Many ethical dilemmas arise in nursing because of conflicts between patients, health care professionals, and institutions. To understand these conflicts, the following areas are explored: (1) personal value systems, (2) peers' and other professionals' behaviors, (3) patients' rights, and (4) institutional and societal issues.

RESEARCH NOTE

Critical care nurses are key care providers in critical care units, environments in which ethical dilemmas frequently occur. M. C. Hough, a doctoral student at Florida State University wondered what factors might assist critical care nurses in ethical decision making. She designed a study to explore and describe ethical decision making in a critical care nursing practice.

A qualitative study design utilizing ethnographic methods was used to accomplish this goal. Data triangulation was accomplished by utilizing three techniques of data collection: (1) open ended, indepth semistructured interviews and probes; (2) participant observation, and (3) document analysis.

Fifteen critical care nurses with various experience and education levels were interviewed to ensure a representation similar to that found in typical clinical practices. Verbatim transcriptions of each tape-recorded interview were analyzed for content using *The Ethnograph*, a computer software program. Participant observation was conducted with a hospital ethics committee; the researcher attended monthly business meetings and requested copies of all ethics consultations for a twelve-month period. Informal short interviews were used to clarify, explain, or describe relevant issues as the researcher attempted to learn what role the ethics committee played as a nontraditional form of education with critical care nurses in the area of ethical decision making.

Document analysis was also conducted of written records of ethics committee consultations over a twelve-month period prior to beginning the research study.

The findings indicated that nurses who had the advantage of an experienced preceptor or coach, particularly during orientation, had the most focused reflection and the least difficulty with sound, systematic, ethical discourse and decision making. Nurses who did not have this coaching had the greatest difficulty identifying and resolving ethical dilemmas in clinical practice. While difficulty was more often seen with nurses with less than five years of experience, the lack of a coach or mentor caused even more senior nurses to experience difficulty with focused reflection.

Hough concluded that institutions could benefit from developing programs to educate critical care nurses about ethical decision making. Such programs would be enhanced by training preceptors to function as coaches during critical care orientation.

From Hough, M. C. (1998). Walking the line: A qualitative study of critical care nursing and the importance of experiential learning in ethical decision making in clinical nursing practice. PhD dissertation, Florida State University, *Dissertation Abstracts*.

Role of Personal Value Systems

Values are important preferences that influence the behavior of individuals. Value systems are learned beliefs that help people choose among difficult alternatives.

As discussed in Chapter 9, each person has a value system. This value system has a beginning foundation in beliefs, purposes, attitudes, qualities, and objects that are important to a child's early caregivers. In time, individuals develop their own value systems. A **personal value system** is a rank ordering of values with respect to their importance to one another.

Value systems vary from individual to individual. Something important to one individual may hold greater or lesser significance to someone else. For example, a clean, neat home means more to some individuals than others.

Variations in value systems become highly significant when dealing with critical issues such as health and illness or life and death. Value systems enable people to resolve conflicts and decide on a course of action based on a priority of importance. In professional nursing, it is not enough to recognize and act on one's values. In addition, one must determine if the value system is ethical. Only after careful reflection can nurses take action based on their personal or professional values.

Identifying your personal value system and its influence on decision making helps you understand your behavior more clearly. In addition, it gives you clues as to why other people's choices are different from your own. The "Childhood Value Messages" exercise in Box 19–2 can help you identify values learned as a child that may still influence you today.

To see how value conflicts can affect health care delivery, consider the following patient-centered situation:

BOX 19–2
Childhood Value Messages

By the time we are about 10 years old, most of our values have already been "programmed." Values are taught to us by family members and friends, through the media, in churches and schools, and by watching other people. What are the value messages you learned as a child?

Recall as many values as you can remember hearing as a child and write them in the space provided. Here are a few examples to get you thinking:

"Nothing worthwhile ever comes easy."

"Life is fatal—you're eternal."

"You can accomplish almost anything you want to if you persevere."

"Clean your plate, there are starving children in China!"

"You are your brother's keeper—reach out to others."

"Tell me the truth and I won't punish you!"

"Get your work done first, then you can play."

Now it's your turn to write some of your childhood values. How many of these values still influence the way you think and act today? Which ones influence you professionally? If you want to explore further:

1. Next to each value on your list, write the person's name who taught or modeled that value.
2. Put a star next to those messages that are still your values today.
3. Put a check next to those messages that you need to alter.
4. How are some of these values still influencing you today? Is this a positive or negative influence?

1. _____
2. _____
3. _____
4. _____
5. _____
6. _____
7. _____
8. _____

Reprinted with permission of Uustal, D. B. (1993). Clinical ethics and values: Issues and insights in a changing health care environment. East Greenwich, R. I.: Educational Resources in Health Care, Inc.

Mrs. Hamid has recently relocated to the United States from Iran. It is important in her religious faith that men not be present during labor and delivery or at anytime when a woman's body is exposed. A female obstetrician is delivering Mrs. Hamid, but complications develop. Her baby's heart rate drops abruptly, and a cesarean delivery is indicated. The only anesthesiologist available in the hospital for this emergency surgery is a man. What action should the nurse take?

Dilemmas Involving Peers' and Other Professionals' Behavior

All practicing nurses participate as members of the health care team. This involves cooperation and collaboration with other professionals. As is true in all situations involving human beings, conflicts can easily develop, particularly in stressful circumstances. These conflicts may be between two nurses, the nurse and physician, the nurse and hospital administration, or the nurse and any other health care professional.

As discussed in the section on personal value systems, conflicts can evolve because of differing value systems. A nurse may believe that assisting with abortions is wrong, whereas the institution in which he or she is employed routinely performs abortions. This creates a conflict between the nurse's value system and the institution's practices.

Some conflicts develop because individuals are not respectful of the human rights of other individuals. Conflicts in human rights often center around one of the ethical principles discussed earlier: justice, autonomy, beneficence, or veracity. In some circumstances, the ethical dilemma may result from a violation of even more basic human rights, those guaranteed by the U. S. Constitution.

At times, health care workers may be incompetent or their actions unethical (Fry, 1997). An incompetent worker may suffer from physical or mental impairment or may be ignorant of standards of care. Unethical actions result when health care workers break basic norms of conduct toward others, especially the patient, whatever the reason.

A serious issue today is the large number of nurses and other health care professionals impaired by drug dependence or other addictions. Deciding how and when to confront a suspected drug user may result in an ethical dilemma. Fortunately, some employers and state nurses associations have developed plans to assist impaired nurses in getting the help they need and make provisions for them to return to the profession once they are far enough along in their recovery process. Your state nurses association can provide information on specific programs for impaired nurses in your state.

To understand the ethical dilemmas that can result from conflict between peers, consider the following nurse-centered situation:

Miss Corbin, RN, works on a surgical floor. She has just assisted in the transfer of Mr. Hudson to his room from the postanesthesia unit after surgery and noticed that he was resting comfortably. Miss Corbin sees a nurse colleague drawing up a pain medication. The nurse colleague returns to the medicine room 10 minutes later with an empty syringe. Miss Corbin asks, "Who needed pain medication?" "Mr. Hudson," the colleague replies, "He was in pain after surgery." Confused, Miss Corbin checks Mr. Hudson's room and learns from his wife that he has not asked for or received pain medication. What should Miss Corbin do now?

Conflicts Regarding Patients' Rights

Years ago, health professionals, particularly physicians, were considered "all-knowing" experts. Few patients questioned the physician, let alone demanded their basic human rights. Now consumers of health care are increasingly demanding to have a say in matters affecting their health care. A *Patient's Bill of Rights* (American Hospital Association, 1992) outlines currently accepted **patients' rights** (see Box 3–5). The patient's relationship with the physician as well as the relationship between the patient and hospital are discussed.

Many other specialty groups have developed published lists of rights. Examples include *Declaration of the Rights of Mentally Retarded Persons, Dying Person's Bill of Rights, Pregnant Patient's Bill of Rights, Rights of Senior Citizens,* and the *United Nations Declarations of the Rights of the Child.* As consumers have become more aware of their rights, conflicts between patients, health care professionals, and institutions have developed. Many of the rights demanded by consumers are their legal as well as moral rights and have been upheld by the judicial system.

It is beyond the scope of this chapter to discuss all rights due patients. Many have been identified, however, including informed consent, the right to die, privacy, confidentiality, respectful care, and information concerning medical condition and treatment. In addition, patients have the right to be informed if any aspect of treatment is experimental. Based on that knowledge, they have the right to refuse to participate in research projects.

Patient Self-Determination Act

Another safeguard for patients, the Patient Self-Determination Act, gives patients the legal right to determine how vigorously they wish to be treated in life or death situations. The Patient Self-Determination Act forces individuals to think about the type of medical and nursing treatment they want if they become critically injured or ill. When questions arise, the patient is often unconscious or too sick to make decisions or communicate personal wishes.

This act, which went into effect in December 1991, calls for hospitals to abide by patients' **advance directives.** Advance directives are legal documents that indicate the wishes of individuals in regard to end-of-life issues. The Patient Self-Determination Act specifies that any organization receiving Medicare or Medicaid funds must inform patients of state laws regarding directives, document the existence of directives in the patient's medical record, and educate the community about directives.

Advance directives were designed to ensure individuals the rights of autonomy, refusal of medical intervention, and death with dignity (Norman and

Pinkham, 1994). Critically ill individuals can remain in charge of their own end-of-life decisions if their advance directives are carried out.

Families should talk about how each member wishes critical situations to be handled. Individual preferences can then be understood, and family members, caregivers, and courts should not need to be involved. Often the first time a patient learns about advance directives is upon admission to a health care facility. The question then arises as to who is responsible for discussing this sensitive issue with the patient. The ideal time for patients to make difficult end-of-life decisions is well in advance of the need (Fig. 19–1).

Advance directives have not been uncontroversial. One problem is that states have passed different legislation, and there is no guarantee that one state will honor another's advanced directives. Another problem sometimes arises when a person is designated as the proxy to decide about medical treatment if the patient cannot do so. In some situations, persons have been named as proxies without their knowledge. Conflict still arises among caregivers in honoring certain advance directives.

Figure 19–1

To avoid unwanted, life-prolonging interventions, patients must make end-of-life decisions early, discuss them with family members and caregivers, commit them to writing in advance directive documents, and periodically review and renew them (Courtesy of Memorial Hospital, Chattanooga, Tennessee).

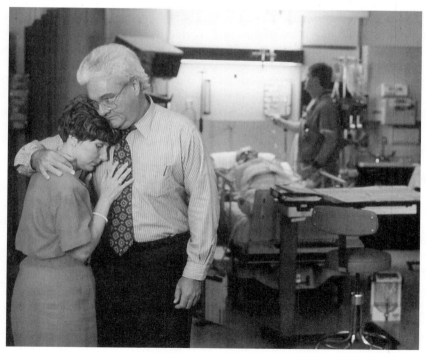

The following case illustrated a conflict related to patients' rights:

> A 28-year-old quadriplegic man is admitted to the hospital with pneumonia and severe pressure ulcers. He asks not to be given antibiotics and to be allowed to die with dignity. At the insistence of the hospital administration, the physician orders intravenous antibiotics. What is the nurse's responsibility?

More information about patient rights and the Patient Self-Determination Act is found in Chapter 20.

Conflicts Created by Institutional and Societal Issues

Nurses experience ethical dilemmas when they disagree with the policies of their institution; conflicts can thus develop. Controversial health care policies at the local, state, or national level can also interfere with the nurse's ability to implement care safely and effectively.

Grave concerns over health care have centered around its cost. The rising cost of health care over the past 25 years has prompted worry by individuals, groups, and communities as well as governmental officials. All health care agencies are stressing cost-containment measures to survive. At times, cost-containment policies conflict with the value system of the nurse, whose goal is to provide high-quality, individualized patient care.

Other institutional and societal concerns can result in ethical dilemmas for the nurse whose personal value system does not support the policies set forth by those in authority. Examples include policies concerning access to health care for the elderly, children, and persons with acquired immunodeficiency syndrome (AIDS).

Nurses today work in many settings, of which the scope and complexity vary significantly from large multiservice medical complexes to small clinics or offices. All organizations, however, that receive governmental funds are subject to public scrutiny and accountability. Ethical dilemmas between nurses and the organizations that employ them may develop over policies dictated by the organizations or mandated by governmental agencies.

This chapter's News Note describes one family's conflict with health care professionals regarding end-of-life decisions.

Ethics committees were created to assist with ethical dilemmas in institutional settings. Ethics committees are multidisciplinary groups charged with the responsibility of providing consultation and emotional support in situations in which difficult ethical choices are necessary. Cases needing consideration are referred to the committee by those desiring help, usually clinical caregivers such as physicians and nurses.

The following vignette illustrates an ethical conflict between a nurse and the employing institution:

> Dina McLeod is a nurse working in a critical care unit. All beds in the unit are full. For the past two days, Miss McLeod has been assigned to care for a 92-

N E W S   N O T E

"A Troubling Death: Wishes of Terminally Ill Patients are Often Ignored, New Study Says"

Perry Elfmont knew he had heart problems. And, as a physician, he knew the questionable future he could face should he suffer a heart attack.

So, like many Americans, he wrote a "living will" saying that he didn't wish to be resuscitated when the inevitable time arrived that his heart would stop.

That time came in May 1994, when he was 88. After he awoke one morning seeming disoriented, his wife, Sabrina, took him to the hospital. She went home 14 hours later to rest—but not before reminding a doctor and nurse about her husband's living will.

Yet she returned the next morning to a horrifying sight. Her husband, whose heart had stopped during the night, had been revived despite his wishes. He was connected to numerous tubes and his hands were restrained "because, the nurses said, he wanted to pull them out," she recalls.

Now her husband, who once spoke five languages, no longer can read, speak or recognize anyone. He lies in bed or sits listlessly, not reacting to anything. His wife is bitter. "No one has the right to change a person's living will," she says.

A quarter century after the living will movement began, many people like Elfmont are unable to achieve their goal of dying with dignity.

A new study, financed by the Robert Wood Johnson Foundation and published in the *Journal of the American Medical Association,* found that almost half of all seriously ill hospital patients who asked their doctors to issue do-not-resuscitate orders for them did not get their wish—at least initially.

The result, in many cases, is a now familiar litany of lives senselessly prolonged by futile treatment of seriously ill patients who spend their final days in pain or twilight existences.

The study found that even an organized effort to improve in-hospital communications about patients' wishes—by using nurses as liaisons between patients and doctors—had little effect.

What's a person to do? While improved long-range answers are being thought out, experts say, most individuals could make better use of the tools we already have. These include writing out your wishes before a medical emergency arises, aggressively informing family members, doctors and religious counselors about these wishes and—most important—naming at least one trusted surrogate to vigorously represent you should you become incapacitated.

Fewer than one-third of Americans have even prepared advance directives spelling out their wishes. "There is a tremendous amount of denial, discomfort and fear on the part of the public and doctors," says Robert Butler, M. D., professor of geriatrics at Mt. Sinai School of Medicine in New York.

Denial leads many people to wait until the last minute—often, when they're sick or unable to think clearly—to fill out advance directives.

Preparing the required forms can be relatively easy: the AARP, American Bar Association, and American Medical Association have jointly prepared a patient guide that includes a model living will and healthcare power of attorney. Instructions and forms also can be obtained from Choice in Dying, a New York–based nonprofit group (http://www.choices.org).

These organizations also can help you make sure your documents are consistent with the laws of the state (or states) in which you reside. That's important because state laws vary on some significant issues.

Once you've written an advance directive, insist it be in a prominent spot in your medical records.

Arthur Caplan, director of the Center for Bioethics at the University of Pennsylvania, recommends updating your directive every couple of years. "People will not trust a document you filled out 10 years ago as much as one you just signed," he notes.

Caplan has another bit of advice: "Never fill out an advance directive alone." The reason: Your loved ones should know your wishes so that they can become forceful advocates for you when you're facing death. Moreover, doctors are more comfortable stopping aggressive treatment when families are united behind the decision.

Besides lining up your family members, try to gauge whether your physician or health maintenance organization would honor your wishes to accept death rather than fight it beyond a point you consider appropriate.

If your doctor won't discuss the issue, he or she may also have trouble letting you die when the time comes.

To assess a caregiver's familiarity and comfort with letting people die with dignity, "ask whether they know the nuts and bolts of how do you die at home," suggests Joanne Lynn, M. D., director of

(*continued*)

the Center to Improve the Care of the Dying at George Washington University and codirector of the study.

Lynn suggests asking "if people who are dying sometimes have to be in pain." A doctor knowledgeable about pain management and comfortable with it, she explains, should confidently answer "no," while one who focuses only on fighting death might give a less definite response.

Having a personal physician who supports your views can enhance your chances of dying with dignity. Even if the attending physician isn't your own doctor, he or she is more likely to act as you wish if that action is backed by a doctor who knows you, according to William Prip, program associate for Choice in Dying.

You should also discuss your wishes with your religious counselor, who may be present when you are seriously ill. And warn your attorney, suggests Robert Veatch, director of the Kennedy Institute of Ethics at Georgetown University.

The mere act of involving your lawyer puts a physician on notice that you are serious about having your wishes honored, he argues.

And experts increasingly emphasize the importance of appointing representatives, with properly executed powers of attorney, to make sure your wishes are carried out.

"A living will may be too vague to guide practitioners," argues Robert Harootyan, a senior research associate at AARP who formerly headed a study by the congressional Office of Technology Assessment on "Life-Sustaining Technologies and the Elderly." "Having a health-care proxy who is legally appointed removes a lot of ambiguity and vagueness," he says.

But be careful whom you appoint to be your representative. Make sure he or she appreciates your values—whether you'd sacrifice extra months of life in order to die at home, for instance. And make sure that he or she is physically able to represent you forcefully.

Still, even if you have taken all these steps, you can't be sure that your wishes will be fulfilled.

Many authorities say the ultimate solution will be to fundamentally change the American way of dying—among other things, by making it easier for people to die at home or in hospices rather than in hospitals.

"We're a victim of our own success," says William Knaus, M. D., chairman of the Department of Health Evaluation Sciences at the University of Virginia School of Medicine, and a study codirector. "A lot of this technology is very useful, and we have wanted to make sure it is widely available.

"Now we have to make it just as easy," he adds, "to get pain relief, comfort and dignity at the end of life as it is to get high-technology care."

Reprinted with permission of Conte, C. (1996). A troubling death: Wishes of terminally ill patients are often ignored, new study says. *AARP Bulletin*, 37(1), 4–5.

year-old woman critically ill with heart failure. The patient has no financial resources of her own, and no family member has seen her since she was admitted from a nursing home. She remains in very critical condition. Suddenly, orders come for the elderly woman to be transferred to a bed on a regular nursing unit. As she is being moved out of the intensive care unit, a state senator's son in a diabetic coma is admitted to her recently vacated bed. What is the nurse's responsibility?

Ethical Decision Making

Nurses encounter situations daily that require them to make professional judgments and act on those judgments. The judgments or decisions are often made in conjunction with other persons involved in the situation: patients, families, and other health care professionals. When an ethical decision is made, everyone must respect and value the perspective held by others. Through respectful collaboration, the best decision can be reached in even the most difficult dilemma. Notice that it is suggested that the best decision will be made. In an ethical dilemma, there is not a right or wrong answer. Instead, we search for the best answer.

Ethical Decision-Making Model

Whether involved in a collective or individual decision, nurses need to be knowledgeable about the steps in **ethical decision making,** listed in Table 19–1. Various models of ethical decision making have been developed. Each model is unique to some degree, but the models do share commonalities. Although the models all have steps, they are not intended to be rigid processes for decision making. Instead, ethical decision making is a process in which ideas are thoroughly examined to determine the best solution to a difficult situation.

The following steps can be used in ethical decision making.

1. Clarify the Ethical Dilemma

What is the specific issue in question? Who owns the problem and should actually make the decision? Who is affected by the dilemma? Determine the ethical principle or theory related to the dilemma. Are there value conflicts? What is the time frame for the decision?

2. Gather Additional Data

After clarifying the ethical dilemma, in most instances more information needs to be gathered. It is important to have as many facts as possible about the situation. Make sure you are up-to-date on any legal cases related to the situation because ethical and legal issues often overlap.

3. Identify Options

Most ethical dilemmas have multiple solutions, some of which are more feasible than others. The more options that are identified, the more likely it is that an acceptable solution can be identified. Brainstorm with others and consider every possible alternative.

TABLE 19-1
Comparison of Nursing Process and Ethical Decision-making Model

Nursing Process	Ethical Decision-making Model
Assess	Clarify the ethical dilemma
	Gather additional data
Analyze	Identify options
Plan	Make a decision
Implement	Act
Evaluate	Evaluate

4. Make a Decision

To make a decision, think through the options that are identified and determine each option's impact. Ethical principles and theories may help determine the significance of each option. When confronted with an ethical dilemma, a decision should be made. Refusing to make a decision is not a responsible professional behavior.

5. Act

Once a course of action has been determined, the decision must be carried out. Implementing the decision usually involves working collaboratively with others.

6. Evaluate

Unexpected outcomes are common in crisis situations that result in ethical dilemmas. It is important for decision makers to determine the impact an immediate decision may have on future ones. It is also important to consider whether a different course of action might have resulted in a better outcome. If the action accomplished its purpose, the ethical dilemma should be resolved. If the dilemma has not been resolved, additional deliberation is needed.

Case Study: Administration of Pain Medication

Mr. Johnson is a 56-year-old white male admitted with the diagnosis of acute myocardial infarction (MI) and cardiogenic shock. He has a history of severe coronary artery disease (CAD) and has suffered several MIs over the past three years. The patient has an advanced directive and a do-not-resuscitate (DNR) order on his chart. When the nurse assesses the patient, he is short of breath and diaphoretic with a blood pressure of 69/36 and heart rate of 162. His respirations are labored and rapid at 42. Mr. Johnson is mentally alert and states he is having crushing midsternal chest pain radiating into his jaw and down his left arm. He is crying and requesting that the nurse give him something for the pain. There is an order for IV morphine sulfate, 2 to 10 mg for pain every one to two hours as needed. The nurse on the off-going shift refused to give the IV morphine because of the patient's compromised status and the fear of further depressing his respiratory and cardiac status. After receiving the report from his evening nurse, you enter the patient's room and find his wife and one of his sons. They are upset and demand you administer the IV pain medication immediately. **What do you do?**

    1. Clarify the Ethical Dilemma. The specific issue is the patient's right of autonomy versus your duty related to beneficence (to do good) and nonmaleficence (to do no harm). Mr. Johnson clearly owns the problem and appears alert enough to make a decision. Obviously, his wife and son are also affected by Mr. Johnson's pain, as is anyone who provides care to him. The dilemma needs to be resolved quickly because of the extent of the pain.

    2. Gather Additional Data. A review of the medical record indicates that the patient has a do-not-resuscitate order. One of your experienced colleagues tells you about the double effect doctrine and the condition that must be met to justify its use. You realized that giving the medication to relieve the chest pain may further compromise the patient's already critical condition.

3. Identify Options. Options include (1) asking someone else to care for Mr. Johnson with intention of avoiding the dilemma; (2) refusing to medicate Mr. Johnson and let him continue in pain; (3) medicating Mr. Johnson with 2 to 10 mg of morphine sulfate; and (4) asking for an order for a medication with fewer side effects.

4. Make a Decision. You determine that to allow your patient to be in severe pain is unacceptable. Morphine sulfate is without question the drug of choice. You think through the principle of double effect and realize the proposed action of administering the medication to relieve pain is intrinsically good. You only intend the good effect (relieving pain) but realize there is potential for the undesired and unintended effect (premature death) from giving the morphine sulfate. You discuss the situation with the patient and his family, indicating both positive and negative consequences of giving the pain medication. You are honest enough to indicate that the morphine sulfate may cause him to stop breathing. Mr. Johnson, his family, and you decide that it is appropriate to administer the medication.

5. Act. You proceed to administer the diluted IV morphine sulfate slowly over a 10-minute period, frequently checking Mr. Johnson's blood pressure. After a total of 6 mg of morphine is given, he states that the pain has been relieved.

6. Evaluate. It would be important to determine if the intended effect was achieved and also to identify any unintended effects. The patient's and family's satisfaction with the decision is also important. **Note:** This situation is based on a real life case. The patient lived for another five hours free of pain. He and his family visited throughout the remaining five hours of his life and reminisced about past family memories. The patient, his wife, and son all expressed much appreciation for the relief of pain.

Summary of Key Points

- The terms *morals* and *ethics* are often used interchangeably. Technically, however, morals reflect what is done in a situation, whereas ethics are concerned with what should be done.
- It is important that nurses are familiar with ethical theories and principles, moral development, and decision-making models to participate actively in resolving ethical dilemmas.
- Codes of ethics, developed by the profession's members, are important to the development of the profession.
- The ANA *Code for Nurses* (1985) serves as a guideline for nurses regarding ethical behavior.
- The history of the *Code for Nurses* is reflective of nursing's history as a profession.
- Ethical dilemmas occur in all areas of nursing practice.
- Dilemmas often occur owing to conflicts between personal value systems, patients, health care professionals, institutions, and society.
- Ethical decision-making models are helpful in determining the best action to take concerning an ethical dilemma.

Critical Thinking Questions

1. What is the difference between morals and ethics? Give an example of each from your own value system.
2. How can the American Nurses Association's *Code for Nurses* be used by the bedside nurse?
3. Compare the American Nurses Association's *Code for Nurses* with the *International Council of Nurses Code for Nurses*. How are they similar, and how are they different?
4. Select an ethical theory or principle that is most congruent with your approach to ethical dilemmas. Use it as a basis for resolving the ethical dilemmas in this chapter. How well does it hold up under these test conditions?
5. Discuss your reactions to the following questions in a small group:
   A. Mrs. Otto has recently undergone extensive surgery for gynecological cancer. The day after surgery, she asks for more pain medication than the physician has prescribed. You call for an order to increase the pain medication dosage, but she still complains every two hours that she cannot tolerate the pain. What should be done?
   B. Mrs. Loriz suffers from severe chronic pain, the cause of which has not been definitely diagnosed. Her husband has brought her into the emergency department for the fifth time this month asking for narcotic relief from the pain. In tears she states, "A shot of Demerol is the only thing that takes the edge off." She threatens suicide if she is sent home without some help. The physician has ordered a placebo. What is the nurse's responsibility?
   C. You are caring for a neonate in intensive care who needs a minor emergency operative procedure. The resident on call immediately begins the procedure in the unit without any anesthesia. The infant is intubated and makes no sound, but she becomes very restless and her pulse rises significantly. You believe that she is experiencing severe pain. What should you do?

Web Resources

American Association of Critical Care Nurses, http://www.aan.org

American Nurses Association, http://www.ana.org

American Society for Bioethics and Humanities, http://www.asbh.org

Biomedical and Health Care Ethics Resources, http://www.ethics.ubc.ca/papers/biomed.html

Bioethical Services of Virginia, Inc., http://www.members.aol.com/bsvinc

Center for Bioethics, http://www.med.upenn.edu/bioethics

Center for Bioethics and Human Dignity, http:www.bioethic.org

Center for Bioethics at Stanford University, http://stanford.edu/dept/scbe

Center for Biomedical Ethics at Case Western Reserve University, http://www.cwru.edu/csru/Dept/med/bioethics.html

Centers for Ethics and Humanities in the Life Sciences (Michigan State University), http://www.chm.msu.edu/chm html/chm ethics.html

Choice in Dying, http://www.choices.org

Consortium Ethics Program at the University of Pittsburgh, http://www.pitt.edu/"caj3/cep.html

International Council of Nurses, http://www.icn.ch/index.html

Johns Hopkins University's Bioethics Institute, http://www.med.jhu.edu/bioethics _institute

National Abortion and Reproductive Rights Action League, http://www.naral.org

National Right to Life, http://www.nrlc.org

Nursing Ethics Network, http://www.bc.edu/bc_org/avp/son/ethics/nen.html

Provincial Health Ethics Network (of Alberta), http://www.ualberta.ca/"ethics/bethics.htm

RNWeb: Ethics Online Resources File, http://www.rnweb.com/ethics.html

University of Alberta's Bioethics Center, http://gpu.srv.ualberta.ca/"ethics/bethics.htm

University of Buffalo Center for Clinical Ethics and Humanities in Health Care, http://wings.buffalo.edu/faculty/research/bioethics/index.html

University of Pennsylvania's Center for Bioethics, http://www.med.upenn.edu/bioethic

University of Toronto Joint Centre for Bioethics, http://www.utoronto.ca/jcb

Virginia Bioethics Network, http://www.med.virginia.EDU/ed.programs/gpo/ethics/vbn.html

References

American Hospital Association (1992). *A patient's bill of rights.* Chicago: American Hospital Association.

American Nurses Association (1976). *Code for Nurses with interpretive statements.* Kansas City, Mo.: American Nurses Association.

American Nurses Association (1985). *Code for nurses with interpretive statements.* Kansas City, Mo.: American Nurses Association.

Aroskar, M. A. (1995). Envisioning nursing as a moral community. *Nursing Outlook,* 43(3), 134–138.

Arras, J., and Hunt, J. (1977). *Ethical issues in modern medicine.* Palo Alta, Calif.: Mayfield publications.

Beauchamp, T. L., and Childless, J. F. (1994). *Principles of biomedical ethics* (4th ed.). New York: Oxford University Press.

Burkhardt, M. A., and Nathaniel, A. K. (1998). *Ethics and issues in contemporary nursing.* Albany, N. Y.: Delmar.

Chally, P. S. (1990). Theory derivation in moral development. *Nursing and Health Care,* 11(6), 302–306.

Chally, P. S. (1995). Nursing research: Moral decision making by nurses in intensive care. *Plastic Surgical Nursing,* 15(2), 120–124.

Chulay, M., Guzzetta, C., and Dossey, B. (1997). *Critical care nursing.* Stamford, Conn.: Appleton & Lange.

Conte, C. (1996). A troubling death: Wishes of terminally ill patients are often ignored, new study says. *AARP Bulletin,* 37(1), 4–5.

Davis, A. J., Aroskar, M. A., Liaschenko, J., and Draegh, T. S. (1997). *Ethical dilemmas and nursing practice* (4th ed.). Stamford, Conn.: Appleton & Lange.

Foote, P. (1993). Virtues and vices. In C. Sommers and F. Sommers, *Vice and virtue in everyday life: Introductory readings in ethics* (3rd ed.) (pp. 250–265). Orlando, Fl.: Harcourt Brace & Company Reprint, Berkley, Calif.: University of California Press.

Fowler, M. D. (1992). A chronicle of the evolution of the code for nurses. In G. B. White (Ed.), *Ethical dilemmas in contemporary nursing practice* (pp. 149–154). Washington, D. C.: American Nurses Publishing.

Fowler, M.D. (1999). Relic or resource? The *Code* for Nurses. *American Journal of Nursing,* 99(3), 56–57.

Frankena, W. K. (1998). *Ethics* (2nd ed.). Englewood Cliffs, N. J.: Prentice-Hall.

Fry, S. T. (1997). Protecting patients from incompetent or unethical colleagues: An important dimension of the nurse's advocacy role. *Journal of Nursing Law,* 4(4), 15–22.

Gilligan, C. (1982). *In a different voice: Psychological theory and women's development.* Cambridge, Mass.: Harvard University Press.

Gilligan, C. (1987). Moral orientation and moral development. In E. Kittay and D. Meyers (Eds.), *Women and moral theory* (pp. 19–33). Totowa, N. J.: Rowman & Littlefield.

Gilligan, C., and Attanucci, J. (1988). Two moral orientations: Gender differences and similarities. *Merrill-Palmer Quarterly,* 34(3), 223–231.

Gilligan, C., Brown, L., and Rogers, A. (1988). *Psyche embedded: A place for body, relationships, and culture in personality theory* (Monogr. No. 4). Cambridge, Mass.: Harvard University, Laboratory of Human Development.

Hough, M. C. (1998). Walking the line: A qualitative study of critical care nursing and the importance of experiential learning in ethical decision making in clinical nursing practice. PhD dissertation, Florida State University, *Dissertation Abstracts.*

Husted, G. L., and Husted, J. H. (1995). *Ethical decision making in nursing* (2nd ed.). St. Louis: Mosby.

International Council of Nurses. (1973). *International Council of Nurses code for nurses.* Geneva, Switzerland: International Council of Nurses.

Jameton, A. (1984). *Nursing practice: The ethical issues.* Englewood Cliffs, N. J.: Prentice-Hall.

Kant, I. (1985). The categorical imperative. In J. Feinburg (Ed.), *Reason and responsibility: Readings in some basic problems of philosophy* (6th ed.) (pp. 540–547). Belmont, Calif.: Wadsworth. 1959, Reprint, Kant, I. *Foundations of the metaphysics of morals,* trans. L. W. Beck (pp. 31–49). Indianapolis: Bobbs-Merrill.

Kohlberg, L. (1986). A current statement on some theoretical issues. In S. Modgil and C. Modgil (Eds.), *Lawrence Kohlberg: Consensus and controversy* (pp. 485–546). Philadelphia: Falmer Press.

Kohlberg, L. (1976). Moral stages and moralization: The cognitive developmental approach. In T. Lickona (Ed.), *Moral development and behavior* (pp. 31–53). New York: Holt, Rinehart & Winston.

Kohlberg, L. (1973). Continuities and discontinuities in childhood and adult moral development revisited. In L. Kohlberg (Ed.), *Collected papers on moral development and moral education.* Cambridge, Mass.: Moral Education Research Foundation.

Mill, J. S. (1985). Utilitarianism. In J. Feinburg (Ed.), *Reason and responsibility: Readings in some basic problems of philosophy* (6th ed.) (pp. 503–515). Belmont, Calif.: Wadsworth (original work published 1863).

Mitchell, P. R., and Grippando, G. M. (1993). *Nursing perspectives and issues* (5th ed.). Albany, N. Y.: Delmar.

Norman, E. M., and Pinkham, D. B. (1994). Advance directives: Understanding their impact on care. In O. L. Strickland and D. J. Fishman (Eds.), *Nursing issues in the 1990s* (pp. 267–279). Albany, N. Y.: Delmar.

Scott, P. A. (1995). Aristotle, nursing, and health care ethics. *Nursing ethics,* 2(4), 279–285.

Silva, M. C. (1990). *Ethical decision making in nursing administration.* Norwalk, Conn: Appleton & Lange.

Thompson, J. B., and Thompson, H. O. (1990). *Professional ethics in nursing.* Malabar, Fl.: Robert E. Krieger.

Tschudin, V. (Ed.) (1993). *Ethics: Nurses and patients.* London: Scutari Press.

Uustal, D. B. (1993). *Clinical ethics and values: Issues and insights in a changing health-care environment.* East Greenwich, R. I.: Educational Resources in HealthCare, Inc.

Veins, D. C. (1989). A history of nursing's code of ethics. *Nursing Outlook,* 37(1), 45–49.

Legal Aspects of Nursing

*Virginia Trotter Betts**

20

Key Terms

Administrative Law
Advance Directives
Assault
Battery
"Captain of the Ship"
   Doctrine
Civil Law
Common Law
Competency
Confidentiality
Criminal Law
Delegation
Documentation
Duty of Care
Duty to Report
Expert Witness
Informed Consent
Law
Legal Authority
Licensure
Licensure by Endorsement

Malpractice
Managed Care
Mutual Recognition Model
National Practitioner
   Data Bank
Negligence
Patient Self-Determination Act
Prescriptive Authority

Privileged Communication
Proximate Cause
Respondeat Superior
Risk Management
Standard of Care
Standard of Nursing Practice
Statutory Law
Tort

Learning Outcomes

After studying this chapter, students will be able to:

- Describe the components of a model nurse practice act.
- Discuss the authority of state boards of nursing.
- Explain the conditions that must be present for malpractice to occur.
- Identify nursing concerns related to delegation, assault and battery, informed consent, and confidentiality.
- Describe strategies nurses can use to protect themselves from legal actions.

Professional nurses have many complex and interesting relationships with the law that are important to identify and understand. This is an area that is both extremely important and constantly changing. Therefore, nursing education programs sometimes offer required or elective courses in law as applied to nursing. "Nursing and the law" is also of the most popular continuing education topics for nurses. This chapter highlights key issues in the law for professional nurses to develop interest in and to study further, which is essential to maintain a working knowledge of the law as it relates to professional nursing practice.

* The author wishes to acknowledge the contributions of Frances I. Waddle and Sara E. Hart to the preparation of this chapter.

American Legal System

The purpose of the law in the United States is found in the Preamble to the U. S. Constitution: to assure order, protect the individual person, resolve disputes, and promote the general welfare. To achieve these broad objectives, the law concerns itself with the legal relationships between persons and the government.

United States law evolved from centuries-old English **common law.** Common law is decisional or judge-made law. Every time a judge makes a legal decision, the body of common law expands.

In addition to common law, there are **statutory laws,** which are laws established through formal legislative processes. Every time the U. S. Congress or a state legislature passes legislation, the body of statutory law expands.

An important distinction to understand is the difference between civil and criminal law. **Civil law** involves issues between individuals, whereas **criminal law** involves public concerns against unlawful behavior that threatens society.

All law in the United States flows from the U. S. Constitution and must conform to its principles. The Constitution provides for division of powers through the establishment of three branches of government: judicial, executive, and legislative. The chief functions of the judicial branch are to resolve legal disputes, interpret statutory laws, and amend the common law. The executive branch implements laws through governmental agencies. The legislative branch may delegate authority to governmental agencies to create **administrative law** to meet the intent of a statute. Both federal and state administrative laws have the force and effect of statutory law. The legislative branch makes statutory laws and speaks most directly for the people.

The word **law** is defined as the sum total of man-made rules and regulations by which society is governed in a formal and binding manner (Hemelt and Mackert, 1982). It encompasses the actions of the legislative branch in enacting statutes, the executive branch in administering the statutes through rules, and the judicial branch in interpreting statutes and rules.

Professional nurses need to be aware of a wide array of legal issues. Nurses must be particularly aware of the statutory authority governing nursing practice, executive authority of state boards of nursing, the civil law areas of torts, privacy rights, and the evolving common law related to health care. The remainder of this chapter focuses on these key areas.

Nursing as a Practice Discipline

Disciplines such as nursing, medicine, dentistry, law, and many others are regulated by the individual states. The practitioners of these disciplines cannot legally practice without a license. The purpose of licensing certain professions is to protect the public safety. The statute that defines and controls nursing is called a nurse practice act. All 50 states and several U. S. territories have nurse practice acts.

Statutory Authority of State Nurse Practice Acts

Nurses, as health care providers, have certain rights, responsibilities, and recognitions through various state laws, or statutes. The nurse practice act in each state does at least four things:

1. Defines the practice of professional nursing.
2. Sets the educational qualifications and other requirements for licensure.
3. Determines the legal titles and abbreviations nurses may use.
4. Provides for disciplinary action of licensees for certain causes.

In many states, nurse practice acts also define the responsibilities and authorities of the state board of nursing. Thus, the nurse practice act of each state is the most important statutory law affecting nurses (Fig. 20–1).

Once the law regarding nursing practice is established, the legislative branch delegates authority to an executive agency, usually the state board of

Figure 20–1
The nurse practice act and other state rules and regulations are vital documents that affect the legal practice of nursing. Every professional nurse should have current copies of these documents and be familiar with their contents (Photo by Fielding Freed).

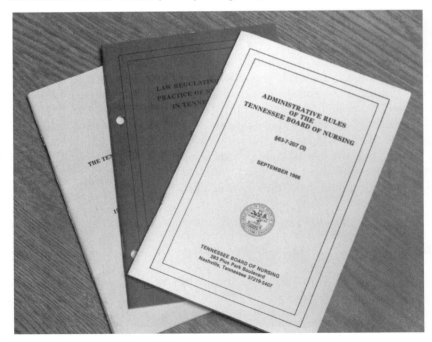

nursing. State boards of nursing are responsible for enforcing the nurse practice acts in the various states. The state board of nursing promulgates rules and regulations that flesh out the law. The statutory law plus the rules and regulations promulgated by the state board of nursing give full meaning to the nurse practice act in each state.

Nurse practice acts are revised from time to time to keep up with new developments in health care and changes in nursing practice. State nurses associations are usually instrumental in lobbying for appropriate updating in nurse practice acts.

Because of the importance of practice acts to professional nurses, the American Nurses Association (ANA) has developed suggested language for the content of state nurse practice acts. The document *Model Practice Act* was published in 1996 to guide state nurses associations seeking revisions in their nurse practice acts (American Nurses Association, 1996a). The guidelines encourage consideration of the many issues inherent in a nurse practice act and the political realities of each state's legislative and regulatory processes. Through this document, the ANA recognizes the great importance of the nurse practice act and urges that the following content be included:

1. A clear differentiation between advanced and generalist nursing practice.
2. Authority for boards of nursing to regulate advanced nursing practice, including authority for prescription writing.
3. Authority for boards of nursing to oversee unlicensed assistive personnel.
4. Clarification of the nurse's responsibility for delegation to and supervision of other personnel.
5. Support for mandatory licensure for nurses while retaining sufficient flexibility to accommodate the changing nature of nursing practice.

The ANA document provides a broad definition of the practice of professional nursing and appropriate professional practice activities. It incorporates aspects of technical nursing practice and identifies technical activities (American Nurses Association, 1996a).

The model nurse practice act guidelines recognize the baccalaureate degree with a major in nursing (bachelor of science in nursing, or BSN) as the minimum educational credential for the professional nurse. There has been extensive debate about the need to change the minimum educational qualifications for professional nursing practice. In the early 1980s and again in 1995, the ANA reaffirmed its long-standing position that the baccalaureate degree should be the minimum educational qualification for professional nursing practice and the associate degree the minimum educational qualification for technical nursing practice.

To date, only North Dakota has fully implemented these changes in the minimum educational qualifications for nurses. Many state nurses associations, however, consider such changes a priority for future nurse practice act modifications.

Executive Authority of State Boards of Nursing

Both federal and state laws provide for the executive branch of government to administer and implement laws. The state executive, or governor, generally delegates the responsibility for administering the nurse practice act to an executive agency, the state board of nursing. In most states, the state board of nursing consists of registered nurses (RNs), licensed practical nurses (LPNs), and consumers, all of whom are generally appointed to the board by the governor.

The state board of nursing's authority is limited. It can adopt rules that clarify general provisions of the nurse practice act, but it does not have the authority to enlarge the law.

State boards of nursing usually have three functions:

1. Quasiexecutive—authority to administer the nurse practice act.
2. Quasilegislative—authority to adopt rules necessary to implement the act.
3. Quasijudicial—authority to deny, suspend, or revoke a license or to otherwise discipline a licensee or to deny an application for licensure.

Each of these functions is as broad or as limited as the state legislature specifies in the nurse practice act and related laws.

State boards of nursing may be independent agencies in the executive branch of state government or part of a department or bureau such as a department of licensure and regulation. Some state boards have authority to carry out the nurse practice act without review of their actions by other state officials. Others must recommend action to another department or bureau and receive approval of the recommendation before the decision is finalized.

Licensing Powers

The **licensure** process is a police power of the state, which, through the legislative branch, determines what groups are to be licensed and the limitations of such licenses. Licensure laws may be either mandatory or permissive. A mandatory law requires any person who practices the profession or occupation to be licensed. A permissive law protects the use of the title granted in the law but does not prohibit persons practicing the profession or occupation if they do not use the title. All states now have a mandatory licensure law for the practice of nursing.

Just as the state has the power to issue a nursing license based upon established criteria, so does it retain the power to discipline a licensee for performing professional functions in a manner that is dangerous to patients or the general public. Discipline may include sanctions such as license suspension or revocation arising from unsafe, uninformed, or impaired practice by the nurse licensee.

Historically, the nursing profession has demonstrated a commitment to the rehabilitation of nurses whose practice is below standard because of impairment by psychological dysfunction or substance abuse and misuse. In

1990, the ANA published suggested state legislation that included a Nursing Disciplinary Diversion Act (American Nurses Association, 1990). This publication recommended a diversion procedure, such as a peer assistance program to combat substance abuse, as a voluntary alternative to the traditional disciplinary actions of suspension or revocation of a license. In 1999, 37 state boards of nursing had nondisciplinary alternative programs (disciplinary diversion processes) to assist impaired nurses to return to safe nursing practice. Additionally, 23 boards also provided alternative programs for psychiatric and mental health problems (National Council of State Boards of Nursing, 1999a).

In most states, state boards of nursing have the authority to enforce minimum criteria for nursing education programs. The practice act usually stipulates that an applicant for licensure must graduate from a state-approved nursing education program as a prerequisite to being admitted to the licensure examination.

State approval is different from national accreditation; many nursing education programs achieve accreditation by nationally recognized accrediting bodies. Although many other professions and occupations require graduation from a nationally accredited educational program as a prerequisite of licensure, only state approval is required in nursing.

Licensure Examinations

Since 1944, most state boards of nursing have participated in a cooperative effort to assist in the interstate mobility of nurses, both registered nurses and licensed practical nurses. Because nurse licensure examinations are national examinations, they facilitate this system, called **licensure by endorsement.** Endorsement means that registered nurses or licensed practical nurses or licensed vocational nurses (LVN) can move from state to state without having to take another licensing examination. If they submit proof of licensure in another state and pay a licensure fee, they can receive licensure in the new state by endorsement. Licensure by endorsement is not available to all practice disciplines. Nursing's plan serves as a national model for other licensed professions and occupations.

Until 1978, the national nursing licensing examination was developed by the ANA's Council of State Boards of Nursing, and the National League for Nursing served as the testing service. In 1978, the National Council of State Boards of Nursing (NCSBN) was established and continued the activities of the ANA Council of State Boards. Through the NCSBN, each state still participates in the licensing process through test development and adoption of a minimum passing score.

The nurse licensure examinations are now called the National Council Licensure Examination for Registered Nurses (NCLEX-RN) and the National Council Licensure Examination for Practical Nurses (NCLEX-PN). The test was traditionally administered by paper and pencil; however, the state boards of nursing and the NCSBN began administering them by computerized adaptive testing (CAT) in 1994. The test plan for the NCLEX-RN licensure examination provides for the examination to measure critical thinking and nursing competence in all phases of the nursing process.

Trends in Licensure

The climate for licensure of health professions became increasingly unstable in the mid- to late 1990s, largely because of dramatic alterations in the financing and delivery of health services following the 1994 failure of health care reform. Federal and state governments indicated interest in examining all types of deregulation, and licensure of health professionals has no immunity to regulatory changes.

The Pew Charitable Trust funded extensive projects examining health care work force regulations, which may, over time, create a variety of regulatory schemes in different jurisdictions. The nursing community needs to be vigilant in the analysis of each proposal for regulatory change. Nursing has much to gain or lose in terms of its scope, authority, and accountability for practice should deregulation occur (Pew Health Professions Commission, 1995).

In 1998, 24 state boards of nursing were issuing a separate license for one or more categories of advanced practice nurses (APNs), and every state reported having some form of recognition for advanced practice nurses (National Council of State Boards of Nursing, 1999a).

Currently, nurses sometimes practice across state boundaries both by physically crossing state lines to provide nursing care in person and by being physically present in one state while providing nursing care to a patient in another state through electronic means (telehealth). In response to the increasing practice of telehealth and because of other regulatory pressures, the National Council of State Boards of Nursing has endorsed a **mutual recognition model** for nursing licensure. The mutual recognition model would allow a registered nurse to have one license (in the state of residency) yet practice in other states without additional licenses. While practicing in another state the nurse would be subject to that state's laws, scope of practice, and discipline. Each state that wishes to participate will have to pass legislation to allow the board of nursing to enter into the interstate compact. At the end of the 1999 legislative session, five states (Arkansas, Maryland, North Carolina, Texas, and Utah) had enacted this legislation (National Council of State Boards of Nursing, 1999b).

Special Concerns in Professional Nursing Practice

Nurses make decisions daily that affect the well-being of their patients. They often know personal information about patients and are in positions of great trust. Several areas of nursing practice are particularly fraught with legal risk. They include malpractice, delegation, assault and battery, informed consent, and confidentiality. Each of these areas is discussed.

Malpractice

Malpractice is the greatest legal concern of health care practitioners. To understand malpractice, it is necessary first to understand the legal concepts of torts and negligence. **Torts** are civil wrongs against a person and may be either intentional or unintentional. There must be harm resulting from the action, but the harm may be physical, emotional, or economic. An intentional tort refers to willful or intentional acts that violate another person's rights or property.

Negligence is the failure to act as a reasonably prudent person would have in specific circumstances. For example, if in burning yard debris on a windy day a man sets fire to his neighbor's garage, the neighbor may charge negligence. A reasonably prudent person would not have started a yard fire on a windy day, and an injury (the burned garage) can be shown to be a direct result of his failure to act prudently. The differences between negligence and intentional torts are summarized in Table 20–1.

Malpractice is negligence applied to the acts of a professional. In other words, malpractice occurs when a professional fails to act as a reasonably prudent professional would under specific circumstances. Malpractice is classified as an unintentional tort. This means that it is not necessary to prove that the professional intended to be negligent. In malpractice, both doing things that should not be done (commissions) and not doing things that should be done (omissions) may be the basis of legal actions.

When a patient brings a malpractice claim against a nurse defendant, evidence is presented to the jury to determine whether the elements of liability are present. At question is whether the nurse met the prevailing **standard of care.**

TABLE 20–1
Differences between Negligence and Intentional Torts

Negligence	Intentional Torts*
Intent	
May occur without any intent to act.	Requires an intent to interfere with another's rights; a hostile motive not required.
Proof of Damages	
Requires proof of a specific injury.	Proof of actual injury not required.
Duty or Standards of Care	
Relevant; usually involves expert witnesses.	Not needed.
Consent	
Not necessarily a defense.	Always may be a defense.

*Examples of intentional torts include defamation (libel or slander), invasion of privacy, assault and battery, false imprisonment, and intentional infliction of emotional distress. From Aiken, T. (1994). *Legal, ethical, and political issues in nursing.* Philadelphia: F. A. Davis.

The nursing standard of care is what the reasonably prudent nurse, under similar circumstances, would have done. It is a peer standard of care that reflects not excellence but a minimum standard of "do no harm." The nursing standard of care is decided by a jury on a case-by-case basis and is developed through use of **expert witness** testimony; documents, including national **standards of nursing practice;** the patient record; and other pertinent evidence such as the direct testimony of the patient, the nurse, and others.

The prerequisite of a malpractice action is twofold: The defendant (nurse) has specialized knowledge and skills and through the practice of that specialized knowledge causes the plaintiff's (patient's) injury. For a plaintiff patient to prove that the nurse defendant is liable for the injury, all elements of a cause of action for negligence must be proved. The elements are the same for any professional accused of malpractice. The elements necessary for a malpractice action are as follows:

1. The professional nurse has assumed the **duty of care** (responsibility for the patient's care).
2. The professional nurse breached the duty of care by failing to meet the standard of care.
3. The failure of the professional nurse to meet the standard of care **proximately caused** the injury.
4. The injury is proved.

Setting forth all elements of a malpractice action requires a high degree of proof. Monetary damages are awarded when a patient plaintiff prevails. These are based on proven economic losses, such as time missed from work or out-of-pocket health care costs and on remuneration for pain and suffering caused by the injury. In the case of a death, the next of kin can become the plaintiff on behalf of the deceased patient.

In the past, some malpractice lawsuits involved nurses, but the physician or hospital defendants were traditionally called on to pay damages even when the substandard care was provided by nurses. In these instances, physicians were implicated through the "**captain of the ship**" **doctrine.** This doctrine implies that the physician is in charge of all patient care and thus should be responsible financially. Hospitals were implicated through the legal theory of **respondeat superior,** which attributes the acts of employees to their employer. As nurses obtain more credentials and their expertise, autonomy, and authority for nursing practice increases, however, liability for nursing care will correspondingly rise. Nurses are expected to be defendants more often in the future (Sweeney, 1991).

A review of malpractice cases in which the liability of the nurse has been successfully litigated showed the categories of cases as follows:

1. The nurse failed to carry out the medical order.
2. The nurse carried out an order incorrectly.
3. The nurse implemented a faulty medical order.
4. The nurse failed to make an accurate assessment.
5. The nurse failed to act on an assessment.

6. The nurse failed to report inadequate patient care.
7. The nurse failed to secure adequate care for a patient.
8. The nurse abandoned a patient needing care.

Some examples of malpractice that involved professional nurses were covered in the popular press. One such highly publicized case involved a number of nurses at a Massachusetts hospital who carried out a physician's faulty order and gave two different cancer patients overdoses of chemotherapy (Trossman, 1999). Another example is an operating room nurse who failed to follow well-established hospital policy for identifying and preparing patients for surgery. This breach of procedure resulted in the removal of one patient's only func-tioning kidney (*Holbrooks v. Duke Hospital, Inc.*, 305 SE^2 69, 1983). Although physicians and facilities are also involved in both of these cases, the nurses are likely to be named as codefendants because they too fell below the stan-dard of care, and "but for" their actions, these serious injuries would not have occurred.

The lesson to be learned from such malpractice cases is that professional nurses must carefully consider the legal implications of practice and be willing and capable of conforming to professional standards and all legal expectations.

Delegation

Delegation, that is, "empowering one to act for another," is an issue gaining increasing importance in nursing practice. The ability to delegate has gener-ally been reserved for professionals because they hold licenses that sanction the entire scope of practice for a particular profession. Professional nurses, for example, may delegate independent nursing activities and delegated medical functions to other nursing personnel. State nurse practice acts do not give del-egatory authority to licensed practical or vocational nurses.

Professional nurses retain accountability for acts delegated to another per-son and are responsible for determining that the delegate is competent to per-form the delegated act. Likewise, the delegate is responsible for carrying out the delegated act safely. The professional nurse remains legally liable, how-ever, for the nursing acts delegated to others unless the delegate is a licensed professional whose scope includes the assigned act.

Delegatory acts must also be considered from the standpoint of their eth-ical implications. The *Code for Nurses* states, "The nurse exercises informed judgment and uses individual competence and qualifications as criteria in seeking consultation, accepting responsibilities, and delegating nursing activ-ities to others" (American Nurses Association, 1985). An important point is that nurses are ethically bound to refuse to accept acts that are not within their area of expertise, even if a physician or hospital authority requests that they accept them.

Delegation is an important liability and one not fully appreciated by many practicing nurses. The professional nurse's primary legal and ethical consid-eration must be the patient's right to safe, effective nursing care. Box 20–1 contains the American Nurses Association's *Basic Guide to Safe Delegation*.

BOX 20-1
American Nurses Association Basic Guide to Safe Delegation

Delegation: Defining the Term

The ANA defines delegation as "The transfer of responsibility for the performance of an activity from one individual to another, with the former retaining accountability for the outcome." Delegation can also be differentiated as direct or indirect.

- Direct delegation comes about when the nurse determines which tasks can be delegated and to whom to delegate.
- Indirect delegation provides that tasks or activities from an approved list contained within the policies and procedures of the facility can be carried out by the LPN/LVN or unlicensed assistive worker.

In either case, the nurse is still obligated to assess the competence of the individual carrying out the assignment.

Delegation: Determining the Appropriate Delegate

Key issues must be addressed in determining when, and to whom, to delegate. In addition to state laws and institutional policies that guide the nurse, the following steps help to reinforce the decision-making process about delegation:

- Assess the patient's status and needs and the appropriateness of delegating tasks to another caregiver. Then evaluate available staff for skills and competence before determining the delegate—the person receiving the delegation.
- Educate the delegate about what is to be done. It is vital that the nurse demonstrate the task or procedure and then observe the delegate's ability to perform safely and appropriately. The nurse must document the training, observations, and competence of the delegate and keep the documentation available and updated for legal protection.
- Communicate expectations of both performance and outcomes as well as receptivity to questions and concerns. Be certain also to inform the delegate which situations require asking for immediate assistance.
- Observe the delegate directly the first time any task or procedure is done. In addition, make certain to reassess competencies from time to time. Most important of all, the nurse must always be available to assist the delegate should the need arise.

Reprinted with permission of American Nurses Association (1995). *ANA basic guide to safe delegation.* Washington, D. C.: American Nurses Association.

Assault and Battery

Assault and battery is an intentional tort that is often the basis for legal action against a nurse defendant. **Assault** is a threat or an attempt to make bodily contact with another person without the person's consent. Assault precedes battery; it causes the person to fear that a battery is about to occur. **Battery** is the assault carried out, the unpermissible, unprivileged touching by one person of another. Actual harm may or may not occur as a result of assault and battery.

If, for example, a nurse threatens a patient with a vitamin injection if he does not eat his meals, the patient may charge assault. Actually giving the patient a vitamin injection against his will leaves the nurse open to charges of battery, even if there is a physician's order. It is important to remember that patients have the right to refuse treatment, even if the treatment would be in their best interest. Both by common law and by statute, **informed consent** is required in the health care context as a defense to battery (*42 United States Code* 1395 cc., 1990).

Informed Consent

All patients should be given an opportunity to grant informed consent before treatment unless there is a life-threatening emergency. Three major conditions of informed consent include the following:

1. Consent must be given voluntarily.
2. Consent must be given by an individual with the capacity and competence to understand.
3. The patient must be given enough information to be the ultimate decision maker.

Informed consent is a full, knowing authorization by the patient for care, treatment, and procedures and must include information about the risks, benefits, side effects, costs, and alternatives. Consumers of health care need a great deal of information and should be told everything that they would consider significant in making a treatment decision (*Canterbury v. Spence,* 464 F^2 772, 1972).

For informed consent to be legally valid, elements of completeness, competency, and voluntariness are evaluated. Completeness refers to the quality of the information provided. **Competency** takes into account the capability of a particular patient to understand the information given and make a choice. Voluntariness refers to the freedom the patient has to accept or reject alternatives. When patients are minors, are under the effects of drugs or alcohol (including preoperative medications), or have other mental deficits, it is questionable that competency to consent exists.

The role of nurses in informed consent, unless they are themselves primary providers, is to collaborate with the primary provider, most often a physician. A nurse may witness a patient's signing of informed consent documents but is not responsible for explaining the proposed treatment (Fig. 20–2). The nurse is not responsible for evaluating whether the physician has truly explained the significant risks, benefits, and alternative treatments. Professional nurses are responsible for determining that the elements for valid consent are in place, providing feedback if the patient wishes to change consent, and communicating the patient's need for further information to the primary provider.

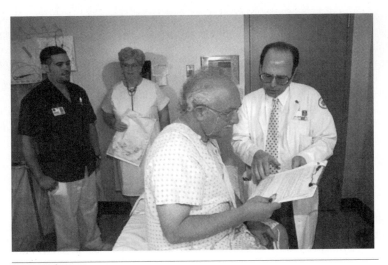

Figure 20–2

Professional nurses may be called upon to witness a patient's signing of informed consent documents. The primary provider, however, is responsible for providing necessary information to the patient or legal guardian. (From: Leahy, J. M., Kizilay, P. E.: Foundations of Nursing Practice, 1998. W.B. Saunders Company, Philadelphia.)

Confidentiality

Confidentiality is both a legal and an ethical concern in nursing practice. Confidentiality is the protection of private information gathered about a patient during the provision of health care services. The *Code for Nurses* states, "The nurse safeguards the client's right to privacy by judiciously protecting information of a confidential nature" (American Nurses Association, 1985).

The *Code* acknowledges exceptions to the obligation of confidentiality. The exceptions include discussing the care of patients with others involved in their direct care, quality assurance activities, and when the law demands disclosure (American Nurses Association, 1985). The *Code* also recognizes the need to disclose information without the patient's consent when the safety of innocent parties is in question (*Tarasoff v. Board of Regents of the University of California,* 551 P^2 334, 1976).

Although some professions have statutorily protected **privileged communication,** nurses are usually not included in such statutes. Thus, nurses may be ordered by a court to share information without the patient's consent. The principle of confidentiality is protected by state and federal statutes, but there are exceptions and limitations. It is essential for the professional nurse to understand these legal limitations.

In certain situations, through statute and common law, there has developed the antithesis of confidentiality—the **duty to report** or disclose. These laws require nurses and other health professionals to report child abuse, gunshot wounds, certain communicable diseases, and threats toward third parties. These laws vary by state and may be the responsibility of institutions providing health care services and not of an individual practitioner.

Evolving Legal Issues and the Nurse

Because of the dynamic nature of nursing and health care, legal issues affecting nursing practice are also evolving. Specific legal issues that illustrate the changing nature of nursing practice are related to role changes, supervision of assistive personnel, payment mechanisms, and a new law, the Patient Self-Determination Act. Each of these issues is briefly discussed.

Role Changes in Health Care

Just as a nurse's knowledge base and the nurse's accountability for nursing practice have increased over time, so has the need to expand the **legal authority** for nursing practice. Even though the definitions and parameters of nursing outlined in nurse practice acts may seem to be an issue of concern only to nurses, this is not the case.

Nurses have found that as they worked through their state nurses associations to modify and update these acts, they met significant political resistance. This is due, in part, to the defensiveness of organized medicine, which often views an expansion of nurses' domain as a diminishment of physicians' roles or as a threat to physicians' economic base.

Professional nurses realize that it is important for a state nurse practice act to reflect nursing practice accurately and to keep up with changes in health care delivery as they occur. Otherwise, nurses have questionable legal basis for practice. Health care is becoming more specialized, so nursing specialties and subspecialties are increasing. Advanced practice nurses set the pace for evolving nursing practice, and the nurse practice act must support their ability to offer nursing services to consumers in various settings. Many functions defined as advanced practice have been absorbed into the statutory scope of professional nursing practice.

Prescriptive Authority

An important role addition for advanced practice nurses is **prescriptive authority.** Prescriptive authority is defined as the legal acknowledgment of prescription writing as an appropriate act of nursing practice. The ANA supports prescriptive authority for advanced practice nurses, as distinguished from generalist registered nurses (American Nurses Association, 1990).

Several questions about prescriptive authority that nurses should consider include does the state recognize prescriptive authority for nurses? If so, is the state board of nursing the state regulatory authority for this practice? Does the law require physician collaboration or supervision or written protocols? What are the parameters for prescribing controlled substances, if any?

In 1999, advanced practice nurses had some type of prescriptive authority in all fifty states. This authority ranged from completely independent authority with no collaborative requirements in the District of Columbia, to a pilot study in Ohio granting limited prescriptive authority to specific advanced practice nurses (American Academy of Nurse Practitioners, 1999). Most states require advanced practice status, the collaboration or supervision of a physician, and prescription writing protocols (American Nurses Association, 1995a).

In some states, nurses in advanced practice, such as nurse-midwives, nurse practitioners, and nurses in private practice, have not been supported by timely changes in the nurse practice act. For example, nurses in a women's health practice in Missouri were sued for practicing medicine without a license. After intense litigation, their practice was supported by the Missouri Supreme Court. The court found "legislative intent" in the nurse practice act not to limit nursing practice except to protect the public. The nurses in question were well credentialed and were practicing with the knowledge and support of the Missouri Board of Nursing and the Missouri Nurses Association, so the safety of the public was not in question (*Sermchief v. Gonzales,* 660 SW^2 683,1983).

This is only one example of the legal exposure nurses face when their state's nurse practice act is not updated periodically to support explicitly an expanded scope of practice. Working within the state nurses association to expand the evolving scope of nursing practice appropriately ensures the growth of the profession and increases the number of primary care providers needed by the public.

Supervision of Unlicensed Assistive Personnel

Another evolving legal issue is the role expansion of unlicensed assistive personnel or limited licensed (licensed practical/vocational nurses) personnel within health care institutions. Nurse aides (i.e., unlicensed assistive personnel) are increasingly being substituted for nurses, thus creating greater risks to patients and enlarging the liability of nurses, who supervise their work. Court decisions indicate that lack of professional nurse supervision poses a significant risk to patients, institutions, and nurses alike (Politis, 1983).

The substitution of unlicensed personnel for registered nurses is a strategy used by health care facilities to hold down costs. Such substitution is ill advised because it jeopardizes quality of care and places the registered nurse at increased risk for patient injury liability because of acts performed by unlicensed assistive personnel. It is questionable whether, in the long-term, professional nursing care is actually more expensive than care provided by unlicensed personnel, who are less likely to do patient teaching and recognize complications.

In 1992, the ANA issued a *Position Statement on Registered Nurse Utilization of Unlicensed Assistive Personnel.* This statement indicated that the ANA recognizes that unlicensed assistive personnel provide support services that assist the registered nurse in providing nursing care (American Nurses Association, 1992). The statement identified the need to clarify the activities that should be in the domain of the registered nurse and those that can be safely delegated. Additional materials were developed by the ANA to provide registered nurses and health care facilities guidance on utilization of unlicensed assistive personnel in the workplace (American Nurses Association, 1996b).

Historically, organized nursing has opposed the licensure or legal recognition of nurse aides and other nursing support personnel. This position needs further study, however, following congressional action mandating training and state registration of nurse aides in Medicaid-certified and Medicare-certified nursing facilities and Medicare-certified home health agencies. In 1998, only 15 state boards of nursing regulated some aspect of the federally mandated requirements (National Council of State Boards of Nursing, 1999a). Federal law allows the state Medicaid agency to contract with a state board of nursing to operate the required nurse aide registry; however, only the Medicaid agency can enter a finding of patient abuse, neglect, or misappropriation of patient property by individuals on the nurse aide registry.

Payment Mechanisms for Nurses

As discussed in Chapter 5, nurses are increasingly practicing in nontraditional roles and settings. Many professional nurses are both capable of and interested in offering nursing services as private practitioners, but current payment mechanisms may limit such activities. Nurses are concerned about offering services for which consumers are unable to obtain reimbursement from their insurance carriers, and third-party reimbursement has traditionally been limited to care provided by physicians.

Over the years, nurses have supported state and federal legislation to provide direct and indirect payments to nurses for nursing services rendered (American Nurses Association, 1991). A major step toward reimbursement of advanced practice nurses came with the passage of the 1997 Balanced Budget Act. This legislation authorized nurse practitioners and clinical specialists to bill the Medicare program directly for nursing services furnished in any setting, regardless of whether the setting is rural or urban. Advanced practice nurses may now bill Medicare at 85 percent of the physician rate for Medicare Part B services.

Changes in state insurance laws were enacted in many states to achieve direct payment for nursing services from private insurance companies. This means that consumers of health care may choose to receive services from physicians, nurses, or other qualified health professionals and receive insurance reimbursement for the chosen professional's fees. Nurses are concerned that these changes are often not implemented or that nurses are paid less for similar services when provided by other health care professionals.

Laws are often passed that are not implemented. This occurs when the group affected by the law, for example, the insurance industry, is unwilling to implement the changes and no "watchdog" agency is created to ensure that changes occur. For example, federal legislation was enacted requiring state Medicaid agencies to pay certain nurses (nurse practitioners, nurse-midwives, and nurse anesthetists) directly for services provided to Medicaid recipients.

As with the laws affecting private insurers, these requirements have not been implemented in every state. Nurses may need to seek legal remedies to require implementation of policies mandated by federal law (*Nurse Midwifery Associates v. Hibbett,* 918 Fed² 605, 1990).

Following the failed 1994 efforts to overhaul the entire health care system, health care finance nevertheless underwent dramatic changes. One change, discussed in Chapter 16, was from fee-for-service provider reimbursement to capitation. Additionally, many individual and group insurance plans changed from indemnity plans to **managed care** plans, such as health maintenance organizations (HMO) and preferred provider organizations (PPO). As of 1998, 53 percent of the nation's Medicaid recipients were enrolled in some form of managed care plan (Health Care Financing Administration, 1999).

These shifts have posed new challenges for nurses because they are often not included on HMO and PPO provider panels. As a result of these new challenges, the ANA and state nurses associations are working to ensure that nurses are included on managed care panels, in "any willing provider" clauses, and in all federal insurance programs as appropriate providers of basic plan services.

Patient Self-Determination Act

As mentioned in Chapter 19, the federal **Patient Self-Determination Act** (PSDA) became effective December 1, 1991. This act applies to acute care and long-term care facilities that receive Medicare and Medicaid funds and encourages patients to consider which life-prolonging treatment options they desire and to document their preferences in case they should later become incapable of participating in the decision-making process. Written instructions recognized by state law that describe an individual's preferences in regard to medical intervention should the individual become incapacitated is called an **advance directive.**

This act was passed partly in response to the U. S. Supreme Court's decision in *Cruzan v. Director Missouri Department of Health* (110 Supreme Court 2841, 1990), which was viewed as limiting an individual's ability to direct health care when unable to do so. The PSDA requires the health care facility to document whether the patient has completed an advance directive.

The PSDA's basic assumption is that each person has legal and moral rights to informed consent about medical treatments with a focus on the person's right to choose (the ethical principle of autonomy). The act does not create any new rights, and no patient is required to execute an advance directive.

According to the PSDA, acute care (hospitals) and long-term care facilities must:

1. Provide written information to all adult patients about their rights under state law.
2. Ensure institutional compliance with state laws on advance directives.
3. Provide for education of staff and the community on advance directives.
4. Document in the medical record whether the patient has an advance directive.

There have been a number of widely publicized cases wherein families and providers disagreed about whether to terminate life support mechanisms (See

News Note, Chapter 19). Widespread education of the public about advance directives should result in fewer such legal and ethical dilemmas in the future. Documentation of the existence of advance directives and use of them in planning care is an important patient advocacy role for nurses and is a legal requirement that needs careful implementation in clinical settings.

Preventing Legal Problems in Nursing Practice

Although the range of potential "hot spots" for health care litigation may seem enormous, there are a number of effective strategies that professional nurses can use to limit the possibility of legal action.

Practice in a Safe Setting

To be truly safe, facilities in which nurses work must be committed to safe patient care. The safest situation is one in which the agency:

1. Employs an appropriate number and skill mix of personnel to care adequately for the number of agency patients at all levels of acuity.
2. Has policies, procedures, and personnel practices that promote quality improvement.
3. Keeps equipment in good working order.
4. Provides orientation to new employees, supervises all levels of employees, and provides opportunities for employees to learn new procedures consistent with the level of health care services provided by the agency.

In addition to an active quality improvement program, each health care organization should have a **risk management** program. Risk management seeks to identify and eliminate potential safety hazards, thereby reducing patient and staff injuries. Common areas of risk include patient falls, failure to monitor, failure to ensure patient safety, improper performance of a treatment, failure to respond to a patient, medication errors, and failure to follow hospital procedure (Aiken, 1994).

Communicate with Other Health Professionals

The professional nurse must have open and clear communication with nurses, physicians, and other health care professionals. Safe nurses trust their own assessments, inform physicians and others of changes in patients' conditions, and question unclear or inaccurate physicians' orders. A key aspect of communication essential in preventing legal problems is keeping good patient records. This written form of communication is called **documentation.** Current and descriptive documentation of patient care is essential, not only to quality care but also to protecting the nurse. Assessments, plans, interventions, and evaluation of the patient's progress must be reflected in the patient's clinical record if malpractice is alleged.

The clinical record, particularly the nurse's notes, provides the core of evidence about each patient's nursing care. No matter how good the nursing care, if the nurse fails to document it in the clinical record, in the eyes of the law the care did not take place.

Meet the Standard of Care

The most important protective strategy for the nurse is to be a knowledgeable and safe practitioner and to meet the standard of care with all patients. Meeting the standard of care involves being technically competent, keeping up-to-date with health care innovations, being aware of peer expectations, and participating as an equal on the health care team.

In addition to being current with the nursing literature, professional nurses must use national standards of practice as parameters for care giving, care planning, and care evaluation (American Nurses Association, 1998). The ANA has promulgated generic and specialty standards of nursing practice. These national standards can be used by quality improvement programs in individual hospitals in establishing their own "local" standards of nursing care.

Carry Professional Liability Insurance

Despite the efforts of dedicated professionals, at times mistakes are made, and, unfortunately, patients are injured. It is essential for nurses to carry professional liability insurance to protect their assets and income, should they be required to pay monetary compensation to an injured patient. Nursing students should also carry insurance, and most nursing education programs require that they do so.

Professional liability insurance policies vary. Generally, they provide up to $1 million coverage for a single incident and up to $3 million total. The amount of coverage depends on the nurse's specialty. Nurse-midwives, for example, pay much higher liability insurance premiums than do psychiatric nurses because a nurse-midwife's potential for being sued is greater. Most policies also provide the defendant nurse with a defense attorney (American Association of Nurse Attorneys, 1984).

Professional liability insurance is available through most state nurses associations, nursing students associations, and private insurers. Group policies, such as those available through professional associations, are usually less expensive than individual policies and are an important benefit of association membership. Box 20–2 displays information about the two main types of professional liability policies.

Liability and the National Practitioner Data Bank

The Health Care Quality Improvement Act (Public Law 100-177) was passed by Congress in 1986. It established a **National Practitioner Data Bank** (NPDB) to encourage identification and discipline of health care practitioners who engage in unprofessional behavior. An additional purpose was to restrict the ability of those practitioners to move from state to state without disclosing problems of damaging or incompetent practice. The act requires that certain things be reported to a national data bank: any malpractice payments made to any licensed

BOX 20–2
Basic Types of Professional Liability Insurance Policies

Occurrence Policies
Cover injuries that occur during the period covered by the policy.

Claims-made Policies
Cover injuries only if the injury occurs within the policy period and the claim is reported to the insurance company during the policy period or during the "tail." A tail is an uninterrupted extension of the policy period and is also known as the extending reporting endorsement.

health practitioner, any licensure action taken by a licensing body, any clinical privilege suspension or revocation by a health care facility, and any clinical society censureship action. The NPDB affects nurses in two major ways:

1. Malpractice payments made on behalf of a nurse are reported to the NPDB and copied to the state board of nursing.
2. An inquiry to the NPDB is required when nurses apply for hospital privileges and is required every two years for renewal of hospital privileges.

In 1998 the NPDB annual report stated that over the history of the database, registered nurses have been responsible for only 2,520 malpractice payments. This constitutes only 1.6 percent of all malpractice payments made. Approximately two-thirds of those payments were for nonspecialized registered nurses. The remaining one-third of the claims were for advanced practice nurses. This includes nurse anesthetists, who were responsible for 24.3 percent of all nurse payments and nurse-midwives, who were responsible for 4.1 percent of all nurse payments. The NPDB reported that problems with the monitoring of patients and implementation of nursing care have been responsible for the majority of payments for nonspecialized nurses, followed by obstetrical and surgical problems. In 1998, the median malpractice payment for all types of nurses was $83,300 and the mean was $290,053 (National Practitioner Data Bank, 1999).

Promote Positive Interpersonal Relationships

Even in the face of untoward outcomes from a health care provider, it is usually only the disgruntled patient that sues. Therefore, the best strategy for the professional nurse is prevention of legal actions through positive interpersonal relationships.

Prevention includes giving personalized, concerned care; including the patient and the family in planning and implementing care; and promoting positive, open interpersonal relationships that value the psychosocial aspects of care. The professional nurse who uses self as a therapeutic agent and acknowledges the holism of the patient is likely to prevent most legal problems. Box 20–3 summarizes the important steps nurses can take to avoid legal problems in professional practice.

BOX 20-3

Guidelines for Preventing Legal Problems in Nursing Practice

- Practice in a safe setting.
- Communicate with other health professionals.
- Delegate wisely.
- Meet the standard of care.
- Carry professional liability insurance.
- Promote positive interpersonal relationships.

Summary of Key Points

- Nurses must recognize that the law is a system of rules that governs conduct and attaches consequences to certain behavior.
- Consequences include civil or criminal action or both.
- Nursing practice is limited by the definition of practice in the state nurse practice act and the qualifications for licensure to practice nursing in that state.
- The law is dynamic and must be responsive to society's needs.
- Advances in technology have increased the possibility for legal actions involving nurses.
- Technological advances have increased concern about informed consent and patients' right to direct the care they choose to receive or refuse.
- Many nurses possess inadequate knowledge of legal issues that affect nursing practice every day. These issues deserve increased attention by nurses in all areas of practice.

Critical Thinking Questions

1. Using your state's nurse practice act, describe the scope of practice of the registered nurse. When was the last time the law was modified? Does it accurately reflect current nursing practice?
2. Read the section of the nurse practice act relating to advanced practice. What parameters, if any, do nurses have in the areas of practice and prescription writing in your state?
3. Go to the college library and browse through back issues of the *Journal of Nursing Law*. What kinds of legal issues do you find involving nurses?
4. Explain the Patient Self-Determination Act to your family and friends. What questions do they have about an advance directive? Find out what the laws regarding advance directives are in your state.
5. When interviewing for a position, what questions should you ask to determine whether it is a legally safe setting in which to practice?

Web Resources

American Academy of Nurse Practitioners, http://www.aanp.org

American Bar Association Health Law Site, http://www.abanet.org/health

Findlaw Legal Search Engine, http://www.findlaw.com

Health Care Financing Administration, http://www.hcfa.gov

National Council of State Boards of Nursing, http://www.ncsbn.org

National Practitioner Data Bank, http://www.hrsa.dhhs.gov/bhpr/dqa

Patient Self-Determination Act, http://www.springnet.com/ce/m710a.htm

References

Aiken, T. (1994). *Legal, ethical and political issues in nursing.* Philadelphia: F. A. Davis.

American Academy of Nurse Practitioners (1999). *Nurse practitioner prescriptive authority.* Washington, D. C.: American Academy of Nurse Practitioners. Available from http://www.aanp.org/prescrip.htm

American Association of Nurse Attorneys. (1984). *Demonstrating financial responsibility for nursing practice.* Baltimore, Md.: American Association of Nurse Attorneys.

American Nurses Association (1985). *Code for nurses.* Kansas City, Mo.: American Nurses Association.

American Nurses Association (1990). *Suggested state legislation: Nurse practice act, nursing disciplinary diversion act, prescriptive authority act.* Kansas City, Mo.: American Nurses Association.

American Nurses Association (1991). *Pacesetter,* 18(2), Kansas City, Mo.: ANA Council of Psychiatric/Mental Health Nursing.

American Nurses Association (1992). *Position statement on registered nurse utilization of unlicensed assistive personnel.* Washington, D. C.: American Nurses Publishing.

American Nurses Association (1995a). *Analysis and comparison of advanced practice recognition with medical reimbursement and insurance reimbursement.* Washington, D. C.: American Nurses Publishing.

American Nurses Association (1995b). *Capital update.* (vols. 13 and 14). Washington, D. C.: American Nurses Publishing.

American Nurses Association (1996a). *Model practice act.* Washington, D. C.: American Nurses Publishing.

American Nurses Association (1996b). *Registered professional nurses and unlicensed assistive personnel* (2nd ed.). Washington, D. C.: American Nurses Publishing.

American Nurses Association (1998). *Standards of clinical nursing practice* (2nd ed.). Washington, D. C.: American Nurses Association.

Health Care Financing Administration (1999). *Medicaid managed care penetration rates by state.* Baltimore, Md.: Health Care Financing Administration.

Hemelt, M., and Mackert, M. E. (1982). *Dynamics of law in nursing and health care.* Reston, Va.: Reston Publishing.

National Council of State Boards of Nursing (1999a). Profiles of member boards—1998. Chicago: National Council of State Boards of Nursing.

National Council of State Boards of Nursing (1999b). Mutual recognition: Frequently asked questions. Chicago: National Council of State Boards of Nursing. Available from http://www.ncsbn.org/files/mutual/mrfaq.asp

National Practitioner Data Bank (1999). *1998 annual report*. Washington, D. C.: Author.

Pew Health Professions Commission. (1995). *Critical challenges: Revitalizing the health professions for the twenty first century*. San Francisco: Pew Health Trust.

Politis, E. (1983). Nurses' legal dilemma: When hospital staffing compromises professional standards. *University of San Francisco Law Review, 3*, 109–126.

Sweeney, S. (1991). Medical negligence: Proving nursing negligence. *Trial, 91*(5), 34–40.

Trossman, S. (1999). ANA, MNA support Dana-Farber nurses facing disciplinary action. *The American Nurse, 31*(2).

Nurses and Political Action

*Virginia Trotter Betts**
Judith K. Leavitt

21

Key Terms

Adjudicate
Balance of Power
Electoral Process
Executive Branch
General Election
Judicial Branch
Knowledge-Based Power
Latent Power
Legislative Branch
Nurse Activist
Nurse Citizen
Nurse Politician
Pay Equity
Policy
Policy Outcomes
Political Action Committees
  (PACs)

Politics
Position Power
Power Grabbing
Power Sharing

Powers of Appointment
Primary Election
Referendum
Separation of powers

Learning Outcomes

After studying this chapter, students will be able to:

- Differentiate between politics and policy.
- Explain the concept of personalizing the political process.
- Cite examples of sources of both personal and professional power.
- Describe how nurses can become involved in politics and policy development at the levels of citizen, activist, and politician.
- Explain how organized nursing is involved in political activities designed to strengthen professional nursing and influence health care policy.

H ave you ever known a nurse member of Congress? Or a nurse mayor? Did you know that a nurse was responsible for developing the federal system for health care financing? Nurses have served as heads of the Social Security Administration and Planned Parenthood of America and as chief of staff for the majority leader in the U. S. Senate. Nurses have held major leadership roles in government, professional and community organizations, and the workplace. This chapter discusses the political process, describes how nurses can become politically active, and explains some of the ways in which nurse leaders have achieved positions of power and influence.

Politics: What It Is and What It Is not

Politics is more than what is happening in Washington, D. C. It is part of our daily lives, both personal and professional. Ultimately, politics refers to the

* The author wishes to acknowledge the contributions of Cheryl Peterson and Sara E. Hart to the preparation of this chapter.

processes that influence the outcome of decisions among people. People often speak of politics with negative overtones. In fact, politics is neither good nor bad. It is the *outcome* of the political process that may be judged as positive or negative.

Politics is defined as the allocation of scarce resources. *Allocation* implies that decisions are made about how to use these scarce resources. Who distributes the resources, the amount of resources allocated, and who receives the allocated resources are all based on the application of politics to gain power.

Scarce connotes limits. There are never enough resources for everyone who wants or needs them. Resources usually indicate money. *Resources*, however, can also be people, time, status, power, and programs—any number of precious assets that are limited.

Policy is defined as the principles and values that govern actions directed toward given ends; policy statements set forth a plan, direction, or goal for action. Policies may be laws, regulations, or guidelines that govern behavior in government, workplaces, schools, organizations, and communities. Although different from politics, policy is *shaped* by politics (Mason and Leavitt, 1998).

Politics (i.e., influencing the allocation of scarce resources) affects the development and implementation of policy. During the 1995–1996 balanced budget debate, congressional Republicans argued that the federal budget must be balanced within seven years (by the year 2002) through significant policy changes to slow the growth of domestic programs such as Medicare and Medicaid. The Clinton administration and many Democrats agreed that although there was a need for a balanced budget, the Republican-proposed Medicare and Medicaid changes would overburden the constituencies that these programs serve. This debate was not only about the allocation of scarce federal revenue but was also an attempt to change the role of the federal government in health and human service programs. The passage of the Balanced Budget Act of 1997 has had, and will continue to have, major repercussions throughout the health care delivery system.

Policy has significant impact on the practice of nursing. The ability of the individual nurse to provide care is affected by innumerable public policy decisions. As discussed in Chapter 20, state licensure of a registered nurse (RN) derives from legislation that defines the scope of nursing practice. The defined scope determines what a nurse legally can and cannot do. For example, giving intravenous medication and performing physical assessments are now well accepted as falling within the scope of nursing practice. Twenty-five years ago, these activities were within the scope of the medical practice act rather than the nursing practice act, but as a result of nursing education and nursing's political influence on public policy, these changes were realized.

Regulations developed to implement legislation also affect practicing nurses and their work environments. For example, the protocols for administering and documenting the administration of narcotic drugs are promulgated by a regulatory agency of the federal government. The rules that define nurses' authority to order or administer narcotics depend on how regulations are written. If nurses do not actively participate in developing regulations, policy outcomes are likely to restrict rather than enhance nursing authority for regulated activities.

Broader issues affecting the nursing profession are also political in nature. Issues of **pay equity,** or equal pay for work of comparable value, are of concern to nurses because nurses have historically been underpaid for services. One of the first cases demonstrating the inequality of nursing salaries involved public health nurses in Colorado. They brought a case against the city of Denver, stating that they were paid considerably less than city tree trimmers and garbage collectors. The nurses demanded just compensation for their work by demonstrating that nursing requires more complex knowledge and is of greater value to society than tree trimming.

As a result of this suit, recognition of nursing's low pay was brought to public attention in such a way that public support was mobilized for increasing nursing salaries. This was an example of political action by nurses that resulted in both **policy outcomes** (regulations that expanded comparable pay issues to other jobs) and professional outcomes (salary increases for the individual nurse).

"The Personal Is Political"

Women involved in the feminist movement in the 1960s coined the phrase "The personal is political." The statement recognized that each individual—woman or man—could use personal experience to understand and become involved in broader social and political issues. It enabled individuals who did not consider themselves political to gain insight into what needed to be changed in society and how they could help bring about the change. It gave each individual power and resulted in people becoming involved in the political process—usually for the first time.

This premise of personalizing the political process has become a fundamental activity for organized nursing. Nurses at the grassroots level become involved in advocating for legislation and supporting candidates for elective office because they understand the relationship between public policy and their professional and personal lives. The American Nurses Association (ANA) is actively involved in federal legislation, regulation, and electoral politics. The ANA and many of the state nurses associations have government relations experts on their staffs, as do many other nursing and health organizations, such as the American Association of Colleges of Nursing, the American Hospital Association, and numerous specialty nursing organizations. They engage in lobbying to advocate for the professional concerns of their members (Fig. 21–1). Contemporary nursing leaders recognize that "being political," both through professional associations and as individuals, is a professional responsibility essential to the practice and promotion of the nursing profession.

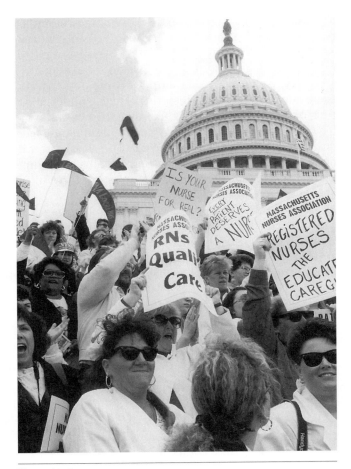

Figure 21–1
Nurses gathered on the grounds of the Capitol building in Washington,
D. C. for the historic Nurses' March on Washington—March 25, 1995. Issuing
a wake-up call to consumers and lawmakers, the 25,000 nurses rallied and
marched through Washington in a display of nursing unity (Photo courtesy
of the American Nurses Association).

Politics and Power

Politics connotes power. Without power, there cannot be influence. To be effective in influencing the outcome of decisions, an individual must ask, "Who has the power?" "How is it used?" "How can it be mobilized?"

There are numerous kinds of power. There is **position power,** such as that inherent in being a dean, vice-president for nursing, or chief executive of a company. There is **knowledge-based power,** such as the way information can be used by an expert to affect an outcome. There is power in numbers; a group is almost always more influential than an individual. There is power related to wealth. Wealth itself is a resource and provides access to other significant resources. There has always been power accorded to whomever belongs to the dominant race, gender, or class in a community or nation.

Latent power is untapped and underused. As the largest group of health providers, nurses have had latent power. Although there are more than 2.5 million nurses in the United States, nurses have only recently recognized the potential power that such numbers suggest. One in 44 women voters is a nurse. How powerful nursing's voice could be if that power were used wisely in the voting booth. The power of nursing knowledge has also been underused. No other group of health care providers spends as much time as nurses in direct patient contact. Nurses know what patients need and can use this knowledge to develop policies for meeting those needs both in the clinical setting and in the community. More nurses are using their expertise to participate in the development of health policy, share knowledge with legislators, and serve in community organizations to develop health services.

Power is neither good nor bad; how it is used gives it value. If, for example, nurses use the power of persuasion to motivate patients to take prescribed medication, they are using the power of position and knowledge positively.

Power is not given; it must be taken. The taking of power converts latent power into action. Nurses are beginning to recognize that to have power they must want it, and they must use it. Use of power is a hallmark of political activity.

There are differences in the way women and men have traditionally used power. The traditional male model of power has been described as **power grabbing.** It involves hoarding power and control, taking it from others, or wielding it over others. Women more often use **power sharing,** which is a process of equalizing resources, knowledge, or control. It is important to recognize that these two ways of using power are neither good nor bad. The most effective power brokers are those who can use both methods and know which is most effective in a given situation.

The *Woodhull Study on Nursing and the Media* (1997) analyzed more than 2,000 health-related articles from 16 major news publications. Recognizing that communication media are the most effective ways in which to send a message to a large audience, this study recommended that the nursing profession be proactive in promoting and establishing ongoing dialogue with representatives of these media. Effective utilization of media is a powerful political tool for influencing both the public and those who hold elective offices (Sigma Theta Tau, 1997).

Different media provide different ways to influence opinions. For example, talk radio has proved to be very influential. Talk radio hosts advocate certain opinions, often with little factual information. By controlling who gets to talk, they can control the kind of information and the level of feeling expressed and eliminate opposing viewpoints. Prior to the 1994 elections, when the Republican Party took control of both houses of Congress, the majority of talk radio supported the Republican agenda. It is believed that their collective messages influenced the outcomes of the elections.

Television can be a forceful medium for visual influence, particularly advertisements. In 1994, the demise of President Clinton's national health care reform efforts was directly affected by television ads sponsored by the health insurance industry. Despite initial support for national health care reform by Fortune 500 companies, health professional organizations, and major industries, the "Harry and Louise" advertisements were forceful enough to create a climate of fear and distrust about legislating health care. The power of those ads was partially credited with the defeat of federal health care legislation.

The print media are effective in disclosing detailed information supportive of a legislative issue. During the 1993–1994 health care reform debate, there were more than 300 articles in newspapers across the United States focusing on nurses, especially nurses in advanced practice. Most were the result of news releases from the ANA's department of communications and other nursing organizations. Nursing's goal was to educate the public about the important role of nurses in delivering health care as well as to gain support for legislation that would enable these nurses to be directly reimbursed. The news articles were successful on both counts.

In 1995, during the flurry of hospital mergers and restructuring in the health care industry, nursing organizations used paid advertisements on television and in selected newspapers to counter hospital industry attempts to eliminate nursing positions. For example, the ANA'S "Every Patient Deserves a Nurse" campaign raised public awareness of the need for adequate numbers of registered nurses for patient care. The strategy was to support legislative and regulatory measures that would ensure patient safety and job security for registered nurses.

The power of the media affects both legislators and the public. It is a tool that nurses will use even more widely in the future.

A Lesson in Civics Comes Alive

No American student completes secondary school without one or more courses in civics or American government. Many students find these courses dull and irrelevant to their lives. To many adults, however, American government is vibrant and fascinating. To affect governmental processes successfully, it is important that nursing and other health professions clearly understand how government works.

Three Branches of Government

The framers of the U. S. Constitution had a major objective—the **separation of powers**—to prevent the aggregation of power in any one person or branch of government. Thus, they set out a government with three branches—legislative, executive, and judicial—and a mechanism of checks and balances for each. As intended by the founding fathers, U. S. history reveals a waxing and waning of the powers of each branch, depending on the personalities of incumbents, contemporary social problems, and world events.

Under the Constitution, each branch of the federal government has separate and distinct functions and powers. The function of the **legislative branch,** which includes the House of Representatives and the Senate, is to deliberate and enact laws. Examples of legislative powers include setting and collecting taxes, overseeing commerce, declaring war, defining criminal offenses, coining money, and amending the Constitution. The legislative branch, particularly the House of Representatives, is assumed to be the government's closest link to the people and more susceptible to change through social pressure.

The chief function of the **executive branch** of government is to administer the laws of the land. At the federal level, power is vested with the president, who has a wide variety of governmental departments and employees (the bureaucracy) to carry out executive functions. The president has extensive **powers of appointment** (judges, ambassadors, agency heads) and is commander-in-chief of the armed forces. The president recommends legislation, gives the State of the Union report, and approves or vetoes the legislation of Congress, contributing to the balance of power.

The role of the **judicial branch** is to **adjudicate,** or decide, "cases or controversies" of particular matters. The judicial branch is divided into the federal and state court systems. The greatest power of the courts is to provide judicial review over governmental activities to uphold the privileges of the Constitution. The Supreme Court is the ultimate legal authority of the land and reviews decisions from lower courts.

The **balance of power** among the three branches of government is illustrated in Figure 21–2. Notice that all three branches are involved in the legislative process.

Three Levels of Government

Government in the United States is organized at federal, state, and local levels. The Constitution established the relative powers of federal and state governments and the rights of the individual. The Constitution identified specific powers of the federal government as matters of national interest needing uniform policies and reserved all other powers for the states. States, in turn, have developed their own constitutions and delineated power relationships with local communities and between branches of state government.

Exclusive powers of the federal government include declaring war, making treaties, administering postal services, and developing relationships with foreign powers. State and local governments maintain internal order, regulate domestic relationships, and protect the people. Currently, both the federal and the state governments can tax and spend and promote health. In times of shrinking resources, programs that are considered to be costly, such as health services, may be shifted to state control, calling into question the federal government's role in ensuring uniform access to health services throughout the United States.

All levels of government are expected to maintain their activities within the parameters of the Constitution. The Bill of Rights serves to promote and protect the rights of the individual from governmental intrusion.

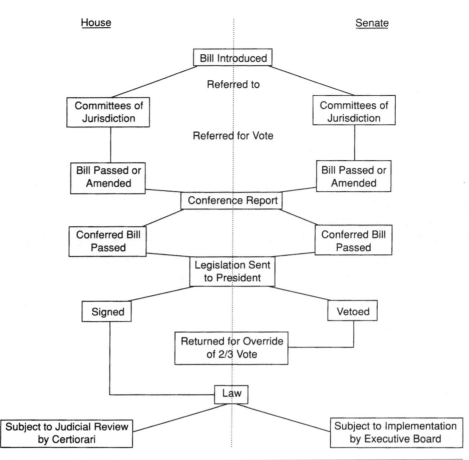

Figure 21–2
Legislation and the balance of power.

Electoral Process

The process of electing public officials to office is known as the **electoral process.** Governmental elections for the most part focus on selecting local, state, and federal legislators and executive branch leaders such as the president, governor, and mayor. Federal judges are appointed, although in some states judges are elected by the people.

In recent elections the American public appeared to be skeptical of politicians, the traditional political parties, and the entire electoral process. This was clearly shown in 1992 when Ross Perot of the United We Stand America Party (subsequently The Reform Party) received 19 percent of the votes cast for president. This was the highest percentage received by an independent or third-party candidate since the early 1900s (Congressional Quarterly, 1993). Many voters viewed the strong third-party showing as a message to long-term politicians and the traditional parties that they were not in touch with voters outside Washington, D. C.

Voter discontent was again evident in the 1994 and 1996 election cycles when only 38 percent and 36 percent, respectively, of eligible people voted. In 1994, congressional Democrats lost majority control of both the House of Representatives and the Senate. Democrats in the House of Representatives lost 52 seats, giving Republicans control of the House for the first time since 1954 (Healy, 1994). However, in 1998 the Democrats won back five seats in the House and had no gains or losses in the Senate. The 1998 elections established a narrow margin in the House of Representatives with 223 Republican seats and 211 Democratic seats (Neal and Morin, 1998). This near balance between the parties in the House created a sluggish legislative session in 1999. Clearly, voters were trying to send a message to Congress, but the exact meaning of that message was difficult to interpret.

During the 1994 election, members of third parties, such as United We Stand America, not only affected the outcome of the elections but also shaped the issues that were discussed as part of a "change agenda." Heretofore the process of getting elected to office has occurred primarily through the two major parties—the Democratic and Republican parties. Third parties have become active in different regions at different times. Some of the more familiar third parties are the Reform Party (formerly United We Stand America), Right to Life, Conservative, Green, Socialist, Communist, and Rainbow Coalition parties. Other than Ross Perot's United We Stand America Party, none of the other third-party organizations has yet played a major role in national elections. At the state level, however a third-party organization, the Reform Party, was successful. Their candidate, former professional wrestler Jesse Ventura, won a gubernatorial campaign in Minnesota in 1998 with a voter turnout of 61 percent.

In most states, citizens declare party affiliation when registering to vote. There are three major types of elections: primary and general elections and referendums.

Primary elections are those in which a party is choosing among several party-affiliated candidates for a particular office. The outcome of primary elections is the selection of a party's candidate for a particular office. In most states, voters may vote only in the primary of the party in which they are registered.

In **general elections,** all registered voters may vote. They need not vote a "straight party ticket"; that is, the voter can choose a candidate from any party on the ballot. Unless there is a tie or a challenge to the general election, the outcome is the selection of a governmental official such as a governor, senator, or president. Length of service as an elected official depends on the office. For example, U. S. senators serve six-year terms, and members of the House of Representatives serve two-year terms.

A referendum occurs when registered voters are asked to express directly their preferences on a policy issue. Usually these issues are referred to the public either by a legislative body or by civic activists who have gathered enough signatures to require a vote. For example, a county commission may seek a referendum on raising property taxes to support school reform. Activist groups may seek a state referendum on gay rights, assisted suicide, or other controversial issues.

Working on a campaign, raising money for a candidate, or running for office requires strict adherence to election laws. Rules vary from locality to locality and state to federal elections. Information about election regulations is available through local boards of election and from the National Election Commission.

Health Care Legislation and Regulation

Many issues facing nursing professionals can best be addressed through public policy, which requires that nurses influence government. The key questions for nurses to ask when seeking governmental intervention to improve nursing practice and health care are "Where can we play?" and "Where can we win?" The options to consider are the judicial, administrative, or legislative arenas.

There are local, state, and federal courts, all of which require standing (a *material* interest in the outcome of a case) to seek a judicial remedy. There are mayors, governors, presidents and their staffs and department heads who make key decisions about how to implement (or not implement) health policy. Most often, nurses have sought legislative remedies for changes in health care policy. Historically, nurses have best learned to be effective with legislative branch relationships. The nursing profession has now broadened its focus to use the other two branches more effectively.

There have been three major eras in health policy development in the United States. As you learned in Chapter 16, the era extending from post–world War II through the 1960s served to increase health services dramatically and expand health delivery capacity. The 1970s and 1980s focused on enhanced research, technology development, and concerns about escalating costs in acute care. During the 1990s, several different issues were predominant, including comprehensive health care reform addressing access, cost, and quality of health care. When attempts at comprehensive reform were unsuccessful, a dramatic restructuring of the health care payment and delivery systems to decrease aggregate health care costs followed.

Unfortunately, the nursing profession was not well organized politically during the time of expanding health care capacity and access. Despite being the only health provider group in favor of the Medicare/Medicaid programs of the 1960s, nurses were not included as reimbursable providers. Times have changed, however. Nurses have increased their political savvy. Through the well-orchestrated efforts of the ANA, other professional organizations, state nurses associations, and **political action committees** (PACs), nurses are now participating much more effectively in both governmental and electoral politics. Nursing PACs raise and distribute money to candidates who support the organization's stand on certain issues, and nurses' endorsements of candidates have become a valued political asset for many local, state, and federal candidates.

Influencing Public Policy

Nurses can make a difference in health policy outcomes. Through the political process, nurses influence policy by identifying health problems as policy problems, by formulating policy through drafting legislation with legislators and providing formal testimony, by lobbying governmental officials in the executive and legislative branches to make certain health policies a priority for action, and by filing suit as a party or as a friend of the court to implement health policy strategies on behalf of consumers.

Capitol Update, a newsletter published by the ANA, reports on the progress of nursing's influence with the president, members of Congress and their staffs, and the regulatory agencies that set policy for health programs. Such activity reflects the work of both ANA members and staff. The ANA's political activity in Washington, D. C., is mirrored throughout the United States by other nursing organizations and by state nurses associations conducting similar work with their state governments.

Two of nursing's major political activist programs are the Senator Coordinator and Congressional District Coordinator (SC-CDC) Networks and Nurses Strategic Action Teams (NSTAT). The SC-CDC Networks were developed by the ANA in 1985 and have been replicated on the state level by many state nurses associations. The purpose of the 535 member SC-CDC Network is to ensure that each member of Congress has a well-briefed professional nurse as an ongoing contact on matters of health and workplace legislation. This network seeks to enhance communication between nurses and members of Congress to educate legislators on matters of concern to the nursing profession. This one-on-one network has been a valuable instrument in helping the ANA achieve its legislative agenda.

During the health care reform debate of 1993–1994, grassroots efforts to influence Congress were highly visible. The ANA invested significant resources to develop NSTAT. In 1996, NSTAT consisted of approximately 40,000 state nurses association members who voluntarily mobilized using telephones, faxes, and mail to advocate for specific issues vital to nursing. NSTAT is effective because of the thousands of well-timed, well-targeted messages sent to members of Congress.

Organized activity in identifying, financially supporting, and working for candidates who are committed to nursing and "nurse-friendly" issues has dramatically increased in the last decade. Again, this electoral process is an essential function of the professional association. No better example of the interrelationship of nursing, public policy, and political action exists than the 1992 presidential election and its aftermath. In August 1992, the ANA-PAC endorsed the Clinton/Gore ticket at a nationally televised rally in California. Thousands of nurses were present along with patients and their families. The ANA became the first national health care organization to support Clinton's candidacy publicly, and nurses throughout the United States worked visibly and diligently during the campaign.

That early and visible political support meant that nursing enjoyed unprecedented access to the White House during the Clinton Gore administration. Nurses were involved significantly in the development of the president's Health Security Act of 1993, and nurses were included as qualified providers in that historic federal proposal. Despite the failure of the 103rd Congress to pass comprehensive health reform legislation in 1994, nursing achieved visibility, influence, and inclusion as a force in national health policy. As nursing united through the development of *Nursing's Agenda for Health Care Reform,* the latent power of nursing became evident to the public, to policymakers, and to nurses themselves.

Nurses working at the state level are also making their presence felt. In 1994, the Maine State Nurses Association endorsed Jill Goldthwait, a registered nurse running as an Independent for election to the Maine State Assembly. After a successful race, state senator Goldthwait entered the Maine Assembly and carried significant influence with Maine's newly elected Independent governor. Senator Goldthwait agreed to be the key sponsor of Maine State Nurses Association legislation to give advanced practice nurses prescriptive authority and to enter into a collaborative practice with physicians.

This landmark legislation passed the state senate and assembly and was signed into law in June 1995. Thus, nursing political action through a state nurses association contributed to the election of a nurse politician, which, in turn, led directly to nursing's public policy ideal—independent practice and reimbursement for advanced practice nurses in Maine.

Individual nurses can make a difference in policy development and elections and by speaking out for nursing and becoming policymakers. Either by election or by appointment, nurses need to be *making* health decisions, not just influencing them. Getting elected or appointed requires visibility, expertise, energy, risk taking, and a belief that policy and politics are critically important in achieving nursing's goals.

Getting Nurses Appointed

Becoming a policymaker involves either being elected or being appointed to office. Appointments are made by the chief executive of a city, county, or state or the nation. They are usually made in response to the expertise and visibility of the individual appointee and to the power and influence of that appointee's membership in an organization that supported the elected official.

For example, after the 1992 elections, the ANA was asked to submit names of nurses for appointment to positions in the executive branch and to influential policymaking boards. The ANA began the Federal Appointments Project and worked with outstanding nurses throughout the United States to assemble a professional/political resume that would make them highly competitive for significant positions. Almost 500 nurses eagerly became part of the project, and many were successful. During the Clinton Gore administration's first term, Dr. Myra Synder served on the Department of Health and Human Services transition team; Dr. Christine Gebbie was appointed as the first national AIDS policy coordinator; Dr. Shirley Chater was appointed as director of the Social Security Administration; and Pat Montoya and Pat Ford-Roegner became regional directors of the Department of Health and Human Services.

The ANA and the nursing community worked closely with the Clinton Gore administration throughout its first term. Again in the 1996 election, ANA-PAC endorsed the Clinton Gore ticket and continued a close working relationship on health care and health care workplace safety. During President Clinton's second term Dr. Beverly Malone, ANA president from 1996 to 2000, and Marta Prado were appointed to the President's Advisory Commission on Consumer Protection and Quality in the Health Care Industry (1998), from which the Patient's Bill of Rights concept was developed (Fig. 21–3); Dr. Mary Wakefield was also appointed to the Advisory Commission as well as the Medicare Payment Advisory Commission; and Catherine Dodd was appointed regional director of the Department of Health and Human Services. In 1998, the role of senior advisor on nursing and policy to the Secretary and Assistant Secretary was created within the Department of Health and Human Services. Virginia Trotter Betts, ANA president from 1992 to 1996, was the first to be ap-

Figure 21–3
American Nurses Association President Beverly Malone, PhD, RN, FAAN, addresses a 1999 Capitol Hill press conference in support of the federal Patient's Bill of Rights. Minority Leader Tom Daschle (D-SD) and Senator Ted Kennedy (D-MA) also spoke in support of the bill. (Photo courtesy of the American Nurses Association).

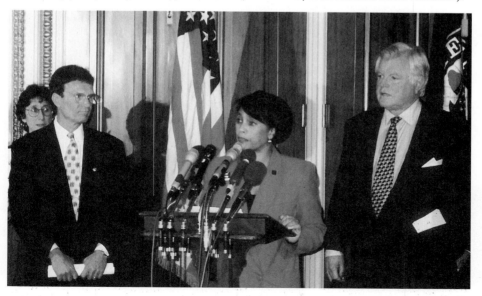

pointed to this key position. Political activism helped secure these and other important federal appointments of nurses.

The same process occurs at the state level. Appointment to many boards, commissions, and key government positions are made by the state executive, usually the governor. Thus, gubernatorial elections are of critical importance to state nurses associations. Qualified nurses who have supported the election of the governor and are known to their state nurses association are encouraged to seek appointments to regulatory bodies such as state boards of nursing. As previously discussed, state boards of nursing, through rules and regulations, make definitive health policy and are highly important to future nursing issues.

Working in a gubernatorial campaign, through the state nurses association or through the candidate's party, can be helpful in securing board of nursing appointments. Boards of health, health and human services commissions, and others all use similar processes of appointment and could benefit from nursing expertise.

Getting Involved

Although nurses are more active at all levels of the political process than ever before, there is still room for improvement. As can be seen in the accompanying Research Note, nurses tend to expect more in the way of political participation from fellow nurses than they themselves actually do. Three levels of political involvement in which nurses can participate are nurse citizens, nurse activists, and nurse politicians. Each level is discussed briefly.

Nurse Citizens

A **nurse citizen** brings the perspective of health care to the voting booth, to public forums that advocate for health and human services, and to involvement in community activities. For example, budget cuts to a school district might involve elimination of school nurses. At a school board meeting, nurses can effectively speak about the vital services that school nurses provide children and the cost-effectiveness of maintaining the position.

Nurses tend to vote for candidates who advocate for improved health care. Here are some examples of how the nurse citizen can be politically active:

- Register to vote.
- Vote in every election.
- Keep informed about health care issues.
- Speak out when services or working conditions are inadequate.
- Participate in public forums.
- Know your local, state, and federal elected officials.
- Join politically active nursing organizations.
- Participate in community organizations that need health experts.
- Join a political party.

RESEARCH NOTE

A New York nurse, Margaret Leonard, wondered about the relationship of area of practice, educational level, and membership in professional organizations to political participation and political expectations of registered nurses (RNs). She hypothesized that nurse educators would have significantly higher levels of political participation and political expectation than clinical nurses, that nurses with master's or doctoral degrees would have higher levels of political participation and political expectation than nurses with baccalaureate or associate degrees or diplomas, and that nurses who were members of the New York State Nurses Association or the Nurses' Association of the Counties of Long Island would have significantly higher levels of political participation and political expectation than nurses who were not members of these professional organizations.

The data collection tool used in this study was the Political Expectations and Participation Questionnaire (PEPQ), which had been previously developed, validated, and established as reliable. It identifies nine politically active roles: voter, campaigner, player, monitor, networker, spokesperson, negotiator, leader, and lobbyist.

Using the PEPQ, Leonard surveyed 108 registered nurses who were attending a nursing association mini-convention. Subjects were 106 women and 2 men ranging in age from 27 to 70 years who had been registered nurses for 2 to 45 years. Most (77 percent) were members of a professional organization.

Leonard found that although there were no significant differences in political expectations between educators and clinical nurses, nurse educators scored significantly higher in political participation than clinical nurses. Levels of political participation were significantly higher for master's or doctorally prepared nurses in all roles except that of spokesperson. Advanced degree nurses had significantly higher levels of political expectations in two areas—voter and

monitor. In terms of organizational membership, subjects who were members of professional organizations had significantly higher levels of participation in campaigner, player, and leader roles. Overall findings confirmed that registered nurses have significantly higher levels of political expectations than levels of participation in all nine politically active roles.

As a result of this study, Leonard recommended that formal coursework in politics be added to nursing curricula to increase the political participation of all nurses and thereby increase nursing's political power. The desired result of increased political participation by nurses is improvement in the health care system to include universal access and reimbursement for services provided by registered nurses.

Adapted with permission of Leonard, M. (1994). Levels of political participation and political expectations among nurses in New York State. *Journal of the New York State Nurses Association*, 25(1), 16–20

Once nurses make a decision to become involved politically, they need to learn how to get started. One of the best ways is to form a relationship with one or more policymakers. Box 21–1 contains several pointers for influencing policymakers.

Nurse Activists

The **nurse activist** takes a more active role than the nurse citizen and often does so because an issue arises that directly affects the nurse's professional life or health care values Fig. 21–4). The need to respond moves the nurse to a higher level of participation. For example, a nurse in private practice who has difficulty getting private insurance companies or health maintenance organizations to honor patients' claims for reimbursement of nursing services may become active in lobbying state legislators for changes in insurance regulations.

BOX 21-1
Communication is the Key to Influence

Cultivate a relationship with policymakers from your home district or state. Communicate by visits, telephone, and letters. Letters need these elements:

- Use personal stationery.
- State who you are (a nursing student or registered nurse and a voter in a specific district).
- Identify the issue by a file number, if possible.
- Be clear on where you stand and why.
- Be positive when possible.
- Be concise.
- Ask for a commitment. State precisely what action you want the policy-maker to take.
- Give your return address and phone number to urge dialogue.
- Be persistent. Follow up with calls or letters.
- If you plan to visit your policymaker on a specific issue, be sure to make your appointment in advance in writing and indicate what issue you are interested in discussing.
- Be quick to thank and praise when policymakers do something you like.

Nurse activists can make changes by:

- Joining politically active nursing organizations.
- Contacting a public official through letters, telegrams, or phone calls.
- Registering people to vote.
- Contributing money to a political campaign.
- Working in a campaign.
- Lobbying decision makers by providing pertinent statistical and anecdotal information.
- Forming or joining coalitions that support an issue of concern.
- Writing letters to the editor of local papers.
- Inviting legislators to visit the workplace.
- Holding a media event to publicize an issue.
- Providing or giving testimony.

Box 21–2 includes some pointers on how to make a difference in health policy development.

Nurse Politicians

Once a nurse realizes and experiences the empowerment that can come from political activism, he or she may choose to run for office. No longer satisfied to help others get elected, the **nurse politician** desires to develop the legislation, not just influence it.

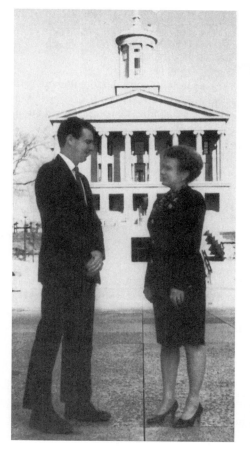

Figure 21–4
The nurse activist has a high level of involvement in selected political issues. (Courtesy of Tennessee Nurses Association. Photograph by Chip Powell).

In 1992, Congresswoman Eddie Bernice Johnson (D-TX) was the first nurse elected to the U. S. House of Representatives. She was reelected in 1994, 1996, and 1998. In 1998, Congresswoman Lois Capps (D-CA) became the third nurse to be elected to the House of Representatives. Congresswoman Capps was a long-time leader in health care and education reforms in her home state. After her election to Congress, she drew on her extensive health care background in her position as cochair of the House Democratic Task Force on Medicare Reform. As a member of Congress, she represented nursing in the Medicare reform debate and advocated for an effective federal Patient's Bill of Rights. In 1998, there were nearly 100 nurse legislators in state government, numerous nurses as local mayors and city council members, and hundreds of nurses appointed to governmental regulatory agencies.

Nurse politicians use their knowledge about people, their expertise about health, their ability to communicate effectively, and their superb organizational skills in running for office. Because the public places a high value on nurses, nurse politicians are trusted. If nurses know how to run a campaign and can raise money, they stand a good chance of being elected.

BOX 21-2

Key Questions for Nurses Who Want to Make a Difference in Health Policy

1. *Know the system.* Is it a federal, state, or local issue? Is it in the hands of the executive, legislative, or judicial branch of government?
2. *Know the issue.* What is wrong? What should happen? Why is it not happening? What is needed: leadership, a plan, pressure, data?
3. *Know the players.* Who is on your side and who is not? Who will make the decision? Who knows whom? Will a coalition be effective? Are you a member of the professional nursing organization?
4. *Know the process.* Is this a vote? Is this an appropriation? Is this a legislative procedure? Is this a committee or subcommittee report?
5. *Know what to do.* Should you write, call, go to lunch, organize a petition, show up at the hearing, give testimony, demonstrate, file a suit?

Once nurses are elected, they can sponsor legislation that reflects their professional experiences. Many of the laws that expand reimbursement for nursing services, funding for services to women and children, occupational safety and health issues, and research on women's health have been sponsored by nurse legislators and supported by nurses working as key legislative staff members.

Political life can be grueling, and the nurse politician must be ready to sacrifice a regular schedule and personal privacy. In addition, adequate financial resources are critical to a successful run for office. Fortunately, more nurses are willing to make this commitment because they believe in their own power and ability to enhance the well-being of the public. Individual nurses and nurse-specific PACs are increasingly willing and able to support nurse candidates financially at all levels of government.

The nurse politician can

- Run for an elected office.
- Seek appointment to a regulatory agency.
- Be appointed to a governing board in the public or private sector.
- Use nursing expertise as a front-line policymaker who can enhance health care and the profession.

We Were All Once Novices

Nurses who have achieved success as leaders started with no knowledge of the political process and no expectation of the greatness they would achieve. Instead, they became involved because some issue, injustice, or abuse of power affected their lives. Instead of complaining or feeling helpless, they responded by taking an active role in bringing about change.

The mark of a leader is the ability to identify a problem, have a goal, and know how to join others in reaching that goal. A leader must know how to ask the right questions, analyze the positive and restraining forces toward meeting the goal, and know how to get and use power. A leader must know how to ask for help and how to give support to those who join the effort. These are the marks of nursing leaders who have been political experts.

A Nurse Who Knew How to Use Political Power

As discussed in Chapter 1, Florence Nightingale, the founder of modern nursing, was the consummate political woman. Her story exemplifies how she learned to use her skills and power to bring about revolutionary change in health care in the nineteenth century. She never anticipated that she would achieve greatness, especially as a nurse—a lifestyle Victorian society considered demeaning to a woman of her social standing.

Nightingale achieved incredible goals through her own intellect and determination and the utilization of the political influence of powerful friends in government. She was a strong-willed person with social and financial power. She had an excellent education and used theoretical knowledge as well as practical experience to learn about care of the sick. She developed and nurtured connections to powerful men (since there were few powerful women at the time other than Queen Victoria). She sought their support and, in turn, supported them when they needed her help.

Nightingale's goals changed as new problems arose because she recognized that being adaptable was a characteristic of leadership. In essence, she used her public support, her connections to people in powerful positions, and her intellectual skills to reach an unparalleled position of leadership. As a result, she was able to gain personal and professional power to move nursing and health care into the modern era. She was the first nurse politician.

Nursing Awaits Your Contribution

You can apply the skills discussed in this chapter. Look to teachers, family, friends, and community leaders whom you admire. What are the qualities they possess that you wish to have? These individuals can offer inspiration, and serve as role models for you to imitate.

You may also choose to form a relationship with a political mentor. A mentor not only serves as a role model but also actively teaches, encourages, and critiques the process of growth and change in the learner. All nurses who have become political leaders have found mentors along the way to guide and support their growth. Your mentor could be a faculty member, such as the adviser to the nursing student organization or honor society, who can teach you leadership skills. Ask for help in running for a class office or student council president. If elected office does not appeal to you, use your political skills to develop a school or community project with other nursing students.

You may have a relative or friend involved in a political campaign who could help you learn about the political process. You might find a problem during a clinical experience that inhibits your ability to provide necessary care or the level of care that you wish to provide. Seek a faculty member or nurse in the clinical facility who can guide you through the process of change.

Watch the communication skills of your role models or mentors. How does your own behavior compare with theirs? What enhances or impedes your progress? Get your friends and peers to join your activity. Seek their help and support. Always thank them and be ready to offer your help and support when they need it.

Summary of Key Points

- Professional organizations and professional nurses have much to offer in formulating policy decisions at federal, state, and local levels and in each branch of government.
- Nursing, once called "the sleeping giant of the health care industry," has awakened.
- Today, organized nursing is involved in politics at many levels in promoting (1) the principles for comprehensive health reform as stated in *Nursing's Agenda for Health Care Reform,* discussed in Chapter 4; (2) reimbursement for professional nurses at federal, state, and local levels and through all reimbursement mechanisms, including managed care; (3) expanding the scope and authority of nursing practice in every jurisdiction. (4) protection of the civil and privacy rights of clients, for example, in the areas of abortion rights, human immunodeficiency virus/acquired immunodeficiency syndrome (HIV/AIDS), and terminal illness; (5) prevention services and primary care services for women, children, and the elderly; and (6) a federally mandated Patient's Bill of Rights.
- Roles and opportunities for women and nurses in the field of policy development and politics are changing, and nursing can benefit from this "window of opportunity."
- Becoming politically active is as easy as signing your name in support of an issue, registering to vote, organizing a project, or speaking out on an issue.
- Political involvement is empowering; one person *can* make a difference.
- The involvement of nurses in the political process benefits nurses, the nursing profession, and the recipients of health care.

Critical Thinking Questions

1. Conduct a class poll. Of those in the class who are eligible to vote, how many are registered? How many voted in the last local, state, or national election? Challenge those not registered to become registered before the end of the current school term.

2. List three types of power. How can nurses use these types of power on behalf of their profession and the health care system?

3. Because nurses have differing personal and political values, it has been a challenge to get them all united behind a single issue or candidate. If you were the president of the American Nurses Association, what techniques would you use to convince the 2.5 million American nurses of to use the power of their numbers, their knowledge, and their commitment?

4. In what types of political issues should nurses take a particular interest? Do you see signs that nurses are actively involved in these issues in your community?

5. Find out whether the members of your state board of nursing are elected or appointed. What is the makeup of the board (how many registered nurses, licensed practical nurses, consumers, and so forth)? Do nurses hold most of the seats on the state board? Are there any other health professionals, such as physicians, on the board of nursing? If so, are there any nurses on the state board of medicine?

Web Resources

American Nurses Association: Links to ANA's legislative branch and to state nursing associations, http://www.nursingworld.org

Department of Health and Human Services: Links to HHS agencies, http://dhhs.gov

Electronic Policy Network: Links to health policy information, http://epn.org/idea/hciclink.html

Health Hippo: Resources for health policy issues, http://hippo.findlaw.com

Thomas: The Library of Congress site for legislative information including links to congressional members' home pages, http://thomas.loc.gov

References

Balanced Budget Act of 1997, Pub. L 105–33 (1997).

Congressional Quarterly (1993). *The 49th annual CQ almanac.* Washington, D. C.: Congressional Quarterly.

Healey, J. (1994). Jubilant GOP strives to keep legislative feet on ground. *Congressional Quarterly Weekly Report.* 52(44), 3210–3215.

Leonard, M. (1994). Levels of political participation and political expectations among nurses in New York State. *Journal of the New York State Nurses Association,* 25(1), 16–20.

Mason, D., and Leavitt, J. (Eds.) (1998). *Policy and politics in nursing and health care* (3rd ed.). Philadelphia: W. B. Saunders.

Neal, T., and Morin, R. (1998). For voters, it's back toward the middle. *Washington Post,* November 5, A33.

President's Advisory Commission on Consumer Protection and Quality in the Health Care Industry. (1998). *Quality first: Better health care for all Americans* (final report to the president of the United States). Washington, D. C.: Government Printing Office.

Sigma Theta Tau International. (1997). *Woodhull study on nursing and the media.* Indianapolis: Center Nursing Press.

Nursing's Future Challenges

Kay K. Chitty

22

Key Terms

Alternative Treatment
Assisted Suicide
Birthrate
Centenarian
Cultural Diversity
Demography
Designer Medicines
Differentiated Practice
Disenfranchised
Distance Learning
Epidemiologist
Euthanasia
Futurist
Genetic Counselor
Heterogeneous
Homogeneous
Human Genome Project
Managed Care

Morbidity Rate
Mortality Rate
Multidrug Resistant Strains
Multiskilled Worker

Nursing Informatics
Shared Governance
Telehealth
Urbanization

Learning Outcomes

After reading this chapter, students will be able to:

- Review societal influences on the nursing profession anticipated during the next decade.
- Recognize the impact that changes in the health care system will have on the practice of nursing.
- Explain trends in nursing education needed to meet society's future nursing needs.
- Describe major issues that the nursing profession must resolve to assure its continuing viability.

As you have seen throughout this textbook, the nursing profession is profoundly affected by changes in society and in the world. As we enter the twenty-first century, it is clear that nursing again faces many challenges, as it has in the past. The challenges nurses face relate to a variety of factors: changes in demographics, unhealthy lifestyles of many Americans, the continued deterioration of the environment, rapid change in the health care system brought about by cost containment initiatives, advances in technology and informatics, cultural diversity within both nursing and the population, blurring of professional boundaries and increasing interdisciplinary collaboration, and issues within nursing itself.

As you learned in Chapter 10, the World Health Organization (WHO) established a goal of health for all by the year 2000. It is now painfully clear that even in the United States, the wealthiest of the industrialized nations, we fell far short of this goal. Millions of Americans still have no health insurance, and many more have less than enough. Infant mortality rates remain unacceptably high. The fitness level of citizens, particularly young people, continues to decline as obesity rates climb at an alarming rate. Smoking in youth continues to increase.

All these negative trends continue even though the United States spends more of its gross domestic product on health than any nation in the world. Complete overhaul of the health care system, believed by many Americans to be essential if these problems are to be addressed, has been stalled in Congress since 1994.

Nursing enjoys high levels of respect and public confidence. It is a profession in heavy demand, and its practitioners enjoy more autonomy than ever. As the health care profession with the highest number of practitioners, nursing has enormous but largely untapped political power that would allow nurses to influence societal changes—rather than simply be influenced by them—if they were unified in their efforts. Yet turf issues continue to divide nurses, weakening their influence at every level.

Everyone is excited about the dawning of the new millennium. The year 2000 represented a milestone for humankind. Most of us remember exactly where we were on New Year's Day 2000 just as older Americans remember where they were when President Kennedy was shot and astronauts first walked on the moon. This chapter explores some of nursing's challenges and opportunities in the new millennium.

Societal Challenges

At least five societal influences are expected to have major impact on the future of the nursing profession: demographic changes, environmental deterioration, unhealthy lifestyles and resulting illnesses, continuing need for cost containment, and regulation of health care. Each of these influences is examined briefly.

Demographic Challenges

Demography is the science that studies vital statistics and social trends. Demographers examine vital statistics such as **birthrates** (births per thousand people), **morbidity rates** (illness), **mortality rates** (deaths), marriages, the ages of various populations, and migration patterns. From this wealth of information, **futurists,** people who predict what will occur, draw conclusions about what these trends mean for the future.

Four demographic trends are particularly important to the future of nursing: the aging population, poverty, the cultural diversity of the population, and urbanization, including increasing levels of violence. Each has implications for nursing.

Aging Population
Estimates vary, but demographers have predicted that the number of people over the age of 75 in the United States by the year 2020 will exceed 21.8 mil-

lion. The number of aging "baby boomers" will create an additional strain on the U. S. health care system. **Centenarians,** people over 100 years of age, represent one of the fastest-growing groups in the United States. The World Future Society predicts that by the end of the twenty-first century, the average life span will approach 100 years (Hendrick, 1995).

Many elderly people are healthy, but the likelihood of illness becomes greater as people age. For example, indications are that by the age of 90, one of two people will develop Alzheimer's disease (Herbert et al., 1995). Clearly, nurses of the future must be prepared to work effectively with the rising numbers of elderly patients.

Ethical issues such as **euthanasia** and **assisted suicide** will become increasingly important as technology enables people to sustain life far beyond the point of useful, meaningful existence. Society's views of assisted suicide and euthanasia are changing, as evidenced by the fact that juries have acquitted Dr. Jack Kevorkian of charges of murder in the assisted deaths of several terminally ill people as well as by the passage of an assisted suicide referendum in Oregon. The future will bring further changes in these attitudes.

Poverty

Even though the United States is considered the world's wealthiest nation, the number of Americans living below the poverty line is increasing. This is particularly true of women, children, and the elderly. The gap between the "haves" and the "have-nots" in the United States is widening, creating discontent and disillusionment.

When basic needs for food, clothing, and shelter are unmet or uncertain, health care becomes a luxury. Children's immunizations, prenatal care for pregnant women, nutritious meals, and a variety of other health-maintaining factors are neglected. Poor people tend to put off seeking care until illness is advanced and thus harder to treat. Conditions that can be prevented often are not because of lack of education, poor sanitation, crowded living conditions, improper shelter, homelessness, and a host of other poverty-related factors.

Poverty will continue to create increasing numbers of **disenfranchised** people, that is, people who have no power in the political system, with limited access to health care. As their numbers grow, both federal and state governments will implement more strategies that limit health care expenditures for these vulnerable populations.

Nursing, as a profession, values providing care to all people, regardless of social and economic factors. The increasing numbers of medically disenfranchised people and pressure to limit health care expenditures will collide to create an intense values conflict for nurses of the future.

Cultural Diversity

Cultural diversity refers to the array of people from different racial, ethnic, religious, social, and geographic backgrounds who make up a particular entity. Some countries, such as Japan, are **homogeneous** in culture. This means the citizens have similar cultural beliefs and practices.

Others, such as the United States, have a **heterogeneous** cultural mix. This means that the cultural beliefs and practices of the citizens are quite different.

Immigration to the United States from Southeast Asia, Central America, Mexico, and the islands of the Caribbean has increased in recent years as a result of civil unrest, wars, and poor economic conditions (Fig. 22–1). People from these countries are the latest wave of newcomers to the United States and join the European-Americans, African-Americans, and others whose ancestors came to this country in the twentieth century. Each group has its own nutritional practices, health beliefs, folk remedies, and conventional wisdom about health and sickness.

Nurses need to take cultural beliefs, values, and practices into consideration when planning and implementing nursing care for individuals of diverse cultural backgrounds. Culturally competent care will be more important in the future than ever before. Speaking a second language, particularly Spanish, will be an important skill that will increase nurses' marketability.

The nursing profession itself will become increasingly diverse as its membership reflects a heterogeneous society. This will create the need for nurses to understand, respect, and value the contributions of co-workers of all cultural backgrounds.

Figure 22–1

Immigration to the United States from Southeast Asia, Central America, Mexico, and islands of the Caribbean is expected to continue in the next decade, contributing to sweeping demographic changes (Courtesy of *Tennessee Nurse*, photo by Thomas Sconyers).

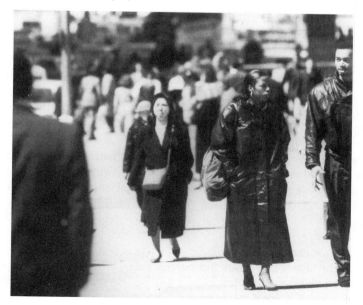

Urbanization

Urbanization, that is, people moving from rural, farming areas to cities, has increased since the time of the industrial revolution. That trend continues today and is expected to go on well into the new century.

As cities grow, suburbs flourish, and most people who can afford to do so move away from the business centers of cities. Decaying inner cities with large populations of poor people create major social problems such as homelessness, drugs, gangs, single-parent households, mental illness, violence, and crime. Despite the increase in public-private partnerships designed to revitalize inner cities and programs formulated to deal effectively with urban issues, social problems continue to grow and spill over into the suburbs and rural areas, creating further social changes. Nurses of the future will be increasingly confronted with health problems resulting from these social phenomena.

Violence is of particular concern to members of the nursing profession. Violence is present in our homes, workplaces, schools, and communities, causing untold chaos and loss. Violence is becoming a major public health problem in the United States and elsewhere, and we see the results in offices, clinics, and trauma units. Because the nursing profession cannot turn a blind eye to this problem, we will see nurses as individuals and as a professional group increasingly take action against the rising tide of violence to protect basic societal principles.

Environmental Challenges

Every newspaper, news magazine, and television news program brings disturbing reports of the deterioration of our environment. Major environmental tragedies, such as a nuclear power plant incident in Japan and floodwaters spreading effluent from hundreds of pig farms in eastern North Carolina, overshadow the less dramatic but insidious gradual decline in the quality of the world's air, water, and plant and animal life.

Acute and chronic respiratory diseases are increasing, as are debilitating allergic reactions to chemicals in the environment and cancers of all types (Fig. 22–2). Reports of holes in the ozone layer, accidental lead and mercury poisonings, toxic shellfish beds, truckloads of pesticides spilling into streams and rivers, and accidental release of radioactive steam from nuclear power plants occur with distressing regularity.

Epidemiologists, who study the origins of diseases, believe that there is a relationship between environmental decline and increases in certain diseases, including epidemic diseases such as Hantavirus and Ebola virus. Emerging diseases and **multidrug resistant strains** of organisms currently under control, such as tuberculosis, will increasingly challenge health care resources.

Humans are responsible for destroying the environment, and the more human beings there are, the faster the environment will decline. Overpopulation contributes to the deterioration of the world's environment, yet, other than China, few countries are dealing effectively with issues of overpopulation.

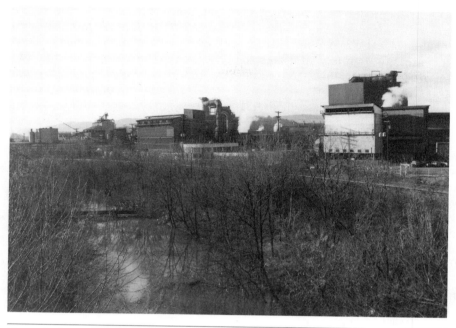

Figure 22–2

This manufacturing plant, while providing jobs to scores of workers, has polluted the air and the ground around it and a nearby stream (Photo by Kelly Whalin).

In October 1999 the world population reached the record number of 6 billion people. The United Nations has projected that the world's population will increase to 2.5 times its present size by the end of the twenty-first century (*Newsweek,* 1992). This represents a total of 13 billion people, more than twice as many human beings as have ever lived. Feeding, immunizing, and caring for this many human beings threatens to destroy the economic, social, and medical systems of the world.

At the first Earth Summit Conference held in Rio de Janeiro in 1992, the analogy of the overloaded lifeboat was frequently used. World overpopulation and over consumption by wealthy nations threaten to deplete the resources and destroy the environment of the entire world, not just overpopulated countries. The related problems of environmental deterioration and overpopulation are health care issues that future nurses will face, and there are no easy answers.

Lifestyle Challenges

Despite the focus on wellness in contemporary American society, unhealthy lifestyles still predominate; this trend shows no signs of changing. Every year public health officials report that there are more obese Americans than ever, even though obesity has long been known to predispose people to a number of illnesses.

Futurists predict that Americans will eat more meals in restaurants in the future, but ordering a nutritious, well-balanced meal in a restaurant is a major challenge, even to people with a working knowledge of nutritional science. In a distressing sign that indicates acquiescence to the fast-food mentality of many families, nutritional consultants are now being hired by public school districts to teach cafeteria workers how to make nutritious school lunches look and taste more like fast foods. Apparently, many modern children refuse to eat anything else.

As a result of pressure from health-conscious consumers, many of whom are now aging "baby boomers," some restaurant chains have introduced grilled foods and other "low-fat" items. Upon examination, however, the fat content of some of these foods is unacceptably high. Restaurant owners report that even when they include low fat meals on the menu, few people order them. The majority of regular menu items are still loaded with animal fats, long known to cause cardiovascular disease, and sodium, known to aggravate a variety of health conditions. A taco salad, for example, can contain as many as 30 g of fat.

Yet another lifestyle issue is tobacco use. Smoking continues to increase among the young, especially females and minorities, both of whom are targeted for higher levels of marketing by tobacco companies. For decades, smoking has been known to cause lung cancer, emphysema and other chronic lung diseases, low-birth-weight babies, and a host of other health problems. The incidence of lung cancer in older women has exceeded breast cancer, long the leading killer in this age group. The use of smokeless tobacco is rising, creating unhealthy oral mucous membranes and predisposing users to oral cancer. All these trends ensure that tobacco-related illnesses and deaths will rise in the future.

Lack of exercise is another lifestyle issue for Americans of the future, particularly the young. The ready availability of entertainment on television is at least partly to blame. Studies show the more television people of all ages watch, the more likely they are to be overweight. Snacking and television watching go hand in hand. Entire generations of Americans, raised watching several hours of television each day, are unlikely to give up the habit in the future, especially because more channels are added yearly. Others spend hours in front of computer screens or in other sedentary pursuits. These habits are expected to continue in the future.

Lack of exercise is not limited to the young, however. For every middle-aged jogger seen pounding the roadways, legions of sedentary adults remain unseen at home, gradually becoming less fit and more susceptible to disease. Browsing through mail-order catalogs aimed at the affluent middle-aged population reveals a plethora of labor-saving devices being developed and marketed to make Americans even less active in the future.

Advertising affects yet another lifestyle risk factor. With the emphasis on thinness in fashion advertising, many girls and young women resort to unhealthy habits such as starving or binging and purging. Rather than eating sensibly and engaging in exercise to maintain normal weights, they assume bizarre eating habits in the pursuit of the fashionable, if unnatural, degree of gauntness. Barring a dramatic change in the fashion industry, eating disorders and their resulting health hazards will continue to increase.

Another lifestyle issue is stress. The rapid pace of modern life creates stress, yet Americans continue to step up the pace with cellular telephones, fax machines, satellite communications, personal computers, paging devices, "call-waiting" options, and all the other fruits of modern technology. Although many Americans mourn the loss of leisure time, indications are that when given more leisure time, many people spend it working. This evidence indicates that stress-related diseases will increase in the next century.

The twin epidemics of acquired immunodeficiency syndrome (AIDS) and drug abuse are two issues that will profoundly affect the future of nursing. When the AIDS epidemic began in the United States early in the 1980s, many of those affected were homosexual men. A few years later, infection rates among intravenous drug users began to rise. By the mid 1980s, AIDS moved into the general population of heterosexual adults, a trend already seen in other countries and now well established in the United States. The spread of AIDS to adolescents is causing considerable concern.

Even optimists in the medical community no longer predict a vaccine against human immunodeficiency virus (HIV), believing that it will be many years before a vaccine is discovered, if ever. Meanwhile, millions of Americans are already infected, and no cure is on the horizon.

Substance-abusing people suffer more accidents and illness than their nonabusing counterparts, thus requiring more medical and nursing care. They are also more likely to have unprotected sex, putting them at risk for acquiring HIV. Other health risks include hepatitis, noninfectious liver disorders, and kidney failure, among others. Nurses of the future will be called on to provide intensive nursing care to increasing numbers of substance abusers and people with AIDS.

Nurses' own lifestyle choices will come under scrutiny as the issue of HIV and hepatitis infections in physicians, dentists, nurses, and other health care workers becomes a focus of public concern. Nurses will be involved in the development of sound public policies concerning these issues.

Given the predominance of unhealthy lifestyle factors, it is clear that nurses will play an increasingly important role in educating people about wellness and self-care in the years ahead. Nurses will also be instrumental in educating the public about how to be informed consumers of health care services. Nurses will continue to provide nursing care in acute care settings, such as hospitals, to those who choose not to listen.

Cost-containment Challenges

During most of the 1970s, 1980s, and 1990s, governmental budget deficits reached all-time highs. At federal, state, and local levels, governments spent more money than was generated through taxes, and the pressure for health care for the elderly and poor created a significant part of those budgetary problems.

Society's poor, homeless, elderly, substance abusers, AIDS patients, and mentally ill are increasing in number and will increase in the new century. The question yet to be answered is "How can we pay for health care for these vulnerable populations now and in the future when their numbers are expected to increase?"

Federal and state governments are seeking to answer that question. In many states, Medicaid is the largest and fastest-growing single state expense. Although welfare reform efforts have effectively removed thousands from welfare rolls, the aging of America will continue to create huge numbers of Social Security–eligible and Medicare-eligible citizens. The decrease in the ratio of these individuals to the number of those working and paying Social Security and income taxes will place an additional burden on the federal government's budget.

The future will bring hospital closings, pressures from the business community to force changes in health care financing, and significant health care reform, piece by piece if not by sweeping legislative mandate. The nursing profession stands to benefit because nursing has been shown to be a cost-conscious yet high-quality alternative to traditional medical care. In addition, nurses are well equipped to provide managed care. As a profession, nursing is expected to benefit from health care woes in the United States by expanding roles in prevention and community-based nursing.

One cost-effective method of providing basic health care to children is through school nurses. As the burden of providing care continues to shift from federal agencies to state and local agencies, local school boards will recognize the economies to be realized through school nursing. Health care reform will likely provoke a dramatic rise in state-mandated health services for school children. These services will be delivered by school nurses.

Regulatory Challenges

Even if the cost of health care can be contained, health care expenses in the United States will continue to rise owing to the large number of aging Americans and the growing number of impoverished ones. Greater governmental regulation of health care will thus be required.

Nurses will become increasingly active in developing health policies that improve access, quality, and value in the delivery of health services. Legislation mandating the direct reimbursement of nurses for their services will be a feature of most government-funded programs, despite the opposition of organized medicine and hospitals. Private **managed care** programs will increasingly use advanced practice registered nurses to provide primary health care.

Nursing, through its professional associations, will continue to be a player in health care politics in the United States. Nurses will form coalitions with consumer groups to influence consumer-friendly legislation at state and national levels. Individual nurses will become more politically active as voters, campaign workers, community health activists, and political candidates. As nursing's public profile becomes higher, public scrutiny of the profession will increase. Consumers of nursing services will exercise their political power to ensure that nurses and other primary care providers consistently offer first-class health care.

Challenges in Nursing Practice

The societal changes just reviewed will necessarily create changes in nursing practice. Nurses in the next decade will face an ever-widening array of practice opportunities in hospital and community-based health care settings, each of which will bring its own set of challenges.

Challenge of Differentiating Practice Levels

There has been considerable resistance to differentiating levels of nursing practice, even though visionary nursing leaders have pointed out the need to do so for years. **Differentiated practice** means that nurses prepared in associate degree, baccalaureate degree, and higher degree programs should have different, well-defined roles and possibly even different levels of licensure. The competencies of nurses at each level could be clearly demonstrated, and nurses at each level could be held accountable for practice standards at that level. If differentiated practice became a reality, educational programs could be streamlined, employers and consumers could understand the differences, and patient care delivery systems could be reorganized to capitalize on the strengths of each level.

In the past, nurses prepared in diploma and associate degree programs opposed efforts to differentiate educational and practice levels in nursing, believing that they would be disenfranchised. Nursing leaders have been unwilling to take the risk of tacking such a potentially divisive issue. The result is that nursing is the only health care profession for which entry into practice is less than a baccalaureate degree. Many professions currently require a master's degree as the credential for entry into a profession, and educational standards are rising in all fields but nursing. This has hampered nursing in its quest for professionalism and equal status among the health care professions.

In addition to improving educational standards, differentiated practice could help nurses be more cost-effective by determining who is best suited to perform certain nursing actions. Differentiated practice can be realized in the twenty-first century only if practicing nurses are willing to give up the notion that "a nurse is a nurse is a nurse" and acknowledge that different educational programs do and should prepare different types of nursing practitioners. Nurses must be willing to see the larger picture and recognize that advances in the profession benefit all nurses.

Challenges of Cost Containment

During the 1990s, cost-containment initiatives in hospitals eliminated layers of middle-management nurses. This represented a crisis for individual nurse managers but created an opportunity for a stronger voice for nurses involved in direct patient care. Future cost-containment measures will require nurses to demonstrate the cost-effectiveness of the care they provide. The "bottom line" will be an increasing focus of concern in all health care settings, and nurses will need resource management skills more than ever before. Nurses will find that they need business expertise as much as they need clinical expertise.

Increasingly, nurses will work with unlicensed assistive personnel and delegate tasks to deliver patient care. They will need communication, interpersonal, and management skills to make the new partnerships work. **Multiskilled workers** will take their place alongside nurses in all settings. Nurses will be challenged to expand their skills into areas formerly the domain of specialized workers, such as respiratory therapists and physical therapists. This will be essential if nurses are to cope with the periodic variations in supply and demand for traditional nursing positions.

Challenges of Autonomy and Accountability

Shared governance, that is, participation by nurses on strong policymaking hospital committees, is a trend already seen and mandated by accreditation bodies such as the Joint Commission on the Accreditation of Healthcare Organizations (JCAHO). Along with the empowerment of nurses, however, will come increased demand for accountability. Effective nursing care will be measured by patient outcomes. Continuous quality improvement of nursing care will be emphasized more than ever. Nurses must be able to show evidence that the care they provide makes a demonstrable difference in patient outcomes.

As more and more nursing care is provided in community settings, autonomy and accountability will become increasingly important. Additional education and experience are needed by nurses who function independently in homes and other community-based practices. When the supervisory guidance of better-prepared colleagues is not readily available, nurses must assume responsibility for knowing the limits of their expertise and for seeking consultation. Professional nurses of the future will increasingly pursue baccalaureate and advanced degrees to prepare them for autonomous practice.

Challenges of Technology and Nursing Informatics

Technology will continue to advance at a dizzying pace in the twenty-first century. **Nursing informatics,** the organization and use of nursing data, will change nursing practice dramatically. Computerized health information networks (CHINs) will allow immediate access to all patient data needed in refining the plan of care. The increased access to patient data will reinforce the need for patient confidentiality. Voice-activated bedside computers already allow nurses to record patient information literally "at the bedside," rather than making written notes and transferring them to the patient's chart at a later time. This practice will become widespread.

Advances in telecommunications will improve access to medical services for rural and elderly Americans. Nurses and physicians will examine and treat patients who are hundreds of miles away using two-way television systems. They will evaluate and prescribe treatments via telephone. Telemedicine will become routine for those who live in remote areas or are homebound. Nurses will be increasingly involved in **telehealth** in the twenty-first century.

Genetic engineering will become more common as the scientists participating in the **Human Genome Project** complete the mapping and sequencing of a composite set of human genes. This will make it possible to treat and prevent genetically transmitted and genetically predisposed diseases. It will also create ethical dilemmas of gigantic proportions as the ability to clone individuals and predetermine characteristics of human infants becomes a reality. Genetic research will also make possible individualized medications, or **designer medicines.** Designer medicines are drugs tailor-made to treat patients based on their individual genetic makeup.

Nurses will continue to fight the dehumanizing tendency of technological advances such as patient monitoring devices while valuing and providing a holistic, "high-touch" environment for patients. Nurses will realize that advanced technology and traditional nursing values are not mutually exclusive. Patients can have both if nurses stay focused on the patient rather than on the machine or monitor. Advances in technology will bring new ethical dilemmas. Nurses will be more active in exploring ethical aspects of patient care, and their unique ethical perspective will be valued by other professionals. As a result, nurses will sit on ethics committees and serve as ethics consultants in greater numbers. Because of their interpersonal skills and the public perception of trustworthiness, nurses will become **genetic counselors** in increasing numbers (Pesut, 1997).

More Americans will turn away from mainstream medical care and seek **alternative treatments** as they take responsibility for their own health (Fig. 22–3). Nontraditional care such as chiropractic, homeopathy, acupuncture, massage, therapeutic touch, and herbal remedies will become a focus of interest, study, research, practice, and publication (McKenna, 1995).

The Internet will create major changes in the way Americans view health care and their role as partners in their own care. The proliferation of web sites designed to provide reliable medical and health information to the lay public will continue. Nurses will be called upon to educate patients about how to evaluate and use appropriately the information they obtain from these sites.

Challenges of Practice in Community Settings

Community-based primary health care will continue to expand as cost-effectiveness remains a high priority. Nurse-managed clinics will increasingly serve underserved populations in inner city and rural areas. School nurses will be needed in large numbers, as will hospice nurses and those specializing in gerontology and chronic illnesses. For nurses who are willing to work outside traditional settings and their own "comfort zones," there will be no end to the available opportunities.

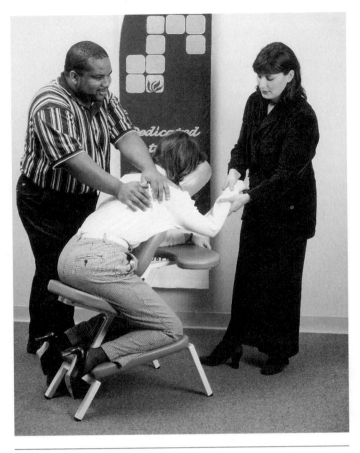

Figure 22–3
Alternative treatments such as massage therapy are appealing to more Americans as they take responsibility for their own health (Courtesy of Memorial Hospital, Chattanooga, Tennessee).

Flexible scheduling and job sharing will increase in all professions and will become commonplace in nursing. Nurse entrepreneurship will flourish in the future owing to changes in restrictive legislation, the resourcefulness and self-confidence of better-educated nurses, and the trust the public places in the nursing profession. Increasing numbers of nurses will own clinics and other health-related businesses, such as independent practice associations, free-standing wellness programs, dialysis care services, and worksite health programs.

Challenges of Cultural Competence

Providing culturally competent nursing care will become even more important in the future as the nation's demographics continue to change. Nurses of the future must recognize that cultural sensitivity begins with one's fellow health care providers. If relationships within the team are strained by insensitivity and prejudice, patient care cannot be culturally sensitive. Meaningful dialogue must become a vehicle for building relationships within the work group. A united team will be capable of providing respectful, understanding, and dignified care to patients.

Effective nursing leaders of the future will provide cultural support groups and mentoring to ensure that "faculty, providers, students, patients, and others can become less inhibited about individuals who are culturally different. They can foster the courage to engage in conversations, to get to know each other, to share our worldviews, to speak out, and to trust that interactions about our specific and particular culture, on a personal level, will make a difference" (Gary, Sigby, and Campbell, 1998, p. 277). Nurses who are unable or unwilling to become culturally aware, culturally sensitive, and culturally competent will unnecessarily limit their career potential.

Challenges of Maintaining a Healthy Work Environment

No profession is free from hazards, and no work place can ever assure absolute security. Nursing is no exception to this sad fact of contemporary life. Occupational health hazards in nursing range from needlestick injuries and possible infection with hepatitis and HIV, to exposure to chemicals such as disinfectants and chemotherapeutic agents.

Hazards also include latex allergy, a growing concern for nurses, with a prevalence rate of 10 percent in frequent glove users (Rogers, 1997). Injuries from accidents and back strain also occur too frequently, with pain, disability, lost income, absenteeism, and decreased productivity only a few of the results.

Shift work itself is a hazard to nurses, causing a variety of physical and psychological problems, including exhaustion, depression, interpersonal problems, and accidents. Stress from work overload, inadequate staffing, and the intense feelings generated by caring for acutely ill and dying patients adds to the mix of workplace hazards faced by nurses.

In addition, nurses increasingly find themselves at risk for violence in the workplace. This is not a new phenomenon, but it is being discussed more openly than in the past, as evidenced by the fall 1999 issue of Sigma Theta Tau International's membership publication, *Reflections,* being devoted entirely to the issue of workplace violence.

Among the articles in that issue of *Reflections* was a report of a 1997 survey by the Colorado Nurses Association's Task Force on Violence, which conducted a seven-state survey examining nurse safety. There were 586 respondents, one-third of whom disclosed "that they were victims of workplace violence in 1996. Most nurses indicated patients were the assailants. . . . Yet half of the nurses acknowledged that violence went unreported at work" (Carroll and Goldsmith, 1999, p. 26).

Assuring nurses of a healthy work environment is a major challenge for the next decade (Disch, 1997). It is not, however, a problem that nurses can expect will be solved by others. Clearly, nurses of the future must themselves take positive, effective, united action to ensure the basic dignity and safety of practicing nurses everywhere. They must demand and use safer needlestick devices and disposal containers; high-efficiency ventilation systems; alternatives to latex gloves and products; adequate housekeeping support; adequate lifting assistance with devices or additional personnel; reduction or elimination of shift rotation; and appropriate occupational safety and health training. Nurses themselves must use impeccable handwashing techniques and personal protective equipment such as gloves, gowns, and masks. And they must demand that adequate security be provided to protect them against violent patients and family members.

Challenges in Nursing Education

As the profession of nursing matures, more nurses will recognize the value of bachelor's degrees for beginning professional practice and master's degrees for advanced practice. More nurses will pursue doctoral degrees to prepare for leadership roles in research and theory development. In response, colleges of nursing will expand flexible educational programs to improve access. They will also develop differentiated levels of nursing education that correspond to differentiated levels of practice.

Challenges of Outcome-based Education

The quality of educational programs will continue to be judged by student competencies, that is, what students can actually do as a result of education. Nursing educational programs will monitor their graduates' activities and achievements as professional nurses. They will be required to report on graduates' accomplishments as part of the accreditation process. The emphasis on accountability of nursing education programs will increase as measures of competence in graduates are refined.

Just as nursing practice is being challenged to measure patient outcomes and adopt evidence-based practice, nursing education will be challenged to develop student outcomes and adopt evidence-based education. Faculty will modify age-old teaching/learning strategies and adopt new pedagogies proven effective through research. Passive learning, such as lectures, will be deemphasized. Critical thinking, independent decision making, and creative problem solving will assume even greater importance, fostered by role playing, simulations, and group problem solving (Huston and Fox, 1998). Faculty will be required to document evidence-based teaching as part of accreditation processes.

Accreditation of nursing education programs will become more difficult to achieve as national accrediting bodies come under increasing pressure to raise standards and to apply standards consistently. Substandard programs will be closed in increasing numbers. This will strengthen nursing.

Challenges of Diversity

In the twenty-first century, students in nursing education programs will reflect the demographics of the United States and become more diverse than ever before. More men, older students, and students with degrees in other fields will come into nursing because of the emotional rewards and professional image it offers. Student bodies will become more culturally diverse, reflecting the diversity of the nation's population.

Access to education for nontraditional and traditional students will be an even greater issue. Schools will expand nontraditional curricula that enable adults to work and go to school simultaneously. Nursing courses delivered by **distance learning** technologies, such as telecommunications and satellite linkages, will increase access for students living in remote areas. Cost-minded legislators will require that state-supported schools offer fully articulated programs in order to qualify for state funding. Schools that fall behind in distance learning offerings will have difficulty filling their classes as more and more students seek non-residential education.

Changes in demographics will affect the content of curricula as well as the methods by which content is delivered. As the population ages, the need for nurses prepared in gerontology, chronic disease management, and hospice care will give emphasis to educational programs at both undergraduate and graduate levels. Curricula will emphasize community-based care instead of traditional hospital-based care. Educational programs will develop and expand multicultural courses. Foreign languages will again become a graduation requirement in baccalaureate programs. International educational opportunities will increase as the global village concept becomes a reality. Every nursing program will have the provision of culturally competent care as an outcome criterion for its graduates.

Challenges of Technology and Nursing Informatics

Technological advances and the growth of nursing knowledge will create the need for informatics expertise in nursing education as well as in nursing practice. Computer competence will not suffice for nurses of the future. Students will need to master sophisticated information systems to use the wealth of available knowledge to improve patient care.

Faculty will be challenged to keep pace with students' acquisition of knowledge from the World Wide Web. Students of the future will become increasingly active in obtaining information from a vast array of sources available to them at the touch of a computer key. This will enable students to be more engaged in their own learning process and foster active learning.

Nursing faculty will be required to practice the profession actively to keep up with rapidly changing technologies. Students will be incorporated into faculty practices to obtain clinical experience. In this regard, nursing education will resemble medical education.

It will be impossible for nursing education programs to include in their curricula everything nurses of the future need to know. All nurses must be educated to become lifelong learners. They must be taught to expect change and be prepared to adapt or retool their skills quickly to respond to health care marketplace demands (Huston and Fox, 1998).

Licensing examinations will change to reflect the expansion of nursing knowledge and the increase in community-based practice and resulting autonomy. Licensure at multiple levels will become a reality. Employers of new graduates will expect to provide internships designed to enable novices to make the transition from student to practicing nurse effectively.

Challenges of Collaboration

As nurses acquire more education, the resulting self-confidence will enable them to develop collaborative relationships on an equal footing with physicians and other highly educated health care professionals. This will enable nurses to be more assertive in patient advocacy and will improve patient care and strengthen the profession.

Nursing faculty, nurse managers, and practicing nurses will join forces to strengthen educational experiences and mentorships for tomorrow's nurses. They will collaborate on clinical research that demonstrates the effectiveness of nursing care in terms of patient outcomes. They will collaborate with other nurses and consumer groups to remove regulatory restrictions that impede advanced clinical practice.

Nurse educators will recognize the need to treat students as professionals in training and will transform nursing education attitudes from controlling students to collaborating with them. This will create a new generation of empowered nursing professionals.

Disciplinary boundaries are becoming blurred as knowledge from all disciplines is brought to bear on problems of mutual concern, such as breast cancer, domestic violence, and AIDS. Nursing must become more interdisciplinary in its focus. Only nurses with a strong sense of personal and professional identity will be able to enter fully into multidisciplinary collaboration. Those nurses who understand the value of collaboration will become the managers of care using a case-management model, and they will thrive.

Challenges of Reforms in Health Care and Higher Education

Due to health care reform and cost-containment initiatives, nurses of the future will need to be well versed in the costs, budgeting, and financing of health care. Business education will be increasingly emphasized, particularly at the graduate level, as nurses pursue entrepreneurial and intrapreneurial roles. Nursing faculty will either return to school to prepare themselves to teach business courses or will create interdisciplinary alliances with business schools to provide nursing students with the necessary business courses.

Higher education will undergo public scrutiny and reform. It already suffers from serious underfunding. As governmental grants are reduced or eliminated to help balance the national budget, educational programs will experience budgetary constraints. By the mid-1990s, several nursing education programs, including some well-regarded ones, had closed as a result of funding shortfalls. In many universities, autonomous schools and colleges of nursing were combined with health and human service programs into one administrative unit to save money. This often weakened the nursing program's voice on the campus. Budgets for operating expenses, equipment, and faculty salaries were underpar in many locations even though the demand for nursing education remained high.

For a time, it appeared that hospitals could be a source of support for nursing education programs, but with their own significant budgetary constraints, it is unlikely that this will be a long-term solution. Hospitals, however, will support nursing education for as long as possible with financial aid to students, subsidies of faculty salaries, joint appointments of faculty, and other forms of assistance.

Graduate education programs will change to produce practitioners who can meet consumer demands. Changes in hospital-based nursing practice will force a reexamination of the clinical nurse specialist and nurse practitioner roles (Williams and Valdivieso, 1994). The need for efficiency and cost-effectiveness will lead to a revision of advanced practice models, and educational programs will combine the two roles and emphasize community-based practice.

Curricula at all levels will be standardized and streamlined to reduce cost and confusion and improve student mobility. The trend toward use of multiskilled workers will force nursing faculty to identify unique aspects of nursing and to educate students for broader roles in the delivery of patient care (Blayney, 1994).

In the next decade, many long-time nursing faculty, educated at the master's level during the nurse-traineeship funding heyday of the 1960s, will retire. There will be no one to replace them because younger nurses are not entering teaching owing to the lag of nursing education salaries behind those in practice settings. There will be a serious shortage of nursing faculty in the twenty-first century that will force a major curriculum reform in nursing education programs. This will be a positive step for nursing.

A Challenge to the Entire Nursing Profession: Unity

Most of the important issues the nursing profession will face in the next decade cannot be resolved by any one group of nurses. They will require the attention of the entire profession, working in a united manner through nursing's professional associations. Even though collective power is the only way nursing will effectively resolve these issues, fewer than 10 percent of all nurses belong to their professional association. As the largest health care profession in the United States, with over 2.5 million registered nurse members, nursing can and should have a powerful voice and presence at every table where substantive health care issues are discussed. But nurses have historically been unwilling to throw their support behind their professional organizations. They have allowed issues of educational background, political philosophies, abortion, and other concerns to divide them.

If you think for a moment about other groups to which you belong, for example a political party, church, or parent-teacher association, you do not expect to agree with every position taken by the organization or its leaders. Nurses seem to have such an expectation of their professional association, however, and use that as a reason for lack of unity. With nursing and society becoming increasingly diverse, nurses of the future must become more tolerant of differences and work hard to find common ground with their colleagues in the profession. If we fail to do so, nursing will not prosper.

You, the readers of this book, are the future of the nursing profession. You represent our best hope for building nursing into an even more powerful force for good. Look around at the other members of your class. Whether there are 25 students or 100, you can accomplish far more working together than you can working in isolation. So it is with nursing's future: We can accomplish far more by working collectively. All nurses, individually and as a profession, will benefit from the resulting unity.

Summary of Key Points

- Societal changes are likely to occur in the first decade of the twenty-first century in the following areas: demographics, the environment, lifestyles, and economics and governmental regulation of health care.
- Both nursing practice and nursing education will be affected by these changes.
- Nursing roles will be differentiated.
- Nursing practice will become more community based.
- Nurses will be able to demonstrate that the care they provide makes a positive difference in patient outcomes.
- Nurses will continue to provide a warm, humanizing influence on patient care in potentially dehumanizing high-tech environments.
- Effective nurses will become culturally competent.
- The major challenges for nursing education will be: to respond to societal changes rapidly with appropriate curricular modifications; to produce a steady supply of well-prepared graduates in the face of an aging faculty; rapidly changing technology; increasing cultural diversity of students and patients; and lack of human and budgetary resources in higher education.
- Joining professional associations is the best way for nurses of the future to unite to solve the challenges facing the profession.

Critical Thinking Questions

1. As the number of elderly Americans rises, the rate of chronic illness also rises. What challenges does this present for nurses of the future?
2. Take a position on the statement, "Nurses of the future will have an impact

on the environment that exceeds that of the ordinary citizen." Be prepared to defend your position.

3. Describe economic issues that will affect nurses of the future. How can you begin now to prepare yourself to deal with these issues?

4. Initiate a classroom debate on the issue "HIV-positive nurses should not be limited in how they practice nursing."

5. As a class, brainstorm ways a school health nurse could improve pupils' health status. Then design an educational program to prepare school nurses. Compare your curriculum with that of an existing school health nurse program.

6. Interview faculty members to identify components of your educational program that will prepare you for the culturally competent nursing needed in the twenty-first century. Report your findings to the class.

Web Resources

Alternative medicine, http://www.wellweb.com

Cultural competence, http://www.tcns.org

Emerging diseases/drug-resistant organisms, http://www.cdc.gov/ncidod/eidtopics.htm

Human genome research, http://www.nchgr.nih.gov

Latex allergy, http://www.nysna.org/protected/npalerts/npalertl4.htm

Occupational health and safety, http://www.healthcaresafety.com

Telehealth, http://www.telehealth.hrsa.gov and http://www.nursingworld.org/readroom/tele2.htm

Violence in the workplace, http://www.cdc.gov/niosh/violcont.html and http://www.nursingworld.org/dlwa/osh/wp5.htm

References

Blayney, K. D. (1994). The future of multiskilling. Paper presented at the national conference, *Multiskilling and the Allied Health Workforce,* cosponsored by the Connelly Allied Health Education Center, Methodist Hospital, Indianapolis, Ind., and the Health Resources and Services Administration, Bureau of Health Professions, Washington, D.C.

Carroll, V., and Goldsmith, J. (1999). One-third of nurses are abused in the workplace. *Reflections*, 25(3), 24–27.

Disch, J. M. (1997). The future of nursing. *Image: Journal of Nursing Scholarship,* 29(3), 225.

Gary, F. A., Sigsby, L. M., and Campbell, D. (1998). Preparing for the 21st century: Diversity in nursing education, research, and practice. *Journal of Professional Nursing,* 14(5), 272–279.

Hendrick, B. (1995). The coming millennium. *The Atlanta Journal/The Atlanta Constitution.* July 16, A12.

Herbert, L. E., Scherr, P. A., Beckett, L. A., Chown, M. J., Funkstein, H. H., and Evans, D. A. (1995). Alzheimer's disease. *JAMA,* 273(17), 1354–1359.

Huston, C. J., and Fox, S. (1998). The changing health care market: Implications for nursing education in the coming decade. *Nursing Outlook,* 46(3), 109–114.

McKenna, M. A. J. (1995). Going mainstream. *The Atlanta Journal/The Atlanta Constitution.* May 17, C8.

Newsweek. (1992). Why Rio will make history. June 15, 33.

Pesut, D. J. (1997). The future, virtue-ethics, and Sigma Theta Tau. *Reflections,* 23(3), 56–59.

Rogers, B. (1997). Is health care a risky business? *The American Nurse,* 29(5), 5.

Williams, C. A., and Valdivieso, M. N. (1994). Advanced practice models: A comparison of clinical nurse specialist and nurse practitioner activities. *Clinical Nurse Specialist,* 8(6), 311–318.

Epilogue

You, our readers, are inheriting a rich legacy of achievement and progress in the nursing profession. While appreciating the accomplishments of those who paved the way for us, let us not lose sight of the fact that much remains to be done. As health care professionals, you will be challenged to lead your communities in addressing the complex issues of health care costs, access to health care for the disenfranchised, and other not-yet-imagined concerns. You will be part of the solution.

It is the hope of all the nurses who have participated in preparing this textbook that through this book you were stimulated to develop values, beliefs, knowledge, professionalism, and desire to become a nursing leader of the future and a positive force for change in the nursing profession.

You can begin to exert your influence to improve the profession by evaluating this book. If you are willing to help in this way, please e-mail me and I will send you a brief questionnaire. You can also tell me anything else you would like to share about the helpful and unhelpful aspects of the current edition. With your help we can continue to improve it to better meet the needs of future students.

KayKChitty@aol.com

Appendices

Appendix A
The Code for Nurses

1. The nurse provides services with respect for human dignity and the uniqueness of the client unrestricted by considerations of social or economic status, personal attributes, or the nature of health problems.
2. The nurse safeguards the client's right to privacy by judiciously protecting information of a confidential nature.
3. The nurse acts to safeguard the client and the public when health care and safety are affected by the incompetent, unethical, or illegal practice of any person.
4. The nurse assumes responsibility and accountability for individual nursing judgments and actions.
5. The nurse maintains competence in nursing.
6. The nurse exercises informed judgment and uses individual competence and qualifications as criteria in seeking consultation, accepting responsibilities and delegating nursing activities to others.
7. The nurse participates in activities that contribute to the ongoing development of the profession's body of knowledge.
8. The nurse participates in the profession's efforts to implement and improve standards of nursing.
9. The nurse participates in the profession's efforts to establish and maintain conditions of employment conducive to high-quality nursing care.
10. The nurse participates in the profession's effort to protect the public from misinformation and misrepresentation and to maintain the integrity of nursing.
11. The nurse collaborates with members of the health professions and other citizens in promoting community and national efforts to meet the health needs of the public.

Reprinted with permission of American Nurses Association (1985). *Code for nurses with interpretive statements.* Washington, D. C.: American Nurses Association.

Appendix B
Sample Critical Path for Congestive Heart Failure

† CATHOLIC HEALTH
  INITIATIVES

Memorial Health Care System

2525 deSales Avenue   Chattanooga, TN 37404
2051 Hamill Road   Hixson, TN 37343

CARETRAC   DRG: 127

Diagnosis/Procedure: CHF

Allergies: _____

Target LOS 4 ——
M&R LOS 1 ——
10/09/99

Date begun/ Initials	Target date/ Initials	Expected Outcomes Patient or significant other will:	Date met/ Initials
		Verbalize understanding of Advance Directive information.	
		Spirituality needs addressed with patient/family.	
		Be free from Injury/Falls.	
		Verbalize understanding of Fall Prevention program.	
		Verbalize understanding of follow-up care.	
		Verbalize understanding of symptoms, treatment options and complications/ risks associated with treatment.	
		Verbalize understanding of how to manage nutrition and hydration to facilitate optimal health and comfort in the presence of disease and/or treatment.	
		Verbalize understanding of pain scale and report relief and/or absence of pain.	
		Verbalize understanding of safe and effective use of medications, including dosage, administration times and actions.	
		Maintain adequate gas exchange as evidenced by stable respiratory status.	
		Demonstrate knowledge of signs and symptoms of disease process (sob, wheezing, chest pain etc).	
		Demonstrate an appropriate increase in activity level.	
		Demonstrate/verbalize knowledge of activity limitations and safety precautions.	
		Patient/family/caregiver verbalizes an understanding of the progression of increasing activity level.	
		Demonstrate understanding of available and appropriate outpatient resources for continuance in rehabilitation.	
		Describe: 1) Best time to weigh daily. 2) Reason for daily weights. 3) Action to take if weight increased by 3–5 pounds.	
		Verbalize s/s to report to MD after discharge (weight gain of 3–5 pounds, SOB with normal activity, inability to lie flat to sleep).	
		Verbalize knowledge of specific risk factor modifications and available resources (smoking, diet, exercise, stress reduction).	

*CARETRACS DO NOT REPRESENT A STANDARD OF CARE. THEY ARE GUIDELINES FOR CONSIDERATION
WHICH MAY BE MODIFIED ACCORDING TO THE INDIVIDUAL PATIENT NEEDS.*

† CATHOLIC HEALTH
  INITIATIVES

Memorial Health Care System

2525 deSales Avenue   Chattanooga, TN 37404
2051 Hamill Road   Hixson, TN 37343

CARETRAC   DRG: <u>127</u>

Diagnosis/Procedure: <u>CHF</u>

Allergies: _____

Page <u>2</u> of <u>5</u>

Target LOS 4 ——
M&R LOS 1 ——
10/09/99

Date Begun/ Initials	Target date/ Initials	Expected Outcomes Patient or significant other will:	Date met/ Initials

Potential barriers to learning: (reflect actions taken for barriers in the 'Comments' below)
☐ None   ☐ Specific Barrier: Describe on line below

_____

Educational packet(s) reviewed with patient/family:
☐ Heart Failure
Continuing Educational Needs Identified:
☐ Post surgical care   ☐ S&S of recurring problems   ☐ Pain Management
☐ Medications   ☐ Equipment/supply use   ☐ Diet & Nutrition
☐ Disease Process   ☐ Community resources   ☐ Self Care Needs
Patient/Family response to educational materials:
☐ Verbalized understanding ☐ Agree with continuing education plan
Comments:

_____

_____

_____

Form faxed to: _____ **on discharge.** _____ **(initial)**

CARETRACS DO NOT REPRESENT A STANDARD OF CARE. THEY ARE GUIDELINES FOR CONSIDERATION
WHICH MAY BE MODIFIED ACCORDING TO THE INDIVIDUAL PATIENT NEEDS.

Memorial Health Care System

2525 deSales Avenue   Chattanooga, TN 37404
2051 Hamill Road   Hixson, TN 37343

CARETRAC   DRG: 127 _____

Diagnosis/Procedure: CHF _____

Allergies: _____

Date or Time →			
Time frame → Phase →	Admission	Day 1	Day 2
CONSULTS REFERRALS	Chaplaincy Care manager Pharmacy Nutrition services Cardiology consult Cardiac rehab	Chaplaincy Care manager Cardiac rehab Consider home health care post discharge	Care Manager Cardiac rehab
NUTRITION	_____ gm Na diet Assess need for fluid restriction	_____ gm Na diet Continue fluid restriction	_____ gm Na diet Reevaluate need for fluid restriction
ACTIVITY SAFETY	Fall risk precautions Bedrest with BSC	Fall risk precautions Up in chair for meals Cardiac rehab phase I	Fall risk precautions Bath with assist only Up in chair for meals Cardiac rehab phase I
ASSESSMENTS DEMOGRAPHICS	Age specific needs addressed Physical assessment Cardiac Monitor Vital signs I&O Q 8 hrs Daily weight Immunization status evaluation Discharge planning Pain Scale 0–10	Assess for activity tolerance Cardiac Monitor Vital signs I&O Q 8 hrs Daily weight Discharge planning Pain Scale 0–10	Assess bowel pattern Cardiac Monitor Vital signs I&O Q 8 hrs Daily weight Assess availability of accurate scales for home use Discharge planning Pain Scale 0–10
TREATMENTS	IV site care 02 per protocol Turn, cough, and deep breathe Oral care	IV site care 02 per protocol Turn, cough, and deep breathe Elevate legs when OOB	IV site care 02 per protocol Elevate legs when OOB
DIAGNOSTIC LAB	Comprehensive metabolic panel Digoxin Level CPK & MB CBC EKG Chest x-ray If diabetic: FSBS 7-11-4-9	Basic metabolic panel	Basic metabolic panel

MEDICATION	INT
	IV diuretics
	Ace inhibitors
	Digoxin
	If diabetic and eating—begin
	  home diabetic meds:
	  (i.e., insulin/oral agent)
		INT
		IV or PO diuretics
		Ace inhibitors
		Digoxin
		Low dose beta blocker
			INT
			PO diuretics
			Ace inhibitors
			Digoxin
			Low dose beta blocker

EDUCATION	Educate pt/family on fall risk
	  precautions
	Orient to room/patient brochure
	Patient education pkt. given
	Advance directives
	Plan of care
	Disease process
	Pain management
		Educate pt/family on fall risk
		  precautions
		Pain management
		S/S of CHF
		Daily weights
		Low Na diet
		Medication compliance
		Exercise
			Educate pt/family on fall risk
			  precautions
			Pain management
			S/S of CHF
			Daily weights
			Low Na diet
			Medication compliance
			Exercise

CARETRACS DO NOT REPRESENT A STANDARD OF CARE. THEY ARE GUIDELINES FOR CONSIDERATION
WHICH MAY BE MODIFIED ACCORDING TO THE INDIVIDUAL PATIENT NEEDS.

\# Related to Outcome   * See narrative notes

Memorial Health Care System

2525 deSales Avenue   Chattanooga, TN 37404
2051 Hamill Road   Hixson, TN 37343

CARETRAC DRG: 127

Diagnosis/Procedure: CHF

Allergies: _____

Target LOS 4 ——
M&R LOS 1 ——
10/09/99

Date or Time →			
Time frame → Phase →	Day 3	Day 4	
CONSULTS REFERRALS	Care manager Cardiac rehab	Care manager Cardiac rehab Reconsult pharmacy for home meds	
NUTRITION	If diet intake poor, consult Nutrition Services	If diet intake poor, consult Nutrition Services	
ACTIVITY SAFETY	Fall risk precautions Bath with minimal assistance Ambulate in room with assistance Cardiac rehab phase I	Fall risk precautions Bathes self Ambulate in hall Cardiac rehab phase I	
ASSESSMENTS DEMOGRAPHICS	Assess bowel pattern Cardiac monitor Vital signs I&O Q 8 hrs Daily Weight Discharge planning Pain Scale 0–10	Assess bowel pattern Cardiac monitor Vital signs routine I&O Q 8 hrs Daily weight Pain Scale 0–10	
TREATMENTS	IV site care 02 per protocol	IV site care	
DIAGNOSTIC LAB	Consider repeat chest x-ray Digoxin level if indicated If blood glucose stable, FSBS 7 & 4	Consider repeat chest x-ray Basic metabolic panel if indicated	
MEDICATION	IV access PO meds Ace inhibitors Digoxin Low dose beta blockers	IV access PO meds Ace inhibitors Digoxin Low dose beta blockers	
EDUCATION	Educate pt/family on fall risk precautions Pain management S/S of CHF Daily weights Low Na diet Medication compliance Exercise Smoking cessation	Educate pt/family on fall risk precautions Discharge instructions and meds Follow-up appt(s)	

CARETRACS DO NOT REPRESENT A STANDARD OF CARE. THEY ARE GUIDELINES FOR CONSIDERATION WHICH MAY BE MODIFIED ACCORDING TO THE INDIVIDUAL PATIENT NEEDS.

Related to Outcome   * See narrative notes

PRINTED 00-Jan-13 08:50by BRAGGET, NADINE M

Memorial Health Care System

2525 deSales Avenue   Chattanooga, TN 37404
2051 Hamill Road   Hixson, TN 37343

CARETRAC   DRG: 127 _____

Diagnosis/Procedure: CHF _____

Allergies: _____

Target LOS 4 ——
M&R LOS 1 ——
10/09/99

SIGNATURE SHEET   **List current consultant's specialty and Full Name here.**

Initials	Name/Title	Initials	Name/Title	Initials	Name/Title

*CARETRACS DO NOT REPRESENT A STANDARD OF CARE. THEY ARE GUIDELINES FOR CONSIDERATION
WHICH MAY BE MODIFIED ACCORDING TO THE INDIVIDUAL PATIENT NEEDS.*

Sample Critical Path (CareTrac) for congestive heart failure (CHF). Courtesy Memorial Health Care System, a
member of Catholic Health Initiatives, Chattanooga, Tenn.

Appendix C
State Boards of Nursing

Alabama Board of Nursing
RSA Plaza, Suite 250
770 Washington Avenue
Montgomery, AL 36130–3900
Phone: (334) 242–4060
FAX: (334) 242–4360
http://www.abn.state.al.us/

Alaska Board of Nursing
Department of Commerce and Economic
   Development
Division of Occupational Licensing
3601 C Street, Suite 722
Anchorage, AK 99503
Phone: (907) 269–8161
FAX: (907) 269–8196
http://www.dced.state.ak.us/occ/pnur.htm

Arizona State Board of Nursing
1651 E. Morten Avenue, Suite 150
Phoenix, AZ 85020
Phone: (602) 331–8111
FAX: (602) 906–9365
http://www.azboardofnursing.org/

Arkansas State Board of Nursing
University Tower Building
1123 S. University, Suite 800
Little Rock, AR 72204
Phone: (501) 686–2700
FAX: (501) 686–2714
http://www.state.ar.us/nurse

California Board of Registered Nursing
400 R Street, Suite 4030
Sacramento, CA 95814–6239
Phone: (916) 322–3350
FAX: (916) 327–4402
http://www.rn.ca.gov/

Colorado Board of Nursing
1560 Broadway, Suite 880

Denver, CO 80202
Phone: (303) 894–2430
FAX: (303) 894–2821
http://www.dora.state.co.us/nursing/

Connecticut Board of Examiners for Nursing
Division of Health Systems Regulation
410 Capitol Avenue, MS# 12HSR
P.O. Box 340308
Hartford, CT 06134–0328
Phone: (860) 509–7624
FAX: (860) 509–7553
http://www.state.ct.us/dph/

Delaware Board of Nursing
861 Silver Lake Blvd
Cannon Building, Suite 203
Dover, DE 19904
Phone: (302) 739–4522
FAX: (302) 739–2711

District of Columbia Board of Nursing
Department of Health
825 N. Capitol Street, N. E., 2nd Floor
Room 2224
Washington, D. C. 20002
Phone: (202) 442–4778
FAX: (202) 442–9431

Florida Board of Nursing
4080 Woodcock Drive, Suite 202
Jacksonville, FL 32207
Phone: (904) 858–6940
FAX: (904) 858–6964
http://www.doh.state.fl.us/mqa/nursing/
   rnhome.htm

Georgia Board of Nursing
237 Coliseum Drive
Macon, GA 31217–3858
Phone: (912) 207–1640
FAX: (912) 207–1660
http://www.sos.state.ga.us/ebd-rn/

Hawaii Board of Nursing
Professional and Vocational Licensing Division
P. O. Box 3469
Honolulu, HI 96801
Phone: (808) 586-3000
FAX: (808) 586-2689

Idaho Board of Nursing
280 N. 8th Street, Suite 210
P. O. Box 83720
Boise, ID 83720
Phone: (208) 334-3110
FAX: (208) 334-3262
http://www.state.id.us/ibn/ibnhome.htm

Illinois Department of Professional Regulation
James R. Thompson Center
100 West Randolph, Suite 9-300
Chicago, IL 60601
Phone: (312) 814-2715
FAX: (312) 814-3145
http://www.state.il.us/dpr/

Indiana State Board of Nursing
Health Professions Bureau
402 W. Washington Street, Room W041
Indianapolis, IN 46204
Phone: (317) 232-2960
FAX: (317) 233-4236
http://www.ai.org/hpb

Iowa Board of Nursing
RiverPoint Business Park
400 S. W. 8th Street, Suite B
Des Moines, IA 50309-4685
Phone: (515) 281-3255
FAX: (515) 281-4825
http://www.state.ia.us/government/nursing/

Kansas State Board of Nursing
Landon State Office Building
900 S. W. Jackson, Suite 551-S
Topeka, KS 66612
Phone: (785) 296-4929
FAX: (785) 296-3929
http://www.ink.org/public/ksbn/

Kentucky Board of Nursing
312 Whittington Parkway, Suite 300
Louisville, KY 40222
Phone: (502) 329-7000
FAX: (502) 329-7011
http://www.kbn.state.ky.us/

Louisiana State Board of Nursing
3510 N. Causeway Boulevard, Suite 501
Metairie, LA 70003
Phone: (504) 838-5332
FAX: (504) 838-5349
http://www.lsbn.state.la.us/

Maine State Board of Nursing
158 State House Station
Augusta, ME 04333
Phone: (207) 287-1133
FAX: (207) 287-1149
http://www.state.me.us/pfr/auxboards/nurho
me.htm

Maryland Board of Nursing
4140 Patterson Avenue
Baltimore, MD 21215
Phone: (410) 585-1900
FAX: (410) 358-3530
http://dhmh1d.dhmh.state.md.us/mbn/

Massachusetts Board of Registration in Nursing
239 Causeway Street
Boston, MA 02114
Phone: (617) 727-9961
FAX: (617) 727-1630
http://www.state.ma.us/reg/boards/rn/

Michigan CIS/Office of Health Services
Ottawa Towers North
611 W. Ottawa, 4th Floor
Lansing, MI 48933
Phone: (517) 373-9102
FAX: (517) 373-2179
http://www.cis.state.mi.us/bhser/genover.htm

Minnesota Board of Nursing
2829 University Avenue S. E., Suite 500
Minneapolis, MN 55414

Phone: (612) 617–2270
FAX: (612) 617–2190
http://www.nursingboard.state.mn.us/

Mississippi Board of Nursing
1935 Lakeland Drive, Suite B
Jackson, MS 39216
Phone: (601) 987–4188
FAX: (601) 364–2352

Missouri State Board of Nursing
3605 Missouri Blvd.
P.O. Box 656
Jefferson City, MO 65102–0656
Phone: (573) 751–0681
FAX: (573) 751–0075
http://www.ecodev.state.mo.us/pr/nursing/

Montana State Board of Nursing
Arcade Building, Suite 4C
111 North Jackson
Helena, MT 59620–0513
Phone: (406) 444–2071
FAX: (406) 444–7759
http://www.com.state.mt.us/License/POL/
   index.htm

Nebraska Health and Human Services System
Department of Regulation and Licensure,
   Nursing Section
301 Centennial Mall South, P. O. Box 94986
Lincoln, NE 68509–4986
Phone: (402) 471–4376
FAX: (402) 471–3577
http://www.hhs.state.ne.us/crl/nns.htm

Nevada State Board of Nursing
1755 East Plumb Lane, Suite 260
Reno, NV 89502
Phone: (775) 688–2620
FAX: (775) 688–2628
http://www.state.nv.us/boards/nsbn/

New Hampshire Board of Nursing
78 Regional Drive, BLDG B

P.O. Box 3898
Concord, NH 03302
Phone: (603) 271–2323
FAX: (603) 271–6605
http://www.state.nh.us/nursing/

New Jersey Board of Nursing
124 Halsey Street, 6th Floor
P.O. Box 45010
Newark, NJ 07101
Phone: (973) 504–6586
FAX: (973) 648–3481
http://www.state.nj.us/lps/ca/medical.htm

New Mexico Board of Nursing
4206 Louisiana Boulevard, N. E., Suite A
Albuquerque, NM 87109
Phone: (505) 841–8340
FAX: (505) 841–8347
http://www.state.nm.us/clients/nursing

New York State Board of Nursing
State Education Department
Cultural Education Center, Room 3023
Albany, NY 12230
Phone: (518) 474–3845
FAX: (518) 474–3706
http://www.nysed.gov/prof/nurse.htm

North Carolina Board of Nursing
3724 National Drive
Raleigh, NC 27602
Phone: (919) 782–3211
FAX: (919) 781–9461
http://www.ncbon.com/

North Dakota Board of Nursing
919 South 7th Street, Suite 504
Bismark, ND 58504
Phone: (701) 328–9777
FAX: (701) 328–9785
http://www.ndbon.org/

Ohio Board of Nursing
17 South High Street, Suite 400
Columbus, OH 43215–3413

Phone: (614) 466–3947
FAX: (614) 466–0388
http://www.state.oh.us/nur/

Oklahoma Board of Nursing
2915 N. Classen Boulevard, Suite 524
Oklahoma City, OK 73106
Phone: (405) 962–1800
FAX: (405) 962–1821

Oregon State Board of Nursing
800 N. E. Oregon Street, Box 25, Suite 465
Portland, OR 97232
Phone: (503) 731–4745
FAX: (503) 731–4755
http://www.osbn.state.or.us/

Pennsylvania State Board of Nursing
124 Pine Street
P.O. Box 2649
Harrisburg, PA 17101
Phone: (717) 783–7142
FAX: (717) 783–0822
http://www.dos.state.pa.us/bpoa/nurbd.htm

Rhode Island Board of Nursing
Registration and Nursing Education
Cannon Health Building
Three Capitol Hill, Room 104
Providence, RI 02908
Phone: (401) 222–3855
FAX: (401) 222–2158

South Carolina State Board of Nursing
110 Centerview Drive, Suite 202
Columbia, SC 29210
Phone: (803) 896–4550
FAX: (803) 896–4525
http://www.llr.state.sc.us/bon.htm

South Dakota Board of Nursing
4300 South Louise Ave., Suite C–1
Sioux Falls, SD 57106–3124
Phone: (605) 362–2760
FAX: (605) 362–2768
http://www.state.sd.us/dcr/nursing/

Tennessee State Board of Nursing
426 Fifth Avenue North
1st Floor—Cordell Hull Building
Nashville, TN 37247
Phone: (615) 532–5166
FAX: (615) 741–7899
http://170.142.76.180/bmf-bin/BMFproflist.pl

Texas Board of Nurse Examiners
333 Guadalupe, Suite 3–460
Austin, TX 78701
Phone: (512) 305–7400
FAX: (512) 305–7401
http://www.bne.state.tx.us/

Utah State Board of Nursing
Heber M. Wells Bldg., 4th Floor
160 East 300 South
Salt Lake City, UT 84111
Phone: (801) 530–6628
FAX: (801) 530–6511
http://www.commerce.state.ut.us/

Vermont State Board of Nursing
109 State Street
Montpelier, VT 05609–1106
Phone: (802) 828–2396
FAX: (802) 828–2484
http://vtprofessionals.org/nurses/

Virginia Board of Nursing
6606 W. Broad Street, 4th Floor
Richmond, VA 23230
Phone: (804) 662–9909
FAX: (804) 662–9512
http://www.dhp.state.va.us/

Washington State Nursing Care Quality
    Assurance Commission
Department of Health
1300 Quince Street S. E.
Olympia, WA 98504–7864
Phone: (360) 236–4740
FAX: (360) 236–4738
http://www.doh.wa.gov/hsqa/hpqad/Nursing/

West Virginia Board of Examiners for
   Registered Professional Nurses
101 Dee Drive
Charleston, WV 25311
Phone: (304) 558–3596
FAX: (304) 558–3666
http://www.state.wv.us/nurses/rn/

Wisconsin Department of Regulation
   and Licensing
1400 E. Washington Avenue
P. O. Box 8935

Madison, WI 53708
Phone: (608) 266–2112
FAX: (608) 267–0644
http://www.state.wi.us/

Wyoming State Board of Nursing
2020 Carey Avenue, Suite 110
Cheyenne, WY 82002
Phone: (307) 777–7601
FAX: (307) 777–3519
http://commerce.state.wy.us/b%26c/nb/

Appendix D
NANDA-approved Nursing Diagnoses 1999–2000

Pattern 1: Exchanging

Altered nutrition: More than body
requirements
Altered nutrition: Less than body requirements
Altered nutrition: Risk for more than body
requirements
Risk for infection
Risk for altered body temperature
Hypothermia
Hyperthermia
Ineffective thermoregulation
Dysreflexia
Risk for autonomic dysreflexia
Constipation
Perceived constipation
Colonic constipation
Diarrhea
Bowel incontinence
Risk for constipation
Altered urinary elimination
Stress incontinence
Reflex urinary incontinence
Urge incontinence
Functional urinary incontinence
Total incontinence
Risk for urinary urge incontinence
Urinary retention
Altered tissue perfusion (specify type: renal,
cerebral, cardiopulmonary, gastrointestinal,
peripheral)
Risk for fluid volume imbalance
Fluid volume excess
Fluid volume deficit
Risk for fluid volume deficit
Decreased cardiac output
Impaired gas exchange
Ineffective airway clearance
Ineffective breathing pattern
Inability to sustain spontaneous ventilation
Dysfunctional ventilatory weaning response
Risk for injury
Risk for suffocation

Risk for poisoning
Risk for trauma
Risk for aspiration
Risk for disuse syndrome
Latex allergy response
Risk for latex allergy response
Altered protection
Impaired tissue integrity
Altered oral mucous membrane
Impaired skin integrity
Risk for impaired skin integrity
Altered dentition
Decreased adaptive capacity: Intracranial
Energy field disturbance

Pattern 2: Communicating

Impaired verbal communication

Pattern 3: Relating

Impaired social interaction
Social isolation
Risk for loneliness
Altered role performance
Altered parenting
Risk for altered parenting
Risk for altered parent/infant/child attachment
Sexual dysfunction
Altered family processes
Caregiver role strain
Risk for caregiver role strain
Altered family processes: Alcoholism
Parental role conflict
Altered sexuality patterns

Pattern 4: Valuing

Spiritual distress (distress of the human spirit)
Risk for spiritual distress
Potential for enhanced spiritual well-being

Pattern 5: Choosing

Ineffective individual coping
Impaired adjustment
Defensive coping
Ineffective denial
Ineffective family coping: Disabling
Ineffective family coping: Compromised
Family coping: Potential for growth
Potential for enhanced community coping
Ineffective community coping
Ineffective management of therapeutic
  regimen: Individuals
Noncompliance (specify)
Ineffective management of therapeutic
  regimen: Families
Ineffective management of therapeutic
  regimen: Community
Effective management of therapeutic regimen:
  Individual
Decisional conflict (specify)
Health-seeking behaviors (specify)

Pattern 6: Moving

Impaired physical mobility
Risk for peripheral neurovascular dysfunction
Risk for perioperative positioning injury
Impaired walking
Impaired wheelchair mobility
Impaired transfer ability
Impaired bed mobility
Activity intolerance
Fatigue
Risk for activity intolerance
Sleep pattern disturbance
Sleep deprivation
Diversional activity deficit
Impaired home maintenance management
Altered health maintenance
Delayed surgical recovery
Adult failure to thrive
Feeding self-care deficit
Impaired swallowing
Ineffective breast-feeding
Interrupted breast-feeding
Effective breast-feeding

Ineffective infant feeding pattern
Bathing/hygiene self-care deficit
Dressing/grooming self-care deficit
Toileting self-care deficit
Altered growth and development
Risk for altered development
Risk for altered growth
Relocation stress syndrome
Risk for disorganized infant behavior
Disorganized infant behavior
Potential for enhanced organized infant
  behavior

Pattern 7: Perceiving

Body image disturbance
Self-esteem disturbance
Chronic low self-esteem
Situational low self-esteem
Personal identity disturbance
Sensory/perceptual alterations (specify: visual,
  auditory, kinesthetic, gustatory, tactile,
  olfactory)
Unilateral neglect
Hopelessness
Powerlessness

Pattern 8: Knowing

Knowledge deficit (specify)
Impaired environmental interpretation
  syndrome
Acute confusion
Chronic confusion
Altered thought processes
Impaired memory

Pattern 9: Feeling

Pain
Chronic pain
Nausea
Dysfunctional grieving
Anticipatory grieving
Chronic sorrow
Risk for violence: Directed at others

Pattern 9: Feeling (continued)

Risk for self-mutilation
Risk for violence: Self-directed
Post-trauma syndrome
Rape-trauma syndrome

Rape-trauma syndrome: Compound reaction
Rape-trauma syndrome: Silent reaction
Risk for post-trauma syndrome
Anxiety
Death anxiety
Fear

Reprinted with permission of the North American Nursing Diagnosis Association (1999). *Nursing diagnoses: Definitions and classification, 1999–2000.* Philadelphia, Pa.: North American Nursing Diagnosis Association.

Glossary

AACN American Association of Colleges of Nursing.

Acceptance See Nonjudgmental acceptance.

Accountability Responsibility for one's behavior.

Accreditation A voluntary review process of educational programs or service agencies by professional organizations.

Action language A developmental phase in language development of older infants that consists of reaching for or crawling toward a desired object or of closing the lips and turning the head when an undesired food is offered.

Active collaborator Engaged as a participant with another person.

Active listening A method of communicating interest and attention using such signals as good eye contact, nodding, and encouraging the speaker.

Acuity Degree of illness.

Acute illness Sudden, steadily progressing symptoms that subside quickly with or without treatment, such as influenza.

Adaptation A change or coping response to stress of any kind.

Adaptation model A conceptual model that focuses on the patient as an adaptive system; that is, one that strives to cope with both internal demands and the external demands of the environment.

Adjudicate To decide or sit in judgment, as in a legal case.

Administrative law Law created by a governmental agency to meet the intent of statutory law.

Advance directives Written instructions recognized by state law that describe individuals' preferences in regard to medical intervention should they become incapacitated.

Advanced degrees Degrees beyond the bachelor's degree; master's and doctoral degrees.

Advanced practice Nursing roles that require either a master's degree or specialized education in a specific area.

Aesthetics Branch of philosophy that studies the nature of beauty.

Affective goal Effort directed toward a change in a patient's feelings, values, or belief system.

Alternative educational programs Programs other than basic nursing programs, such as baccalaureate programs for registered nurses and the New York Regents' External Degree Program.

Alternative treatment Treatment other than traditional Western medical treatment.

Altruism Unselfish concern for the welfare of others.

Ambulatory care Health services provided to those who visit a clinic or hospital as outpatients and depart after treatment on the same day.

ANA Position Paper A 1965 paper published by the American Nurses Association concluding that baccalaureate education should become the basic foundation for professional practice.

Analysis The second step in the nursing process during which various pieces of patient data are analyzed. The outcome is one or more nursing diagnoses.

Ancillary workers Nonprofessional auxiliary health care workers, such as nursing assistants.

Anxiety A diffuse, vague feeling of apprehension and uncertainty.

Applied science Use of scientific theory and laws in a practical way that has immediate application.

Appropriateness A criterion for successful communication in which the reply fits the circumstances and matches the message, and the amount is neither too great nor too little.

Articulation An educational mobility system providing for direct movement from a program at one level of nursing education to another without significant loss of credit.

Assault A threat or an attempt to make bodily contact with another person without the person's consent.

Assessment The first step in the nursing process involving the collection of information about the patient.

Assisted suicide Suicide by a person with help from another person, such as a health care provider.

Associate degree program The newest form of basic nursing education program leading to the associate degree (AD), consisting of three or fewer years, and usually offered in technical or community colleges.

Association An organization of members with common interests.

Authority Possessing both the responsibility for making decisions and the accountability for the outcome of those decisions.

Autonomy Self-governing; freedom from the influence of others.

Baccalaureate degree program Basic nursing education offered in four-year colleges and universities leading to the bachelor of science in nursing (BSN).

Balance of power A distribution of forces among the branches of government so that no one branch is strong enough to dominate the others.

Ball, Mary Ann (1817–1901) A Civil War woman who cared for the wounded and was known as "Mother Bickerdyke."

Barton, Clara (1821–1912) A famous Civil War nurse and founder of the American Red Cross.

Basic program Any nursing education program preparing beginning practitioners.

Battery The unpermissible, unprivileged touching of one person by another.

Belief The intellectual acceptance of something as true or correct.

Beneficence The ethical principle of doing good.

Benner, Patricia Nursing theorist who proposed seven domains of nursing practice based on her research into the nature of nurses' knowledge.

Mother Bickerdyke Affectionate nickname given by soldiers to Mary Ann Ball, a Civil War lay nurse.

Biculturalism A term used to describe nurses who learn to balance the ideal nursing culture they learned about in school and the real one they experience in practice, using the best of both.

Bioethics An area of ethical inquiry focusing on the dilemmas inherent in modern health care.

Biomedical technology Complex machines or implantable devices used in patient care settings.

Birthrate   The number of births in a particular place during a specific time period, usually given as a quantity per 1,000 people in a year.

Breckinridge, Mary   Founder of the Frontier Nursing Service in 1925.

BRN   Baccalaureate registered nurse, a term sometimes used to describe a registered nurse who has returned to school to earn a bachelor's degree.

Brown Report   A 1948 report recommending that basic schools of nursing be placed in universities and colleges and that efforts be made to recruit large numbers of men and minorities into nursing education programs.

Cadet Corps   A World War II, government-created entity designed to rapidly increase the number of registered nurses being educated to assist in the war effort.

Capitation   A cost management system in which a certain amount of money is paid to a provider annually to take care of all of an individual's or group's health care needs.

"Captain of the ship" doctrine   A legal principle that implies that the physician is in charge of all patient care and, thus, should be financially responsible if damages are sought.

Caring   Watching over, attending to, and providing for the needs of others.

Case management   Systematic collaboration with patients, their significant others, and their health care providers to coordinate high quality health care services in a cost-effective manner with positive patient outcomes.

Case management nursing   A growing field within nursing in which nurses are responsible for coordinating services provided to patients in a cost-effective manner.

Case manager   An individual responsible for coordinating services provided to a group of patients.

CCNE   Commission on Collegiate Nursing Education, an arm of the American Association of Colleges of Nursing.

Centenarian   A person who has reached the age of 100 or more years.

Certificate of need (CON)   A cost-containment measure requiring health care agencies to apply to a state agency for permission to construct or substantially add to an existing facility.

Certified nurse-midwife   A nationally certified nurse with advanced specialized education who assists women and couples during uncomplicated pregnancies, deliveries, and postdelivery periods.

Certified Registered Nurse Anesthetist (CRNA)   A nationally certified nurse with advanced education who specializes in the administration of anesthesia.

Certification   Validation of specific qualifications demonstrated by a registered nurse in a defined area of practice.

Change agent   An individual who recognizes the need for organizational change and facilitates that process.

Chief executive officer (CEO)   The senior administrator of an organization.

Chief nurse executive   The senior nursing administrator of an organization.

Chief of staff   A physician in a health care facility, generally elected by the medical staff for a limited term, who is responsible for overseeing the activities of the medical staff organization.

Chronic illness   Ongoing health problems of a generally incurable nature, such as diabetes.

Civil law   Law involving disputes between individuals.

Clarification   A therapeutic communication technique in which the nurse seeks to understand a patient's message more clearly.

Clinical coordinator   See Clinical director.

Clinical director   Middle management nurse who has responsibility for multiple units in a health care agency.

Clinical judgment   The ability to make consistently effective clinical decisions based on theoretical knowledge, informed opinions, and prior experience.

Clinical ladder   Programs allowing nurses to progress in the organizational hierarchy while staying in direct patient care roles.

Clinical nurse specialist   A nurse with an advanced degree who serves as a resource person to other nurses and often provides direct care to patients or families with particularly difficult or complex problems.

Closed system   A system that does not interact with other systems or with the surrounding environment.

Coalition   A temporary alliance of distinct factions.

Code for Nurses   A statement of the nursing profession's code of ethics.

Code of ethics   A statement of professional standards used to guide behavior and as a framework for decision making.

Cognitive   Pertaining to intellectual activities requiring knowledge.

Cognitive goal   Effort directed toward a desired change in a patient's knowledge level.

Cognitive rebellion   A stage in the educational process wherein students begin to free themselves from external controls and to rely on their own judgment.

Collaboration   Working closely with another person in the spirit of cooperation.

Collective action   Activities undertaken by or on behalf of a group of people who have common interests.

Collective bargaining   Negotiating for improved salary and work conditions.

Collegiality   The promotion of collaboration, cooperation, and recognition of interdependence among members of a profession.

Common law   Law that comes about as a result of decisions made by judges in legal cases.

Communication   The exchange of thoughts, ideas, or information; a dynamic process that is a primary instrument through which change occurs in nursing situations.

Community-based nursing   Nursing care provided for individuals, families, and groups in a variety of settings, including homes, workplaces, schools, and other places.

Community health nursing   Formerly known as public health nursing; a nursing specialty that systematically uses a process of delivering nursing care to improve the health of an entire community.

Competency   Refers to the capability of a particular patient to understand the information given and to make an informed choice about treatment options.

Concept   An abstract classification of data; for example, "temperature" is a concept.

Conceptual model or framework   A group of concepts that are broadly defined and systematically organized to provide a focus, a rationale, and a tool for the integration and interpretation of information.

Confidentiality   Assuring the privacy of individuals participating in research studies or being treated in health care settings.

Congruent   A characteristic of communication that occurs when the verbal and nonverbal elements of a message match.

Consultation   The process of conferring with patients, families, or other health professionals.

Consumerism   A movement to protect consumers from unsafe or inferior products and services.

Contact hour   A measurement used to recognize participation in continuing education offerings, usually equivalent to 50 minutes.

Context   An essential element of communication consisting of the setting in which an interaction occurs, the mood, the relationship between sender and receiver, and other factors.

Continuing education (CE) Informal ways, such as workshops, conferences, and short courses, in which nurses maintain competence during their professional careers.

Continuous quality improvement (CQI) A management concept focusing on excellence and employee involvement at all levels of an organization.

Contracts Documents agreed to by workers and management that include provisions about staffing levels, salary, work conditions, and other issues of concern to either party.

Copayment The portion of a provider's charges that an insured patient is responsible for paying.

Coping The methods a person uses to assess and manage demands.

Coping mechanisms Psychological devices used by individuals when a threat is perceived.

Cost containment An attempt to keep health care costs stable or increasing only slowly.

Criminal law Law involving public concerns against unlawful behavior that threatens society.

Critical paths Multidisciplinary care plans.

Cross-functional team People from all parts of an organization who contribute to a particular activity and outcome.

Cross-training Preparing a single worker for multiple tasks that formerly were performed by multiple specialized workers.

Cultural assessment The process of determining a patient's cultural practices and preferences in order to render culturally competent care.

Cultural care, theory of A nursing theory focusing on the importance of incorporating a patient's culturally determined health beliefs and practices into care.

Cultural competence The integration of knowledge, attitudes, and skills that enhance cross-cultural communication and appropriate interactions with others.

Cultural diversity Social, ethnic, racial, and religious differences in a group.

Culturally competent care Nursing care that incorporates knowledge, attitudes, and skills that enhance cross-cultural communication and appropriate interactions with others.

Culture The attitudes, beliefs, and behaviors of social and ethnic groups that have been perpetuated through generations.

Culture of nursing The rites, rituals, and valued behaviors of the nursing profession.

Curtis, Namahyoke The first trained African-American nurse employed as a military hospital nurse during the Spanish-American War of 1898.

Data Information or facts collected for analysis.

Davis, Mary E. One of the founders of the *American Journal of Nursing.*

Deaconess Institute A large hospital and planned training program for deaconesses established in 1836 by Pastor Theodor Fliedner at Kaiserswerth, Germany.

Decentralization An organizational structure in which decision-making authority is shared with employees most affected by the decisions rather than being retained by top executives.

Deductible The amount individuals must pay out-of-pocket before their health insurance begins to pay for health care.

Deductive reasoning A process through which conclusions are drawn by logical inference from given premises; proceeds from the general case to the specific.

Defining characteristics Signs and symptoms of disease.

Delegate To refer a task to another.

Delegation The practice of assigning tasks or responsibilities to other persons.

Demographics The study of vital statistics and social trends.

Demography The science that studies vital statistics and social trends.

Deontology The ethical theory that the rightness or wrongness of an action depends on the inherent moral significance of the action.

Dependency The degree to which individuals adopt passive attitudes and rely on others to take care of them.

Dependent intervention Nursing actions on behalf of patients that require knowledge and skill on the part of the nurse but may not be done without explicit directions from another health professional, usually a physician, dentist, or nurse practitioner.

Designer medicines Pharmacological agent developed for an individual, based on his or her genetic makeup.

Developmental theory A theory in which growth is defined as an increase in physical size and shape to a point of optimal maturity.

Diagnosis Identification of a disease or condition.

Diagnosis-related groups (DRGs) A method of classifying and grouping illnesses according to similarities of diagnosis for reimbursement purposes.

Dietitian Bachelor's-educated nutrition expert who specializes in therapeutic diet preparation and nutrition education.

Differentiated practice Nursing practice at two levels, professional and technical, with differences in both educational preparation and clinical responsibilities.

Diploma program The earliest form of formal nursing education in the United States, diploma programs are usually based in hospitals, require three years of study, and lead to a diploma in nursing.

Disease A pathological alteration at the tissue or organ level.

Disenfranchised The state of having no power or no voice in a political system.

Disseminate Publish or widely distribute scientific information, such as the findings of a research study.

Dissonance Lack of harmony.

Distance learning The process of taking classes and earning academic credit through technological means such as televised or online classes. The teacher and student may be many miles apart.

Dix, Dorthea L. A Boston schoolteacher, devoted to the care of the mentally ill, who served as the first superintendent of the Women Nurses of the Army during the Civil War.

Dock, Lavinia A well-known early twentieth-century nurse who was actively involved in women's rights issues and the suffragette movement.

Documentation Written communication about patient care, usually found in the patient record.

Dominant culture Mainstream culture that contains one or more subcultures.

Double effect Ethical concept encompassing the belief that there are some situations when it is necessary to inflict potential harm in an effort to achieve a greater good.

Duty of care The responsibility of a nurse or other health professional for the care of a patient.

Duty to report The requirement, according to state law, for health professionals to report certain illnesses, injuries, and actions of patients.

Economic and general welfare Employment issues relating to salaries, benefits, and working conditions.

Educative instrument A tool for increasing the knowledge and power of another person.

Efficiency A criterion for successful communication that consists of using simple, clear words timed at a pace suitable to participants.

Electoral process   The procedures that must be followed to select someone to fill an elected position.

Elliott, Francis Reed   The first African-American nurse accepted by the American Red Cross Nursing Service in 1918.

Empathy   Awareness of, sensitivity to, and identification with the feelings of another person.

Entrepreneur   A person who sees a need for, organizes, manages, and assumes responsibility for a new enterprise or business.

Environment   All the many factors, such as physical or psychological, that influence life and survival.

Epidemiologist   A scientist who studies the origins and transmission of diseases.

Epistemology   The branch of philosophy dealing with the theory of knowledge.

Ethical decision making   The process of choosing between actions based on a system of beliefs and values.

Ethics   The branch of philosophy that studies the propriety of certain courses of action.

Ethnocentric   The belief that one's own culture is the most desirable.

Euthanasia   The act of putting to death painlessly a person suffering from an incurable disease; mercy killing.

Evaluation   Measuring the success or failure of the outputs and consequently the effectiveness of a system. It is the final step in the nursing process wherein the nurse examines the patient's progress to determine if a problem is solved, is in the process of being solved, or is unsolved. In communication theory, the analysis of information received.

Evidence-based practice   Using research findings as a basis for practice rather than trial and error, intuition, or traditional methods.

Exacerbation   Reemergence or worsening of the symptoms of a chronic illness.

Executive branch   The branch of government responsible for administering the laws of the land.

Experimental design   Research design that provides evidence of a cause-and-effect relationship between actions.

Expert witness   An individual called upon to testify in court because of special skill or knowledge in a certain field, such as nursing.

Extended care   Medical, nursing, or custodial care provided to an individual over a prolonged period of time.

Extended family   A term used to describe nonnuclear family members such as grandparents, aunts, and uncles.

External degree program   An alternative program in which learning is independent and is assessed through highly standardized and validated examinations.

External factors   Impact on individuals of the values, beliefs, and behaviors of the significant people around them.

False reassurance   A nontherapeutic form of communication.

Famous trio   Three famous schools of nursing founded in 1873: the Bellevue Training School, the Connecticut Training School, and the Boston Training School.

Feedback   The information given back into a system to determine whether or not the purpose of the system has been achieved. A major element in the communication process.

Feminism   The study of gender inequalities; belief in the value and equality of women.

Flexibility   A criterion for successful communication that occurs when messages are based on the immediate situation rather than preconceived expectations.

Flexible staffing   A mechanism whereby nurses work at times other than the traditional hospital shifts.

Flexner Report   A 1910 study of medical education that provided the impetus for much-needed reform.

Ford, Lorretta   With Dr. E. K. Silver, founded the nurse practitioner movement in the United States in the mid-1960's.

Formal socialization   The process by which individuals learn a new role through what others purposely teach them.

For-profit agency   A health care agency that is established to make a profit for the owners or stockholders.

Franklin, Martha   Founder, in 1908, of the National Association of Colored Graduate Nurses (NACGN).

Frontier Nursing Service   Founded in 1925, the Frontier Nursing Service provided the first organized midwifery service in the United States.

Functional nursing   A system of nursing care delivery in which each worker has a task, or function, to perform for all patients.

Futurist   An individual who studies trends and makes predictions about the future.

Galileo   An Italian physicist and astronomer who lived from 1564 to 1642.

Gatekeeper   An individual, generally a primary care physician, who controls patients' access to diagnostic procedures, medical specialists, and hospitalization.

General election   An election in which all registered voters may vote and may choose a candidate from any party on the ballot.

General systems theory   A theory promulgated by Ludwig von Bertalanffy in the late 1930s to explain the relationship of a whole to its parts.

Generalizable   Research findings that are transferable to other situations.

Generic master's degree   An accelerated master's degree in nursing for people with nonnursing bachelor's degrees.

Generic nursing doctorate   A doctoral degree program designed for individuals who are not already registered nurses and who possess baccalaureate degrees in other fields.

Genetic counseling   Health and reproductive advice given to individuals based on their genetic makeup.

Goldmark Report   A major study of nursing education published in 1923 and named *The Study of Nursing and Nursing Education in the United States.*

Goodrich, Annie   Served as assistant professor of nursing at Teachers College, head of the Army School of Nursing (formed in 1918), president of the American Nurses Association, and first dean of the school of nursing at Yale University.

Governmental (public) agency   An agency primarily supported by taxes, administered by elected or appointed officials, and tailored to the needs of the communities served.

Grass-roots activism   The involvement of a large number of people, generally widely dispersed, who are concerned about a particular issue.

Growth   An increase in physical size and shape to a point of optimal maturity.

Hardiness   A personality characteristic that enables people to manage the changes associated with illness and to have fewer physical illnesses resulting from stress.

Health   An individual's physical, mental, spiritual, and social well-being; a continuum, not a constant state.

Health behaviors   Choices and habitual actions that promote or diminish health.

Health beliefs   Culturally determined beliefs about the nature of health and illness.

Health Care Financing Administration (HCFA)   The federal agency charged with the responsibility of overseeing the Medicare and Medicaid systems.

Health care network A corporation with a consolidated set of facilities and services for comprehensive health care.

Health maintenance Preventing illness and maintaining maximal function.

Health maintenance organization (HMO) A network or group of providers who agree to provide certain basic health care services for a single predetermined yearly fee.

Health promotion Encouraging a condition of maximum physical, mental, and social well-being.

Health promotion model A theoretical nursing model that uses illness prevention and health promotion as a basic framework.

Helping professions Professions such as social work, teaching, and nursing that emphasize meeting the needs of clients.

Henderson, Virginia An influential twentieth-century nursing author and theorist who was widely known for her nursing textbooks, insightful definition of nursing, and identification of 14 basic patient needs.

Henry Street Settlement A clinic for the poor founded by Lillian Wald and her colleague, Mary Brewster, on New York's Lower East Side.

Heterogeneous Composed of parts of different kinds.

High-level wellness Functioning at maximum potential in an integrated way within the environment.

High-tech nursing Nursing care that involves the use of technologies such as monitors, pumps, and ventilators.

High-touch nursing Nursing care that involves the use of interpersonal skills such as communication, listening, and empathy.

Hill-Burton Act A 1946 federal law that called for and funded surveys of states' needs for hospitals, paid for planning hospitals and public health centers, and provided partial funding for constructing and equipping them.

Hippocrates (400 B.C.) A Greek physician who believed that disease had natural, not magical, causes; known as the father of medicine.

Holism A school of health care thought that espouses treating the whole patient: body, mind, and spirit.

Home health agency An organization that delivers various health services to patients in their homes.

Home health nursing Rapidly growing field of nursing in which nursing care is provided to patients in their own homes.

Homeostasis A relative constancy in the internal environment of the body.

Homogeneous Composed of parts of the same or similar kinds.

Hospice An agency that provides services to terminally ill patients and their families.

Human caring, theory of Nursing theory emphasizing the nurturing aspects of professional nursing through which curative strategies are implemented.

Human Genome Project A scientific project designed to map the genetic structure of composite human DNA.

Human motivation Abraham Maslow's conceptualization of human needs and their relationship to the stimulation of purposeful behavior.

Humanistic nursing care Care that includes viewing professional relationships as human-to-human rather than nurse-to-patient.

Hypothesis A statement predicting the relationship among various concepts or events.

Illness An abnormal process in which an individual's physical, emotional, social, or intellectual functioning is impaired.

Illness prevention All activities aimed at diminishing the likelihood that an individual's physical, emotional, social, and intellectual functions become impaired.

Implementation A stage of the nursing process during which the plan of care is carried out.

Incongruent Confusing form of communication that occurs when the verbal and nonverbal elements of a message do not match.

Independent intervention Actions on behalf of patients for which the nurse requires no supervision or direction.

Inductive reasoning The process of reasoning from the specific to the general. Repeated observations of an experiment or event enable the observer to draw general conclusions.

Inertia Disinclination to change.

Informal socialization The process through which individuals learn a new role by observing how others behave.

Informatics nurse A nurse who combines nursing science with information management science and computer science to manage and make accessible information nurses need.

Information technology Hardware and software used to manage and process information.

Informed consent The process of asking individuals who are scheduled to undergo diagnostic procedures or surgery or who are potential research subjects to sign a consent form after describing the procedures and risks involved and ensuring their privacy.

Infrastructure Basic support mechanisms needed to ensure that an activity can be conducted.

Input The information, energy, or matter that enters a system.

Institutional review board A committee that ensures that research is well designed and ethical and does not violate the policies and procedures of the institution in which it is conducted.

Institutional structure The way in which the workers within an agency are organized to carry out the functions of the agency.

Interdependent intervention Actions on behalf of patients in which the nurse must collaborate or consult with another health professional before carrying out the action.

Interdisciplinary team Group composed of individuals representing various disciplines who work together toward a common end.

Internal factors Personal feelings and beliefs that influence an individual.

Internalize The process of taking in knowledge, skills, attitudes, beliefs, norms, values, and ethical standards and making them a part of one's own self-image and behavior.

Internship An apprenticeship under supervision.

Irrational belief A fixed idea that is not affected by information to the contrary.

Issues management Assisting a group to resolve a particular question to which there are significant differences of opinion.

Job hopping Moving rapidly from job to job.

Johnson, Dorothy Nursing theorist who proposed a system of nursing based on observation of patient behavior.

Judicial branch The branch of government that decides cases or controversies on particular matters.

Justice An ethical principle stating that equals should be treated the same and that unequals should be treated differently.

King, Imogene Nursing theorist who proposed a theory of goal attainment.

Knowledge-based power Authority or control based upon the way information is used to effect an outcome.

Knowledge technology   The use of computer systems to transform information into knowledge and to generate new knowledge; expert systems.

Latent power   Untapped ability.

Law   All the rules of conduct established by a government and applicable to the people, whether in the form of legislation or custom.

Learned resourcefulness   An acquired ability to use available resources in one's behalf.

Legal authority   A group of people in whom power is vested by law, such as the powers vested in state boards of nursing by nursing practice acts.

Legislative branch   The branch of government consisting of elected officials who are responsible for enacting the laws of the land.

Leininger, Madeleine   Nurse theorist best known for her theory of cultural care.

Levine, Myra   Nursing theorist who proposed a model based on principles of wholeness, adaptation, and conservation.

Licensure   The process by which an agency of government grants permission to qualified persons to engage in a given profession or occupation.

Licensure by endorsement   A system whereby registered nurses or licensed practical/vocational nurses can, by submitting proof of licensure in another state and paying a licensure fee, receive licensure from the new state without sitting for a licensing examination.

Lobby   An attempt to influence the vote of legislators.

Logic   The field of philosophy that studies correct and incorrect reasoning.

Long-term care   Care provided to individuals, such as people with Alzheimer's disease, who require lengthy assistance in the maintenance of activities of daily living.

Long-term goals   Major changes that may take months or even years to accomplish.

Lysaught Report   A 1970 report entitled *An Abstract for Action* that made recommendations concerning the supply and demand for nurses, nursing roles and functions, and nursing education.

Mahoney, Mary Eliza   America's first African-American "trained nurse," who lived from 1845 to 1926.

Malpractice   An unintentional tort that occurs when a professional fails to act as a reasonably prudent professional would under specific circumstances.

Managed care   A process in which an individual, often a nurse, is assigned to review patients' cases and coordinate services so that quality care can be achieved at the lowest cost.

Managed care organization (MCO)   Any of a number of organizations that attempt to coordinate subscriber services to ensure quality care at the lowest cost.

Mandatory continuing education   The requirement that nurses complete a certain number of hours of continuing education as a prerequisite for relicensure.

Maslow, Abraham   An American humanistic psychologist who formulated a theory of human motivation in the 1940s.

Maximum health potential   The highest level of well-being that an individual is capable of attaining.

Medicaid   A jointly funded federal and state public health insurance that covers citizens below the poverty level and those with certain disabling conditions; established in 1965.

Medical paternalism   The attitude that health care providers know best and that "good" patients simply follow directions without asking questions.

Medicare   A federally funded form of public health insurance for citizens 65 years of age and above; established in 1965.

Members   In professional associations, members may be either individuals, agencies such as schools of nursing, or other associations. For example, in the ANA, the members are the state associations, whereas in the NLN, members may be either individuals or organizations.

Mentor   An experienced nurse who shares knowledge with less experienced nurses to help advance their careers.

Message   An essential element of communication consisting of the spoken word, plus accompanying nonverbal communication.

Metaparadigm   The most abstract aspect of the structure of knowledge; the global concepts which identify the phenomena of interest for a discipline.

Metaphysics   The branch of philosophy that considers the ultimate nature of existence, reality, and experience.

Milieu   Surroundings or environment.

Model   A symbolic representation of reality.

Modeling   An informal type of socialization that occurs when an individual chooses an admired person to emulate.

Montag, Dr. Mildred   Originator, in 1952, of the concept of associate degree nursing education.

Moonlighting   The practice of working a second job after the regular one.

Moral development   The ways in which a person learns to deal with moral dilemmas from childhood through adulthood.

Morals   Established rules or standards that guide behavior in situations in which a decision about right and wrong must be made.

Morbidity rate   The incidence or occurrence of a certain illness in a particular population during a specific period of time, usually given as a quantity of 1,000 people in a specific year.

Mortality rate   The number of deaths in a particular population during a specific period of time, usually given as a quantity of 1,000 people in a specific year.

Multidrug resistant strains   Microorganisms, such as tuberculosis, which have become immune to the effects of drugs that formerly were effective against them.

Multiskilled worker   Individual who has been cross-trained to perform a number of tasks formerly performed by a series of specialized workers.

Mutuality   Sharing jointly with others.

Mutual recognition model   A system whereby a registered nurse could be licensed in the state of residency yet practice in other states, after being recognized by them, without additional licenses.

National Practitioner Data Bank   A national clearinghouse containing reports of adverse incidents involving physicians, nurses, and other health care providers that may be useful to potential employers or patients.

NCLEX-PN   National Council Licensing Examination for Practical Nurses, the examination graduates of practical nursing programs must take to become licensed to practice as licensed practical nurses (LPNs) or licensed vocational nurses (LVNs).

NCLEX-RN   National Council Licensing Examination for Registered Nurses, the examination graduates of basic nursing programs must take to become licensed to practice as registered nurses (RNs).

Negligence   The failure to act as a reasonably prudent person would have in specific circumstances.

Neuman, Betty   Nursing theorist who developed a systems model of nursing.

Newman, Margaret   Nursing theorist who developed a theory of health as expanding consciousness.

Newton, Isaac   English philosopher and mathematician who lived from 1642 to 1727.

Nightingale, Florence   Nineteenth-century English woman known as the founder of modern nursing and nursing education.

NLN   National League for Nursing.

NLNAC   The National League for Nursing Accreditation Commission.

Nonexperimental design   Research design in which the research subjects are not influenced in any way.

Nonjudgmental   An attitude that conveys neither approval nor disapproval of patients' beliefs and respects each person's right to his or her beliefs.

Nonjudgmental acceptance   An attitude that conveys neither approval nor disapproval of patients or their personal beliefs, habits, expressions of feelings, or chosen lifestyles.

Nonmaleficence   To inflict no harm or evil.

Nonverbal communication   Communication without words; consists of grooming, clothing, gestures, posture, facial expressions, tone and loudness of voice, and actions, among other things.

North American Nursing Diagnosis Association (NANDA)   Group working since 1970 to establish a comprehensive list of nursing diagnoses.

Not-for-profit agency   An organization that does not attempt to make a profit for distribution to owners or stockholders. Money made by such organizations is used to operate and improve the organization itself.

Nuclear family   Term used to describe a mother and father and their children.

Nurse activist   A nurse who works actively on behalf of a political candidate or certain legislation.

Nurse anesthetist   A nurse with specialized advanced education who administers anesthetic agents to patients undergoing operative procedures.

Nurse citizen   A nurse who exercises all the political rights accorded citizens, such as registering to vote and voting in all elections.

Nurse executive   The top nurse in the administrative structure of a health care organization.

Nurse manager   Also known as a head nurse, a nurse manager is in charge of all activities in a unit, including patient care, continuous quality improvement, personnel selection and evaluation, and resource (supplies and money) management.

Nurse-midwife   A nurse with advanced specialized education who assists women and couples during uncomplicated pregnancies, deliveries, and postdelivery periods.

Nurse-patient relationship   The mode of connection between a nurse and patient.

Nurse politician   A nurse who runs for political office.

Nurse practice act   Law defining the scope of nursing practice in a given state.

Nurse practitioner   A nurse with advanced education who specializes in primary health care of a particular group, such as children, pregnant women, or the elderly.

Nursing   The provision of health care services, focusing on the maintenance, promotion, and restoration of health.

Nursing diagnosis   A process of describing a patient's response to health problems that either already exist or may occur in the future.

Nursing informatics   The branch of nursing that manages knowledge and data through technology with the goal of improving patient care.

Nursing information system   A software system that automates the nursing process.

Nursing Interventions Classification (NIC)   A classification system describing more than 400 treatments that nurses perform in all specialties and all settings.

Nursing orders   Actions designed to assist the patient in achieving a stated patient goal.

Nursing Outcomes Classification (NOC)   A system of patient outcomes sensitive to nursing interventions.

Nursing process   A cognitive activity that requires both critical and creative thinking and serves as the basis for providing nursing care. A method used by nurses in dealing with patient problems in professional practice.

Nursing research   The systematic investigation of events or circumstances related to improving nursing care.

Nutting, Adelaide M.   An early twentieth-century nurse activist, first professor of nursing in the world, and a cofounder of the *American Journal of Nursing.*

Objective data   Factual information obtained through observation and examination of the patient or through consultation with other health care providers.

Occupation   A person's principal work or business.

Occupational health nurse   A nurse specializing in the care of a specific group of workers in a given occupational setting.

Open-ended question   An inquiry that causes the patient to answer fully, giving more than a "yes" or "no" answer.

Open posture   Bodily position, squarely facing another person, with arms in a relaxed position.

Open system   A system that promotes the exchange of matter, energy, and information with other systems and the environment.

Orem, Dorothea   Nursing theorist known for her model focusing on patients' self-care needs and nursing actions designed to meet patients' needs.

Orientation phase   The beginning phase of a nurse-patient relationship in which the parties are getting acquainted with one another.

Orlando, Ida   Nursing theorist who proposed a theory of nursing process.

Outcome criteria   Patient goals.

Out-of-pocket payment   Direct payment for health services from individuals' personal funds.

Output   The end result or product of a system.

Palmer, Sophia   First editor of the *American Journal of Nursing.*

Paramedical   Having to do with the field of medicine; generally used to describe ancillary workers such as emergency medical technicians.

Parish nurse   A specialized nurse that focuses on the promotion of health within the context of the values, beliefs, and practices of a faith community.

Parse, Rosemarie   Nursing theorist who proposed a theory of human becoming.

Patient acuity   Assessment of the degree of illness of a particular patient or group of patients, used to determine staffing needs.

Patient advocate   One who promotes the interest of patients. A nursing role.

Patient classification system (PCS)   Identification of patients' needs for nursing care in quantitative terms.

Patient-focused care   A system that emphasizes coordinating patient care to maximize patient comfort, convenience, and security.

Patient interview   A face-to-face interaction with the patient in which an interviewer elicits pertinent information.

Patient Self-Determination Act   Effective December 1, 1991, this law encourages patients to consider which life-prolonging treatment options they desire and to document their preferences in case they should later become incapable of participating in the decision-making process.

Patients' rights   Responsibilities that a hospital and its staff have toward patients and their families during hospitalization.

Pay equity   Equal pay for work of comparable value.

Peer review process   The process of submitting one's work for examination and comment by colleagues in the same profession.

Pember, Phoebe   A Southern nurse during the Civil War who was made Matron of the huge Chimborazo Hospital in Richmond.

Pender, Nola   A nurse theorist best known for her health promotion model of professional nursing.

Perception   The selection, organization, and interpretation of incoming signals into meaningful messages.

Person   An individual—man, woman, or child.

Personal payment   Direct payment for health services from individuals' personal funds.

Personal space   The amount of space surrounding individuals in which they feel comfortable interacting with others; usually culturally determined.

Personal value system   The social principles, ideals, or standards held by an individual that form the basis for meaning, direction, and decision making in life.

Petry, Lucille   The first woman appointed to the position of Assistant Surgeon General of the United States Public Health Service in 1949.

Pew Health Professions Commission   One of three major national groups that in 1993 issued reports or studies of nursing education in the United States.

Phenomenon   An occurrence or circumstance that is observable.

Phenomenological inquiry/research   A qualitative research approach focusing on what people experience in regard to a particular phenomenon, such as grief, and how they interpret those experiences.

Philosophy   The study of the truths and principles of being, knowledge, or conduct.

Physician hospital organization (PHO)   A separate corporation formed by a hospital and a group of its medical staff for the purpose of joint contracting with managed care organizations and businesses.

Planning   The third step in the nursing process that begins with the identification of patient goals.

Point-of-care technology   Information system used for entering patient data directly from the bedside.

Point-of-service organization (POS)   A hybrid preferred provider organization in which the consumer selects service providers within the defined network or may go outside the network and pay a higher deductible or copayment.

Policy   The principles and values that govern actions directed toward given ends. Policy sets forth a plan, direction, or goal for action.

Policy development   The generation of principles and procedures that guide governmental or organizational action.

Policy outcome   The result of decisions made by governmental or organizational leaders who choose a certain course of action.

Political action committees (PACs)   Groups that raise and distribute money to candidates who support their organization's stand on certain issues.

Politics   The area of philosophy that deals with the regulation and control of people living in society; in government, the allocation of scarce resources.

Population   The entire group of people possessing a given characteristic, such as all brown-eyed people over the age of 65.

Position power   Authority and control accorded to an individual who holds an important role in an organization, profession, or government.

Power grabbing   Hoarding control, taking it from others, or wielding it over others.

Power sharing   A process of equalizing resources, knowledge, or control.

Powers of appointment   The authority to select the people who serve in positions such as judges, ambassadors, and cabinet officials.

Practical nurse program   A one-year educational program preparing individuals for direct patient care roles under the supervision of a physician or registered nurse.

Preceptor   A teacher; in nursing, usually an experienced nurse who assumes responsibility for teaching a novice.

Preferred provider organization (PPO)   A form of HMO that contracts with independent providers such as physicians and hospitals for a negotiated discount for services provided to its members.

Premium   The amount paid for an insurance policy, usually in installments.

Primary care   Basic health care, including promotion of health, early diagnosis of disease, and prevention of disease.

Primary election   An election in which voters who are declared members of a political party choose among several candidates of that same party for a particular office.

Primary nursing   A system of nursing care delivery in which one nurse has responsibility for the planning, implementation, and evaluation of the care of one or more clients 24 hours a day for the duration of the hospital stay.

Primary source   The patient is considered a primary source of data about himself or herself.

Private insurance   Insurance obtained from a privately owned company, as opposed to public or governmental insurance.

Private practice   Nursing practice, engaged in by nurses with advanced education, that is usually provided on a fee-for-service basis, similar to medical practice.

Privileged communications   The principle that information given to certain professionals is so confidential in nature as not even to be disclosed in court.

Problem solving   A method of finding solutions to difficulties specific to a given situation and designed for immediate action.

Profession   Work requiring advanced training and usually involving mental rather than manual effort.

Professional   A person who engages in one of the professions, such as law or medicine.

Professional accountabilities   A basic set of responsibilities of all professional nurses regardless of practice setting.

Professional association   An organization consisting of people belonging to the same profession and thereby having many common interests.

Professional boundary   The dividing line between the activities of two professions.

Professional governance   The concept that health care professionals have a right and a responsibility to govern their own work and time within a financially secure, patient-centered system.

Professional practice advocacy   Includes activities such as education, lobbying, and advocating individually and collectively to advance a profession's agenda.

Professionalism   Professional behavior, appearance, and conduct.

Professional review organization (PRO)   Organizations that review Medicare hospital admissions and Medicare patients' lengths of stay.

Professional socialization   The process of developing an occupational identity.

Proposition   A statement about how two or more concepts are related.

Prospective payment system (PPS)   A cost-containment mechanism wherein providers, such as physicians and hospitals, receive payment on a per case basis, regardless of the cost of delivering the services.

Protocol   A written plan specifying the procedure to be followed.

Provider   A deliverer of health care services: hospital, clinic, nurse, or physician.

Proximate cause   Action occurring immediately before an injury, thereby assumed to be the reason for the injury.

Psychomotor goal   Effort directed toward a change in motor skills or actions by a patient.

Pure science   Summarizes and explains the universe without regard for whether the information is immediately useful; also known as "basic science."

Qualitative research   Answers questions that cannot be answered by quantitative designs and that must be addressed by more subjective methods.

Quality management   See Total quality management.

Quantitative research   Research that is objective and uses data-gathering techniques that can be repeated by others and verified. Data collected are quantifiable; that is, they can be counted, measured with standardized instruments, or observed with a high degree of agreement among observers.

Receiver   An essential element of communication consisting of the person receiving the message.

Reengineering   Radical redesign of business processes and thinking to improve performance.

Referendum   An election resulting from registered voters being asked by a legislative body to express a preference on a policy issue.

Reflection   A communication technique that consists of encouraging patients to think through problems for themselves by directing questions back to the patient.

Reflective thinking   The process of evaluating one's thinking processes during a situation that has already occurred, as opposed to evaluating one's thinking during the situation as it occurs.

Registered nurse (RN)   An individual who has completed a basic program for registered nurses and successfully completed the licensing examination.

Rehabilitation services   Those activities designed to restore an individual or a body part to normal or near-normal function following a disease or an accident.

Reliable   Yielding the same values dependably each time an instrument is used to measure the same thing.

Reality shock   The feelings of powerlessness and ineffectiveness often experienced by new nursing graduates.

Remission   A period of chronic illness during which symptoms subside.

Replication   Repeating a research study as closely as possible to the original.

Research process   Prescribed steps that must be taken to plan and conduct meaningful research properly.

Research question   A statement, question, or hypothesis that a research study is designed to answer.

Resocialization   A transitional process of giving up part or all of one set of professional values and learning new ones.

Resolution   A written position on an issue presented to the voting members of an association for their consideration, discussion, and vote.

Respondeat superior   Legal theory that attributes the acts of employees to their employer (Latin term).

Retrospective reimbursement   Insurance payment made after services are delivered.

Richards, Linda   In 1873, she became the first "trained nurse" in the United States.

Risk management   A program that seeks to identify and eliminate potential safety hazards, thereby reducing patient injuries.

RN-to-BSN education Programs enabling registered nurses who hold associate degrees or diplomas in nursing to acquire baccalaureate degrees in nursing.

Robb, Isabel Hampton An outstanding turn-of-the-century American nurse who was instrumental in forming the forerunners of the National League for Nursing and the American Nurses Association as well as cofounding the *American Journal of Nursing*.

Role A goal-directed pattern of behavior learned within a cultural setting.

Role model An individual who serves as a model of desirable behavior for another.

Role strain Stress created by difficulty experienced in adjusting to a life or occupational roles.

Rogers, Martha Nursing theorist who developed a model known as the "science of unitary human beings."

Roy, Sister Callista Nursing theorist who developed an adaptation model based on general systems theory.

Salary compression A phenomenon in which pay increases are limited during an individual's career, so that the salary of a veteran nurse may be little higher than that of a recently hired novice nurse.

Sample A subset of an entire population that reflects the characteristics of the population.

Sanger, Margaret Founder of the first birth control clinic in the United States in 1916 and an ardent proponent of women's rights to use contraception.

Scales, Jessie Sleet Became the first African-American public health nurse in 1900.

School nurse Nurse specializing in the care of school-age children or adolescents and practicing in school settings.

Scientific discipline A branch of instruction or field of learning based on the study of a body of facts about the physical or material world.

Scientific method A systematic, orderly approach to the gathering of data and the solving of problems.

Secondary care An intermediate level of health care performed in a hospital having specialized equipment and laboratory facilities.

Secondary source Sources of data such as the nurse's own observations or perceptions of family and friends of the patient.

Self-actualization A process of realizing one's maximum potential and using one's capabilities to the fullest extent possible.

Self-awareness Understanding of one's own needs, biases, and impact on others.

Self-insurance An individual or business who pays for care directly rather than purchasing insurance.

Self-care model Nursing theoretical model based on the concept of ability to care for self.

Self-directed work team A method of decentralizing decision making using cross-functional groups united around common goals.

Self-efficacy A belief in self as possessing the ability to perform an activity, such as administering daily insulin.

Sender An essential element of communication consisting of the person sending a message.

Separation of powers Under the Constitution, each branch of the federal government has separate and distinct functions and powers.

Set A group of circumstances or situations joined and treated as a whole.

Sex-role stereotyping The practice of automatically and routinely linking positive or negative characteristics to either males or females.

Shared governance See Professional governance.

Short-term goals   Specific, small steps leading to the achievement of broader, long-term goals.

Sign   Outward evidence of illness visible to others, such as a rash.

Skill mix   The ratio of registered nurses to licensed practical nurses and nursing assistants in a hospital unit.

Socialization   The process whereby values and expectations are transmitted from generation to generation.

Social services   Services designed to assist individuals and families in obtaining basic needs, such as housing, food, and medical care.

Somatic language   Language used by infants to signal their needs to caretakers, such as crying; reddening of the skin; fast, shallow breathing; facial expressions; and jerking of the limbs.

Spellman Seminary   Site of the first nursing program for African-Americans, founded in Atlanta, Georgia, in 1886.

Staff nurse   The bedside nurse who cares for a group of patients but has no management responsibilities for the nursing unit.

Stage theory   A theory that views human development as a series of identifiable stages through which individuals and families pass.

Standard of care   What the reasonably prudent nurse, under similar circumstances, would have done.

Standard of nursing practice   Those nursing actions that are generally agreed upon, by nurses, as constituting safe, effective patient care.

Statutory law   Law established through formal legislative processes.

Stereotypes   Prejudiced attitudes developed through interactions with family, friends, and others in an individual's social and cultural system.

Stereotyping   Erroneous belief that all people of a certain group are alike.

Stress   Any emotional, physical, social, economic, or other factor that requires a response or change.

Stressors   Stimuli that tend to disturb equilibrium.

Subacute care   A level of care between hospital-based acute care and long-term residential care.

Subjective data   Information obtained from patients as they describe their needs, feelings, and strengths, and their perceptions of the problem.

Subjects   The individuals who are studied in a research project.

Subsystems   The parts that make up a system.

Supervision   The initial direction and periodic inspection of the actual accomplishment of a task.

Suprasystem   The larger environment outside a system.

Symptom   An indication of illness felt by the individual but not observable to others, such as pain.

System   A set of interrelated parts that come together to form a whole.

Systems theory   See General systems theory.

Taylor, Susie   A young, African-American Civil War nurse who knew and was influenced by Clara Barton; lived from 1848 to 1912.

Team nursing   A system of nursing care delivery in which a group of nurses and ancillary workers are responsible for the care of a group of patients during a specified time period, usually 8 to 12 hours.

Telehealth   The practice of providing health care by means of telecommunication devices such as telephone lines or televisions.

Termination phase   The final phase of the nurse-patient relationship wherein a mutual evaluation of progress is conducted.

Tertiary care   Specialized, highly technical level of health care provided in sophisticated research and teaching hospitals.

Tertiary source   Sources of data including the medical records and health care providers, such as physical therapists, physicians, or dietitians.

Theory   A general explanation scholars use to explain, predict, control, and understand commonly occurring events.

Therapist   Any of several health care workers with differing educational backgrounds who work with patients with specific deficits; examples include physical therapists and occupational therapists.

Third-party payment   Payment for health services by an entity other than the patient or the provider of services.

Tort   A civil wrong against a person; may be intentional or unintentional.

Total quality management (TQM)   Management philosophy and activities directed toward achieving excellence and employee participation in all aspects of that goal.

Transcultural nursing   Nursing care that is based on the patient's culturally determined health values, beliefs, and practices.

Transmission   The expression of information verbally or nonverbally.

Truth, Sojourner   A famous African-American nurse and former slave who was an abolitionist and underground railroad agent during the Civil War; lived from 1797 to 1881.

Tubman, Harriet Ross   An African-American Civil War nurse who helped more than 300 slaves to freedom on the underground railroad; lived from 1820 to 1913.

Unitary human beings, science of   A nursing theory developed by Martha Rogers.

Universal care   Provision of health care to all people.

Unlicensed assistive personnel   Individuals who are not extensively educated or licensed but provide direct patient care under the supervision of licensed personnel.

Urbanization   The process of population migration to cities.

Utilitarianism   An ethical theory asserting that it is right to maximize the greatest good for the happiness or pleasure of the greatest number of people.

Valid   Measuring what it is intended to measure, as in a valid test question or research instrument.

Values   The social principles, ideals, or standards held by an individual, class, or group that give meaning and direction to life.

Ventilation   The verbal "letting off steam" that occurs when people talk about concerns or frustrations.

Veracity   Truthfulness.

Verbal communication   All language whether written or spoken; represents only a small part of communication.

Value ethics   Ethical beliefs and behaviors that arise from the character of the decision maker.

Voluntary (private) agency   An agency supported entirely through voluntary contributions of time and/or money.

Wald, Lillian   Founder of the Henry Street Settlement and public health nursing in the United States. She later formed the National Organization of Public Health Nurses (1912), marking the beginning of specialization in nursing.

Watson, Jean   Nursing theorist who emphasizes human caring as a focus of nursing.

Whistle blower   A person who speaks out against unfair, dishonest, or dangerous practices by a company or agency.

Whole system shared governance   Involving people at all levels in decision making within the organization.

Woodhull Study   A comprehensive 1997 study of nursing in the print media.

Worker's compensation   A federally mandated insurance system covering workers injured on the job.

Work ethic   A belief in the importance of work; an appreciation for the characteristics employers desire in employees and a commitment to providing it.

Working phase   The middle phase of the nurse-patient relationship wherein goals are achieved.

Workplace advocacy   Ensuring that workers have a voice in the issues that concern them, either through collective action or other effective means.

Yale School of Nursing   The first school of nursing in the world to be established as a separate university department with an independent budget and its own dean, Annie W. Goodrich.

Index

Note: Page numbers in *italic* indicate illustrations; those followed by t refer to tables.